library

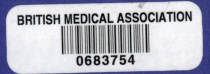

CONGENITAL ANOMALIES OF THE KIDNEY, URINARY AND GENITAL TRACTS

CONGENITAL ANOMALIES OF THE KIDNEY, URINARY AND GENITAL TRACTS

Second Edition

F. Douglas Stephens AO DSO MB MS FRACS

Emeritus Professor, Urology and Surgery, Northwestern University, Chicago, USA
Honorary Consultant Surgeon to the Royal Children's Hospital, Melbourne
Honorary Senior Research Fellow, Royal Children's Hospital Research Foundation, Melbourne
Formerly Consultant Paediatric Surgeon, Royal Women's Hospital, Melbourne, Australia

E. Durham Smith AO MD MS FRACS FACS

Honorary Consultant Surgeon to the Royal Children's Hospital, Melbourne, Australia

John M. Hutson BS MD(Monash) MD(Melb) FRACS, Editor

Director, Department of General Surgery, Royal Children's Hospital and Professor of
Paediatric Surgery, University of Melbourne, Australia

With contributions from
Iekuni Ichikawa, Justin Kelly,
Fumiyo Kuwayama, Yoichi Miyazaki and John C. Pope IV

MARTIN DUNITZ

© 1996, 2002 Martin Dunitz Ltd, a member of the Taylor and Francis group

First published in the United Kingdom in 1996
by Isis Medical Media Ltd

Second edition published in 2002
by Martin Dunitz Ltd, The Livery House, 7–9 Pratt Street, London NW1 0AE
Tel.:   +44 (0) 20 74822202
Fax.:   +44 (0) 20 72670159
E-mail: info@dunitz.co.uk
Website: http://www.dunitz.co.uk

A CIP record for this book is available from the British Library.

ISBN 1 901865 18 5

Distributed in the USA by
Fulfilment Centre
Taylor & Francis
7625 Empire Drive
Florence, KY 41042, USA
Toll Free Tel.:   +1 800 634 7064
E-mail: cserve@routledge_ny.com

Distributed in Canada by
Taylor & Francis
74 Rolark Drive
Scarborough, Ontario M1R G2, Canada
Toll Free Tel.:   +1 877 226 2237
E-mail: tal_fran@istar.ca

Distributed in the rest of the world by
ITPS Limited
Cheriton House
North Way
Andover, Hampshire SP10 5BE, UK
Tel.:   +44 (0)1264 332424
E-mail: reception@itps.co.uk

Always refer to the manufacturer's Prescribing Information before prescribing drugs cited in this book.

Page layout and design by Expo Holdings Malaysia
Image reproduction by Expo Holdings Malaysia
Printed and bound in Spain by Grafos SA Arte Sobre Papel.

Contents

I   NORMAL AND ABNORMAL EMBRYOLOGY OF THE CLOACA

II   INTRINSIC ANOMALIES OF THE URETHRA

III   THE BLADDER

IV   THE URETER

Contributors

Iekuni Ichikawa MD PhD, Departments of Pediatrics and Medicine, Vanderbilt University Medical Center, Nashville, Tennessee, USA, and Department of Pediatrics, Tokai University School of Medicine, Isehara, Japan

Justin Kelly MB BS FRACS, Senior Surgeon, Royal Children's Hospital, Melbourne, Australia

Fumiyo Kuwayama, Department of Pediatrics, Tokai University School of Medicine, Isehara, Japan

Yoichi Miyazaki, Department of Pediatrics, Vanderbilt University Medical Center, Nashville, Tennessee, USA

John C. Pope IV, Department of Urological Surgery, Vanderbilt University Medical Center, Nashville, Tennessee, USA

Foreword

Pediatric urological surgery has developed in spectacular fashion in recent decades. Conditions resulting in severe hydronephrosis are now corrected with confidence and with generally good results. One stage techniques of hypospadias repair are generally employed even in very severe cases. Most patients with exstrophy, even cloacal exstrophy, are now continent after some form of reconstruction. The list goes on and on. Present results would have been deemed spectacular, even a few years ago. How did all these advances come about? Increasing numbers of pediatric urologists and pediatric surgeons with a urological 'bent' have thought and worked very hard to devise solutions to what had been unmanageable problems. Quite simply, they were able to build on careful painstaking studies of the pathoembryology of these conditions. Douglas Stephens has been preeminent in elucidating how these complex anomalies occur. He carefully dissected hundreds of aborted and stillborn fetuses, measured everything, and was gradually able to deduce what went wrong, and when, to cause a specific anomaly or syndrome.

Durham Smith brought tremendous surgical skill to bear on these problems. He devised many of the surgical solutions in use today. John Hutson is of a younger generation, and has refined both the investigative techniques and the surgical solutions and is known especially for his research in cryptorchidism.

Successful correction of congenital anomalies obviously requires a thorough understanding of the problem and the pathologic anatomy. That is the strength and purpose of this book — to summarize and recapitulate in comprehensible fashion the cause of each disease. Much new research has been interdigitated with the classic studies. Conclusions are clearly stated and summarized. The text includes sections on each organ in the urinary tract, starting, appropriately, with the cloaca. Many of the severe anomalies of the lower tract have occurred by 7 or 8 weeks gestation, as the cloaca is forming and reconstituting itself into a separate urinary tract and rectum. Numerous important events occur at that time including the formation of the ureteral bud, its separation from what will become the Wolffian duct, the induction of the orifice of the ureteral bud into the bladder, etc. It is the disruption of the microanatomy and the timing and sequence of these events that results in ectopic ureter, reflux, ureterocele, urethral valves and the prune belly syndrome. Obviously this is a very important section. Happily, it is clearly written and well illustrated to give the anatomist and the surgeon useful insights into what went wrong. Several tables list the array of anomalies seen in each area, and the attention is given to outlining the principles of diagnosis and surgical correction.

The section on hypospadias and the urethra in boys describes the myriad conditions that affect these organs in systemic fashion. Hypospadias is seen usually to be an arrest in the development of the penis, rather than an abnormality. The gradations in chordee, hypospadias and related conditions are described systematically, and with this understanding logical surgical correction evolves in successive steps. Many of the rare anomalies of the penis are illustrated and their causes and treatment discussed. The pathoembryology of urethral valves is covered in this section, with new insights into causation and many illustrations of unusual lesions. Cowper's duct anomalies are covered here. A chapter on the anterior urethra describes and discusses diverticula, anterior valves and the valve of Guérin. Megalourethra is seen to have diverse etiologies.

The section on the bladder describes its formation, the development of the trigone, the take–up and migration of the ureteral orifices, and the derangements resulting in congenital diverticula and reflux. New insights into the formation of ureteroceles are examined. The effect of nearby diverticula on the intravesical ureter are well illustrated. Exstrophy is thoroughly discussed and a new operation based on a clearer understanding of the pathoembryology is described.

The ureteral bud induces the permanent kidney, spilling over 120 different kinds of cells into the renal blastema to organize development. Proper timing and proper anatomic alignment are both essential. This section describes the morphology of the process and shows how some derangements occur. Many relate to the site of the ureteral bud as it is taken up into the bladder. Thus, the position of the ureteral orifice is the key to understanding the cause of many renal anomalies. This section is very well illustrated with many diagrams which clarify the arguments. Duplex kidneys are explained. The site of duplicated orifices give special insight into the effect of the ureteral bud upon developing renal parenchyma. Persistent mesonephric ducts are described and ectopic vasa are explained. The pathology of the various types of megaureter are extensively discussed as are practical means of differentiating them. There are specific chapters dealing with the effect of reflux and of obstruction on the ureter, and of dilatation alone. The abnormalities of the ureter and renal segment seen in conjunction with ureterocele are examined in a new light. More rational modes of therapy can then be developed.

The section on the kidney deals with its embryogenesis in detail, and explores the effect of aberrant or persistent fetal vessels on the collecting system. The study of fused kidneys gives rise to many insights into renal development. The condition of each segment of a duplicated kidney is correlated with the position of the orifice of the subtending ureter, allowing one to explain differences in renal development. The kidneys in boys with valves reveal that severe obstruction reduces the number of nephron generations. This chapter describes various forms of renal dysplasia, and supports the conclusion that there are many causes of such dysplasia. These are then classified in a way that is simple, and helpful to the urologist engaged in the treatment of such patients.

A new development in embryology has been the realization that fetal compression can cause many anomalies. This notion is thoroughly explored as it pertains to the urinary tract. The final section is the triad or prune belly syndrome. Again, the method is to carefully study the developmental anatomy. This allows one to infer the causes of the syndrome and how bladder and kidney development is deranged. The effect on the testes is used to introduce a timely overview of the descent of the testes and the causes of cryptorchidism.

The last portion of the book consists of nomograms, graphs and tables giving normal values by age and by surface area. These data are often very useful and are surprisingly hard to find. Finally, syndromes with a renal component, of which there are hundreds, are listed together with the associated anomalies. At least one reference is given for each syndrome. References abound throughout the text.

In summary, this is a book of great importance. It allows the anatomist or surgeon to understand a great deal about the genesis of the condition that he is studying or treating. Such understanding is very important in successful therapy.

Lowell R. King MD
Professor and Head,
Pediatric Urology Section
Division of Urologic Surgery
Duke University Medical Center
Durham, North Carolina, USA

Foreword

The 'Definitive Work' is a hackneyed and over–used phrase in reviews of books and rarely means what it says. Very few books deserve the term and it surely could never be used to describe two books by the same author on the same topic over a period of 35 years. Yet I insist that this is a true example of such an accolade. We have regarded Douglas's 1963 *Congenital Malformations of the Rectum, Anus and Genitourinary Tracts* as the ultimate reference source that provided either the up-to-date view of the problem or at least a Stephens' theory that often as not challenged all previous ideas; never did we find a statement to the effect that 'little is known on this topic'. Up to the time of the publishing of this present volume I have felt that his previous work was as fresh and timely, with very few exceptions, as it has been the day of its printing.

Now Douglas Stephens has done it again with this mammoth review of his life's work, compiled with love and devotion during a career that has spanned so many developments and innovations in paediatric urology and surgery. He describes specimens that have lurked in jars, some for half a century during which time his painstaking dissections with copious and detailed notes have paid off to the advantage of all of us. His methodology must be compared with that of John Hunter.

Together with his lifelong colleague, Durham Smith and their protegee, John Hutson, Douglas has presented to us a catalogue of all that can go wrong developmentally with the contents of a child's pelvis and beyond. Over the years Douglas Stephens and his co-workers have put forward theories, perhaps the best example being the **Bud Theory** to explain the association of reflux and abnormal development of the kidney, that were well before their time and yet simple, convincing and, of course, now so acceptable.

It is pleasing to see that the truly revolutionary work of John Hutson on the undescended testis which has advanced our knowledge so significantly is included in this volume.

On a more personal note, the publication of this book will give enormous pleasure to the multitude of fans and friends of Douglas Stephens, and I would claim to be just one of these, who have sat in admiration at his feet and in his audiences for more years than many of us would want to admit.

Robert H. Whitaker MD MChir FRCS
Lecturer in Anatomy, University of Cambridge, UK
Formerly Consultant Paediatric Urologist, Adenbrooke's Hospital, Cambridge, UK

Preface to the second edition

Since the First Edition of this book in 1996, our understanding of the embryology and anatomy of the urinary tract has increased rapidly. To keep the book contemporary and yet allow it to remain a priceless reference work of studies going back fifty years, we have retained it in its original format but added three new chapters at the end.

The most significant change in the text is in the title, which now includes the word 'kidney'. This reflects the fact that over one quarter of the book is about renal development, but this had previously been omitted from the title. We hope that the addition of the word 'kidney' in the title will bring the text to the attention of nephrologists and other specialists interested in renal development and maldevelopment. This is particularly so because Chapter 40 has been written by Professor Iekuni Ichikawa and colleagues from Vanderbilt University Medical Center, Nashville TN, USA and Tokai University School of Medicine, Isehara, Japan. Drs Miyazaki, Pope, Kuwayama, Stephens and Ichikawa have together written a crucial chapter linking the anatomy and embryological work in the first thirty-nine chapters with current knowledge on the molecular biology of renal development. They show in a very elegant manner that the bud theory of ureteric development, first proposed by Mackie and Stephens in 1975, is strongly supported by recent evidence from molecular biology. The discovery of the angiotensin type 2 receptor, and its role in ureteric bud and metanephric development, has been a crucial link between the painstaking anatomical studies of Douglas Stephens and co-workers and the sudden explosion in recent years of molecular biology. Professor Ichikawa has visited Melbourne several times to discuss the embryogenesis of the kidney and urinary tract with Douglas Stephens, and to study our collection of specimens. We thank Iekuni and his colleagues for contributing such an important chapter to this revised edition.

In Chapter 41, Douglas Stephens continues on where he left off in Chapter 36, with a detailed analysis of deformation in early embryogenesis. This chapter describes in detail the current knowledge about deformity in the amniotic sac in early embryogenesis, as well as clearly outlining the evidence supporting transient compression of the embryo by a shrunken embryonic sac. It may be that this is a much more important cause of embryonic deformation than has been appreciated previously.

Chapter 42 describes the pathological anatomy and surgical principles of radical soft tissue mobilization in the treatment of epispadias and exstrophy of the bladder. This chapter departs from the aim of the main part of the book, to understand the embryogenesis of the urogenital tract. It has been included because of the significant advances which have been demonstrated by Justin Kelly in the management of exstrophy, when the pathological anatomy is understood well enough to allow radical soft tissue mobilization. This chapter is a very practical one and will be of immense value to urogenital surgeons faced with the difficult problem of bladder exstrophy. In the first edition of the book, Justin Kelly contributed a few pages to Chapter 12 on the anomalies of the bladder, giving a brief introduction to the anatomy and principles of his repair by radical mobilization. Now, in Chapter 42, he gives a complete description of the anatomy of each type of epispadias and exstrophy, along with a practical guide for the surgeon, explaining the principles of his new operation to mobilize the anterior attachments of the levator ani and the external urethral sphincter, and bring these together around the urethra. This operation is a revelation in three-dimensional anatomy of the pelvis, and will revolutionize our ability to treat children with exstrophy. Justin Kelly is possibly the first person to understand fully the anatomical derangement of the pelvic floor in bladder exstrophy, and to use this knowledge to devise this totally revolutionary operation to correct the abnormality. This chapter needs to be read by all pediatric urologists.

John M. Hutson

Preface to first edition

In this book we have collected together the original studies by ourselves and co-workers on the dysmorphology and embryogenesis of congenital anomalies of the urinary and genital tracts and the combined cloacal defects of the rectum and anus. The book is an extension of an earlier publication entitled *Congenital Malformations of the Urinary Tract* (1983), which was limited to the study of the urinary tract.

These studies include not only the classification of visceral abnormalities but also the pathological anatomy, pathoembryology, radiology and in some instances the surgery of the abnormal organs. They provide a practical understanding of the abnormalities posed to clinicians in charge of the foetus, baby or child. Many extra defects of the urogenital tracts including hypospadias, superior and supernumerary kidneys, the vagaries of the vas deferens and seminal vesicles and new facets of old problems have been added to those described in the previous book. The original studies by one of us (J.M.H.) on the Descent and Nondescent of the Testes and Intersex Problems are also important additions. Furthermore the very exciting newly appreciated abnormal anatomy of vesical exstrophy sphincter musculature as discovered by our surgeon colleague Justin H. Kelly is briefly introduced. We have included also Appendix 1, entitled *Forgetmenots* which is a record of standard measurements and terms of normal and abnormal organs and the chronological development of the urogenital organs. Appendix 2, *Syndromes with a Renal Component* by Cyril Chantler MA MD FRCP, Principal, Guy's and St Thomas's Hospital, London, is again reproduced with permission. This is a helpful source for reference when a clinician is faced with babies with multiple anomalies.

Most of these chapters are a life time record of a research program conducted by one of us (F.D.S.) in close association with many members of a changing team of Australian and international colleagues. The book is unique in that it is primarily concerned with the pathoembryology and surgical anatomy of paediatric lesions. The book is not primarily a textbook of detailed therapy, although in a number of sections surgical options are provided on the basis of our understanding of the pathology and natural history of the conditions. We recognize that many recent studies of embryological development of normal cloacal subdivision and observations of anorectal anomalies in porcine embryos offer new ideas on the pathoembryology. However, we have been able to explain the development of the myriad of defects better by the earlier descriptions of embryology and our own reconstructive embryology deduced from studies of specimens of abnormal human foetuses and babies.

During the past 50 years these studies have been conducted at the Royal Children's and Royal Women's Hospitals in Melbourne, at the Hospital for Sick Children, Great Ormond Street in London and at Children's Memorial Hospital, Chicago. E. Durham Smith, Robert Fowler, John M. Hutson and Justin H. Kelly in Melbourne have continuously made contributions many of which are included in this book. At the Hospital for Sick Children in London, one of us (F.D.S.) had the opportunity to work and study with the late Sir Denis Browne, T.T. Higgins and Dr Martin Bodian and at the Children's Memorial Hospital, Chicago with Lowell R. King, Casimir F. Firlit and John Raffensperger and many other colleagues, senior and junior. In producing this book we have included a large number of papers or parts of papers by many co-workers and acknowledgements have been made in the text and as footnotes to each chapter where appropriate.

The authors make a point of classifying congenital anomalies into malformations and deformations of which the latter are described in Chapter 36. Very many abnormalities cannot be accounted for by gene inheritance or the result of chromosomal defects or pathogens and the 'deformation' theory provides a very plausible explanation for many external and internal genito-urinary, cloacal and spinal defects.

The chapters cover a great many topics, regular and irregular, common and rare, which are of prime interest to all urologists and paediatric surgeons. Radiologists, pathologists, embryologists, anatomists and nephrologists would find this a helpful reference book. The concept of 'deformation' should be of considerable interest to geneticists and dysmorphologists in their quests for explanations of a large number of anomalies.

F. Douglas Stephens
E. Durham Smith
John M. Hutson

Acknowledgements

In 1993, a book entitled *Congenital Malformations of the Urinary Tract* was published by Praeger Scientific. This book contained the results of relevant urological research projects undertaken by myself and co-workers up until 1981. Since then many more research projects have been completed and are now included in *Congenital Anomalies of the Urinary and Genital Tracts*. This more recent work has been published in journals or books and is now integrated either in slightly altered form to fit the present text or verbatim into this book as new or expanded chapters. The names of the contributors and publishers to these chapters are acknowledged in footnotes to the relevant chapters, legends, tables and in the reference list.

In the immediate post World War II years, I received a Nuffield Foundation Fellowship grant to study paediatric surgery at the Hospital for Sick Children, London, U.K. where I had the opportunity to work with the late Sir Denis Browne, Mr T.T. Higgins and Dr Martin Bodian. This association further stimulated my interest in the embryology and pathology of congenital anomalies, which became an obsession. At the Royal Children's Hospital in Melbourne and the Children's Memorial Hospital in Chicago, I have been freely advised by my pathologist colleagues everywhere. We acknowledge the help given by Dr Leo Cussen, previously pathologist at the Royal Children's Hosptial, Melbourne in the research program, with the late Daniel Lenaghan, Urologist, on the aetiology of vesicoureteral reflux, renal dysmorphology and on mensuration of the urinary tract which appear in 'Forgetmenots', Appendix 1.

During my long association with the Royal Women's Hospital, Melbourne, I have had the privilege of studying normal and abnormal babies in their first few weeks of life and also many in the postmortem state.

Since the introduction of ultrasonography, we have learnt much from colleagues at the Royal Women's Hospital about the living foetuses and have studied those that have aborted in the early stages of development. We are especially grateful to successive heads of the Department of Pathology, Drs Denys Fortune and Andrew Oster, and their staff, all of whom have given guidance and facilities for study.

The text has also incorporated extracts from the following books with kind permission of the publishers:

Embryology of the Cloaca and Embryogenesis of Anorectal Malformations. In *Anorectal Malformations in Children: Update 1988*. F.D. Stephens, E.D. Smith and N.W. Paul (eds). March of Dimes Birth Defects Foundation – New York. *National Foundation – March of Dimes*. Birth Defects, Original Article Series, Volume 24, Number 4.

Embryology and Pathoembryology of the Urinary Tract. In *Reconstructive Urology*, Volume 1, 1993. G. Webster, R. Kirby, L. King and B. Goldwasser (eds). Blackwell Scientific Publications – Boston.

E. Durham Smith, my friend and colleague of many years, and co-author of two other books entitled *Anorectal Malformations in Children*; Chicago Year Book, 1971 and *Anorectal Malformations in Children: Update 1988*; Alan R. Liss publishers for March of Dimes—Birth Defects Foundation, edited this book. His special knowledge and expertise of the research projects and publications made it possible for him to integrate the new work into old and new chapters.

John M. Hutson, who received very valuable training in research in Professor Patricia Donahoe's Department of Paediatric Surgical Research at the Harvard Medical School, Boston contributed Chapters 38 and 39. These chapters reflect an overview of later research work of the members of his unit in the Royal Children's Hospital, Melbourne on the mechanism of descent of the testes and congenital intersex states.

Professor Cyril Chantler MA MD FRCP, Principal, Guy's and St Thomas's Hospital, London has again given permission to include *Syndromes with a Renal Component* as Appendix 2. This was first published in *Pediatric Nephrology*,

M.I. Ruben and J.M. Barratt (eds), Baltimore: The Williams and Wilkins Co, was reprinted in *Congenital Malformation of the Urinary Tract* and is included in the current volume.

This book stems from research studies conducted by one of us (F.D.S.) first at the Hospital for Sick Children, Great Ormond Street, London, then at the Royal Children's and Royal Women's Hospitals, Melbourne, and later at Children's Memorial Hospital, Chicago. In the past nine years further research projects were conducted again at the Royal Children's Hospital Research Foundation and Royal Women's Hospital in Melbourne. The authors wish to acknowledge the help provided by members of the staff of these great hospitals and the members of the boards of the hospitals for providing clinical and research facilities. The Nuffield Foundation, The Royal Children's Hospital Research Foundation, the Lucy and Edwin Kretchmer Fund of the Northwestern University Medical School and the March of Dimes—Birth Defects Foundation have provided financial support over the years towards the research and publications described in this book.

It is not possible to acknowledge personally the contributions of all our colleagues, medical, nursing, librarians, artists and illustrators, to whom we owe a debt of gratitude, so we thank them collectively now. However, we make special mention of Librarians of the Gordon Craig Library of the Royal Australasian College of Surgeons, Jane Oliver and Jennifer McGurgan for their invaluable assistance, given freely in tracing references and publications. We express our special appreciation to Veda Currie for her extraordinary skills and devotion to the task. She has dedicated two years of the her life in the preparation of the manuscript of the book. We are exceptionally grateful to her for the superb effort in bringing this whole volume to ISIS Medical Media Publishers. Elizabeth Vorrath and Judy Hayes in the Department of General Surgery, Royal Children's Hospital, Melbourne have been most helpful. Finally, we thank John Harrison and his staff, in particular Judith Bovington for the efficient and pleasant collaboration in the preparation and publication of this book.

Dedication

The authors dedicate this book to our wives, the late Rosalie Stephens, Victoria Stephens, Dorothy Smith and Susan Hutson; and to those parents and children, past, present and future, whom we try to help by publication of the results of our research studies.

Normal and abnormal embryology of the cloaca

I

Normal embryology of the cloaca

The human embryo, by the time it has embedded in the wall of the uterus, has changed in shape from a solid, round ball of cells to a flat disk cushioned by fluid spaces. During the third week, the disk elongates and spreads its 'wings' laterally within its chorionic capsule in the wall of the uterus. Its epiblastic and endoblastic laminae become separated by the intrusion of a third mesoblastic component derived from the cells of the primitive streak. Rapid proliferation of all three laminae causes elongation, and the embryo bends within the chorionic capsule. By this time, the amnion and the yolk sac take up much of the peripheral space, cushion the embryo, and accommodate to the enlarging head and tail folds.

The heart and head rotate ventrally and caudally, preceding ventral rotation of the body stalk, cloacal membrane, and the tail (Fig. 1.1). In between, the wings of the disk spread laterally and ventrally, wrapping around the developing organs of the trunk and converting the disk to a cylinder.

In the fourth week, the chorionic sac expands beneath the uterine epithelium out of the confines of the wall, encroaching on the cavity of the uterus. Provided that chorionic and uterine enlargement continue *pari passu* with the growth of the embryo and fetus, and provided that the amniotic and yolk-sac components function appropriately, the spatial relationship between the embryo and host allows normal growth and development.

Malformations result from genetic, chromosomal, or teratogenic causes, which induce arrests or excesses of embryological processes. Deformations are characterized by alterations in the shape and structure of previously normal parts such as may occur with local pressure upon a limb or organ or spatial disproportion between the chorionic capsule or amniotic sac and the embryo or fetus within (Cohen, 1981).

Often malformations and deformations are clearly distinguishable, but they may occur together in multiple lesions, and some anomalies, such as congenital hip dislocation, may result from either malformation or deformation. Discussion here is devoted chiefly to normal embryology and malformations arising from errors of development.

In Chapter 3, some deformations are described that may be the result of focal pressure on the perineum and pelvic organs. The growing caudal end of the embryo may be arrested or twisted by impact against the capsule in which the embryo or fetus develops, giving rise to multiple pelvic, perineal and spinal deformities. Much has been written concerning the 'caudal regression syndrome'. Resorption of the tail and its vertebrae is a normal process in humans, but resorption of an excess number of the terminal vertebrae and soft-tissue structures may occur, accounting for multiple deformities in this area (Duhamel, 1961). On the other hand, abnormal pressures may be exerted against the developing caudal end, resulting in a 'caudal "suppression" syndrome', accounting for similar lesions (Chapter 36; Stephens, 1981).

The kidney and all the urinary organs of the mature fetus arise near the caudal tip of the human embryo, centred around the cloacal membrane. The cloacal cavity comes into existence when the hind end of the disk, together with the contiguous cloacal membrane, undergoes ventrocraniad flexions of 180°, and the lateral wings wrap around the body stalk (Fig. 1.1). The endoderm of the dorsal wall of the yolk sac is the forerunner of the alimentary canal, and the internal cloaca is the expanded hind end of this endodermal tract. During the fourth and fifth weeks, the complex process of partitioning of the internal and external cloacae into separate urinary and anorectal systems takes place by formation of the urorectal and uroanal septa. These two septa are coronal in orientation and are made up of at least four different components. The septum starts cranially and ends caudally, each component being built sequentially upon the other. Two of the processes divide the internal cloaca, and at least two the external cloaca. Septation takes place concurrently with straightening of the hind end of the body and reverse rotation of the cloacal membrane.

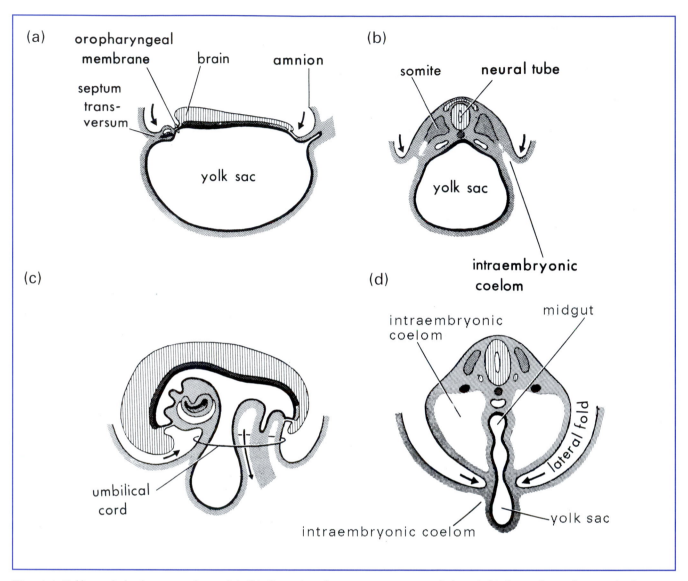

Fig. 1.1 *Folding of the human embryo. (**a**),(**b**) Sagittal and transverse sections of discoid 22-day embryo showing the beginning of folding longitudinally (**a**) and transversely (**b**) (arrows). (**c**) Longitudinal at 28 days. (**d**) Transverse at 26 days. (Reprinted, by permission, after Moore, K.L. (1977), in* The Developing Human. *Philadelphia, Saunders, Fig. 5.1, p. 60.)*

Defects in the partitioning of the cloaca cause errors not only of the visceral tracts but also of the pelvic and perineal muscles and sphincters. Arrest of development or misalignment or overlap of one or more components of the septum account for many of the stereotyped disorders, but others are irregular, and defy classification and may result from deformations.

Partitioning of the cloaca

The cloacal membrane separates the internal from the external cloacae in the transverse plane, and the urorectal and uroanal septa cleave the cloacae in the coronal plane (Fig. 1.2). At the 16-mm crown–rump (six weeks) phase of development, the urorectal septum has come, the cloacal membrane has gone, the internal cloaca is divided and the external cloaca is a deep pit about to be partitioned by the uroanal septum.

The internal cloaca and urorectal septum
At the 4-mm stage (four-week embryo), the internal cloaca is a single chamber, into which issue the large intestine, the postanal gut, the allantois and the wolffian (mesonephric) ducts. This endodermal reservoir contacts the surface ectoderm, forming the cloacal membrane (Fig. 1.3).

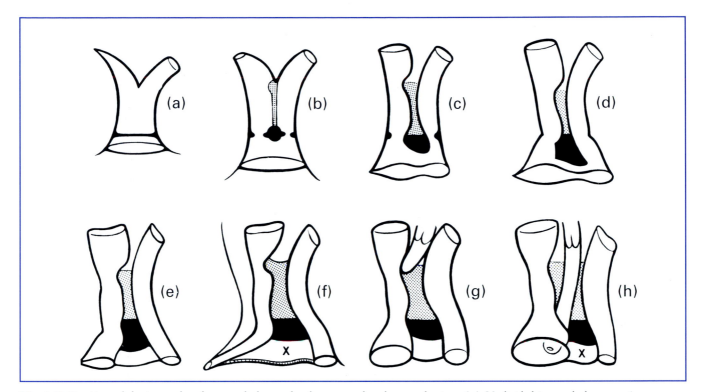

Fig. 1.2 *Partition of the internal and external cloacae by the urorectal and uroanal septa. (**a**) Undivided internal cloaca at 4-mm stage. (**b**) Urorectal septum (hatched area) complete at 16-mm stage. (**c**) Perineal mound (black area) forms the deep part of the uroanal septum which divides the external cloaca. (**d**), (**e**) Inner genital folds now surge medially over the mound to form the perineum as in the female.(**f**) Inner genital folds (X) are further supplemented in the male by overlay of outer genital folds which form the midline perineal raphe.(**g**) In the female, müllerian ducts penetrate posterior wall of the urethra at 36-mm stage. (**h**) Müllerian ducts descend to gain an external opening in the urogenital sinus or vestibule. (Reprinted, by permission, from Stephens, F.D. and Smith, E.D. (1971), Anorectal Malformations in Children. Chicago, Year Book, Fig. 68, p. 119.)*

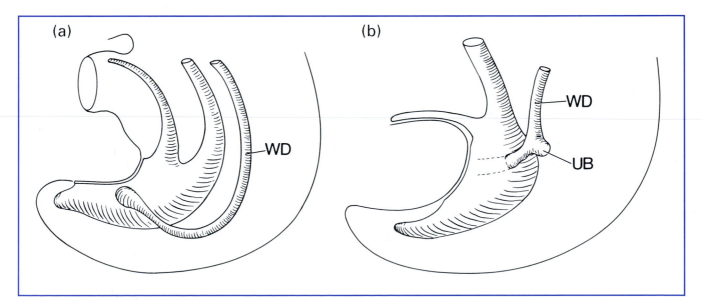

Fig. 1.3 *Internal cloaca. (**a**) At 4-mm stage receiving the allantois, rectum and wolffian ducts. (**b**) Cloacal membrane separates endoderm from ectoderm at 6-mm stage. Note the position of the orifice of wolffian duct (WD) cranial to the original site relative to the cloacal membrane (UB = ureteral bud). (Reprinted, by permission, after Felix, W. (1912), in Manual of Human Embryology, F. Keibel and F.P. Mall (eds). Philadelphia, Lippincott, Figs 605 and 606, p. 875.)*

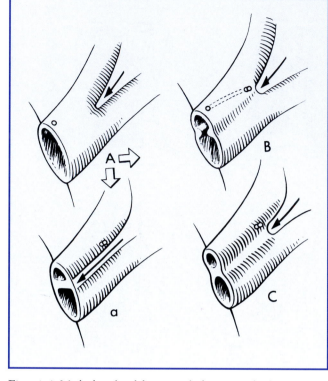

Fig. 1.4 *Methods of subdivision of the internal cloaca. A–a. Subdivision by downgrowth of the urorectal septum to meet the cloacal membrane. **A**, **B**, **C**. Subdivision by downgrowth of urorectal septum (Tourneux's fold) as far as Müller's hillock (verumontanum) and by lateral ingrowths of mesenchyme (Rathke's plicae) caudal to this level. (The dotted lines in **B** represent the line of retraction of the orifices of the wolffian ducts from sites near the cloacal membrane at the earliest stage to the later attained level at the verumontanum.) (Reprinted, by permission, from Stephens, F.D. and Smith, E.D. (1971), Anorectal Malformations in Children. Chicago, Year Book, Fig. 69, p. 120.)*

The partitioning of the internal cloaca begins in the 4-mm (four-week) embryo by the urorectal septum and is completed in the 16-mm (six week) stage. This septum is developed in two parts (Keibel and Mall, 1912a; Stephens, 1953a; Duhamel *et al.*, 1966) (Fig. 1.4).

The cranial part of the septum is a crescentic fold, which settles deeply into the saddle between the allantois and the hindgut, on the cranial aspect of the cloaca. This crescentic spur was claimed by Tourneux to progress caudally until it met the cloacal membrane. Rathke and Retterer (quoted by Duhamel *et al.*, 1966) considered that the septum was formed by the coming together and fusion in the midline of two lateral mesodermal folds or plicae (Fig. 1.5).

There is no controversy amongst embryologists (Patten, 1947; Arey, 1974, Hamilton, Boyd and

Mossman, 1976a;) concerning the progressive craniocaudal march of the septum (Fig. 1.4). Emphasis, however, is placed more on Tourneux's method, although Keibel and Mall (1912a) and Patten (1947) imply that the craniocaudal component is supplemented by that formed from the lateral indentations nearer the cloacal membrane. This combined method of formation of the urorectal septum offers ready explanation of many of the congenital abnormalities of the area. Tourneux's fold partitions the cloaca to the level of the future verumontanum (Müller's tubercle) and Rathke's plicae complete the process to the cloacal membrane. The union of Rathke's plicae forms the septum that was described by James Douglas (1675–1742) and known as the Douglas septum (Thomas, 1964).

The external cloaca

After the formation period of the urorectal septum, between the 4- and 16-mm phases, the urogenital and anal orifices become deeply set in the perineum as the result of the surface build up of mesoderm derived from the primitive streak. This mesoderm creates the anal tubercles posteriorly, the genital folds on either side and the genital tubercle in front where the mesoderm meets on the ventral aspect. The depression so formed is the external cloaca, into which the urethra and rectum open separately.

When the urorectal septum reaches the cloacal membrane, the urogenital and anal membranes anterior and posterior to the septum atrophy, and both systems then issue into the common external cloaca.

The uroanal septum

The process of partitioning now extends caudally into the external cloaca (Fig. 1.5). The uroanal septum, or dividing wall of the external cloaca, is a composite structure. Its deep part, an extension of the urorectal septum, is the perineal mound, and more superficially it is added to by the inward migration and overlap of the genital folds upon the mound. Caudal to the level of the cloacal membrane, the perineal mound forms in continuity with, and as an extension of, the urorectal septum, separating the orifice of the urogenital sinus from the anus. This is the primitive perineum of Keibel and Mall (1912a). It begins to develop at the 16-mm crown–rump

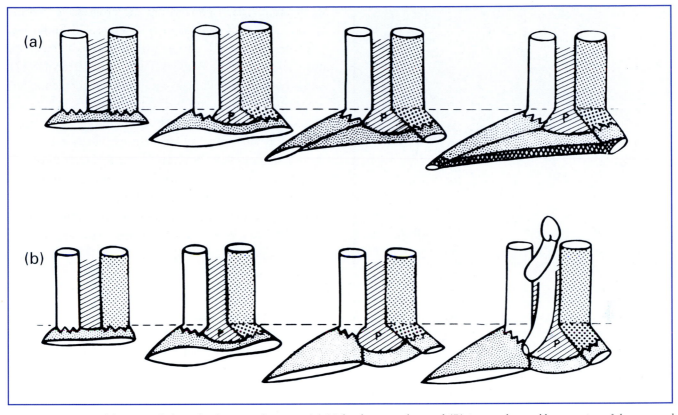

Fig. 1.5 *Partition of the external cloaca by the uroanal septum. (a) Male; the perineal mound (P) is a mushroom-like extension of the urorectal septum into the external cloaca elongating the urethra and creating the bulb. The inner genital folds (stippled) migrate medially over the mound followed by the outer genital folds (cross-hatched) forming the male perineum. The folds extend anteriorly covering the urethra. The anus is also built up and elongated by the mound (P) and inner and outer folds. (b) Female; the perineal mound (P) is covered only by the inner genital folds; the urogenital part of the external cloaca remains open. (Reprinted, by permission, from Stephens, F.D. and Smith, E.D. (1971),* Anorectal Malformations in Children. *Chicago, Year Book, Fig. 71, p. 121.)*

length (six-week embryo), and as it grows caudally, the urethra and rectum elongate with it (Fig. 1.5). The adjoining inner genital folds proliferate to form projecting lateral borders around the whole circumference of the external cloaca. These folds then surge medially over the perineal mound to form the perineum between urinary and anal orifices and to build up and elongate both the urethra and the anal canal (Fig. 1.6). These sex folds develop differentially from the 50-mm (12-week) stage in males and females.

The male urethra

At the 16-mm (six-week) stage, the orifices of the wolffian ducts lie on Müller's tubercle in the future prostatic urethra. The urogenital sinus caudal to the tubercle in its distal half expands sagittally to form the pars phallica and urethral plate which abuts the genital tubercle. The cranial part of the urogenital sinus, the pars pelvina, elongates and becomes the membranous urethra.

The male perineum

In the male, the inner genital folds migrate medially, cover the perineal mound, and tent over the urogenital sinus to form the perineum and bulbous and penile urethra. The outer genital folds also migrate medially, blend into and insinuate beneath the epithelium of the inner folds, and meet in the midline forming the raised-up perineal raphe from the anterior quadrant of the anus to the frenulum of the glans. They enlarge locally to form the scrotum (Fig. 1.7). Further development of the urethra in the glans is described later.

The deep part of the uroanal septum in the male is largely responsible for the anteroposterior length of the perineum, while the superficial components formed by the genital folds add depth.

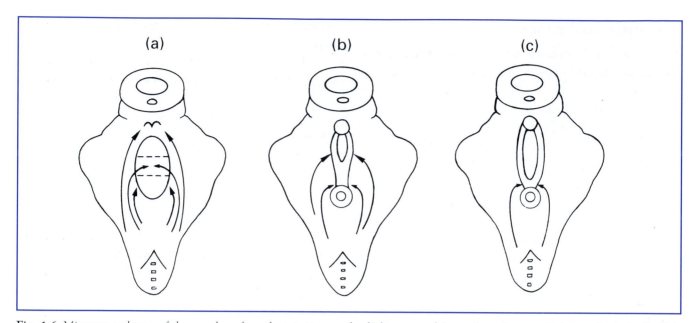

Fig. 1.6 *Migratory pathways of the mesoderm from the primitive streak which separate the anus from the urogenital sinus deeply by Rathke's septum and perineal mound (**a**) (middle arrows) and superficially by the genital folds to form the perineum (**b**, **c**, arrows). The folds advance medially to cover the male urogenital sinus (**b**) but remain lateral as the labia minora in the female (**c**). (Reprinted, by permission, after Duhamel, B. et al. (1966), Des monstruosités aux malformations, in Morphogenèse Pathologique. Paris, Masson et Cie, Figs 103 and 107, pp. 146, 154.)*

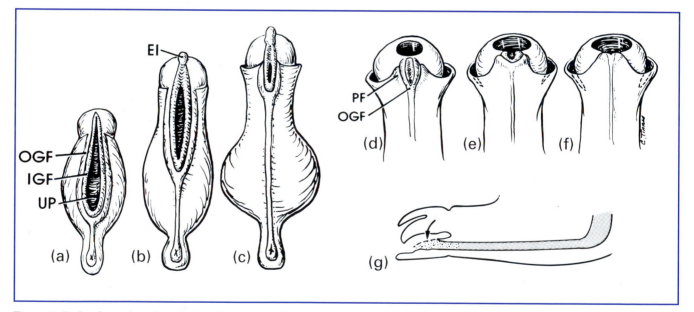

Fig. 1.7 *Embryology of penile and glandular urethra. The inner and outer genital folds cover the urethral plate (UP) and form the raphe (**a**, **b**, **c**). The glandular urethra is a compound of ectodermal pit at tip of glans and open end of the urethral groove. (**d**),(**e**),(**f**) Show further closure of the groove by outer genital and preputial folds, and show also orifice of the central pit in the glans. (**g**) Shows the breakdown (arrow) of the intervening septum to create one orifice, the fossa navicularis and the lacuna magna (OGF = outer genital folds; IGF = inner genital folds; PF = preputial folds; UP = urethral plate; EI = ectodermal tag marking site of ectodermal ingrowth.) Arrow in (**g**) indicates site of 'anastomosis' between the ectodermal pit and the urethral groove. (Reprinted, by permission, from Sommer, J.T. and Stephens, F.D. (1980), Dorsal urethral diverticulum of the fossa navicularis: symptoms, diagnosis and treatment. J. Urol. 124: 94, Fig. 6.)*

The male anal canal

The genital folds enlarge and build up mesenchyme around the external cloaca, but especially around the posterior and lateral quadrants of the anus. Tench (1936) and Bill and Johnson (1958) call these folds in the locality of the anus the 'anal tubercles'; they are, however, no more than specialized areas of differentiation of the inner genital folds. The anal canal is thus elongated by wrappings of first the deep inner genital folds, which meet together covering over the perineal mound and together form the anterior wall of the anal canal. The outer genital folds migrate medially, covering the inner folds, supplementing the anterior quadrants of the anal canal, and forming the perineal raphe which begins on the midpoint of the anus (Fig. 1.5). These anal wrappings and perineal components, when defective, account for anocutaneous, anourethral and rectobulbar fistulas (see Figs 3.1, 3.2 and 3.3).

The female urethra

The whole of the urogenital sinus from Müller's tubercle caudally expands in the sagittal plane and becomes exteriorized to form the vestibule of the vulva. The urethra cranial to Müller's tubercle elongates, forming the whole of the pelvic urethra. The müllerian ducts, which first issue between the orifices of the wolffian ducts at Müller's tubercle, proliferate, invaginate the posterior wall of the sinus, and then migrate caudally to open exteriorly (Fig. 1.5b). They carry in their lateral walls the disintegrating wolffian or Gartner's ducts. The orifice of the fused müllerian ducts lies first cranial to the orifices of Bartholin's glands in the urogenital sinus, but finally lies between them in the vestibule of the vulva, indicating an active caudal migratory progression (Frazer, 1931a).

The female perineum

The perineal mound fills in the deep part of the external cloaca between the urethra and anus, and the inner genital folds cover the mound. The outer genital folds, however, do not take part in the formation of the perineum between the anus and the vestibule. The perineum and anus lack the perineal raphe, and exhibit in the newborn period markings derived from the com-

ponents from which it is formed (Fig. 1.5; see also page 43).

The inner genital folds remain lateral, and the vestibule remains exposed, flanked by the labia minora (inner folds) and the labia majora (outer folds). The genital tubercle at the anterior end of the vestibule remains small, bent on itself, uncanalized, and covered anteriorly by the preputial hood (Fig. 1.8).

The vulva

The uncovered anterior compartment of the external cloaca flanked by the inner and outer genital folds, with the hooded clitoris in front and the fourchette behind, is the vulva. Its floor anterior to the urethra comprises the pars phallica of the urogenital sinus. Its floor posterior to the urethra is occupied by the vagina and the hymen, which is surrounded by the everted posterior wall of the pars pelvina of the urogenital sinus (Fig. 1.8).

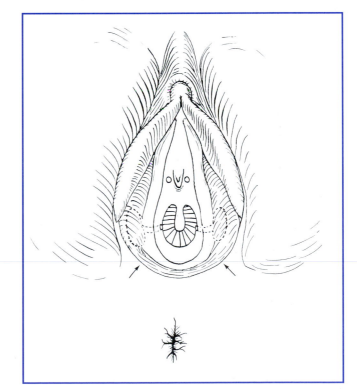

Fig. 1.8 *Vulva showing relationships of labia minora and minoral tails (arrows), labia majora, clitoris and fourchette to the vestibule. Urethra and orifices of Skene's ducts anterior to hymen. Beside the hymen, duct orifices of Bartholin's glands (dotted) which lie between the erectile tissue and the overlying bulbocavernosus muscle. (Reprinted, by permission, from Stephens, F.D. (1983), Congenital Malformations of the Urinary Tract, New York, Praeger, Fig. 1.8, p. 14.)*

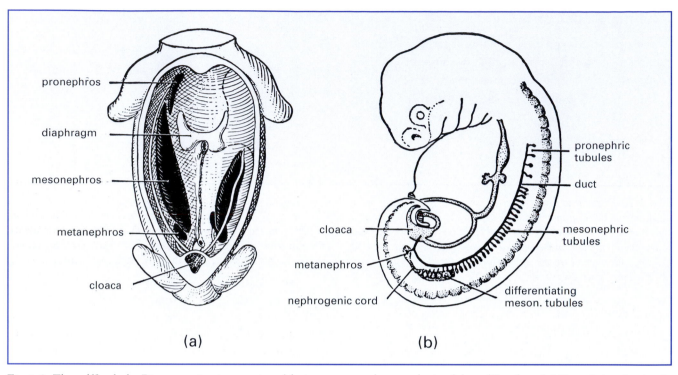

Fig. 1.9 *The wolffian body. Diagrammatic representation of the pro-, meso- and metanephroi and the wolffian duct. (**a**) Ventral view showing the three parts at approximately the five-week stage on the right side of the embryo and a few days later on the left side. (**b**) Lateral view of the embryo showing the three kidneys, the wolffian duct and the internal cloaca. (Reprinted, by permission, from Arey, L.B. (1974), Developmental Anatomy, 7th edn. Philadelphia, Saunders, Fig. 261, p. 296.)*

The female anal canal

The anal tubercles, formed from the inner genital folds, blend with the perineal mound, elongating the anal canal as in the male. The outer genital folds, however, play no part in the development of the anus or perineum.

Incorporation of mesonephric (wolffian) ducts and ureters into the urinary tract

Early in the fourth week, the solid growing end of the wolffian (mesonephric) duct migrating from the thoracic to the hind end along the lateral side of the wolffian body turns medially from the back wall of the embryo across the nephrogenic cord (Fig. 1.9). It courses obliquely around the side wall of the cloaca to enter it anterolaterally near the cloacal membrane. Soon after penetration of the cloacal wall, the duct canalizes. The original entry point of the wolffian ducts is close to the anterior border of the cloacal membrane, and, at the completion of partition of the cloaca, the orifices lie together high on the posterior wall of the

anterior chamber at Müller's tubercle (the future verumontanum in the male) (Fig. 1.10). Rathke folds, which complete the subdivision of the cloaca, carry the duct orifices from lateral to posterior orientations, and atrophy of the roof of the orifice and duct transposes the orifice cranially. The receding ducts leave their mucosal imprints on the membranous urethra as delicate fins converging cranially and forming the central inferior crest.

The ureteric bud on each side arises from the wolffian duct posterior, but close to, the tubercle. The terminal end of the duct to a point just cranial to the bud widens in trumpet shape and exstrophies into the vesicourethral canal, forming the ipsilateral half of the vesical trigone and providing separate entry of wolffian duct into the urethra and of the ureter into the bladder (Fig. 1.10).

At the 30-mm stage, the müllerian ducts, having followed the paths of the wolffian ducts, penetrate the urogenital sinus at Müller's tubercle. They then fuse together and in the male undergo atrophy except for the utriculus masculinus. In the female they grow to form a single vagina, which migrates caudally to the vestibule

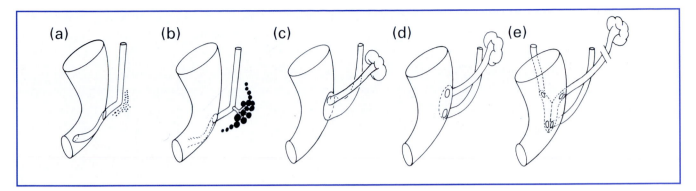

Fig. 1.10 *Diagram to demonstrate the absorption of the terminal end of the wolffian duct, and ureter into the urethra and bladder. (a),(b) Relocation of orifice from original site adjacent to cloacal membrane to upper urethra. (b) Ureteric bud arises from the elbow bend of the wolffian duct and penetrates the contiguous renal blastema. (c) Trumpet expansion of duct up to and a little distance beyond the bud which rotates laterally to an anterior position on the duct. (d) Further expansion and separation of ureter from wolffian duct. (e) Orifices of ureter and wolffian duct (vas deferens) in corner of trigone and urethra, respectively. (Reprinted, by permission, from Stephens, F.D. (1983), Congenital Malformations of the Urinary Tract, New York, Praeger, Fig. 2.6, p. 35.)*

concomitantly with exstrophy of the urogenital sinus (Luthra and Stephens, 1988).

Defects in the partitioning of the cloaca cause errors not only of the visceral tracts but also of the pelvic muscles, perineal muscles and sphincters, and the resulting anomalies follow fairly regular patterns.

Components of pelvic urethra and rectum formed from the internal and external cloaca

Males

Most of the bladder, urethra and rectum down to the level of the verumontanum is derived from that part of the internal cloaca that is divided by Tourneux's fold. The membranous urethra and part of the bulbar urethra, together with the ampulla of the rectum and part of the anal canal, are derived from that part of the internal cloaca partitioned by Rathke's folds. The remainder of the perineal and penile urethra is derived from the external cloaca. The junction between the internal and external cloacal segments of the anal canal is clear-cut and visible by the change in epithelium at the pectineal line, but in the urethra, it is less easily distinguished, because no such change in epithelium occurs. Transverse membranes in the urethra above and below the junction of the membranous and bulbar urethra provide some evidence as to the nature and siting of the urogenital membrane (page 98).

Females

The bladder and urethra down to the external urethral orifice are derived from that part of the anterior subdivision of the cloaca cranial to the original site of Müller's tubercle. The part caudal to Müller's tubercle folds outward and evaginates to form the vestibule within the confines of the external cloaca. The rectum and anal canal are similar in formation to that of the male, with one exception: contribution to the anterior quadrant of the anal orifice by the outer genital folds is lacking in the female.

Pubococcygeal (P/C) line and ischial (I) point

Previous dissection studies of specimens of normal and abnormal pelves of newborn babies and radiographic interpretations of the living counterparts have shown that normal pelvic structures and rectourinary fistula malformations can be conveniently oriented about the ossific centres of the pelvic skeleton.

The pubococcygeal line represents the transverse plane of the pelvis demarcated by the upper surface of the pubis (or the middle of the boomerang-shaped ossific centre of the pubis as viewed in direct lateral radiographs) and the sacrococcygeal junction. The normal midline structures contiguous with this line are the verumontanum, the peritoneal reflection from the rectum to the prostate gland, the external os of the cervix uteri, and in most female babies, the fornix of the pouch of Douglas. The origin of the levatores ani musculature is also very close to this level in the pelvis. This line represents the level to which Tourneux's fold of the urorectal septum descends normally. It also demarcates the level of the common rectoprostatic urethral fistula and provides a landmark about which other high fistulas may be oriented and defined.

The I-point is identified radiographically on direct lateral projection of the pelvis of an infant by the inferior tip of the comma-shaped ossific centre of the ischium. This point demarcates the junctions of pelvis and perineum, and membranous with bulbar urethra and the zone between the pubococcygeal line and the I-point represents Rathke's component of the urorectal septum of the internal cloaca. The I-point is the level of the rectobulbar fistula.

The pubococcygeal line and I-point are embryologically and diagnostically significant in males, but in females, the changes caused by the intrusion and descent of the müllerian ducts renders the interpretations somewhat less reliable. Fortunately, blind terminations of the rectum are very rare in females, and most anomalies can be diagnosed from the external inspections of the fistulas.

An understanding of the deviations from normal of the urorectal septum and the consequent effects on the structure and relations of the pelvic viscera and musculature is essential to the proper appreciation of the distinction between rectal and anal anomalies drawn as long ago as 1904 by Wood Jones. The rectal group of malformations consists of those abnormalities intrinsic in the partitioning of the internal cloaca, whereas the anal group is referable to aberrations of the partitioning of the proctodeal pit, the perineum, and genital folds.

The schemata in Figs 2.1 and 2.2 correlate the usual malformations with their underlying defects in development, and the stages at which such lapses occur in males and females.

The internal cloacal development is similar in males and females until the eighth week (30-mm crown–rump length) when the müllerian ducts enter the urogenital sinus, and in the female continue to enlarge and migrate. Likewise, malformations of the cloaca are similar in both sexes until the müllerian ducts superimpose themselves and continue to develop in the female but undergo atrophy in the male.

Faulty partitioning of the internal or external cloaca results usually in a rectal or anal fistula, which issues in the urinary or genital tracts or onto the skin of the perineum. Less commonly, the rectum or anus ends blindly. These anomalies are termed 'communicating' or 'non-communicating', respectively.

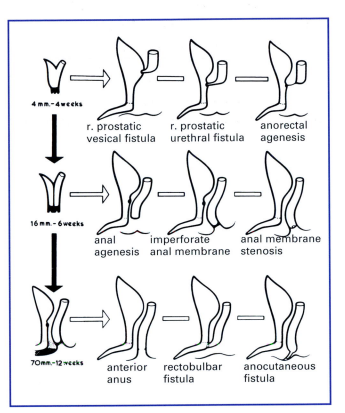

Fig. 2.1 *Embryologic classification of anorectal anomalies in the male. Upper row. Rectoprostatic defects arising from failure of subdivision of cloaca. Middle row. Defects in the formation of the anal pit. Lower row. Malformations derived from concurrent faulty development of the perineal mound (dotted area), causing irregular migration of the anus and of genital folds which causes anterior projection of anal fistula. Black arrow = normal development. White arrow = abnormal development. (Reprinted, by permission, after Stephens F.D. and Smith E.D. (1971), Anorectal Malformations in Children. Chicago: Year Book, Fig. 74, p. 135.)*

Males

Communicating anorectal anomalies
Arrest of formation of the septum
The two parts of the urorectal septum are interdependent in their formation. If Tourneux's fold stops short, Rathke's plicae fail to appear. The rectum then ends at the most distal point of descent of Tourneux's fold and may remain temporarily or permanently in communication with the cloacal cavity by a fine fistula to the bladder or bladder neck. If Tourneux's fold is fully developed, and Rathke's folds do not develop, the rectal fistula issues into the urethra (undivided cloaca) at the level of the verumontanum (Figs 2.3 and 2.5).

Rectoprostatic urethral fistula. The most common rectourinary fistula arising from failure of partition of the internal cloaca occurs at the normal level of the verumontanum. The bladder and urethra cranial to the fistula exhibit normal features; the normal calibre rectum ends

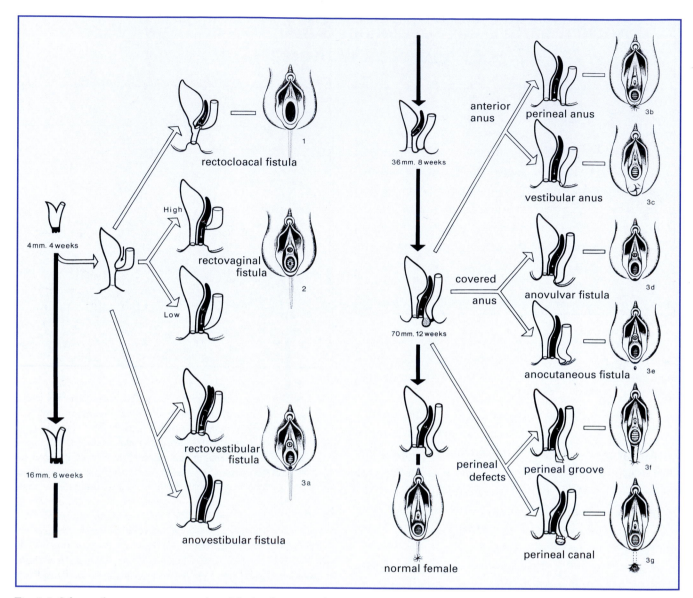

Fig. 2.2 *Schema of communicating anomalies of the female urogenital tracts with rectum and anus. Left column. Stages of development of the normal female pelvic organs (black arrows). Middle column. Congenital abnormalities derived from aberrations of development of the cloaca and perineum (white arrows). Right column. Perineal patterns corresponding with the internal anatomy shown in middle column. 1, rectocloacal fistula—one external orifice; 2, rectovaginal fistula—two external orifices; 3a, rectovestibular and anovestibular fistulas—three external orifices, the fistulas being stenotic and all within the vestibule; 3b, anterior perineal and 3c, anterior vulvar anus—both anomalies exhibiting three external orifices, the anuses being normal in dimensions; 3d, anovulvar fistula and 3e, anocutaneous fistula—both being examples of covered anus, and both exhibiting three orifices, the anal orifice being stenotic and issuing into the fourchette (3d) or perineum close to the fourchette (3e); 3f, perineal groove—three external orifices, the anus being non-stenotic and in continuity with the vestibule by a wet perineal groove; 3g; perineal canal—four external orifices, the anus being normal in appearance and a fine fistulous tract leading from the anterior wall of anal canal to vestibule. (Reprinted, by permission, from Stephens, F.D. and Smith, E.D. (1971), Anorectal Malformations in Children. Chicago: Year Book, Fig. 75, pp. 136, 138.)*

abruptly behind the mid-urethra in a fine fistulous tract, 1 or 2 mm in width and several millimetres in length, which issues into the verumontanum. The prostate gland develops above and lateral to the fistula, but does not develop caudal to the fistula; the ejaculatory ducts open on the verumontanum to either side, and the orifice of

utriculus masculinus is central, either separate from and cranial to the fistula, or sharing the orifice of the fistula.

The utriculus nestles between and cranial to the ejaculatory ducts, which also issue on the verumontanum. The trigone has normal dimensions, and the ureteric orifices are usually normally placed in the lateral cornua.

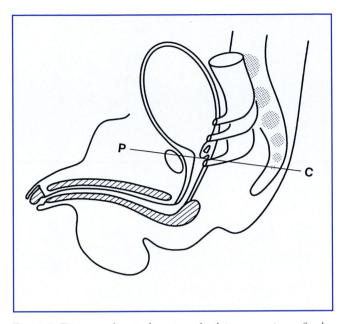

Fig. 2.3 *Diagram of sagittal section of pelvis: rectourinary fistulas resulting from lack of formation of Rathke's component of the urorectal septum. Rectourinary fistula lies at level of pubococcygeal line when Tourneux's fold is fully formed and cranial to it when only partially formed (P–C = pubococcygeal line). (Reprinted, by permission, after Stephens, F.D. (1953), Congenital imperforate rectum, recto-urethral and recto-vesical fistulae. Aust. N.Z. J. Surg. 22: 616, Fig. 1.)*

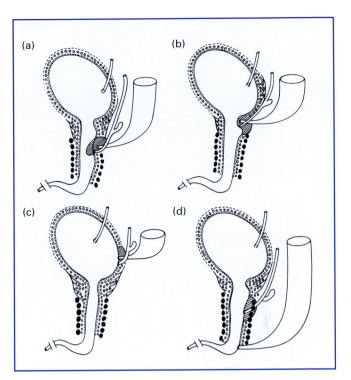

Fig. 2.4 *Urethral sphincters associated with rectourinary fistula abnormalities. (**a**) With rectourethral fistula located at normal level of verumontanum; normal arrangement of internal and external sphincters and smooth muscle of membranous urethra except for the break in continuity posteriorly caused by the tract of the rectal fistula. (**b**) With fistula issuing in region of internal urinary meatus; the internal sphincter was well formed except posteriorly where it was disrupted by prostatic tissue. The external voluntary sphincter surrounded the distal three-quarters of the 'urethra'. (**c**) With fistula issuing into the base of the bladder, the internal and external sphincters and the inner sleeve of smooth muscle were all well formed and resembled the normal anatomy of the female urethra. (**d**) With rectobulbar fistula the sphincters were normally disposed. (Heavy black dots = voluntary sphincter, small circles = circular smooth muscle of bladder, internal sphincter and urethra; dotted lines = internal layer of smooth muscle of bladder and urethra.) (Reprinted, by permission, from Stephens, F.D. (1983), Congenital Malformations of the Urinary Tract, New York, Praeger, Fig. 2.2, p. 32.)*

The bladder, bladder neck and urethra above the rectal fistula have normal musculature. The urethra from the fistula down to the perineal membrane exhibits a well-formed voluntary muscle coat, which rises higher than the fistula on the anterior wall (Fig. 2.4). Inside this circularly arranged voluntary muscle coat lies a sleeve of smooth muscle, which is arranged in two thin layers of inner longitudinal and outer circular muscle. In the membranous urethra, these two layers are as thick as the voluntary coat. The glands and ducts of Cowper in two specimens examined were absent.

The well-formed urethra and internal sphincter and upper tracts above the fistula at this level ensure that gas, meconium and infecting organisms from the rectum do not ascend into the bladder and ureters and are directed distally in the urethra to the exterior.

Rectoprostatic urethral fistulas issuing near internal urinary meatus. The rectal fistula enters the urinary tract at the centre of the verumontanum, which, in this instance, is located at a point close to the internal urinary meatus (Fig. 2.4b); the urethra is ultra-short above the fistula, and the 'urogenital sinus' (or cloacal canal) below it is correspondingly long. The internal

sphincter muscle is somewhat deranged by the ejaculatory ducts, utriculus masculinus and the prostatic ducts, all of which enter the urethra between its muscle bundles. Anomalies of the ureter are common; the ureters may be located ectopically on the trigone or issue into shallow diverticula, and they may be large in calibre, or one or both may be absent.

The pelvic urethra has a long, circular voluntary muscle coat from bladder neck to perineal membrane and an inner sleeve of involuntary muscle composed of two coats, inner longitudinal and outer circular (Fig. 2.4b). At this level of entry into the urinary tract,

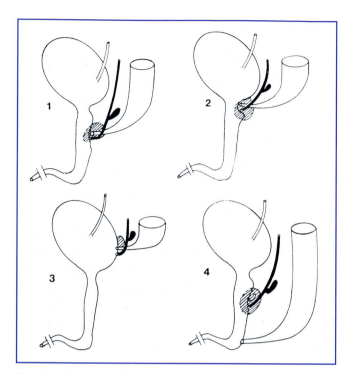

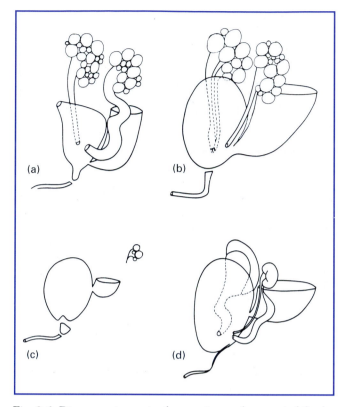

Fig. 2.5 *Diagrams showing relationship of rectal fistulas to the prostate gland and vas deferens in urethra and bladder (1 to 3). Both structures accompany the fistulas at verumontanum, internal urinary meatus, and bladder levels, but do not accompany the fistula at the level of the bulbar urethra (4). Note absence of posterior lobe of prostate when fistula issues at verumontanum. (Reprinted, by permission, from Stephens, F.D. (1983), Congenital Malformations of the Urinary Tract, New York, Praeger, Fig. 2.3, p. 33.)*

Fig. 2.6 *Diagrams representing four specimens of rectovesical fistulas with atresia of the 'urethra': single atresia in lower end (**a**) and upper ends (**b**) of pelvic 'urethra'; double atresia of 'urethra' (**c**); and combination of atresia and stenoses of pelvic 'urethra' (**d**). (Reprinted, by permission, after Magnus, R.V. (1972), Congenital rectovesical fistula and its associated anomalies. Aust. N.Z. J. Surg. 42: 197, Figs 1 (**a, c**), 3 (**a, c**).)*

some of the rectal content discharged through the fistula spills back into the bladder.

The incidence of vertebral defects, such as agenesis or hemigenesis of terminal vertebrae of the spinal column and irregular vertebral defects elsewhere in the spine, increases in those babies in whom the rectal fistula issues in the region of the bladder neck and trigone.

Rectovesical fistula. The rectovesical fistula (Fig. 2.4c) may be narrow and short or up to 2–3 cm in length and enters the bladder in the midline high in the trigone. The ejaculatory ducts issued into the bladder in one specimen at the mouth of the fistula; in this same specimen, one ureter also opened into the mouth of the fistula and the opposite ureter issued onto the trigone 1 cm lateral to the fistula. Around the fistulous tract, some rudimentary prostatic ducts could be identified opening into it. The epithelium in the fistula was chiefly stratified columnar but some plaques of transitional epithelium could be found, in both the fistula and the contiguous rectum.

The prostate gland lacked its posterior lobe when the fistula entered at the verumontanum, was well formed at the bladder neck in all lobes in one example of fistula at the bladder outlet, and was rudimentary and contiguous with the fistula in one example of rectovesical fistula. The orifices of the rectal fistula and vas deferens maintained intimate relationship in those fistulas issuing at or above the mid-pelvic urethra, but when the fistula issued in the bulbar urethra, the wolffian duct and prostate gland were normally situated and separate from the fistula (Fig. 2.5).

The ureteric orifices were located in the cornua of a normal trigone in the specimens with the fistula at and below the mid-pelvis, but were ectopic or absent in specimens with higher level fistulas.

In babies with rectovesical fistulas, the bladder and rectum may be ectatic, the ureters abnormal or absent, the sacrum deficient and the pelvis contracted. The

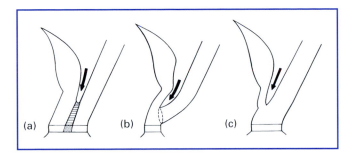

Fig. 2.7 *Rathke's fistula.* (**a**) *Normal urorectal septum, arrow indicates Tourneux's fold and hatching represents Rathke's component.* (**b**) *Rathke fistula due to failure of union of partially formed Rathke's folds which fail to meet in the midline, the orifice of the rectal fistula is large, and extends from verumontanum to bulb.* (**c**) *Very rare variant of* (**b**) *in which the cloacal canal caudal to Tourneaux's fold is rectal instead of urethral. (Reprinted, by permission, from Stephens, F.D. (1983), Congenital Malformations of the Urinary Tract, New York, Praeger, Fig. 2.5, p. 35.)*

'urethra' or cloacal outlet was found by Magnus (1972) to be atretic in seven of 11 specimens dissected, and the urachus was patent in three (Fig. 2.6).

Embryology of septal defects leading to rectourinary fistulas. Because of the common occurrence of rectourethral fistulas in males at the levels of the verumontanum and the bulb and the rarity of fistulae in the membranous urethra between these two levels, some explanation is sought from the manner in which the internal cloaca is subdivided by the urorectal septum. It is for this reason that the two-part urorectal septal cleavage of the internal cloaca is favoured.

The site of entry of the rectal fistula into the urotract does not necessarily coincide with the level of patent rectum when the tract is long. Whereas the levels of patent bowel indicate a spectrum of high to low, no such continuous spectrum of fistula orifice levels was found in the study of postmortem specimens.

Combination of arrest of Tourneux's and Rathke's folds. The rectourethral fistula, which issues at the normal level of the verumontanum, represents the stage of arrest of the urorectal septum when Tourneux's fold is completed at approximately the fifth week (8-mm stage). Rathke's folds fail to complete the septation. The stage is set for normal development of all structures above the verumontanum, including the wolffian ducts, ureters and kidneys and that part of the cloaca which forms the rectal ampulla. Below the level of the verumontanum and point of entry of the fistula, the undivided cloaca (urogenitorectal sinus) is at first a slim,

tubular structure down to the cloacal membrane. It develops in a manner similar to that of the normal urethra, elongating within the pelvis and expanding distally as the pars phallica. The pars pelvina forms the bulbar urethra. The membranous 'urethra' is fully clothed with voluntary external sphincter muscle and an inner sleeve of smooth muscle arranged in two thin layers, inner longitudinal and outer circular (Fig. 2.4d).

The rectal fistula and the lack of the septum derived from Rathke's folds interfere with the development of the posterior lobe of the prostate gland and also the two Cowper's glands, all of which may be lacking. Apart from these deficits, the undivided urogenitorectal sinus, together with the urethra above the fistula, closely resemble the normal urethra anatomically and functionally.

A narrow rectoprostatic urethral fistula may undergo atrophy; the rectum then ends blindly, remaining attached to the cloaca by fibrous tissue in proximity to the prostate gland and ejaculatory ducts (see Fig. 2.1). The term 'anorectal agenesis' has been applied to this particular anatomic defect. Sometimes Tourneux's fold may be more rudimentary; then the rectal fistula, wolffian ducts and prostate gland together open into the urinary system at a higher level, with the production of high rectoprostatic urethral or rectoprostatic vesical fistulas (Fig. 2.5).

Rectal fistulas issuing into the urinary tract in the vicinity of the bladder neck and trigone are examples of arrest of descent of Tourneux's fold at earlier stages than the previously described rectourethral fistula. Again, Rathke's folds fail to develop and the cloaca remains undivided. In each, the fistula, the vasa deferentia (wolffian ducts) and uterus masculinus enter the urinary tract close together at the distal limit of descent of Tourneux's fold. Prostatic ducts and fibromuscular tissue form around the orifice of the fistula high in the 'urethra' or bladder neck. Prostatic development is more rudimentary in the rectovesical fistula anomaly. The undivided cloaca distal to the fistula develops internal and external sphincters arranged in normal anatomical relationship with the bladder neck and urethra (Fig. 2.4).

Partial arrest of Rathke's plicae and full development of Tourneux's fold. The formation of the urorectal septum distal to the verumontanum is dependent on full development of Tourneux's component, and Rathke's contri-

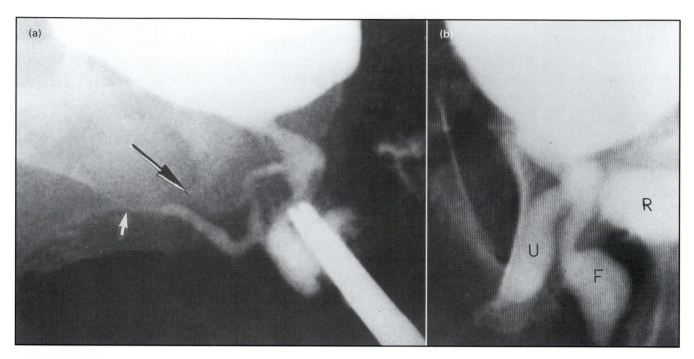

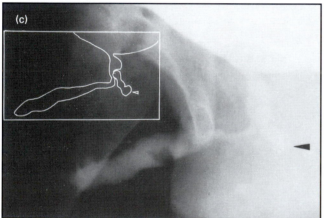

Fig. 2.8 *H-type fistula. Micturition cystourethrograms of the boy R.P. at age 3 months (**a**), 10 years (**b**) and 11 years (**c**). Note the true dimension of the posterior urethra (U) demonstrated at 10 years, as compared with the misleading calibre shown at 3 months. The long tract of the fistula (F) is better shown in (**b**). Note the spillage of opaque medium into the rectum. The phallic microurethra is shown (white arrow) in (**a**). Capacious reconstructed penile urethra and the blind-ending, partially excised fistulous tract alongside the membranous urethra are shown in (**c**). Arrow indicates level of perineal membrane (U = urethra; F = fistula; R = rectum). (Reprinted, by permission, from Stephens, F.D. and Donnellan W. L. (1977), 'H-type' urethral fistula. J. Pediatr. Surg. 12: 95, Fig. 2.)*

bution to the septum is then usually an 'all or none' event; if 'all', the partition of the internal cloaca is complete; if 'none', the anomaly is the rectourethral fistula at the pubococcygeal (P/C) line. Very rarely, however, Rathke's plicae approach the midline but do not meet, resulting in a large rectourethral fistula, the orifice of which is a long, vertical slit in the back wall of the membranous urethra from the verumontanum to the bulbar urethra (Fig. 2.7).

The orifice of this fistula, unlike those previously described, conducts meconium freely through the penile urethra, and is wide enough to admit the infant cystourethroscope or urethral catheter. It is suggested that this very rare anomaly be designated a 'Rathke fistula',

to distinguish it from rectourethral and rectobulbar types. The microanatomy of this rare malformation has not been studied by the present author (F.D.S.).

The cloacal duct of Reichel (Paul Freidrich Reichel, German obstetrician, born 1858) is the eponym applied to a communication between the urethra and rectum alleged to result from failure of the most distal part of a one-part urorectal septum to unite with the cloacal membrane. The fistulas embraced by this term presumably included both the Rathke and the rectobulbar fistulas. In this latter anomaly, the internal cloaca is completely partitioned, the perineal mound fails to develop, and the urethra and rectum gain separate contiguous orifices in the external cloaca but subsequently both orifices become covered over by the genital folds forming the rectobulbar urethral fistula. Rathke fistula fits the definition of the cloacal duct of Reichel, whereas the rectobulbar urethral fistula is more likely to derive from anomalous development of the structures of the external cloaca.

The ureteric migration in normal and rectourinary fistula conditions. The ureters arise as buds from the distal ends of the wolffian ducts at approximately the 4-mm (four-week) stage, when the cloaca is undivided. At first, the bud sprouts where the wolffian duct lifts off the posterior wall and angulates medially towards the internal cloaca. By the processes of trumpeting and absorption of the terminal ends of the wolffian ducts into the vesicourethral canal, the buds achieve independent orifices in the developing vesicourethral canal (see Fig. 1.10). The absorption involves that part of the duct between the cloaca and the bud called the 'common excretory duct' and also a short segment cranial to the bud, thus bringing about a separation of the ureter from the duct (or vas) and, at the same time, adding a wolffian gusset in the bladder neck and trigone. The trumpeting and absorption may also extend for a short distance into the mouth of the ureteric bud. The bud arises at first from the posterior aspect of the duct, then rotates around the expanding duct to lateral and then cranial relationships. Absorption of the expanded duct into the vesicourinary tract gives the ureter separate entry, and its orifice a lateral location, on the trigone far removed from that of the wolffian duct (vas deferens). While the caudal end of the ureter migrates into the bladder, the cranial end and kidney migrate towards the flank (see Fig. 1.10).

The wolffian ducts and ureters were found to be normally formed and located in postmortem specimens exhibiting a rectourethral fistula issuing at or below the normal position of the verumontanum. This reflects the findings in similar anomalies seen in patients.

If the fistula issues at even a slightly higher level in the urethra, or in the bladder neck or trigone, the bud formation, absorption of the wolffian duct segment and the migration of the ureter are more often faulty, giving rise to agenesis or ectasia of the ureter or lateral or medial ectopy of the orifice and renal hypodysplasia. The higher the fistula, the more complex are the anomalies in the upper tracts.

Overlapping of components of the urorectal septum
Heretofore, the anomalies resulting from agenesis or arrest of formation of the two parts of the urorectal septum have been explained. Misalignment of the two parts of the septum, however, leads to other forms of urinary or urorectal anomalies in males and are compounded in their complexity in the female by the superimposed müllerian ducts.

H-type urorectal and urocutaneous fistulas. This rare malformation occurs in males, alone or in combination with other anomalies such as tracheoesophageal fistula or cardiac defects. Urine passes freely via the fistula into the rectum and as 'tear drops' only from the penile urethra. Urine and meconium are discharged from the rectum through the anus into the diaper and the abnormality may pass unnoticed for days. The basic pattern of the urorectal anomaly is recognizable by voiding cystourethrography (Fig. 2.8) and the detailed anatomy has been confirmed by a histoanatomical study of the anomaly from which the following description is derived (Stephens and Donnellan, 1977) (Fig. 2.9).

The urethra from bladder neck to verumontanum was of normal dimensions. At the verumontanum it divided into two channels, the anterior being the continuation of the urethra and the posterior being the urethroanal fistula.

The urethra turned anteriorly at a right angle from the bifurcation and, after a 2-cm course through the prostate gland, turned caudally again at a right angle, traversing the pelvis and perineal membrane as the membranous urethra. Thence it continued in the perineum as the bulbar and penile urethra. The calibre of the urethra was normal as far distally as the perineal membrane. The lumen of the bulbar and penile urethra, however, was mostly microscopic in dimension. The penis and scrotum were outwardly normal.

The tract of the fistula, which continued in line with the proximal urethra, was 3-cm long, as measured radiographically, and slightly wider in diameter than the main urethra. It simulated the main course of the urethra, though it deviated terminally to enter the rectum at the pectinate line (Fig. 2.9).

The rectum and anus were normal in appearance and function except for the orifice of the fistula in the anterior wall on the pectinate line.

The prostate gland consisted of three lobes, two lateral and one caudal, all three being joined at the

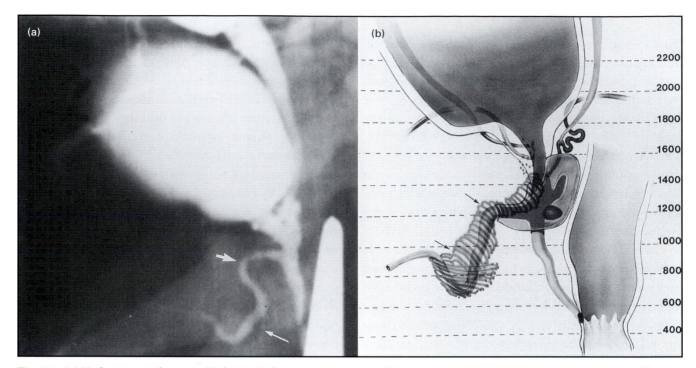

Fig. 2.9 (*a*) *Voiding cystourethrogram of Baby McC. showing prostatic urethra bifurcating into main urethra (upper arrow) and urorectal fistulous tract posteriorly: also reflux of opaque medium into left ejaculatory duct and ureter (lower arrow marks perineal membrane and junction of membranous and bulbar urethra).* (**b**) *Anatomy of the 'H-type' fistula of Baby McC. built up from serial section (10 μm thickness). The bladder leads into the prostatic urethra which divides into a ventral urethra and a dorsal H-fistula. One ureter joins the vas and the ejaculatory duct issues into the prostatic urethra. The other ureter and vas have independent orifices in the bladder neck. The utriculus opens into the urethra cranial to the verumontanum. The prostate is rotated anteriorly and separates the urethra from the fistula. Voluntary muscle of the external urethral sphincter is present throughout the posterior urethra, but is circumferentially disposed only around the membranous urethra (arrows) distal to the prostate gland. Bulbourethralis is caudal to the external sphincter. The fistula tract has no intrinsic voluntary or involuntary sphincter muscle in its walls. (Reprinted, by permission, from Stephens, F.D. and Donnellan, W.L. (1977), 'H-type' urethral fistula. J. Pediatr. Surg. 12: 95, Figs 1B and 3B.)*

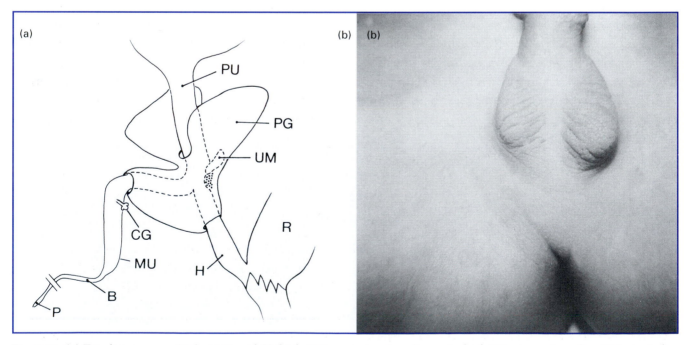

Fig. 2.10 (*a*) *Triradiate prostate of Baby McC. with H-fistula (PG = superior wing of prostatic gland; PU = prostatic urethra; UM = utriculus; H= H-fistula; R = rectum; CG = Cowper's gland, MU = membranous urethra; B = bulbous; and P = penile urethra. (**b**) H-fistula patient with absent perineal raphe and separate scrotal sacs (courtesy of Dr John Smith). ((**a**) Reprinted, by permission, from Stephens, F.D. (1983), Congenital Malformations of the Urinary Tract, New York, Praeger, Fig. 2.9A, p. 38.)*

point of bifurcation of the urethra by a common stalk. The main channel of the urethra grooved the bridge between the lateral lobes, then entered the triradiate stalk and turned anteriorly through the substance of the caudal lobe. The lateral lobes were wing-like, and the caudal lobe was conical and all ducts converged toward the verumontanum, which lay on the posterior wall of the bifurcation. The orifice of the utriculus lay in the verumontanum, and the abnormally sited vasa deferentia and ureters issued ectopically into the urethra above the verumontanum.

The bladder neck and pelvic urethra and fistula were lined by transitional epithelium. Above the prostate gland, the muscle of the urethra was involuntary and heaped to form the internal sphincter at the bladder outlet. Below the prostate gland, the membranous urethra exhibited an inner smooth-muscle coat composed of outer longitudinal and inner circular muscle bundles and a thick outer coat of voluntary muscle arranged circumferentially. The voluntary muscle extended onto the anterior wall of the urethra that tunnelled the prostate gland and could be traced even higher toward the bladder neck (Fig. 2.9). The prostate gland consisted mainly of ducts in a fibromuscular matrix issuing into the main urethra above and below the verumontanum (Fig. 2.10).

Cowper's glands were smaller than normal, and lay high on the side walls of the membranous urethra close to the prostate gland and consisted of a few mucous secreting acini. The duct of each gland was short and entered directly in the membranous urethra (Fig. 2.10a).

The external appearances of the bulbar and penile urethra were usually not abnormal, except for the very small size and calibration of the external meatus. The whole length of the pendulous and bulbar urethra was of microcalibre. In the bulbar urethra, many mucous secreting glands were present in the mucosal crypts.

Variations of the H-type urethrorectal anomaly. The fistula may issue into the rectum higher than the pectinate line or onto the perineum (Fig. 2.11). In one patient (Dr John Smith's patient), the anomaly was similar to that described above except that the fistula issued higher in the rectum and the perineal raphe was entirely lacking on the perineum and penis (Fig. 2.10b). In another (Dr Eugene Carlton's patient), the urethra and rectum lay side by side in the pelvis instead of one behind the other with a short, high fistula between. The external urethral orifice in this baby lay to the side of the anal orifice in the perineum, and the phallic anomalies included penoscrotal transposition and hypospadias. Rice *et al.* (1978) report a patient with a long urethrocutaneous fistula arising from near the bladder neck and tracking to the perineum (Fig. 2.12a) and Lawrence *et al.* (1983) supplied illustrations of the perineum of a patient with a similar though blind-ending urethrosubcutaneous sinus and the excised tract and its histology (Fig. 2.12b, c, d and e). Zimmerman and Mildenberger (1980) reported a case of H-fistula with a double tract from urethra to anus, a widely dilated penile urethra and a stenotic segment in the bulbomembranous zones. Scott (1960), Harrow (1966) and Gehring *et al.* (1973) described an anomaly in which the fistula issued onto the skin of the

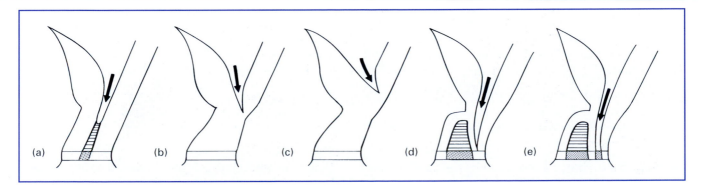

Fig. 2.11 *Aberrations of cloacal septation—urofistulas. Sagittal misalignments of the two parts of the septum; craniocaudal overriding of Tourneux's and Rathke's components. (**a**) The direction of Tourneux's component (arrows) determines the normal alignment, misalignment and absence of Rathke's plicae (**b**, **c**) with rectourethral and rectovesical fistula formation; overlapping of Rathke's component (**d**, **e**) leading to H-type urorectal and uroperineal fistulae respectively (hatching = Rathke's component; cross-hatch = cloacal membrane). (Reprinted, by permission, from Stephens, F.D. (1983),* Congenital Malformations of the Urinary Tract, *New York, Praeger, Fig. 2.10, p. 39.)*

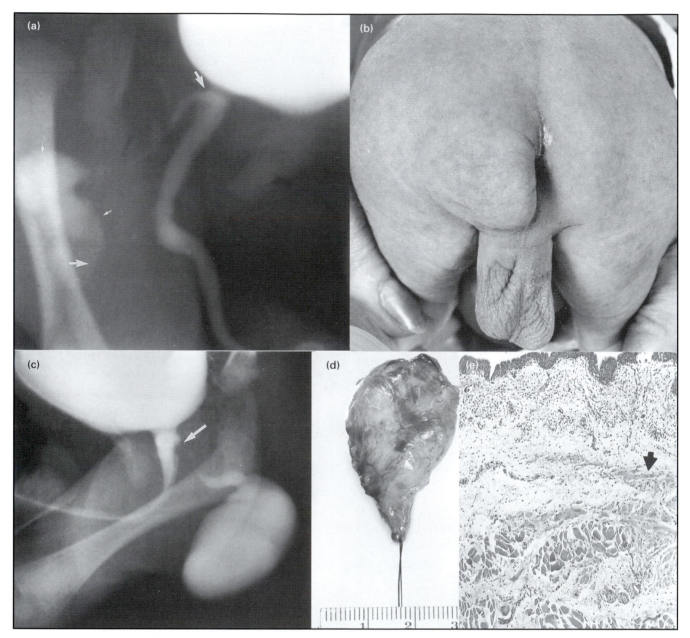

Fig. 2.12 *Variants of the H-fistula. (**a**) Urethrocutaneous fistula; voiding cystourethrogram showing long fine fistula with terminal sacculation tracking from the bladder neck posteriorly to the skin of perineum (large arrows); small arrows mark the cyst-like expansion. ((**a**) Reprinted, with permission, from Rice, P.E., Holder, T.M. and Ashcraft, K.W. (1978), Congenital posterior urethral perineal fistula: a case report. J. Urol. 119: 416.) (**b**) Urethral sinus forming subcutaneous swelling in the left side of perineum. (**c**) Voiding cystourethrogram (catheter visible in urethra and bladder) showing narrow sinus (arrow) arising at the verumontanum (filling defect on posterior wall of urethra) tracking to a blind ending cyst-like structure. (**d**) Photograph of excised sinus. (**e**) Photomicrograph of wall of fistula showing smooth muscle in the wall (arrow). ((**b**) and (**c**) Reproduced, by permission, from Lawrence, D., Howard, E.R. and Harris, R. (1983), A case of congenital urethral duplication cyst and its embryological significance. Brit. J. Surg. 70: 565–6 Figs 1 and 2. (**d**) and (**e**) by courtesy of E.R. Howard.)*

perineum in front of the anus (Fig. 2.11e) and Boisonnat (1961), Effman *et al.* (1976) and Das and Brosman (1977) report the opening on the phallus. In two other patients seen recently by one of the authors (F.D.S.), the phallic urethra was normal in calibre in

one and exhibited a focal stenosis of the bulbar urethra in the other.

Embryogenesis of H-type fistula and ventral duplications of the urethra. In this anomaly, the two parts of the septum, which normally divide the internal cloaca into

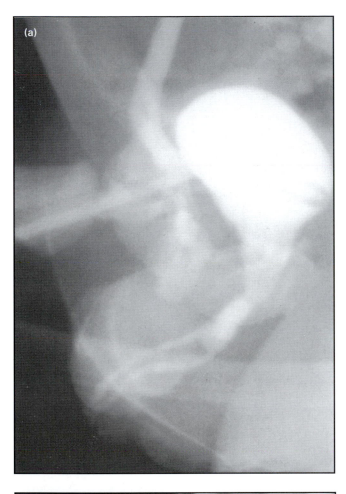

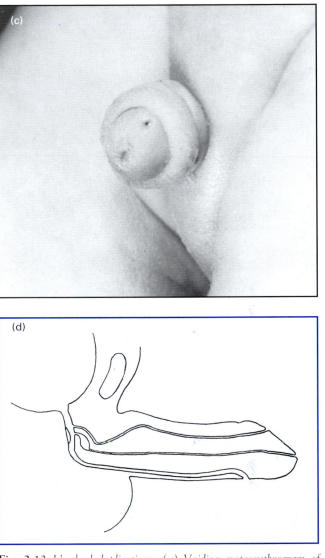

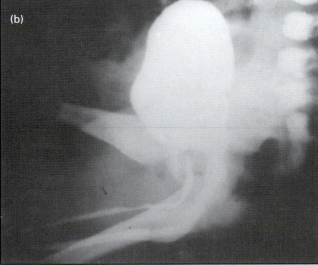

Fig. 2.13 *Urethral duplications.* (**a**) *Voiding cystourethrogram of duplication of the bulbar and penile urethra.* (**b**) *Complete 'tandem' duplication of urethra.* (**c**) *Two urethral orifices on the glans (same patient as shown in (**b**). (**d**) Tracings from radiographs of contrast-filled trifurcated urethra.* (**b**) *and* (**c**) *reprinted, by permission, from Thevathasan, D. (1961), Accessory urethra in the male child: Report of two cases. Aust. N.Z. J. Surg. 31: 134, Figs 1 and 2.* (**d**) *reprinted, by permission, from Schmeller, N.T. and Schermer, H.K.A. (1982), Trifurcation of the urethra. A case report. J. Urol. 127: 545, Fig. 2c.)* ((**a**) *Reprinted, by permission, from Stephens, F.D. (1983), Congenital Malformations of the Urinary Tract, New York, Praeger, Fig. 2.13A, p. 44.)*

urinary and rectal tracts, are misaligned. The direction of Tourneux's fold may determine not only the type of rectal fistula, but also the extent of overlap of the septal components (Fig. 2.11). This fold descends pos-

terior to Rathke's components and continues to grow caudally to the cloacal membrane. The cloacal membrane is thus subdivided by two septa into three membranes: the anal membrane posteriorly, the urogenital

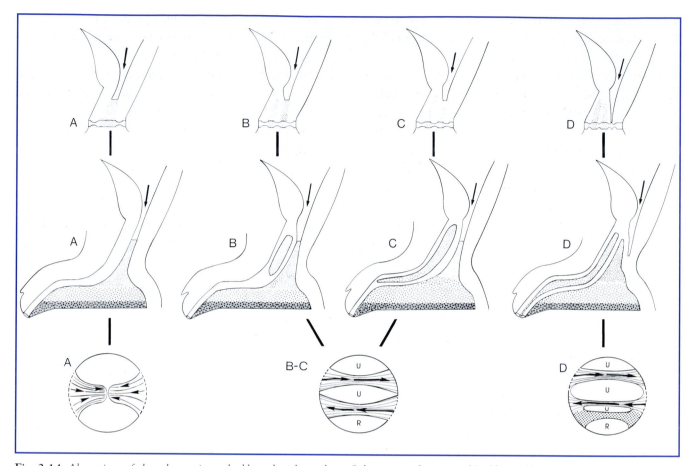

Fig. 2.14 *Aberrations of cloacal septation—double and triple urethras. Sideways misalignment of Rathke's folds. Column A. Coronal midline union of Rathke's plicae, in alignment with Tourneaux's fold completes the normal urorectal partition. Columns B and C. Side-to-side override of Rathke's plicae with alignment of the posterior plica with Tourneux's fold (arrows) creates duplications of the posterior or posterior and anterior urethra (inset B-C). Column D. Combinations of sagittal and side-to-side overriding (inset D) create duplication of urethra with H-type fistula. Thus D may represent a form of triplication of the urethra (compare Fig. 2.13(d)). Fine dots = Rathke's plicae; small circle = inner genital folds; black dots on hatching = outer genital folds. (Reprinted, by permission, from Stephens, F.D. (1983), Congenital Malformations of the Urinary Tract, New York, Praeger, Fig. 2.12, p. 43.)*

membrane anteriorly and in between the small fistula contiguous with the anal membrane. The level of the fistula in the urinary tract is governed by the length of Rathke's component; if it is normal in length, the fistula arises at the level of Müller's tubercle (verumontanum). If longer than normal, the bifurcation may be near the internal urinary meatus (Fig. 2.12a) and if shorter, in the membranous urethra. The level of the opening of the fistula in the anal canal or perineum depends on the extent of caudal growth of Tourneux's fold. The fistula may issue into the rectum, anus or perineum. The wolffian ducts open at, or slightly cranial to, the site of bifurcation on the back wall of the urethra. The double tract described by Zimmerman and Mildenberger (1980) is

extremely rare, and its embryogenesis is puzzling in the extreme.

Overlapping defects of the genital folds which move medially to close in the floor of the urogenital sinus to form the urethra may account for duplications restricted to the ventral aspect of the penis (Fig. 2.13).

Variants of ventral duplications. The ventral channel of the duplex anomaly may be defective, exhibiting degrees of hypospadias or stenosis or ectasia. Junctions of tandem and epispadiac urethras with the ventral urethra occur. The embryology of the junctions in the phallic urethra relates to errors of fusion of the genital folds and is different from the duplication involving both posterior and phallic urethras with an island of tissue between the channels (Fig. 2.13a, 2.14B and C). Triplication occurs when an extra ventral urethra of the H-type fistula coexists (Fig. 2.14D).

Other anomalies may masquerade as a duplication. These are the sinus of Guérin (1864) and its modifications, found distal to the ectopic meatus in patients with hypospadias; some forms of urethral diverticula, which arise as branches from the floor of the bulbar or penile urethra, congenital ectasias of Cowper's duct and acquired fistulous tracts, which arise from inflammation and abscess formations in the urethra.

Side-by-side duplications such as occur with double-bladder and double-penis anomalies and in females are excluded from the description.

The terms that have been used are descriptive in attempts to put together anomalous embryologic processes to explain the many errors of formation. The anomaly exhibiting tandem urethras with two orifices on the unsplit glans separates the epispadiac type from the duplications described by DeVries and Friedland (1974) and Stephens and Donnellan (1977) as H-type fistulas and by Boissonnat (1961), as a 'complete double functional urethra with a single bladder'.

The needs of radiologists and urologists in diagnosis and surgical management of these complex anomalies are better served by practical classifications, such as those of Effman et al. (1976) and Das and Brosman (1977) than those based on theories of embryogenesis.

Besides the anteroposterior overlap of the two parts of the septum creating the H-fistula, the lateral plicae of Rathke may also override from side to side, inducing a further set of malformations that includes duplications of the membranous urethra with extensions of the duplication either towards the bladder neck or distal to the cloacal membrane into the bulbous and penile urethra. These two urethras lie on the ventral aspect of the penis and glans, or one may exhibit hypospadias (Fig. 2.14B and C). There may even be combinations of anteroposterior with side-to-side overlappings of the septa with urethral triplications (Fig. 2.14D).

Dorsal duplications of the urethra. Dorsal duplications of the urethra occur in several formations.

1. A complete or incomplete tandem channel follows closely the normal urethra from glans to bladder. It may join the urethra at some point or end blindly on the way. The glans and prepuce are otherwise normally formed (Fig. 2.13b).

2. An epispadiac type of channel tracks from the dorsum of the penis to the bladder or joins the urethra at some point. The orifice is coronal or toward the base of the penis which is grooved distally, somewhat broadened and sometimes recurved. The ventral urethra may issue normally on the glans or exhibit hypospadias (Fig. 2.13d).

3. A dermoid sinus simulates a urethra but tracks from the base of the penis in front of the pelvic urethra and bladder behind the symphysis pubis to or toward the umbilicus.

Before attempting to explain embryologically the occurrence of these three anomalies, the present concept of the genesis of epispadias without duplication should be mentioned.

Patten and Barry (1952) and others have postulated a posterior shift of the genital tubercle toward the external end of the urorectal septum on the cloacal membrane. The two lateral anlagen of the tubercle fuse behind the urogenital membrane, which breaks down exposing the urogenital sinus epithelium on the dorsal aspect of the glans and penis. If the urogenital sinus encroaches onto the body stalk or if the migration of the lateral mesoderm falls short of the midline, epispadias and exstrophy of the bladder are combined.

If gross misplacement of the anlagen of the genital tubercle is a key factor in the total shift of the urogenital membrane to the dorsal aspects of the genital tubercle, presumably there are intermediate degrees of misplacement that permit the formation of a urethral plate on both the dorsal and ventral aspects of the fused bilateral components of the genital tubercle. The dorsal urethra may be restricted to the phallus, but if diastasis pubis is also a feature, the dorsal urethra exhibits epispadias.

The dorsal urethra of the duplication may be represented by a separate complete urethra or a dimple on the glans, a cord, a sinus or a V-junction with the ventral urethra. If the medial migration of the mesoderm of the abdominal wall also falls short, the dorsal orifice would be at the base of the penis, with a groove in the phallus distally. This urethra may reach the bladder or join the ventral urethra or be represented by a dimple, a cord, or a sinus. Effman *et al.* (1976) measured radiographically the width of the symphysis pubis in 10 examples of patent urethral duplications and found that in the epispadiac type duplications, diastasis of the symphysis pubis was also present.

The dermoid sinus is not a duplex urethra embryologically but an inturned epithelial tube or remnant occurring along the line of fusion of the lateral components of the abdominal wall between the umbilicus and the base of the penis.

Non-communicating anorectal anomalies, in males

Occlusions of the rectum and anus occur embryologically at three levels, namely, at the cranial and caudal ends of the Rathke septum and at the pelvic floor. These three levels correspond to the clinical assessment of high (anorectal agenesis), intermediate (anal agenesis) and low (imperforate anus) non-communicating anomalies in males and females.

Anorectal agenesis and anal agenesis without fistula

Rectoprostatic urethral and rectobulbar fistulas are narrow and usually short and may become occluded spontaneously during the pre- or postnatal development (see Fig. 2.1). The patent rectum then ends abruptly with an anterior beak leading to the site of occlusion, which may connect by a fibrous string to the prostate gland or to the bulb. In some high anomalies, the fibrous string is several centimetres in length, or the patent rectum may float free from any connection with the urinary tract. The anal pit is absent in these anomalies.

Anal agenesis

When the cloaca is completely divided at the 16-mm stage, the anal membrane lies closely approximated to the urogenital membrane. If the anal pit is absent or rudimentary, the rectum remains imperforate, lying in its original location adjacent to the urogenital sinus at the level of the upper border of the bulbocavernosus muscle; on the perineum the pit may be absent or represented only by a shallow blind dimple or pigmented spot (see Fig. 2.1).

Imperforate anal membrane

If the urorectal septum is complete and the anal membrane fails to perforate, septation of the external cloaca and development of the anal canal may take place normally (see Fig. 2.1). The membrane demarcates the rectum from the shallow blind anal pit in the perineum. The membrane, however, may be covered and thickened superficially by the overgrowth of genital folds.

Microperforation of the anal membrane may be a cause of anal stenosis at the junction of the skin-lined anus with mucosa of the rectum. More commonly, however, anal stenosis appears to result from overgrowth of the outer genital folds, which leads to a build up of skin behind, in front of, or sagittally over the anus ('buckethandle anomaly') with constriction of the lumen.

Anorectal atresia

Anorectal atresia is another clear-cut entity that occurs subsequent to initial normal development of the rectum and anus at or about 12 weeks (60-mm crown–rump length). An ischemic accident deprives a part of the rectum or anal canal of its blood supply, leading to stenosis or to total occlusion of a segment. The rectum above and the anal canal below the ischaemic zone connect through a short or long stenotic segment, or, if the occlusion is total, the rectum and anal canal may be separated by a thin membrane, a fibrous cord, or a gap analogous to atresias elsewhere in the intestine. The anus and part of the anal canal caudal to the ischaemic zone have normal clinical features and sphincter anatomy.

Females

Communicating anorectourogenital anomalies
Septal defects of the internal cloaca leading to rectocloacal, rectovesical, rectovestibular and rectovaginal fistulas

The cloacal abnormality, caused by failure of partition into urogenital and rectal compartments, is similar in males and females at the 16-mm stage. The hindgut and urinary systems remain in direct communication. The basic deformity of the internal cloaca is either an arrest or an overlap of the septal components. The müllerian ducts arriving at the site of the verumontanum at the 35-mm stage impose female modifications upon these basic deformities, and the final result depends on the course taken by the müllerian ducts after their point of contact with the cloaca (Fig. 2.15).

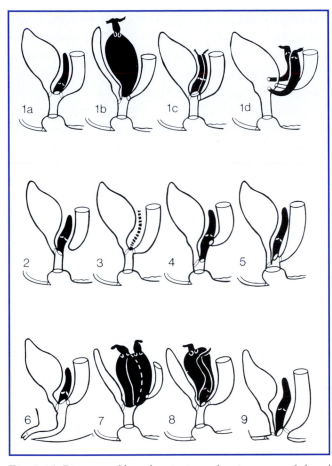

Fig. 2.15 *Diagrams of lateral projections of various types of cloacal malformations. (Reprinted by permission from Stephens, F.D. and Smith, E.D. (1986), Classification, identification, and assessment of surgical treatment of anorectal anomalies. Pediat. Surg. Int. 1: 200–5, Fig. 3.)*

Arrest of the urorectal septum in the female. *Rectocloacal fistula.* In the regular rectocloacal fistula (analogous with male rectoprostatic urethral fistula, Fig. 2.1), the external borders of the vulva appear normal, but the vestibule has only the one central orifice of the cloacal canal (Fig. 2.2 (1)). The anus is absent from the perineum. The cloacal canal is a tube-like structure of slightly larger diameter than that of its external orifice. The vagina enters the vault, the urethra issues on the anterior wall and the rectum enters the posterior aspect of the cloacal canal contiguous with the orifice of the vagina (Fig. 2.2 (1)).

The urethra is short but of normal calibre. The internal urinary meatus, ureteric orifices and trigone may be normally developed. The vagina may be single, the septum between the two müllerian ducts having disap-

peared, or septate because of persistence of part or whole of the septum between the ducts or single because of absence of one müllerian duct. The uterus exhibits a well-formed cervix and cervical canal and, if septate, the uterus is bicornuate and exhibits two cervices (Fig. 2.15).

The rectum at birth is usually normal in dimensions to the point where it turns anteriorly and funnels abruptly to enter the cloacal canal through a moderately stenotic, inelastic orifice. Its smooth-muscle coats do not form sphincters at the site of entry into the cloaca. The levatores ani and the important puborectalis component are present but merged with pubovaginalis and pubourethralis and form a pelvic platform and sling around the back wall of the cloacal canal. The sling elevates and compresses the fistula, affording some sphincteric action on the orifice.

The epithelium of the urethra, vagina and cloaca is transitional in type; in the rectum, it is columnar with goblet cells and crypts, but the fistula itself is lined by stratified columnar epithelium.

Urinary continence can be expected in the rectocloacal anomalies in which the urethra is adequate in length and unimpaired by the müllerian structures. Continence also depends on intact nervi erigentes and sacral roots.

Voiding cystourethrography is necessary to study the reservoir and voiding functions of the bladder and urethra, to assess the degree of continence and length of the urethra and to detect vesicoureteral reflux if present. This procedure, together with excretory urography and endoscopy, should be undertaken in the neonatal period before or shortly after the colostomy operation in order to determine the anatomy, assess function of the bladder and urethra, and give appropriate treatment to other abnormalities that may be present. An appropriate gauge bicoudé catheter is needed to negotiate the urethral orifice, which is tucked up in the anterior wall of the cloacal canal.

The length of the urethra between the internal meatus and the cloacal canal varies from patient to patient and is inversely proportional to the length of the cloacal canal. The intrinsic sphincter anatomy is impaired when the urethra is very short leading to grades of incontinence of urine. The cloacal canal itself is wide in calibre and the muscular wall is incapable of effective urinary sphincter activity. Urinary continence is reliant entirely on the short urethral component, which may be expected to lengthen with growth of the child. In some older patients, this urethral lengthening together with self-training has converted borderline incontinence to satisfactory continence.

Continence may be impaired also by defects of the spinal cord as evidenced by deficiencies of the sacral vertebra and perineal anesthesia. Agenesis of the sacrum involving all vertebrae below S2 portends neuropathic incontinence. Agenesis below S3 is, however, compatible with adequate innervation and continence.

Rectocloacal fistula with short urethra is accompanied more commonly with additional malformations of the urinary and genital tracts. Agenesis of the ureter, lateral ectopy of the ureteric orifice, duplication of the ureter, ectasia of the ureter, renal hypodysplasia, fused kidneys and megacystis may occur. The vagina remains septate and the uterus is then usually bicornuate. If one or both hymens remain imperforate at the vault of the cloacal canal, a large mucocolpos may develop owing to the stimulation of secretion of cervical mucus by maternal oestrogens. Alternatively, the occlusion may first come to notice at the onset of the menarche at puberty. In infancy, the tumour formed by the mucocolpos may compress the bladder and rectum and rise high in the abdomen (Fig 2.15). The ureters become displaced laterally, partially obstructed and dilated.

Instead of the hymen being imperforate, the terminal end of the müllerian duct may remain uncanalized, in which event, the uterus and cervix may be connected with the cloacal canal only by a thick, solid core several centimetres in length.

Rectovesical fistula. Rectovesical fistula (analogous with rectovesical fistula in the male) is rare and usually incompatible with life because of renal defects or malformations of other systems (Fig. 2.16).

The rectum and bladder may both exhibit gross ectasia. The gut ends abruptly in a narrow, fistulous tract which issues on the bladder base near or far from the internal urinary meatus. Wherever the fistula enters the bladder, the müllerian ducts penetrate or issue separately to the side of, or beyond, or into, the fistula. They are completely separate, usually large in dimension and may exhibit terminal occlusion. The ureter may issue close to the orifice of the fistula or lateral to it on a corner of the ipsilateral trigone or in a diverticulum or may be abnormal or absent. Vesicoureteral reflux may occur into one or both ureters. The kidneys are often hypoplastic and dysplastic, fused, ectopic, or malrotated. The cloacal canal or 'urethra' is somewhat elongated and may be

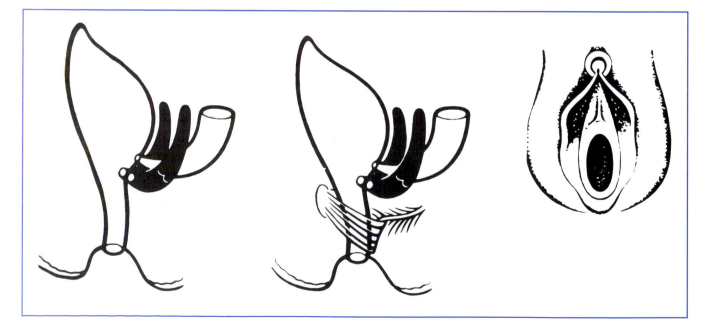

Fig. 2.16 *Rectovesical fistula showing separation of the two müllerian ducts by the fistula which issues into the trigone of the bladder. Also shown is the pubovisceral sling muscle around the cloacal canal and the single introitus of the cloaca in the vulva. (Reprinted, by permission, from Stephens, F.D. and Smith, E.D. (1971), Anorectal Malformations in Children. Chicago, Year Book, Fig. Z-15, App. C, p. 5.)*

focally atretic or stenotic (Fig. 2.6). The urachus may or may not be patent (Magnus, 1972). The muscle coats of the 'urethra' are both involuntary and voluntary sleeves similar to those of the normal female urethra and may subserve continence if the innervation is unimpaired by associated spinal malformations. If the sacrum is deficient, the pelvis is often much contracted and the levator diaphragm is poorly developed.

Rectovestibular and anovestibular fistulas. In rectovestibular and anovestibular fistulas, the urethra and vagina are anatomically normal but the rectum ends in mid-pelvis, funnels acutely to a narrow fistula that issues behind the vaginal wall in the fossa navicularis of the vestibule (Fig. 2.2). If the fistula is short and less than 1.0 cm long, it is called an 'anovestibular fistula'. The sphincters of the bladder and urethra are entirely normal. The intrinsic internal and external sphincter muscles of rectal and anal fistulas are rudimentary, but the components of the levator ani musculature are sound and afford good anorectal continence if preserved by appropriate reconstructive surgery (Fig. 2.17). In the perineum at the site where the anus would normally form,

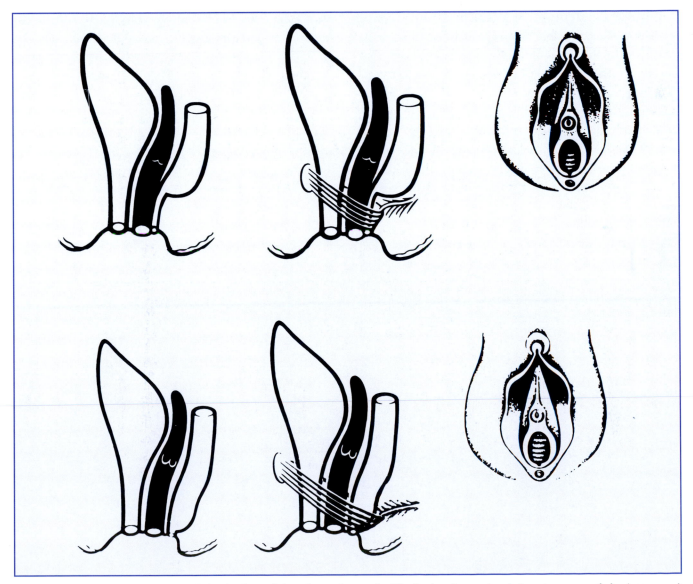

Fig. 2.17 *Rectovestibular and anovestibular fistulas and the puborectalis muscle. The fistula is longer than 1.0 cm in rectovestibular (upper row) and shorter in anovestibular (lower row). The puborectalis muscle is the chief muscle of continence after reconstruction of the anal canal. (Reprinted, by permission, from Stephens, F.D. and Smith, E.D. (1971), Anorectal Malformations in Children. Chicago, Year Book, Fig. Z-22, App. C., p. 6 and Z-29, App. C., p. 8.)*

some voluntary muscle fibres of the rudimentary external sphincter lie in the subcutaneous tissue and pucker the skin if stimulated electrically.

Rectovaginal fistula. In rectovaginal fistula, a rare anomaly, the bladder and urethra are functionally normal, and the vagina is well formed in all respects except for the orifice and entry of the rectal fistula in the posterior wall. The rectum ends abruptly, funnelling anteriorly to an inelastic orifice approximately 1 cm in diameter in full-term babies (Fig. 2.2). Firm stools clog in the rectum, which soon becomes ectatic. A high rectal fistula has no intrinsic rectal sphincters.

External examination of the vulva and vestibule reveal no abnormalities, but meconium or faeces issue from the vagina. The anus is absent from the perineum. The rectal fistula can be identified endoscopically prior to initial colostomy surgery.

Variants of this anomaly include an entry of the fistula into the vagina at a lower level (Fig. 2.2), a septate vagina above the fistula and rectal ectasia. When the orifice is low in the vagina, the fistula is hugged by the puborectalis sling, which affords a good measure of anorectal continence by its sling action at the rectovaginal junction.

Microscopic examination of the muscle in the walls of the rectovaginal fistula reveals a continuous coat of inner circular smooth muscle as far as the orifice in the vagina and an outer longitudinal coat of smooth muscle, which interweaves with the muscle coats of the vagina.

Imperforate hymen in cloacal anomalies. One or both müllerian ducts may remain imperforate or partially obstructed at the site of penetration of the cloacal canal (Fig. 2.18). If maternal hormones in the terminal weeks of pregnancy stimulate the production of mucus in the fetal cervical canal the vagina, cervical canal and uterus fill with mucus, distend and undergo massive dilatation. The urethra and bladder and the rectum are compressed, all being partially obstructed by the tense mucocolpos intervening between them. Hydroureteronephrosis usually develops in both upper urinary tracts. If mucus secretion is not stimulated in the fetus or neonate, the imperforation may remain unnoticed until puberty when the menstrual periods occur. Then periodic pain, absence of overt haemorrhage and an abdominopelvic mass lead to the appropriate diagnosis and management. Menstrual blood flow is blocked and fills the obstructed vagina. If, however, one passage of a double vagina is blocked, but the other is patent, the haematocolpos causes acute exacerbations of pain when periodic menstrual flow occurs from the patent system (Fig. 2.18b).

Atresia of the vagina. The vagina, whether single or one of two separate vaginas associated with cloacal deformities, may exhibit a focal atresia. The segments below and above are connected by a diaphragm or stalk. This

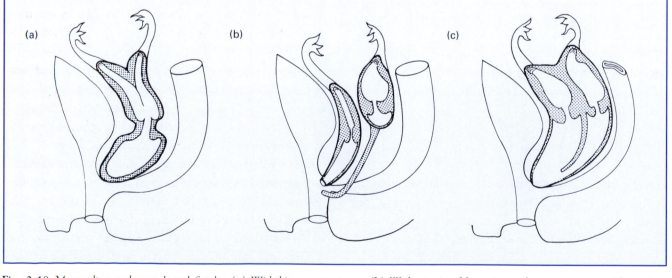

Fig. 2.18 *Mucocolpos and rectocloacal fistula.* (**a**) *With bicornuate uterus.* (**b**) *With atresia of L vagina and separate patent right vagina.* (**c**) *With septate uterus and partial septation of vagina. (Reprinted, by permission, from Stephens, F.D. (1983), Congenital Malformations of the Urinary Tract, New York, Praeger, Fig. 2.17, p. 49.)*

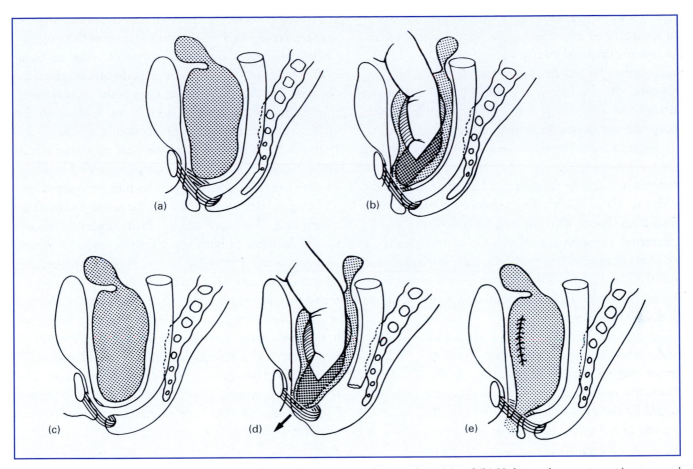

Fig. 2.19 *The principles of Raffensperger's operation for imperforate vagina with mucocolpos.* (**a**) *and* (**b**) *High imperforate vagina with rectum and urethra normally disposed. Abdominal culpotomy and digital bouginage and perineal anastomosis of vagina to vestibule.* (**c**), (**d**) *and* (**e**) *Imperforate vagina accompanying rectocloacal fistula. Abdominoperineal culpoplasty and rectoplasty. Note the puborectalis muscle in the reconstructions.* (*Reprinted, by permission, from Stephens, F.D. (1983),* Congenital Malformations of the Urinary Tract, *New York, Praeger, Fig. 3.9, p. 71.*)

obstruction may give rise to early muco- or late haematometrocolpos.

Decompression may be achieved by perforation of the hymen, if it is thin and accessible externally, or by the Raffensperger technique if the vagina ends at a high level in the pelvis (Fig. 2.19).

A detailed discussion of the significance of vaginal atresia in the Rokitansky Syndrome is included in Chapter 4.

Overlap cloacal septal defects: vaginoanal fistula. Vaginoanal fistula is a rare anomaly that may be the female counterpart of the H-type urethroanal fistula of the male. The vulva and vestibule and the anus in one patient were externally normal. However, inside the vagina, just above the hymen, was a fistulous tract directed posteriorly and caudally to the anal canal where it issued on the pectinate line (Fig. 2.20). The

orifice in the anal canal could be identified by examining the baby placed face down in the frog position. The tract traversed the deep perineum obliquely in the sagittal plane, was more than a centimetre long, and was cleanly dissected with the repair of the rectal and vaginal walls. This very rare malformation in the genitorectal tracts was accompanied by a lung bud deformity, namely agenesis of the right bronchus and lung.

One variant of this overlap cloacal septum malformation occurred in a female baby in whom the vagina was absent and here the bifurcation in the urethra was located at a lower level in the pelvis than the male H-fistula described on page 19. Cranial to the fistula, the urethra was normal in length, and distal to it, the urethra was covered by the genital folds to form a short, bulbar segment (Fig. 2.21). The sphincters of the urethra were cranial to the fistula and normal in

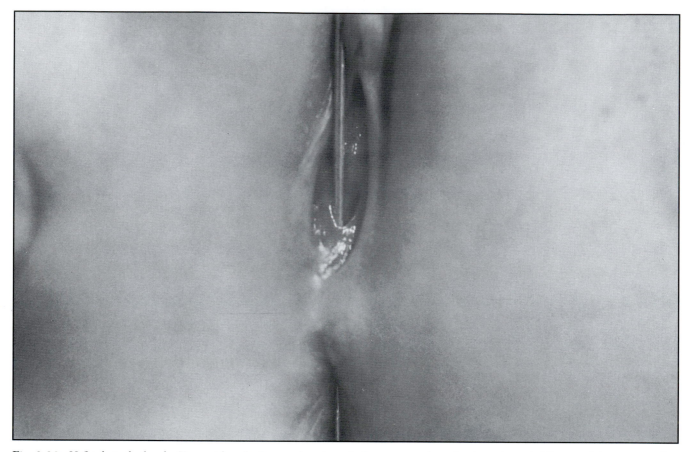

Fig. 2.20 *H-fistula in the female. Tract with probe from vagina above the hymen to pectinate line in anal canal. (Photograph by courtesy of Dr David Collins.)*

function. In this baby, the deformity was one of the components of the VATER syndrome. Two years after the colostomy procedure for the urethro-rectal anomaly and repair of the tracheo-oesophageal fistula, the H-fistula in the urethra and rectum was excised. The 'bulbar' urethra and anterior part of the perineum were laid open down to the fistula, which was dissected free and then detached from the urethra and rectum. The defects in the urethra and rectum were repaired. The vestibule was exteriorized by sewing the cut edges of the floor of the 'bulbar' urethra to the skin and letting in a posterior V-shaped skin flap down to the urethral orifice.

The anatomy of these overlap cloacal defects is only slightly different from the perineal canal, which arises from the back of the vestibule below the hymen and issues into the anal canal at the same site (Fig. 2.22).

Embryology of septal defects leading to rectocloacal, rectovestibular and rectovaginal fistulas

The embryogenesis of the internal cloaca in males and females is similar until at least the 16-mm (six-week) stage when partition by Tourneux's and Rathke's septa is complete, the urogenital and anal membranes have opened, the ureters have achieved a vesical location and the ends of the müllerian ducts approach the urogenital sinus. The müllerian ducts actually penetrate the sinus at about the 23-mm (eighth-week) stage, and from then on, in the female, they grow rapidly and impose female characteristics on future development. Arrest or overlap of the parts of the septum deform the cloaca prior to the arrival of the müllerian ducts which later impose an array of female malformations, the nature of which depends on the intrinsic development and migratory capacity of the ducts.

Arrest of Rathke's septation of the cloaca and formation of rectocloacal and rectovesical fistulas. Failure of formation of Rathke's folds but normal descent and development of Tourneux's fold leads to the initial development of the standard rectourethral fistula. Shortly after, the müllerian ducts migrate caudally in Tourneux's mesenchymal fold to penetrate the cranial wall of the fistula. The cloaca into which the urethra,

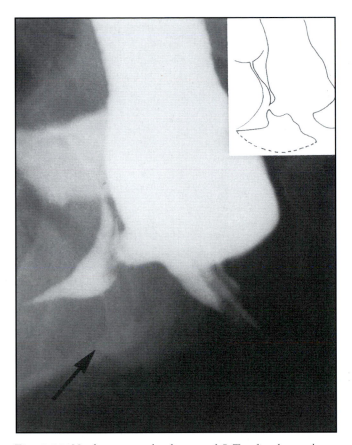

Fig. 2.21 *Urethrogram and cologram of S.T., female, aged two years. Absence of vagina and H-fistula between urethra and anal canal. Perineum covers 'bulb' of urethra which issues at the clitoris; inset outlines urethra, H-fistula and rectum and anal canal (courtesy of Dr Richard Goldstein).*

müllerian ducts, and rectum all issue is called the 'recto-cloacal canal' (Fig. 2.2(1)). The medial walls of the pelvic ends of the two müllerian ducts fuse and resorb, forming one single vagina, or they fuse and remain septate. The pars phallica dilates and exteriorizes into the external cloaca but the pars pelvina remains tubular. In some girls, further exteriorization and widening of the cloacal canal takes place after birth and even later in childhood in the years before puberty, transforming a long, narrow cloacal canal into a short, shallow, wider canal. The walls of the introitus remain somewhat inelastic and constricted, but this rather unyielding ring is readily amenable to surgical correction at puberty. In such patients, the cloacal introitus and canal are an adequate substitute for the vagina.

If the sacrum is well developed, containing most of its vertebrae, the nerves to the bladder and urethra are intact and the upper tracts of the urinary system are usually normally formed. This rectocloacal fistula is the

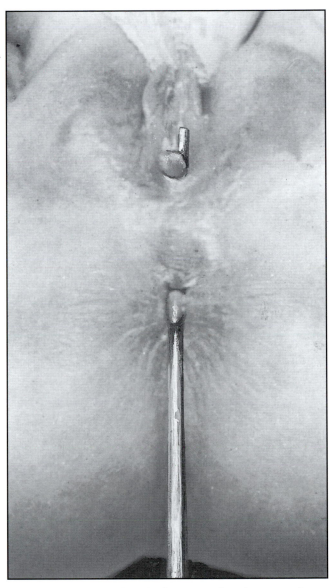

Fig. 2.22 *Perineal canal. Probe depicts tract from fossa navicularis in vestibule below the hymen to the pectinate line in anal canal (small polyp at each end of the tract). Urorectal septum normally formed but uroanal septum defective. (Reprinted, by permission, from Stephens, F.D. and Smith, E.D. (1971), Anorectal Malformations in Children. Chicago, Year Book, Fig. 67a, p. 117.)*

female counterpart of the regular rectoprostatic urethral fistula issuing at the verumontanum in the male (Fig. 2.1).

Arrest of Rathke's and Tourneux's septa
Rectovesical fistula. Failure of Rathke's plicae to develop and complete the cloacal septation caudal to Tourneux's fold accounts for the basic rectourinary fistula. This fistula issues into the urethra, bladder neck, or base or even back wall of the bladder, depending on the length of Tourneux's saddle. The wolffian ducts also traverse the mesoderm of

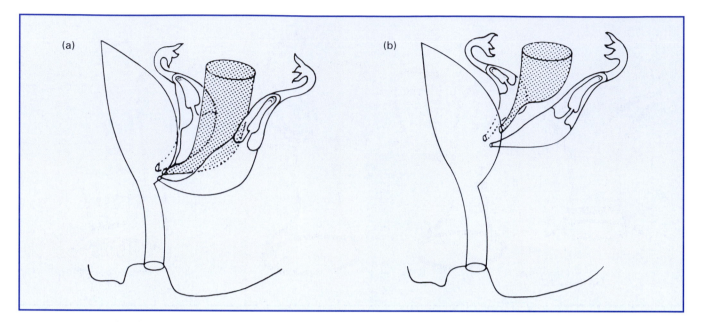

Fig. 2.23 *Rectovesical fistula. The fistula separates the two müllerian ducts which issue separately into the bladder, either (**a**), near the internal meatus, or (**b**), high in the bladder (rectum is shaded). (Reprinted, by permission, from Stephens, F.D. (1983), Congenital Malformations of the Urinary Tract, New York, Praeger, Fig. 2.21, p. 51.)*

Tourneux's fold to gain entry into the cloaca to either side of, and close to, the orifice of the rectal fistula. These abnormally located ducts give origin to the ureteric buds, guide the müllerian ducts to abnormal destinations and then undergo atrophy. The müllerian ducts remain separate and penetrate the bladder to either side of, and slightly distal to, the site of entry of the rectal fistula. The müllerian ducts are large structures but the orifices are very small or the ducts remain imperforate (Fig. 2.23).

Ectasia of the bladder, rectum, or both is common. It may derive from excessive dilatation of either organ after partial partitioning of the cloaca, or from subdivision of a cloaca that was intrinsically ectatic in its initial formation (Brent and Stephens, 1976). The tract of the rectal fistula is terminally very narrow but may be up to several centimetres in length.

The coccyx and sacrum are also frequently deficient, indicating a derangement of the hind end of the body.

In this anomaly, in which the wolffian ducts are aberrant, the nephrogenic cords, which grow caudally with them, may also be malformed and result in combined ureterorenal derangements. The ureters may fail to develop or may have ectopic orifices close to the fistula or lateral to it or even in a paraureteral diverticulum. The kidneys are frequently hypoplastic or dysplastic, and may be ectopic or fused.

Rectovestibular and rectovaginal fistula. These two abnormalities are embryological variants of the standard rectocloacal malformation. The müllerian ducts, instead of arresting at the site of entry into the undivided internal cloaca, undergo further active growth and migration from the pelvis to the perineum. With this advancement, the urethra, vagina and the rectal fistula elongate and all orifices issue into the vestibule (Figs. 2.2 (3a) and 2.24). Alternatively, the actively proliferating fused vaginal bulbs may incorporate the rectum as a rectovaginal fistula into the back wall and advance to the external cloaca. The urethra and vagina elongate in the process, the cloacal canal everts, and the orifices of the urethra and vagina open to the exterior in the vestibule (Fig. 2.2 (2)).

Turner (pers. commun.,1981) describes a rare type of rectovestibular fistula that issues by a narrow stenotic orifice anterior to two separate vaginal orifices in the vestibule. This combination may arise when the right and left ducts remain separate and issue into the cloacal canal beside or just distal to the rectal fistula and advance all together caudally to the vestibule. The urethral orifice lies anterior, with the orifice of the rectal fistula behind it, and the orifices of the two vaginas beside or behind the orifice of the fistula (Fig. 2.25).

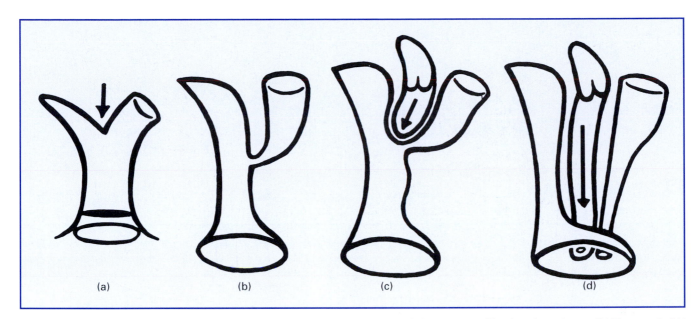

Fig. 2.24 *Stages in the formation of a rectovestibular fistula. (**a**) Internal and external cloaca separated by cloacal membrane. (**b**) Tourneux's fold (arrow in (**a**)) forms a saddle-shaped cleavage of the cloaca as far distally as Müller's hillock. Rathke's folds fail to appear. (**c**) Müllerian ducts descend upon the partially divided cloaca. (**d**) Müllerian ducts migrate down the posterior wall of the undivided cloaca, carrying the attenuated rectal fistula and orifice with them into the undivided external cloaca (short and long arrows in (**c**) and (**d**)). (Reprinted, by permission, from Stephens, F.D. and Smith, E.D. (1971), Anorectal Malformations in Children. Chicago, Year Book, Fig. 72, p. 127.)*

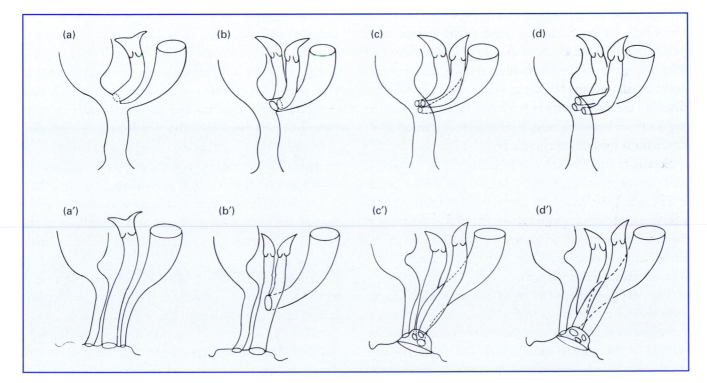

Fig. 2.25 *Diagrams of end results of müllerian duct migration from the urogenital sinus to the exterior depending on exact sites of issue of the ducts relative to the rectocloacal canal. (**a**),(**a'**) Single duct in urethra to rectovestibular fistula. (**b**),(**b'**) Ducts incorporate rectal fistula as a rectovaginal fistula and migrate to vestibule. (**c**),(**c'**) Ducts penetrate urogenital sinus above and contiguous with the rectal fistula and all three migrate to vestibule in same relationship. (**d**),(**d'**) Ducts straddle rectal fistula to open below but contiguous with orifice of rectal fistula, migrate distally and retain posterior relationship to rectal fistula. (Reprinted, by permission, from Stephens, F.D. (1983), Congenital Malformations of the Urinary Tract, New York, Praeger, Fig. 2.23, p. 52.)*

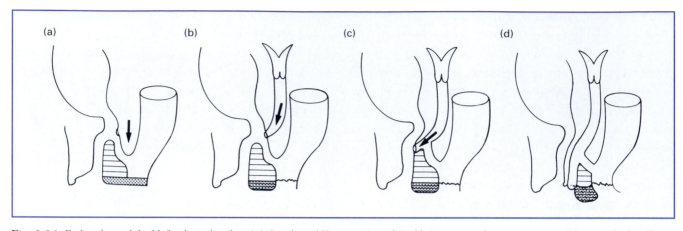

Fig. 2.26 *Embryology of the H-fistula in females.* (**a**) *Overlap of Tourneux's and Rathke's septa at the 16-mm stage.* (**b**) *Arrival of müllerian ducts at the 23-mm stage.* (**c**) *Incorporation of the H-fistula in the vaginal wall.* (**d**) *Müllerian migration progresses to the vestibule, and the fistula connects the vagina above the hymen to the rectum. Transverse hatching indicates Rathke's septum. Dotted areas indicate cloacal membrane in* (**a**) *and perineal mound in* (**b**),(**c**) *and* (**d**). *Arrow in* (**a**) *indicates Tourneux's fold, and arrows in* (**b**) *and* (**c**) *indicate the direction of the müllerian duct migration.* (Reprinted, by permission, from Stephens, F.D. (1983), Congenital Malformations of the Urinary Tract, *New York, Praeger, Fig. 2.24, p. 52.*)

Overlap septal defects in the female. The H-fistula between the back wall of the vagina and pectinate line of the anus is located deep in the perineum in contrast with the pelvic location of the urethroanal H-fistula in the male. Prior to the arrival of the müllerian ducts in the urogenital sinus, the overlap septal deformity of the internal cloaca is similar to that described in the male. However, the müllerian ducts are guided by the wolffian ducts to Müller's tubercle where the urinary tract bifurcates into the urogenital sinus anteriorly and the rectal fistula posteriorly. The müllerian ducts proliferate, incorporate the cloacal attachment of the fistula and descend in the sinus to open to the exterior carrying the fistula part-way with them. In the meantime, the perineal mound and the inner genital folds complete the formation of the perineum superficially (Fig. 2.26) behind the vagina and deepen the tract of the fistula.

Non-communicating anorectourogenital anomalies

Occlusions of the rectum and anus develop at the same embryonic sites in females as in males and in a similar manner (Fig. 2.27). However, they occur less frequently, and the level of occlusion in the mature fetus may be altered. These differences may be explained by the nature and development in the female of the müllerian ducts and perineum.

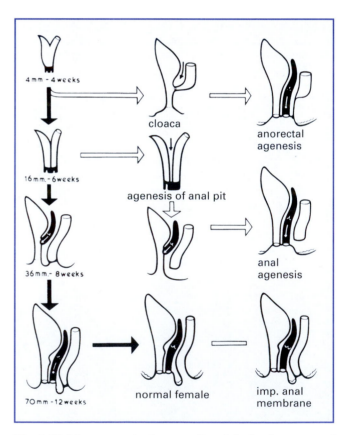

Fig. 2.27 *Non-communicating anomalies of the female rectum and anus. Left column. Stages in normal development. Middle column. Presumed aberrations of stages of development. Right column. The malformations.* (From Stephens F.D. and Smith E.D. (1971), Anorectal Malformations in Children. *Chicago, Year Book, Fig. 76, p. 140.*)

Anorectal agenesis and anal agenesis

The late-coming müllerian ducts wedge between the urinary tract and rectum and impose themselves upon a pre-existing patent or occluded rectourinary fistula. The ducts continue their autonomous development and incorporate the nearby rectal connection in its growing end. The solid end of the fused müllerian ducts canalizes and either incorporates the rectourinary connection into its lumen as a fistula or occludes it. The blind end of the rectum remains attached by a fibrous cord, and, with further migration of the müllerian ducts, the rectum may be carried part-way toward the vestibule.

Imperforate anus

Anal occlusion and stenosis at the normal site are rare in females, because the outer genital folds, which form the labia majora, do not encroach on the perineum and anus as in males. Hence, covering of the anal pit is uncommon. It is likely that persistence or incomplete perforation of the anal membrane accounts for the rare occluded or stenotic anus in the female.

Anorectal atresia

Anorectal atresia, as already described in this chapter, in the male, is an uncommon acquired lesion with similar clinical and morphologic features.

3

Malformations of the external cloaca

Communicating anal anomalies in males

Developmental errors that induce specific communicating and non-communicating defects in the male are summarized in Table 3.1

Table 3.1 *Embryogenesis of cloacal defects in males*

Defect of Tourneux's septum	Rectoprostatic vesical or trigonal fistula (with anorectal agenesis)
Agenesis of Rathke's plicae	Rectoprostatic urethral fistula (with anorectal agenesis)
Defects of Rathke's plicae	Rathke's fistula
Overlap of Tourneux's and Rathke's components of urorectal septum	H-fistula
Agenesis of perineal mound	Rectobulbar fistula
Minimal development of the perineal mound	Rectal fistula to floor of anterior urethra
Moderate development of the perineal mound	Rectocutaneous fistula
Defects of the perineal mound and inner genital folds with fusion of normal or hypertrophic outer genital folds	Anocutaneous fistula and anal stenosis
Defect of anal membrane	Imperforate anal membrane, and membrane stenosis, or anal agenesis

Source: Stephens, F.D. (1988), Embryology of the cloaca and embryogenesis of anorectal malformations. In *Anorectal Malformations in Children* (eds. Stephens, F.D., Smith, E.D. and Paul, N.W.), Vol. 24, No. 4, Table 11.1, p. 207. New York, Alan R. Liss for March of Dimes Birth Defects Foundation.

Rectobulbar fistula (arrest of development of the perineal mound)

The bladder and whole length of the urethra are normal except for the entry of the rectum by a fine fistula into the bulb of the urethra. The anus is absent from the perineum and the patent rectum forms an anterior beak or funnel which turns anteriorly into the bulb of the urethra. The rectal fistula may be very short

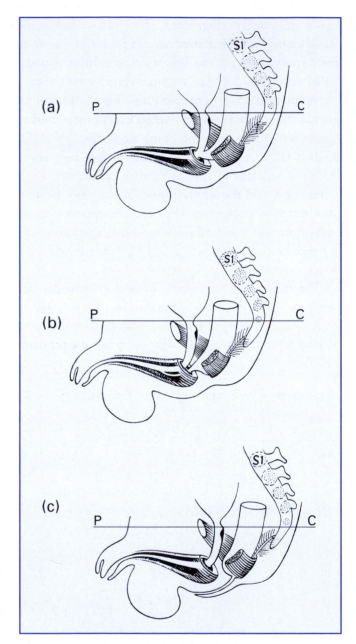

Fig. 3.1 *Rectobulbar fistula in the male child. The corpus spongiosum urethrae is distal to the fistula in the rectobulbar type as in (**a**), or surrounds the track as in (**b**). The puborectalis muscle is related to the rectum in both. The anocutaneous fistula lies caudal to the corpus spongiosum as in (**c**). (The pubococcygeal line P/C is drawn through the ossific centre of the body of the pubis and the sacrococcygeal junction.) (Reprinted, by permission, from Stephens, F.D. (1963), Congenital Malformations of the Rectum, Anus and Genito-Urinary Tracts. Edinburgh, Livingstone, Fig. 25, p. 33.)*

and issue directly into the bulb, or long and narrow running in the fibrous septum that divides the two halves of the corpus spongiosum issuing into the floor of the bulbar urethra anterior to the two ducts of Cowper (Fig. 3.1b). The rectal connection with the bulb may seal off leaving a blind beak demonstrable radiographically (Fig. 3.2). The penis and penile urethra may also be abnormal, exhibiting various forms of hypospadias: (a) the urethra may exhibit hypospadiac anomalies with or without chordee and with or without penoscrotal transposition (Fig. 3.3a); (b) the penis and urethra may be normal except for a urethrocutaneous fistula at some point along the raphe (Fig. 3.3b); (c) the skin and urethral mucosa may co-apt along a segment of the raphe with or without fistula formation and the urethra lacks the spongy tissue in the corpus spongiosum. The perineum may be unusually thin and the fistula and terminal rectum may be covered only by perineal skin and a thin layer of subcutaneous tissue (Fig. 3.3a).

For the rectobulbar fistula without hypospadias and with a well-formed perineum, a colostomy is recommended, followed later by disconnection of the rectobulbar fistula and rerouting of the rectum to the perineum.

Embryogenesis of rectobulbar fistula

At the 16-mm stage, when the subdivision of the internal cloaca is complete, the urogenital and anal pits normally lie closely approximated, but in the mature fetus, the anus lies considerably posterocaudal to its original site. This separation of anus from urethra takes place concurrently with the appearance and interposition of the perineal mound in the depths of the external cloaca.

The perineal mound is the extension of the urorectal septum of the internal cloaca into the external cloaca. It forms the deep part of the perineum. The genital folds bordering the external cloaca grow medially over the mound forming the superficial part of the perineum. With the absence of development of the perineal mound, the anal opening remains co-apting the urethral orifice and both are projected forward in a common urethral canal when the genital folds close in to cover the external cloaca. The rectal orifice is transposed to the bulbar urethra, which receives urine and meconium and conducts them to the external urinary meatus. With rectobulbar fistula malformations, the external meatus may be normally sited or exhibit hypospadias (Fig. 3.4 a,b).

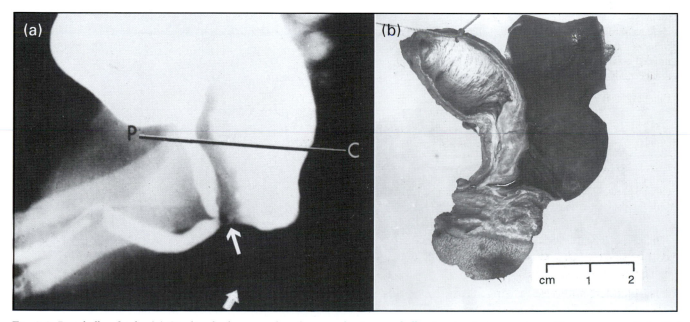

Fig. 3.2 *Rectobulbar fistula.* (**a**) *Combined cologram and urethrogram showing rectobulbar junction (upper arrow, and lower arrow marks level of natal cleft).* (**b**) *Photograph of a specimen of rectobulbar fistula with bristle passing from rectum into bulbar urethra through the narrow communication. P/C = pubococcygeal line.* ((**a**) *reprinted, by permission, after Stephens, F.D. and Smith, E.D. (1971), Anorectal Malformations in Children. Chicago, Year Book, Fig. 102, p. 194.* (**b**) *reprinted, by permission, from Stephens, F.D. (1963), Congenital Malformations of the Rectum, Anus and Genito-Urinary Tracts. Edinburgh, Livingstone, Fig. 24B, p. 32.)*

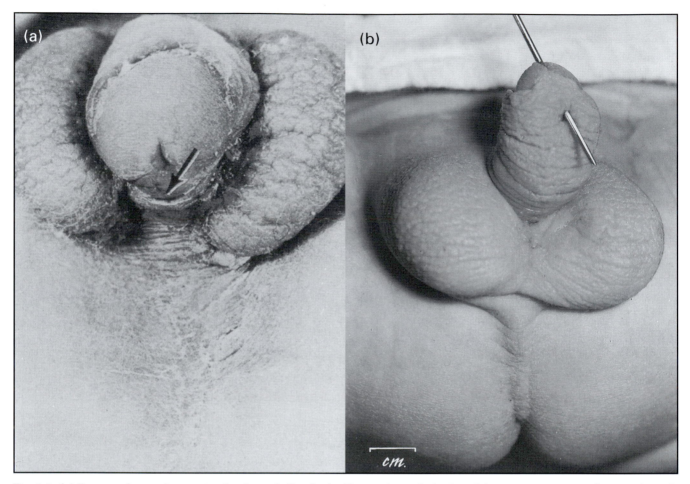

Fig. 3.3 (*a*) *Penoscrotal anomalies associated with rectobulbar fistula. Hypospadias with chordee, cleft scrotum, perineoscrotal meatus (arrow); shallow perineum, absence of raphe.* (*b*) *Rectobulbar fistula (sealed spontaneously). Absence of anal pit, split scrotum, normal penile urethra except for urethrocutaneous fistula (probe). No connection existed between the rectum and urethra but cologram showed a beak-like extension of the rectum sealed off at the bulb of the urethra.* ((*a*) *reprinted by permission, from Stephens, F.D. (1963), Congenital Malformations of the Rectum, Anus, and Genito-Urinary Tracts. Edinburgh, Livingstone, Fig. 24A, p. 32.* (*b*) *reprinted, by permission, from Stephens, F.D. and Smith, E.D. (1971), Ano-Rectal Malformations in Children. Chicago, Year Book, Fig. 31, p. 57.*)

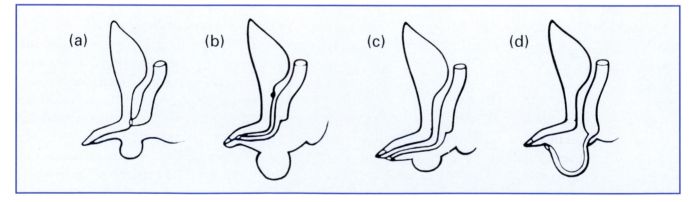

Fig. 3.4 *Rectobulbar, rectocutaneous, and anocutaneous fistulas.* (*a*) *Rectobulbar fistula.* (*b*) *Rectopenile urethral fistula coursing in the central raphe of the corpus spongiosum.* (*c*) *Rectocutaneous fistula contiguous with corpus spongiosum but deep to the scrotum and perineal raphe.* (*d*) *Anocutaneous fistula coursing within the perineal raphe to issue at some point along the raphe. (Reprinted with permission from Stephens, F.D., Smith, E.D. and Paul, N.W. Anorectal Malformations in Children: Update 1988. Birth Defects. Original Article Series, Vol. 24, No. 4, Fig. 11.7, p. 187. New York, Alan R. Liss. for March of Dimes Birth Defects.)*

If the perineal mound is not absent but very deficient, a sliver of the mound interposes itself between the rectal and urethral orifices and when the genital folds close in as they do from behind forward, the rectal canal may be prolonged as a very fine fistula to the floor and mid-part of the bulbar urethra (Kitchen and Stephens, 1971) or to the under surface of the penis (Fig. 3.4c). Aleem *et al.* (1985) prefer to call this latter fistula the perineal canal and male counterpart of the perineal canal in the female.

Anocutaneous fistulas and stenosis

When the perineal mound and inner genital folds are near normal in development but the outer genital folds are hypertrophic and elongated, they may meet behind the anus, forming a skin mound or a thick raphe that may occlude or divide or project the lumen anteriorly. 'Covered anus' is a term sometimes applied to such a process in which the anus is covered.

The anomalies resulting from this exuberant growth of the outer genital folds are anocutaneous stenosis or occlusion, 'bucket-handle' raphe with one or two pin-point orifices to the sides of the raphe, or the anocutaneous fistula projected anteriorly between the inner and outer genital folds to some point along the perineal or penile raphe (Fig. 3.4d).

The genital folds at the posterior site of fusion may be hypertrophic and represented by a sagittal cord of skin across the anal pit, the 'bucket-handle' type, or by a lump encroaching on the pit from in front or behind or by a mass consisting of a combination of all three (see Fig. 3.5). The anal orifice is stenotic, sometimes divided into two minute orifices on either side of the bucket handle, or the orifice may be occluded by the folds or by a persisting anal membrane.

Anterior anus

In this classification, the term 'anterior anus' is restricted to that type of anus that is outwardly and functionally a normal continent anus but that issues to the skin of the perineum at a point anterior to the normal location. This anomaly results from defective posterior migration of the anus, consequent upon a relative shortness of the perineal mound. This anomaly is uncommon, although minor degrees of abnormal anal positioning may pass unrecognized.

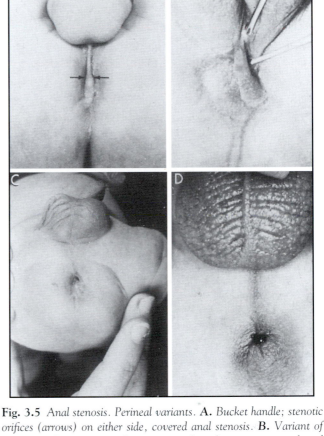

Fig. 3.5 *Anal stenosis. Perineal variants.* **A.** *Bucket handle; stenotic orifices (arrows) on either side, covered anal stenosis.* **B.** *Variant of bucket handle; stenotic orifices on one side and anterior, covered anal stenosis.* **C.** *Anorectal stenosis; circumferential stenosis extending into the rectum (note also phocomelia).* **D.** *Anal membrane stenosis; plug of meconium at the anal membrane. (From Stephens, F.D. and Smith, E. D. (1971), Anorectal Malformations in Children. Chicago, Year Book, Fig. 40, p. 70.)*

Scrotal anomalies and embryogenesis

The scrotum is a baggy, bilateral structure divided into two compartments by a sagittal septum, the external marking of which is the pigmented cutaneous scrotal raphe. The scrotum lies anterior to the perineum and encroaches on the base of the penis, and each pendulous compartment contains the ipsilateral testis.

Scrotal anomalies usually occur in combination with other internal or external cloacal defects. These include anorectal malformations (page 375), penoscrotal hypospadias, and webbed penis and intersex states, penoscrotal translocations, undescended testes, cleft scrotum and vesical exstrophy. It is not proposed to elaborate on these malformations, but one additional rare deformity is described, namely transverse bisection of one side of the scrotum. Here the pigmented rugose redundant skin of one side of the scrotum is interrupted transversely by a smooth skinned depression. The hemiscrotum is bisected usually into two unequal parts and the testis may reside in either. The anterior part may be dislocated laterally, or even onto the anterior abdominal wall, and the other may be positioned normally or posteromedially (see Fig. 36.12).

Bisection may be associated with anal anomalies, such as the covered anus, or with a fine anocutaneous fistula that tracks anteriorly in the perineal and scrotal raphe, or with a rectobulbar fistula.

The manner of closure of the external cloaca and urogenital sinus in the male has been described in Chapter 1. The scrotum is derived from the outer genital folds which lie lateral to the inner folds which border the urogenital sinus between the genital tubercle and the perineal mound. The inner folds migrate, meet and cover over the sinus from behind forward to the corona of the penis. Then the outer folds enlarge, migrate medially between the perineum and base of the penis, over the medial folds to meet in the midline forming a scrotal septum and raphe. Failure to meet creates a double raphe, a groove or a cleft between the two sides and accounts for the longitudinal bisection of the scrotum. Transverse bisections, however, are more difficult to explain on the basis of malformation and in view of some hitherto previously unmentioned associated anomalies, the aetiology may be attributed to perineal deformation rather than malformation (Chapter 36). These associated anomalies are foot and toe deformities such as talipes, overriding toes, pressure dimples on knees and sacral scoliosis or vertebral deficits, all being suggestive of direct or indirect uterine pressure points on the embryo. Pressure transmitted through the knee to the heel of the flexed hind limb on the genital folds may deform the scrotal folds, upset the union of the lateral folds and perineal mound, or compress the lateral folds around the developing anal canal (see Fig. 36.12).

A compression of this nature may result from local disproportion in size of the fetus and chorionic sac or transient oligohydramnios at the six- to eight-week period when the hind limb flexes and the external cloaca differentiates (Smith, 1982a). The resulting pressure deformations include the transverse bisection of the scrotum,

some forms of anocutaneous fistula in the raphe or rectobulbar fistula, and perhaps other defects, such as rotational anomalies of the phallus and the retractile or maldescended testis. Compression of the outer genital folds in the female embryo or fetus by the heel may deform or displace the labium major. A more detailed discussion of the concept of deformations is included in Chapter 36.

Communicating anal anomalies in females

Developmental errors that induce specific communicating and non-communicating anomalies in the female are listed in Tables 3.2

Table 3.2 *Embryogenesis of cloacal defects in females*

Defect of Tourneux's septum	Rectovesical or trigonal (cloacal) fistula; separate müllerian duct orifices in bladder
Agenesis of Rathke's plicae and arrest of müllerian duct migration	Cloaca (rectocloacal fistula); septate or nonseptate vagina
Agenesis of Rathke's plicae, migration of müllerian ducts to vestibule, and incorporation of rectal fistula	Rectovaginal fistula (high and low)
Agenesis of Rathke's plicae, migration of müllerian ducts to vestibule, together with rectal fistula	Rectovestibular or anovestibular fistula
Defect of Rathke's plicae, migration of müllerian duct to vestibule, and incorporation of Rathke's fistula	Rectal fistula at the vaginal introitus
Overlap of Tourneux's and Rathke's septa, müllerian migration to vestibule, and incorporation of fistula into vagina	H-type vaginoanal fistula
Agenesis of perineal mound	Perineal canal
Defect of inner genital folds	Perineal groove
Defect of outer genital fold (abnormal midline perineal fusion)	Anocutaneous fistula and anal stenosis
Defective perineal mound and lack of inner genital folds between vagina and anus	Anterior anus
Defect of anal pit	Anal agenesis, imperforate anal membrane, and anal membrane stenosis

Source: Stephens, F.D. (1988), Embryology of the cloaca and embryogenesis of anorectal malformations. In *Anorectal Malformations in Children* (eds. Stephens, F.D., Smith, E.D. and Paul, N.W.), Vol. 24, No. 4, Table 11.1, p. 207. New York, Alan R. Liss for March of Dimes Birth Defects Foundation.

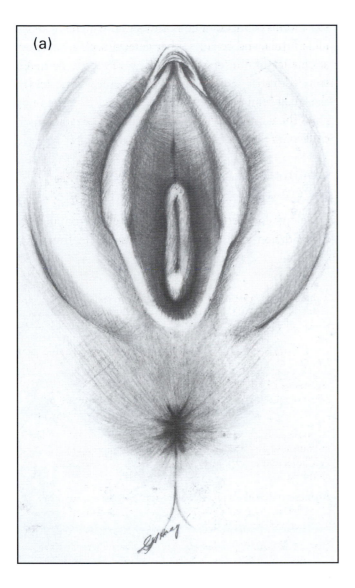

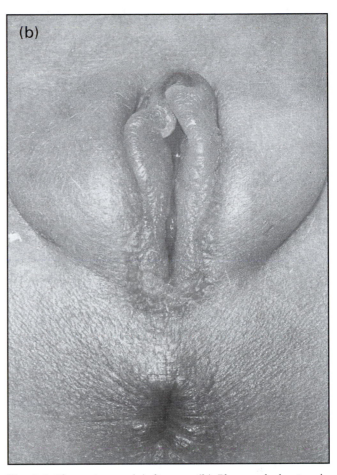

Fig. 3.6 *Flat perineum:* (**a**) *diagram.* (**b**) *Photograph showing the meeting of the minoral tails and smooth flat perineum. (Reprinted, by permission, from Stephens, F.D. (1968), The female anus, perineum and vestibule: Embryogenesis and deformities. Aust. N.Z. J. Obstet. Gynae. 8: 55, Figs. 1A and B.)*

The female perineum and associated anomalies

In the female, the partitioning of the internal cloaca by the urorectal septum is complete at the 16-mm (six-week) stage. The caudal end of the septum proliferates into the external cloaca, forming the central mound or primitive perineum. The inner genital folds bordering the external cloaca now fold inward onto and over the mound, and together they form the perineum. In the vulval zone, however, the inner genital folds remain quite separate. They form the labia minora, which flank the anterior two-thirds of the vulva. Linear extensions called the 'minoral tails' border the posterior one-third of the vulva. These tails converge on and overlie the perineal mound, adding depth to the perineum, the anterior end of which is the fourchette.

The outer genital folds remain even more widely separated and enlarge to form the labia majora and lie lateral to the labia minora, fourchette and perineum.

The normal perineum and fourchette

The labia minora, which were free flaps of skin projecting from the anterior two-thirds of the rim of the urogenital fossa, joined the prepuce of the clitoris anteriorly. Posteriorly, the free labial fringes ended abruptly, and the back one-third of the vestibule and fourchette were bordered by the minoral tails in continuity with the fringes of the labia minora (see Fig. 1.8).

The anus in these premature babies lay 0.5–2.0 cm posterior to the fourchette, sometimes perched on a raised platform, sometimes seated in a cleft.

Examinations were conducted of the perineal area of 62 unselected female babies in the premature babies' ward. Many of the perineums studied displayed temporary markings that were interpreted as representing their embryological components, namely, the genital folds and the perineal mound. The markings of the perineum and genital areas of many of these neonates were clear and indicated the embryological processes. There was some variability in the topography, but it was possible to define three major perineal patterns (Stephens, 1968).

The flat perineum. In 12 babies (Fig. 3.6), the fourchette was an end-to-end junction of the minoral tails, which formed a U border. Posterior to this, the perineum was flat from vestibule to anus. The labia majora were lateral and did not encroach posteriorly beyond the limit of the 'U'.

The convex perineum. In 38 babies (Fig. 3.7), the perineum was an oval, diamond or shield-shaped elevation. In 27, the minoral tails were separated by the perineum, the fourchette being formed mainly by the perineal mound.

The concave perineum. In 12 babies, the perineum exhibited a well-marked central groove from the fourchette leading back to the anus (Fig. 3.8), or exhibited a red, shallow sagittal groove between the vulva and anus bordered by minoral tails (Fig. 3.9). Several perineums were grooved anteriorly, yet raised posteriorly (Fig. 3.9b).

The labia majora

The labia majora lie lateral to the labia minora and the fourchette, but in some, the labia majora extended posteriorly beyond the line of the fourchette or were asym-

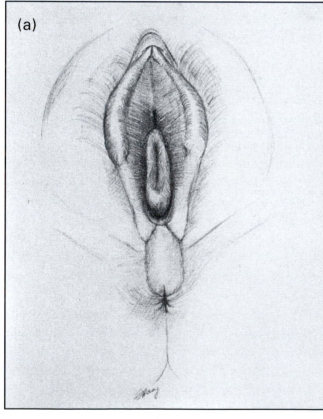

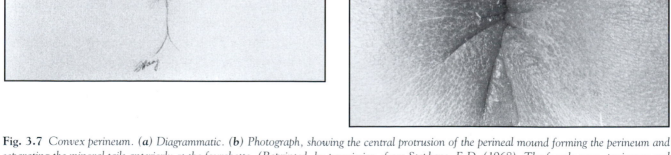

Fig. 3.7 *Convex perineum.* (**a**) *Diagrammatic.* (**b**) *Photograph, showing the central protrusion of the perineal mound forming the perineum and separating the minoral tails anteriorly at the fourchette. (Reprinted, by permission, from Stephens, F.D. (1968), The female anus, perineum and vestibule: Embryogenesis and deformities. Aust. N.Z. J. Obstet. Gynae. 8: 55, Figs 2C and G.)*

(a)

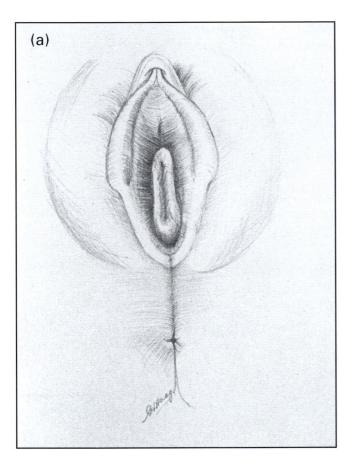

(b)

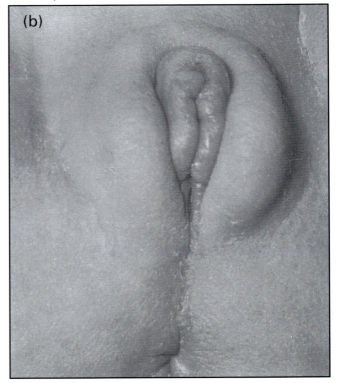

Fig. 3.8 *Concave perineum. (**a**) Diagrammatic. (**b**) Photograph, showing central groove between the fourchette and anus. (Reprinted, by permission, from Stephens, F.D. (1968), The female anus, perineum and vestibule: Embryogenesis and deformities. Aust. N.Z. J. Obstet. Gynae. 8: 55, Figs 3A and E.)*

metrically disposed beside the perineum. Minor variations in disposition are normal. When the perineum was convex, the labia majora were set forward, ending abruptly near the fourchette (Fig. 3.7). If the perineum was concave, they extended in some more posteriorly, even as far as the anus (Figs 3.8 and 3.9).

Abnormal perineums and vulvas

Perineal groove, perineal canal, covered anus and vulval anus

The perineum, being a composite structure formed of the primitive perineal mound and genital folds, may have maximal mound and minimal fold components or vice versa or any combination of both. However, when the major contribution is formed from the mound, the perineum is convex. Perineal deformities in this type are rare. When the mound contribution is minimum, the genital folds assume a major role in the composition and completion of the perineum; if, however, the folds fail to migrate medially, the perineum remains cleft as a per-

ineal groove (Fig. 2.2 (3f) and Fig. 3.9), the floor being the perineal mound and the sides the genital folds; if the cleft is bridged over by the genital folds, it becomes a canal—the perineal canal (Figs 2.22 and 3.10); if the medial migration of the folds affects a greater extent of the external cloaca, the anus may be covered over and its lumen projected anteriorly onto the perineum or vestibule to form the anocutaneous or anovulvar types of female covered anus (Figs 2.2 (3d) and (3e)).

An anterior anus in the female may be either perineal or vulvar in situation, depending on the anteroposterior extent of the perineal mound.

The anterior perineal anus results from inadequate sagittal length of the otherwise normal uroanal septum, and the perineum and fourchette are slender. The vulvar anus results from agenesis of this same septum, and the perineum is absent and the fourchette rudimentary (see Fig. 2.2).

The anterior vulvar anus is an anus by right, supple and normal in calibre, gaining by normal development and

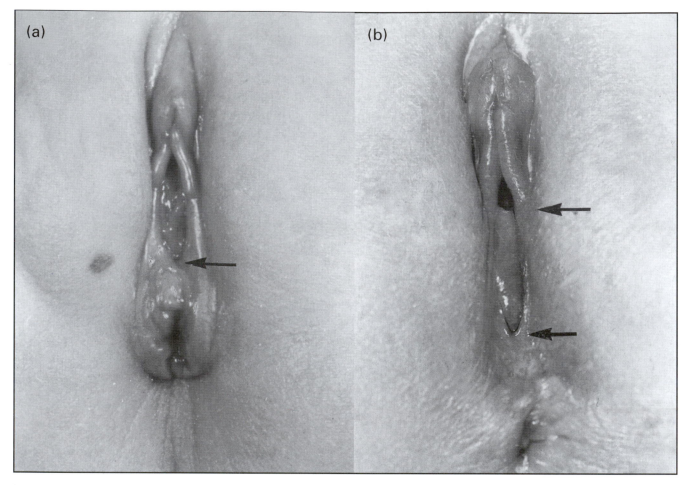

Fig. 3.9 *Perineal groove.* **(a)** *Minoral tails bifurcate bordering the groove and anus and contribute to the fourchette (arrow) partly covering perineal mound in groove.* **(b)** *Minoral tails meet anterior to anus (lower arrow) and rudimentary perineal mound forms the shallow fourchette (upper arrow) and floor of perineal groove (between the arrows).* ((**a**) *reprinted, with permission, from Stephens, F.D. and Smith, E.D. (1971), Anorectal Malformations in Children. Chicago, Year Book, Fig. 66A. p. 115.* (**b**) *reprinted, by permission, from Stephens, F.D. (1968), The female anus, perineum and vestibule: Embryogenesis and deformities. Aust. N.Z. J. Obstet. Gynae. 8: 55, Fig. 4.)*

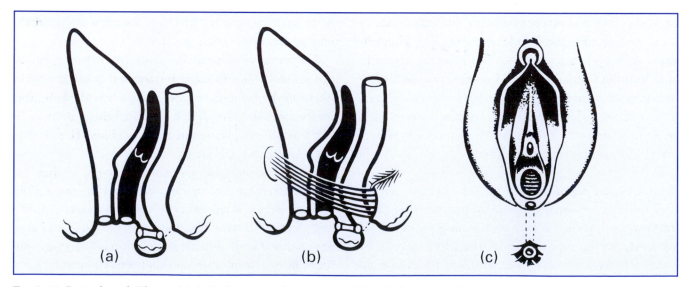

Fig. 3.10 *Perineal canal. The canal links the fossa navicularis in the vestibule with the anal canal at the pectinate line* (**a**) *and* (**c**) *below the chief sphincter of the rectum, the puborectalis muscle* (**b**). *(Reprinted, by permission, from Stephens, F.D. and Smith, E.D. (1971), Anorectal Malformations in Children. Chicago, Year Book, Fig. Z-33, App. C, p. 8.)*

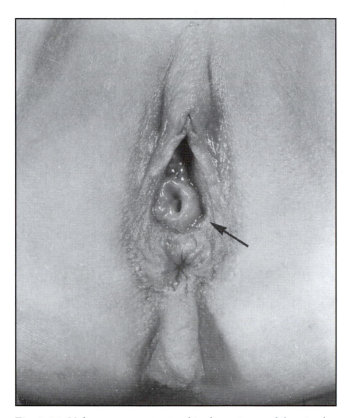

Fig. 3.11 *Vulvar anus: anus normal in dimensions and function but anterior in location. Minoral tails divide and unite behind the anus and also weakly between vagina and anus (arrow) forming rudimentary fourchette. (Reprinted, by permission, from Stephens, F.D. (1968), The female anus, perineum and vestibule: Embryogenesis and deformities. Aust. N.Z. J. Obstet. Gynae. 8: 55, Fig. 10.)*

subdivision of the internal cloaca its rightful entry into the external cloaca. It remains in its abnormal situation because of failure of subdivision of the external cloaca by the uroanal septum (Fig. 2.2 (3c) and Fig. 3.11). The müllerian ducts descend caudally in the urorectal septum to issue into the vestibule wedged between, but quite separate from, the urethra and anus in the unpartitioned external cloaca. The orifice of the rectum is embryologically not a fistula but an anus, albeit abnormal in respect to site and sphincters and epithelium.

H-fistula—anovaginal fistula

The H-fistula between the back wall of the vagina and the pectinate line of the anus is located in the perineum in contrast to the male urethroanal H-fistula, which traverses the pelvis. Prior to the arrival of the müllerian ducts in the urogenital sinus, the overlap septal deformity of the internal cloaca is similar in the female embryo to that described in the male. However, the müllerian ducts are guided by the wolffian ducts to the Müller tubercle where in this anomaly the urinary tract bifurcates into the urogenital sinus anteriorly and the rectal fistula posteriorly. The müllerian ducts proliferate, incorporate the urogenital attachment of the fistula, descend caudally concurrently with the exstrophy of the urogenital sinus, and complete the formation of the vagina, while the perineum and anal canal develop normally. The fistula may connect to the back wall of the vagina or to the vaginal introitus in the vestibule (Fig. 2.27). The anal canal and perineum are otherwise normal, or the anus may exhibit stenosis or other defects pertaining to the genital fold development. These very rare fistulous communications have a different embryogenesis from the rectovaginal fistula and perineal canal described above. Chatterjee (1980) described these rare rectovaginal and perineal canals coexisting with a patent anal canal and preferred the terms 'high' and 'low' H-type fistula, respectively.

Vulval anomalies and adherent labia

Adhesion of the edges of the vestibule forward from the fourchette for a variable distance, perhaps to or including the labia minora, even as far as the clitoris, is a not uncommon circumstance in infancy (Fig. 3.12). The pink lateral edges of the vestibule adhere superficially in the midline to cover in the 'lumen' of the vestibule. This line of fusion is delicate and extremely thin and has a faint bluish appearance. One or more orifices may be present interrupting this blue line, or a single orifice may be tucked up under the clitoris.

The nature of adherent labia (syn. synechia vulvae) is not known. That in some instances it is congenital is likely on the evidence of one family where the baby, the mother and an aunt all had exhibited the condition. It has been shown, however, to be acquired (Dewhurst, 1963; Leungetal, 1993).

This condition may be discovered by the mother, on routine examination by the doctor, or on inspection because of symptoms of wetting or dysuria. It is especially important that this condition be recognized and not confused with absence of the vagina, a misdiagnosis that causes a storm of anxiety and embarrassment.

In babies, lateral pressure with the thumbs unsticks the labia and reveals the normal urethrovaginal anatomy within. Sometimes, minimal bloodshed on the

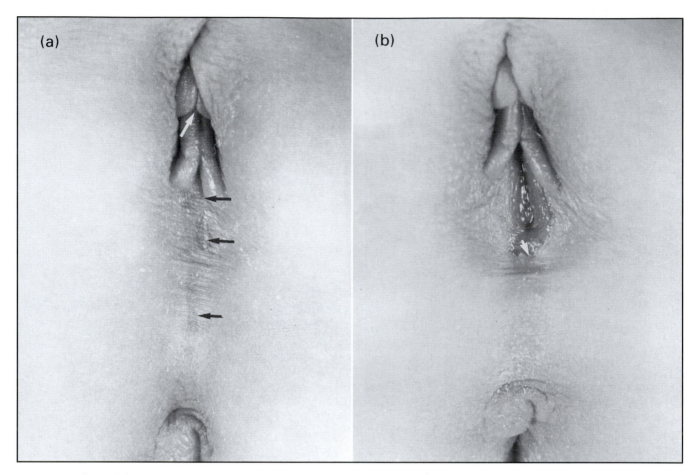

Fig. 3.12 *Adherent labia: in (**a**), line of fusion is indicated by black arrows and orifice is under clitoris (white arrow); in (**b**), arrow marks linear raw edge remaining after separation of adhesions; normal vestibule exposed. (Reprinted, by permission, from Stephens, F.D. (1966), Urethro-vaginal malformations.* Aust. N.Z. J. Obstet. Gynae. 5: 64, Fig. 3.)

edges of the vestibule after separation reveals the fineness of the line of fusion. The mother should be instructed to separate the labia weekly for six months, to prevent spontaneous reformation of the adhesions. Even after this period, re-adherence may creep forward from the fourchette. Regular observation is thus necessary for a year or more. An alternative and sometimes successful method of lysing the adhesions consists of applications of an oestrogen ointment to the line of fusion daily for a few days with re-applications when necessary.

Other less common aberrations of development of the genital folds and perineum distort the vestibule though the vagina itself is normally formed. The vestibule may be covered in part by thick skin displaying a raphe, as in the male. The labia majora may be prolonged backward onto the perineum as in some forms of anterior anus or even behind the anus. Part of one may be disposed laterally on the lower abdominal wall to the side of the mons (Fig. 3.13). This bisection and dislocation of a portion of the labium may be the result of deforming pressures as in the male (Chapter 36). In this female patient, the fourth and fifth sacral vertebrae were deviated to the left, indicating that the pressure of the heel of the flexed limb was transmitted diagonally through the pelvis from the site of the pit shown beside the labium minor to the back of the embryo.

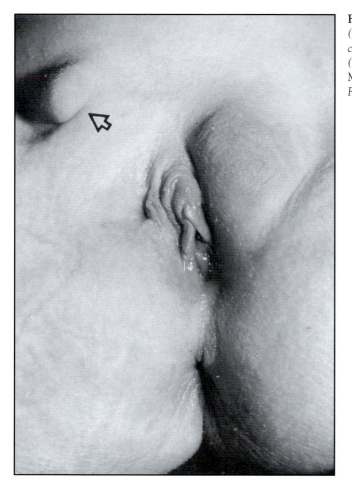

Fig. 3.13 *Ectopic position of labium majus. The right labium majus (arrow) is located on the side of the mons. The normal site is umbilicated. The labia minora and left labium majus are normally formed. (Reprinted, by permission, from Stephens, F.D. (1983), Congenital Malformations of the Urinary Tract, New York, Praeger, Fig. 3.17, p. 76.)*

4

Müllerian and wolffian anomalies

Understanding the variations in the anatomy of the vagina, hydrometrocolpos, urogenital-sinus malformations and the anomalies of the perineum requires a good knowledge of the development of the müllerian and wolffian ducts and the processes that subdivide the external cloaca. The subdivision of the external cloaca by the formation and interposition of the perineum between the anal canal and the urogenital sinus is described in Chapters 1 and 3. Urinary tract anomalies, especially renal agenesis associated with genital tract defects in females, are features of the Mayer–Rokitansky syndrome, described later in this chapter.

Müllerian ducts

Normal development of müllerian ducts

The müllerian ducts form from longitudinal invaginations of the coelomic epithelium on the wolffian ridges of the intermediate cell masses. They remain open cranially, forming the ostium on each side, and lie closely applied but lateral to the wolffian ducts, which precede and guide their actively growing caudal ends to the urogenital sinus. As far as the brim of the pelvis, the müllerian ducts lie lateral to the pilot ducts, but in the pelvis, they turn medially, cross anterior to the wolffian ducts, meet and continue migration side by side to the sinus. They fuse to form the uterovaginal primordium, and the caudal ends penetrate the urogenital sinus between the two openings of the wolffian ducts on the site of the Müllerian tubercle at about the seventh week (the 23-mm stage) (Arey, 1974b). This müllerian eminence is then excavated by small, paired sinovaginal protrusions, which meet the fused müllerian ducts in the wall of the urogenital sinus and form the hymen (Fig. 4.1). (See also embryogenesis of the hymen in Chapter 5.)

The definitive urogenital sinus is initially a tubal structure which widens and turns outward to form the vestibule. The urethral and vaginal orifices descend caudally from the müllerian tubercle as the urogenital sinus everts, both finally issuing externally. The hymen at first

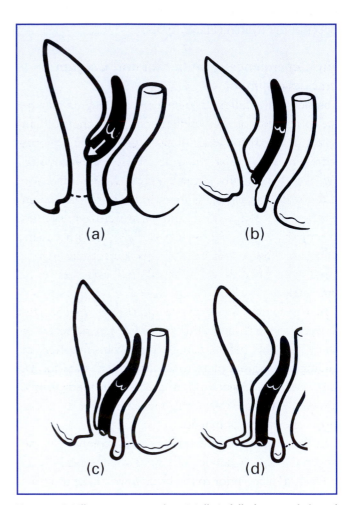

Fig. 4.1 *Müllerian migration from Müller's hillock to vestibule and abnormal states resulting from arrests en route. (**a**) The müllerian ducts penetrate the urogenital sinus in seventh week (23-mm crown–rump length). (**b**) By eversion first of the pars phallica and then pars pelvina, the ducts descend caudally and the urogenital sinus becomes shallow. (**c**) The urethral and vaginal orifices are contiguous. (**d**) With continued eversion the urethra turns anteriorly and its orifice separates from the urethra. (Reprinted, by permission, from Stephens, F.D. (1983), Congenital Malformations of the Urinary Tract, New York, Praeger, Fig. 3.5. p. 68.)*

separates the epithelium of the sinus from that of the vagina, but eventually it disintegrates and the two structures become confluent. In the view of Koff (1933), sinus epithelium streams into and lines the vaginal wall in the distal two-fifths of its extent, but other embryologists regard the hymen as the epithelial demarcation line.

The wolffian ducts, after piloting their müllerian sisters to their destination, undergo atrophy in the female. Sometimes they persist temporarily or permanently, part or whole, as Gartner's ducts, which are incorporated within the lateral walls of the vagina. The orifices of persisting wolffian ducts issue on to the outer aspect of the hymen (Frazer, 1931b).

Interdependence of müllerian and wolffian duct development

Absence of the fallopian tube, uterus or vagina may be due to agenesis of the wolffian body or of the wolffian duct. An intrinsic defect of the müllerian duct alone, however, may cause arrest at any level even when the pilot is normally formed. Arrest during migration of the wolffian duct leads to an arrest of the müllerian duct at the same level and absence of müllerian structures caudally. Arrest may occur at any level from fallopian tube to the hymen. The defects so engendered may be uni- or bilateral and asymmetric or symmetric.

In the female fetus, the wolffian duct degenerates between the 10th and 20th weeks but not normally in its caudal end before completion of its function of guiding the vaginal plate to its ultimate destination in the vestibule. Degeneration may occur prematurely, however, causing errors in the development of the lower part of the vagina or hymen.

In the sexually indifferent stage of development, the urogenital sinus is pelvic. The sinus widens caudally in the sagittal plane prior to the breakdown of the urogenital membrane at six weeks (16-mm stage) to become the pars phallica. This part of the sinus forms the urethral plate, the anterior end of which is contiguous with the genital tubercle.

In the female, the pars pelvina of the sinus then exstrophies to form the vestibule and the fused müllerian ducts migrate caudally along the posterior wall to the exterior. The growing ends of the müllerian ducts are at first solid but later hollow out and lose the septum between them before they descend as one into the vestibule. The hymen of the vagina remains imperforate until about the beginning of the fifth month then breaks down, establishing continuity of the vaginal lumen with the vestibule. The bulbourethral glands and ducts (Bartholin's glands) originally arising between the pars

pelvina and phallica are translocated from pelvis to vestibule by the exstrophy of the pars pelvina and descent of the müllerian ducts. They come to lie to either side of the vaginal introitus in the grooves between it and the labia minora.

While the pars phallica and pars pelvina of the urogenital sinus are relocating, the tract between the bladder neck and the Müller's tubercle elongates to form the whole length of the pelvic urethra. The caudal end of the urethra contiguous with its orifice also everts, but in an anterior direction (Fig. 4.1).

Abnormal development of the müllerian ducts
Defects of septation of uterus and vagina

Aberrations of fusion may lead to degrees of craniocaudal septation of the ureterovaginal canal, varying from the most mild degree affecting the uterine lumen only, uterus subseptus unicollis, without any external evidence of the defect in the uterus, to uterus didelphys with double vagina (Patten, 1947b) (Fig. 4.2).

One or both müllerian ducts may fail to develop or, once started in their migration, may be arrested at any point on their course (Fig. 4.3). Rarely, the ducts may be sagittally instead of coronally oriented (Fig. 4.3) especially when combined in rectocloacal deformities. Absence of both ducts is associated with absence of the vagina and often with renal ectopy.

The ducts that form the vagina may migrate in the normal manner, but develop only as atrophic epithelial tubes of microcalibre, the epithelial walls of which lack the muscle coats. One stillborn baby exhibited this atrophy of the vagina, which was identified histologically from serially cut sections of the pelvic organs. No muscle was present around its epithelial walls, which contained only a thin film of mesenchymal tissue (Fig. 4.3).

The hymen, a septum which should undergo atrophy, may remain imperforate. This may pass unrecognized until puberty, when menstrual pains, absence of 'period' bloodflow, and a mass caused by haematocolpos give rise to acute and intermittent pain. Occasionally, an imperforate hymen may cause symptoms in the newborn infant. Then mucus, secreted by the cervical glands, accumulates in the occluded vagina, compresses and partially obstructs by pressure the urethra and bowel and is readily detected by rectal and abdominal palpation

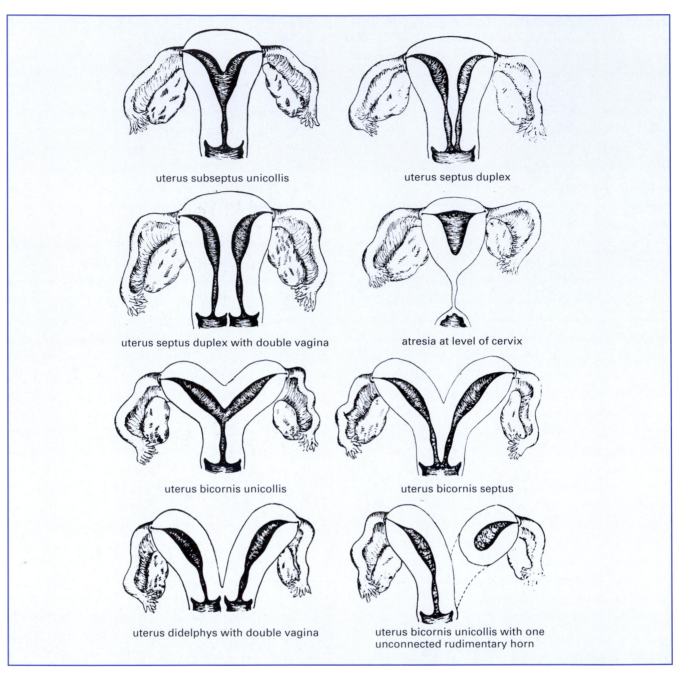

uterus subseptus unicollis

uterus septus duplex

uterus septus duplex with double vagina

atresia at level of cervix

uterus bicornis unicollis

uterus bicornis septus

uterus didelphys with double vagina

uterus bicornis unicollis with one unconnected rudimentary horn

Fig. 4.2 *Schematic diagrams of abnormal fusions of the paired müllerian tubes and atresia with distinguishing terms. (Reprinted, by permission, from Patten, B.M. (1947),* Human Embryology, *London, Churchill, Fig. 367, p. 585. Redrawn by Patten from Stander,* Williams' Obstetrics, *Appleton-Century Co.)*

(Figs 4.3 and 4.4). The hymen bulges in the vestibule and may be pink and fleshy or thin, translucent and blue.

Mid-vaginal occlusion differs from imperforate hymen in that the lumen is blocked by a transversely oriented membrane with normal vagina above and below it. McKusick *et al.* (1964) describe this rare membrane as an inherited malformation as opposed to the imperforate hymen, which is a local non-inheritable development error.

Atresia of the fallopian tract may occur at any level, resulting from vascular accidents during development, or from failure of the solid epithelial growing ends of the ducts to canalize.

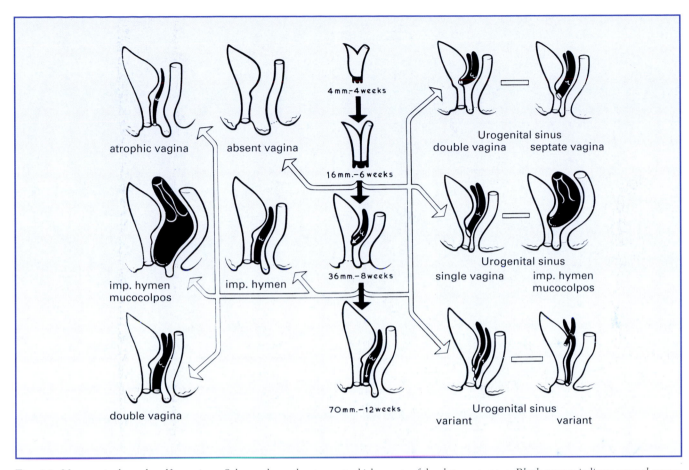

Fig. 4.3 *Uterovaginal canal malformations. Schema shows the stages at which arrests of development occur. Black arrows indicate normal stages, and white arrows depict the corresponding defects. Anterior perineal or vulvar anus may occur in combination with any of the illustrated urogenital defects. Black arrow = normal development. White arrow = abnormal development. (Reprinted, by permission, from Stephens, F.D. (1966), Urethrovaginal malformations. Aust. N.Z. J. Obstet. Gynaec. 5: 64, Fig. 1.)*

Persistence of the urogenital sinus

Arrest of migration of the müllerian ducts from Müller's tubercle to vestibule may occur at any stage (Fig. 4.3). Five patients exhibiting such arrest have been observed and studied over periods ranging from three months to 13 years. The vaginal orifice lay sagittally disposed in the vault of the urogenital sinus, and the urethral orifice was located on the anterior wall of the sinus and contiguous with the hymen. The sinus was relatively long and narrow at birth, and with growth up to and during adolescence, the narrow segment enlarged and everted, thus bringing the urethral and vaginal orifices closer to the surface. The orifice of the urogenital sinus, however, remained stenotic requiring Z-plasty to enlarge it.

Urine storage vagina—urocolpos. Urine storage vagina (Fig. 4.4b) is a variant of the urogenital sinus deformity. The hymen encroaches on the urogenital sinus at the confluence of the vagina with the urethra in the pelvis. The lower or posterior lip of the hymen and adjoining wall form a cusp, which leans across the sinus causing a partial blockage enhanced by contraction of the puborectalis sling muscle. The flow of urine from the urethra is directed up and into the lumen of the vagina. The vagina especially, but also the uterine canal, during late intrauterine life of the fetus, expands to giant dimensions to accommodate the retained urine and mucus (Fig. 4.4b).

The dilated vagina forms a large, palpable, abdominal tumour rising out of the pelvis. A catheter, when passed up the cloacal canal, may enter the vagina, drain a large quantity of urine, and a vaginagram displays a reservoir that resembles, and may be mistaken for, a cystogram. However, an extension of the opaque medium into the cervical canal and uterus with perhaps spillage into the

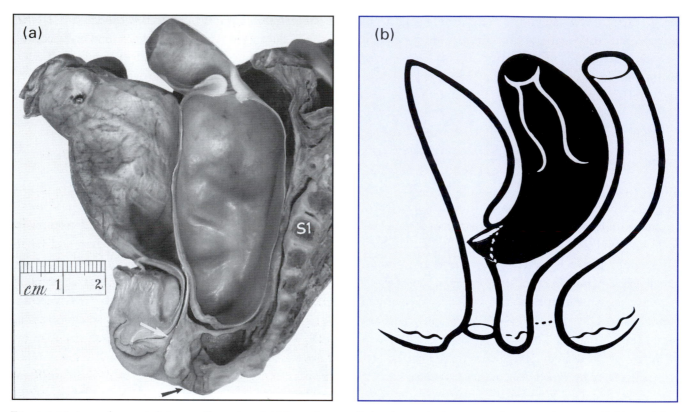

Fig. 4.4 *Variants of urogenital sinus malformation. (**a**) Mucocolpos: müllerian ducts gained contact with urogenital sinus at bladder neck but failed to perforate and descend to vestibule (white arrow). Overdistended vagina expanded into abdominal and pelvic cavities above and below point of contact at bladder neck; black arrow depicts anus. (**b**) Urocolpos: the müllerian ducts perforate the urogenital sinus but the eccentric opening of the hymen creates a valve-like obstruction of the urethra and vagina with uromucocolpos (a). (Reprinted, by permission, from Stephens, F.D. (1966), Urethrovaginal malformations. Aust. N.Z. J. Obstet. Gynaec. 5: 64, Fig. 4.)*

peritoneal cavity via the fallopian tubes are diagnostic signs. Temporary and adequate drainage may be achieved by endoscopic division of the posterior lip of the hymen.

Separated vaginas. Another variant on the sinus theme was seen in two stillborn infants, in each of whom the two vaginas were entirely separate. In the first, two separate vaginas were arranged in line down the back of the sinus. In the other, the müllerian ducts were widely separated: one of these stopped short of the bladder, and the other, somewhat hypoplastic, was very fine and issued in the vestibule between the urethra and anus (Fig. 4.3).

Urorectogenital deformities

If the cloaca remains undivided, the rectum and urinary tract open to the exterior through a common outlet. The müllerian ducts superimpose themselves upon this cloaca, which then resembles the urogenital sinus with a narrow rectal communication added to it. Postnatal development of the congenital urogenital sinus up to and beyond puberty in several children was such that surgery to enlarge the lumen of the sinus was unnecessary and that, if continence of urine was satisfactory, no further reconstructive procedure was necessary. If the rectum is detached from the rectocloacal fistula and rerouted to the perineum, in the fashion described, to conserve the sphincteric control of the levatores ani muscles, the remaining urogenital sinus may develop and enlarge in the years up to puberty. Natural enlargement of the vagina and the urogenital sinus up to and after puberty may be adequate though the external opening of the introitus may need surgical dilatation.

Hydrometrocolpos

In newborn babies, maternal oestrogens stimulate the glands of the cervix uteri to secrete mucus, which normally discharges freely through the introitus. However, if the lumen of the vagina is blocked, the mucus accumulates, and the vagina and uterus enlarge to accommodate it. The hydrometrocolpos forms a tense, hard swelling in the abdomen, extending out of the pelvis to the level of the umbilicus, compressing the urethra, ureters and rectum (Fig. 4.4).

The blockage may be hymenal at the normal site, in the urogenital sinus or at the entry point of the vagina into a rectocloacal canal, or it may be an atresia occurring in the vagina or uterus. If the müllerian ducts are septate or remain separate, as with high rectocloacal fistula deformities, the imperforate hymen or atresia may be unilateral (Figs 2.19 and 4.3).

The imperforate hymen in the normal site can be readily excised, but when located higher in the urogenital sinus, the operation described by Raffensperger and Ramenofsky (1973) is appropriate in the newborn period (Fig. 2.20a and b). For those associated with rectocloacal fistula deformities, the combined rectoplasty and culpoplasty by these same authors is recommended (Fig. 2.20c, d and e). Whereas the levatores ani muscles are protected by the rectum in the operation for the urogenital sinus deformity, this muscle is in jeopardy in the combined operations.

Significance of renal agenesis and müllerian defects

If the ureter and kidney are present it can be assumed that the wolffian and müllerian ducts were together at eight weeks at Müller's tubercle in which event development of the fallopian tube, uterus and upper part of the vagina could form normally thus far. Beyond this level, the lower part of the vagina and hymen may form normally or abnormally depending on further influence exerted by the wolffian duct on the development of the vaginal plate.

If the kidney is absent, the müllerian duct structures and the wolffian duct development may be normal except that the ureteric bud failed to form. If, however, the wolffian duct arrested at some point cranial to the level of bud formation, the kidney would be absent but the migration of müllerian ducts would be correspondingly arrested.

The combination of agenesis of the vagina and uterus with normal fallopian tube and kidney means that the common mesonephric duct at the caudal end of the wolffian duct gave rise to the ureteric bud and became incorporated into the bladder and that müllerian duct migration was due to an intrinsic defect of the müllerian duct or to premature degeneration of the wolffian duct after detachment of the bud.

The Mayer–Rokitansky syndrome: pathogenesis, classification and management*

Agenesis of the vagina in karyotypic female subjects may be accompanied by other defects of the urogenital system. Eight examples are described that exemplify nearly all variants in the group of müllerian and renal anomalies that we identify as the Mayer–Rokitansky syndrome. The association of system defects to errors of formation of the wolffian body is traced. This structure is the progenitor of the gonad and wolffian duct, which although temporary in the female subject, gives rise to the ureter and is the pathfinder of the müllerian system. Errors of formation or premature atrophy of the wolffian duct, or intrinsic müllerian organizers, lead to the array of anomalies in this syndrome. Vaginal agenesis was found to be associated with müllerian, renal or ovarian defects in numerous embryological combinations. A müllerian classification (Fig. 4.5A), was proposed and current diagnostic modalities and techniques of surgery were described by Tarry et al. (1986).

In 1838, Rokitansky described 19 adult autopsy cases of uterovaginal agenesis including three in which unilateral renal agenesis was noted. In 1829, Mayer had described partial and complete duplications of the vagina in four stillborns as an anomaly among many, including cleft lip and limb, and cardiac and urological defects. In 1910, Kuster described several cases with similar genital anatomy and observed that skeletal and renal anomalies were common. Hauser and Schreiner (1961) emphasized the importance of distinguishing between this syndrome and that of testicular feminization in both of which the vaginal development is defective.

The names of these aforementioned authors have been used in various combinations to designate a syndrome. Since these publications, numerous descriptions of müllerian anomalies have been reported in the

Reproduced in part, with permission of the Williams and Wilkins Co., from Tarry, W.F., Duckett, J.W. and Stephens, F.D. (1986), The Mayer–Rokitansky syndrome: pathogenesis, classification and management. J. Urol. 136: 648–52.

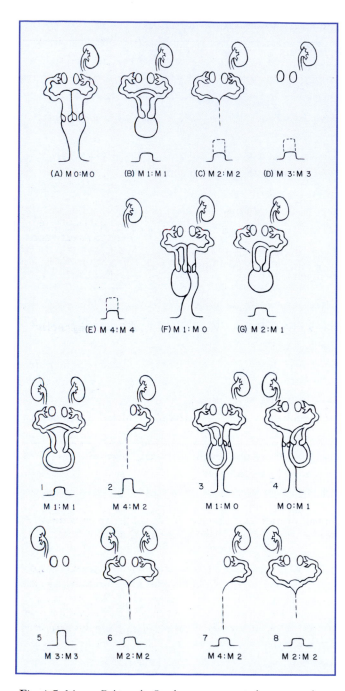

Fig. 4.5 *Mayer–Rokitansky Syndrome, a urogenital anatomy of cases 1–8 (A–G) and müllerian (M) grades. Müllerian (M) system of grading of Mayer–Rokitansky syndrome. Combinations of normal and abnormal features of eight examples of the Mayer–Rokitansky syndrome together with M grading of müllerian systems. M = müllerian defect. Numerals refer to organ status of each side. O, normal right or left vagina and uterus, or duplex vagina and uterus with partial or complete septum. 1, partial or complete absence of vagina. 2, absence of vagina and uterus. 3, absence of vagina, uterus and fallopian tube. 4, absence of vagina, uterus, fallopian tube and ovary. (Reprinted with permission from Tarry, W.F., Duckett, J.W. and Stephens, F.D. (1986) The Mayer–Rokitansky Syndrome: Pathogenesis, classification and management.* J. Urol. 136: 648–52, Fig.1)

literature, some bearing the Mayer–Rokitansky eponym and others designated by embryological (Magee *et al.*, 1979), anatomical (Leduc *et al.*, 1968) and descriptive terms (Spence, 1962; McKusick *et al.*, 1964). Griffin *et al.* (1976), in a report of 14 new cases and an extensive review, included as additional criteria of the syndrome a normal genotype, phenotype and endocrine status, and reiterated the association of anomalies outside of the urogenital system in some cases. They considered that in two affected families in their series the syndrome resulted from a single genetic defect with variable manifestations in other systems. They chose to signify the syndrome by the names Mayer, Rokitansky, Kuster and Hauser, all of whom made significant contributions to the recognition of the association of anomalies.

The Mayer–Rokitansky syndrome is defined as a spectrum of müllerian anomalies, including vaginal agenesis (Smith, 1982b) with or without renal anomalies, in genotypic and phenotypic female subjects with normal endocrine status. The management of patients with this syndrome is shown in Table 4.1 and the embryogenesis with emphasis on the autonomy of development of the two müllerian systems as described by Tarry *et al.* is reiterated herein. Their gynaecological grading of the anomalies of the müllerian systems is based in part on the pathological anatomy described in the following case reports (Fig. 4.6b). The müllerian anomalies associated with malformations of the anorectum or cloacal exstrophy is not included.

Case histories

Case 1

T.D., a mentally retarded one-year-old child, was found to have hydrometrocolpos, septicaemia and normal kidneys. A transverse septotomy failed to improve the clinical status and, therefore, the uterus and vagina were removed. The surgical specimen revealed a dilated uterus and vagina filled with mucus and purulent material. The patient was referred for subsequent management of urinary infection and unilateral vesicoureteral reflux.

Case 2

D.K., a seven-year-old child, had urinary infection, absence of the right kidney and vesicoureteral reflux on the left side. The right ureteral orifice was absent. The vagina was short and blind. At left ureteral re-implantation the right ovary and fallopian tube were noted to be absent. The left fallopian tube and ovary were normal and the tube terminated in a rudimentary midline structure. The patient has had no further reconstruction.

Case 3

K.M., a 10-year-old girl, had lower abdominal pain and a right pelvic mass. An excretory urogram, intravenous pyelogram (IVP),

Table 4.1 *Clinical features, classification and surgical management of Mayer–Rokitansky anomalies of eight patients*

Case no.	Patient age (years)	Presentation	Genital defects	Upper urinary tracts	M Class	Surgery
1	1	Hydrocolpos	Vaginal agenesis	Vesicoureteral reflux	M1, M1	Hysterectomy
2	7	Urinary tract infection	Agenesis of uterus and vagina, absent right ovary and tube	Absent right kidney, left vesicoureteral reflux	M4, M2	Left ureteral implant
3	10	Pain, mass	Uterus didelphys, unilateral vaginal agenesis	Absent right kidney	M1, M0	Marsupialization of blind to patent vagina
4	13	Pain, mass	Uterus, didelphys, unilateral vaginal agenesis	Absent left kidney	M0, M1	Marsupialization of blind to patent vagina
5	17	Amenorrhoea	Agenesis of uterus and upper vagina, tubes hypoplastic	Absent left kidney	M3, M3	Vaginoplasty
6	17	Amenorrhoea	Agenesis of uterus and vagina	Normal kidneys	M2, M2	Sigmoid vaginoplasty
7	17	Amenorrhoea	Rudimentary uterus, vaginal agenesis, right ovary and tube absent	Absent right kidney	M4, M2	McIndoe vaginoplasty
8	19	Amenorrhoea	Agenesis of uterus and vagina	Absent left kidney	M2, M2	McIndoe vaginoplasty

Source: Tarry, W.F., Duckett, J.W. and Stephens, F.D. (1986), The Mayer–Rokitansky syndrome: pathogenesis, classification and management. *J. Urol.* 136: 648, Table 1. Reprinted with permission of the Williams and Wilkins Co.

and ultrasound revealed absence of the right kidney, and dilated uterus and vagina. Exploratory laparotomy revealed uterus didelphys, the right side of which was massively dilated by retained menses. The fallopian tubes, ovaries, and broad and round ligaments were normal. Cystoscopy and vaginoscopy at that time revealed a normal cervix and vagina with a bulge in the lateral wall of the vagina. The right ureteral orifice and hemitrigone were absent. The right blind distended vagina was marsupialized into the right lateral wall of the left vagina.

Case 4

L.U., a 13-year-old girl, had normal menses accompanied by cyclic abdominal pain, and a large pelvic mass was palpable on physical examination. An IVP demonstrated a normal right kidney but no function on the left side. Ultrasonography confirmed absence of the left kidney and revealed two ovaries, two separate uteri and a septate vagina, the left half of which was massively dilated (Fig. 4.6). Cystovaginoscopy confirmed the aforementioned findings as well as the impingement of the left pelvic mass on the apposing wall of the opposite vagina. The haematocolpos was decompressed by marsupialization.

Case 5

M.H., a 17-year-od girl, was investigated because of amenorrhoea. She had a 5-cm blind ending vagina on physical examination and an absent left kidney on an IVP. Laparotomy revealed two normal ovaries but absence of all müllerian structures. A pseudovagina was created by the Frank technique.

Case 6

R.D., a 17-year-old girl, complained of amenorrhoea. On inspection of the vulva the vaginal introitus was absent and no mass was palpable on rectal examination. The IVP was normal. Laparotomy revealed complete uterovaginal agenesis, and normal fallopian tubes and ovaries. Sigmoid vaginoplasty was performed at this operation.

Case 7

R.C., a 17-year-old girl, had amenorrhoea. An IVP revealed a solitary left kidney. At laparotomy the uterus and vagina were found to be rudimentary. Biopsy of the uterine wall revealed myometrium but no endometrial lumen could be identified. The ovary and fallopian tube were absent on the right side and normal on the left side. A vaginoplasty by the McIndoe technique was constructed.

Case 8

S.S., a 19-year-old girl, had amenorrhoea and absence of the vagina. An IVP indicated a healthy right kidney and absent left kidney. On exploration two normal ovaries were identified and two fallopian tubes fused in a midline rudimentary structure. There was no evidence of uterine or upper vaginal development. A McIndoe vaginoplasty was performed.

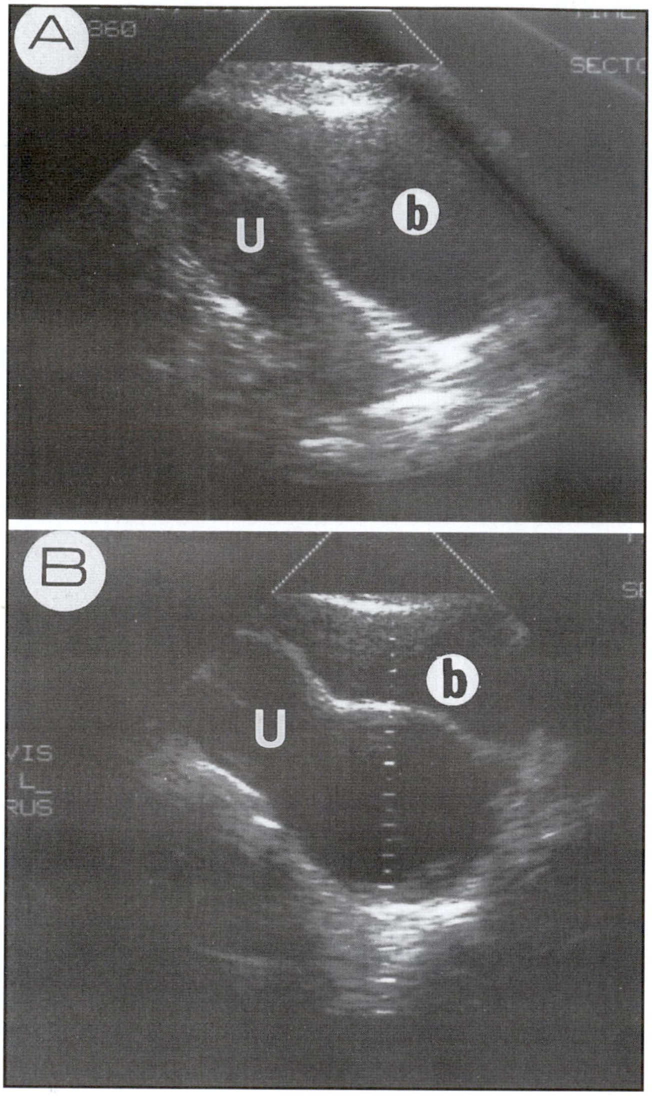

Fig. 4.6 *Sonograms in Case 4.* **A** *Unfused unobstructed right side of duplicate uterus and vagina.* **B** *Left side of same system. Uterus (U) and vagina are extremely dilated. b, bladder.(Reprinted with permission from Tarry, W.F. Duckett, J.W. and Stephens, F.D. (1986) The Mayer–Rokitansky Syndrome: Pathogenesis classification and management. J. Urol. 136: 648–52, Figs 2 and 3.)*

Comment: It was found that when both kidneys were present the müllerian defects were symmetrical. When only one kidney was present the ipsilateral müllerian system developed normally or only in part, and the contralateral system was absent or abnormal in all patients.

Embryology

Normal development of the müllerian ducts. At six weeks of gestation (12-mm crown–rump length) the coelomic epithelium dorsal and lateral to the developing gonad and wolffian (mesonephric) duct invaginates longitudi-

nally to form a furrow. The cranial end of the furrow remains open and develops fimbria, and the lips of the furrow meet to convert it into a tube beneath coelomic epithelium. The distal end of the tube extends caudally in contact with the basement membrane of the wolffian duct as a solid cord, which canalizes as it progresses to the inferior margin of the mesonephros (Gruenwald, 1941). This segment from the ostium caudally forms the fallopian tube. The caudal end of each duct then grows medially in contact with the wolffian duct, and it crosses in front of it to meet and fuse with its opposite number. The two blunt ends of the müllerian ducts migrate caudally side by side, fusing as they go, to penetrate the urogenital sinus between the orifices of the wolffian ducts (eight weeks' gestation, 30-mm). Each müllerian duct migrates and develops independently of the other and usually one ahead of the other (Gruenwald, 1941). Their fusion is a matter of physical proximity and similarity of epithelium. The solid ends of the müllerian ducts fuse, together with the epithelium of the sinus and wolffian ducts, to form the müllerian tubercle. Between 10 and 13 weeks of gestation the co-apting walls of the müllerian ducts fuse to form the uterovaginal canal. The medial septum then disintegrates in a caudocranial direction and the surrounding mesenchyme condenses around the walls.

Two solid epithelial evaginations (sinovaginal bulbs) grow posteriorly from Müller's tubercle to meet the solid tip of the fused müllerian ducts. Epithelial proliferation obliterates the lumen of most of the vagina, and the solid structure that is formed together with the bulbs is called the 'vaginal plate'. With descent of the vaginal bulbs from the high internal to the external vestibular locations, the plate elongates forming an add-on distal segment of vagina. During the same period the urogenital sinus exstrophies into the vestibule, the urethra elongates and the plate canalizes. The hymen remains as a membrane between the urogenital sinus and the canalized vaginal plate. The chronology of these events and the concomitant ureterorenal developments are given in Table 4.2.

Witschi (1970) considered that the müllerian ducts were dependent on, and guided by, the wolffian ducts beyond the point where both ducts penetrate the wall of the urogenital sinus, to the limit of distal migration of the vaginal plate where the hymen is formed. This

Table 4.2 *Timing of events in urinary and genital systems*

Weeks	Crown–to rump length (mm)	Urinary	Genital
4	5	Wolffian duct reaches cloaca, ureteral bud forms	
5	8	Ureter and pelvis forming, kidney migrating to lumbar region	
6	12	Kidney reaches lumbar region, nephrogenesis begins, urorectal septum forming, ureter separated from wolffian duct	Müllerian duct forming
7	17	Collecting tubules forming, urorectal septum complete, urethral membrane ruptures	
8	23		Müllerian ducts cross medial to wolffian ducts
	28		Müllerian ducts meet in midline
	35		Ducts join urogenital sinus
10	40	Kidney secretes	Wolffian duct degenerating
12	56		Uterine horns fused, canalization to cervix region
	66	Ureteral orifice reaches final position in bladder	Sinovaginal bulb migrating distally, uterine and vaginal walls forming from adjacent mesenchyme
16	112		Uterus and vagina recognizable
20	150		Vagina attains lumen, vaginal introitus external, hymen ruptures

Source: Tarry, W.F., Duckett, J.W. and Stephens, F.D. (1986), The Mayer–Rokitansky syndrome: pathogenesis, classification and management. *J. Urol.* 136: 648. Table 2. Reprinted with permission of the Williams and Wilkins Co.

concept corresponds with the first of two extant theories of vaginal canalization, advocated by Felix (1912) and Frazer (1931) in which the müllerian epithelial proliferation forms the entire vagina to the hymen, which has sinus epithelium on its external aspect only. An imperforate hymen is explained easily by this theory. In 1933 Koff proposed that the sinovaginal bulbs formed the entire plate, that the plate hollowed out and that the hymen remained, being composed entirely of urogenital sinus endoderm. This mechanism more readily explains a mid-vaginal transverse septum.

Embryogenesis of müllerian and wolffian anomalies in Mayer–Rokitansky syndrome. In the symmetric anomalies in which both ureters and kidneys were present, the wolffian ducts migrated normally and gave rise to ureteral buds on each side. In Case 1 the wolffian contribution to the vaginal plate failed to induce canalization or complete migration, perhaps because it atrophied too early (10–11 weeks), while in Case 6 premature atrophy (8–10 weeks) may have caused arrest of migration. Symmetric müllerian defects in which one kidney only was present, as in Case 8, may also have resulted from premature atrophy of the wolffian ducts after bud formation on one side and before it on the opposite side. In asymmetric anomalies (Cases 3 and 4) the wolffian duct migration was complete with induction of the kidney and müllerian system on one side but it arrested just short of the site of the ureteral bud on the contralateral side, causing agenesis of the kidney and ureteral bud. The müllerian duct on that side arrested at the same point and failed to fuse lumen to lumen with the opposite duct but recruited mesenchyme to form a mature uterus.

In the remaining three patients with asymmetric anomalies (Cases 2, 5 and 7) the presence of the kidney on one side predicts the former presence of the wolffian duct on that side and the likelihood of premature atrophy as the cause of the müllerian defects. However, on the opposite side agenesis of the wolffian body was the more likely cause of lack of wolffian and müllerian structures (Cases 2 and 7). The gonadal ridge may form independently of the wolffian body as exemplified by the presence of the left gonad but absence of all left wolffian and müllerian organs in Case 5. In Cases 2 and 6, presumably a sinovaginal bulb formed and canalized, and in the absence of the müllerian system, formed into a short vagina without a hymen.

Asymmetric müllerian anomalies are associated regularly with renal malformation (Müller, 1968). Müllerian and wolffian developments proceed independently on each side, and sometimes the ducts of one side descend ahead of those of the opposite side (Gruenwald, 1941). Thus, premature involution of wolffian duct epithelium may prevent a ureteral bud from forming and cause one müllerian duct to arrest higher than the other. Symmetric defects of the müllerian ducts occur without renal involvement if their development is arrested after the ureters bud from the wolffian ducts at four weeks of gestation. Defects in the development of the wolffian duct are thus conducive to müllerian anomalies. In addition, it can be proposed that premature atrophy of normally formed ducts also may lead to symmetric or asymmetric müllerian or vaginal anomalies.

Nomenclature. Vaginal agenesis with shortcomings of müllerian and wolffian development are designated as the Mayer–Rokitansky syndrome. The definition limits the syndrome to these specific anomalies occurring in endocrinologically normal 46XX phenotypic female subjects of all ages. The addition of names of other authors who have contributed to the knowledge and the range of accompanying anomalies to this eponymous title is excessively cumbersome and to be discouraged.

Associated anomalies. Of our eight patients, six had solitary kidneys and vesicoureteral reflux occurred in two. Renal ectopy or agenesis has been reported in 34 and 43 per cent of the patients with the Mayer–Rokitansky syndrome (Müller, 1968; Griffin et al., 1976). Griffin and associates also found from their analysis of 574 case reports that 12 per cent of the Mayer–Rokitansky patients exhibited skeletal anomalies. Ovarian cysts were not seen in our patients but cysts were found in 64 per cent of the patients $\geq$ 20 years old (Girotti and Hauser, 1969).

Genetic defects of the müllerian ducts. None of our patients has a family history suggestive of müllerian anomalies. Such a history or the presence of skeletal, auricular or ocular anomalies suggests one of several known familial disorders (Winter et al., 1968; Pinsky, 1974; Chantler, 1983). Complete müllerian aplasia (Case 5), most often with normal kidneys, may be genetic (Shokeir, 1971; Sarto and Simpson, 1978). Pure fusion defects and symmetric distal vaginal agenesis often are familial with normal or cystic dysplastic kidneys.

Smith (1982b) used the appellation 'Rokitansky malformation sequence' to designate the forms described of müllerian agenesis in any clinical setting, and stated that about 4 per cent of the cases in which ovaries and fallopian tubes are present but which lack the body of the uterus and upper vagina are familial with affected female siblings. The distinction between the familial disorders and the Mayer–Rokitansky syndrome, which is most often a sporadic occurrence, is important for genetic counselling.

Classification of müllerian defects. Monie and Sigurdson reviewed previous classifications of vaginal and uterine anomalies, and evolved a scheme that codes each anomaly of the corpus and cervix of the uterus and vagina (Monie and Sigurdson, 1950). It is couched in Latin terms and omits anomalies of the fallopian tubes, ovary and kidney. It is more applicable to symmetric than asymmetric anomalies.

The müllerian classification as now proposed is comprehensive for the anatomist, gynaecologist and urologist, perhaps easier to recall and incorporates the classes of Monie and Sigurdson (1950) and Müller (1968). It specifies precisely the outcome of müllerian development on each side of the midline. Classification usually will be possible on the basis of physical and ultrasound examinations or laparoscopy, and carries prognostic implications regarding fertility and menstruation.

The grades 0 to 4 refer to the extent of the müllerian systems affected. Each side is graded individually. The letter M refers to müllerian defects. Fortuitously, the M stands for Mayer–Rokitansky as well. The grading is described as follows (Fig. 4.6): grade M0—unilateral system normally formed but unfused or septum retained, M1—vaginal agenesis alone, M2—vaginal and uterine agenesis, M3—müllerian agenesis total and M4—müllerian and ovarian agenesis.

The number of the grade is easy to recall because grade 0 is normal except for septal defects, grade 1 has one müllerian (vaginal) anomaly, grade 2 has two (vaginal and uterine) anomalies, and so on. This system emphasizes the asymmetry that is common, and allows additional qualifications as to laterality and to status of the urinary tract. Our eight cases are classified according to this grading system in Fig. 4.6. It may be convenient to use these grades to describe the müllerian defects in other combined cloacal or exstrophy anomalies.

Management. Before the advent of high-resolution real-time ultrasound, numerous procedures evolved for evaluating patients with the Mayer–Rokitansky syndrome, including standard urographic studies, vaginography (Rock and Jones, 1980), pneumogynaecography (Spasov *et al.*, 1976), laparotomy and, more recently, laparoscopy (Girotti and Hauser, 1969; Casthely *et al.*, 1974). Sonography enables one to demonstrate precise anatomical detail, including visualization of the kidney and bladder, müllerian structures and septae, ovarian cysts and endometriomas (Girotti and Hauser, 1969; Fried *et al.*, 1978; Rosenberg *et al.*, 1982; Kenney *et al.*, 1984). Often the instillation of water into the vagina and rectum can be helpful to clarify the sonographic anatomy. Ultrasound is especially useful to visualize distended obstructed segments of the genital or urinary tract. Because of its benign nature ultrasound is the preferred screening test for pelvic masses, amenorrhoea, dysmenorrhoea, urinary tract infection or a suspected genitourinary anomaly. MRI is now also a very common and useful test.

As shown in Table 4.1, Tarry *et al.* (1986) used a variety of techniques for reconstruction in these patients, which have been described previously (Frank, 1938; McIndoe, 1950, 1959; Leduc-Van Campenhout and Simard, 1968; Raffensperger and Ramenofsky, 1973; Markland and Hastings, 1974; Griffin *et al.*, 1976; Rosenberg *et al.*, 1982). The choice of procedure and patient age at reconstruction are dependent upon individual anatomy, fertility potential, and psychological and social factors (Table 4.1). They found that transvaginal septectomy, or marsupialization for asymmetric hydrocolpos or grade one müllerian agenesis (Cases 3 and 4) was satisfactory, simple and effective (Fig. 4.6). The presence of endometrium and a cervix augurs well for fertility in this group with appropriate surgical management.

Psychological consideration of patients with uterovaginal agenesis may dictate the need for early vaginoplasty, which hitherto has been delayed until just before marriage (Neinstein and Castle, 1983). The patient should be approached with the concept of 'opening up' rather than 'creating' the vagina. She and her parents need counselling regarding fertility and sexual function, and genetic and endocrine status. Several authors have noted that patients presenting with amenorrhoea also complain of dyspareunia or the inability to have vaginal intercourse, although few patients seek help for this complaint primarily (Girotti and Hauser, 1969; Sarto and Simpson, 1978). Behavioural problems of the adolescent patient may be avoided by early appropriate guidance and reassurance.

Formation and malformation of the epididymis

Wolffian duct and the epididymis

All parts of the mesonephros undergo atrophy and with it also the ductules of the nephrons that join the wolffian duct except for those five to 12 that apply themselves to the gonad. These ductules first lose their glomeruli and transform into afferent ductules which anastomose with the efferent ductules emerging from the rete testis towards the upper pole of the testis. These mesonephric afferent ductules undergo extreme elongation and tortuosity forming cones that expand to form the head of the epididymis. They maintain continuity with the mesonephric duct which continues as the sole tortuous convoluted microchannel in the body and tail of the epididymis. The mesonephric duct caudal to the lower pole of the epididymis becomes the non-coiled vas deferens.

Many errors of development befall the duct system inside the testis and epididymis and upper vas deferens. Efferent ducts may be too few (normal 6–12) or fail to connect with the afferent tubules of the wolffian duct or having joined with the afferent ducts they make direct connections without convolutions with the vas (Campbell, 1951). The tortuosities of the microduct in the body and tail may continue caudally converting the normally straight vas deferens into a fine convoluted microduct.

Ipsilateral duplication anomalies of testes and vas deferens

Duplication of an ipsilateral testis may occur as an isolated anomaly of the gonadal ridge or in association with defective müllerian regression.

Isolated anomaly

1. Two small testes of unequal size, in close proximity one above the other and sharing an elongated epididymis and single vas (Boggan, 1933).

2. Two small testes usually of unequal size with separate epididymides and vasa deferentia that join to form a common stem (Pelander *et al.*, 1953).
3. Two small testes, only one of which is complete with epididymis and vas deferens, the other having no connection with the vas (Gauderer *et al.*, 1982).

Theoretically, a transverse division of the longitudinally orientated gonadal ridge explains the anomaly in which two separate testes of small size share the same epididymis and originate from the same gonadal ridge. These testes connect in series with the same wolffian duct. The anomaly of two testes of equal or unequal size, each complete with epididymis and vas joining to form a short or long common stem, however, is perhaps better explained by longitudinal duplication of the gonad and partial or complete duplication of the wolffian duct. Thirdly, the gonadal ridge may divide transversely, one part developing a connection with the afferent ductules of the wolffian duct and the other, usually smaller part fails to connect. Both testes descend toward the scrotum.

The term supernumerary testis implies that two testes arise in the same genital ridge with or without a con-tralateral testis. Polyorchidism means that the individual has three or more testes.

The supernumerary testis with its mate may descend toward or into the ipsilateral scrotum. They may cross to the opposite side and remain intra-abdominal or one or both may enter an inguinal hernial sac without gubernacular attachment and with or without the company of the contralateral testis.

Two otherwise normal testes lodged in the same side of the scrotum but each arising from contralateral gonadal ridges is called 'transverse testicular ectopia' or 'pseudoduplication of the testis' (Gauderer *et al.*, 1982).

Duplication associated with defective müllerian regression

The occurrence of müllerian duct derivatives together with the duplicate testis anomaly was found in 49 per cent of a series of 44 cases of transverse testicular ectopy by Fujita (1980). He considered that müllerian-inhibiting substance may be lacking or the target organ may be resistant to its action in these patients. A further description of this anomaly is given in Chapter 39 (see Fig. 39.4).

Embryogenesis of the hymen and caudal end of the vagina deduced from uterovaginal anomalies*

5

The morphogenesis of the caudal end of the vagina and hymen is controversial amongst embryologists. The urogenital sinus alone or in combination with the müllerian ducts, the wolffian ducts, or all three have been claimed to be the precursors of these organs. Two examples of imperforate hymen in one unit of a duplex vagina associated with ipsilateral ureterorenal anomalies that lend light to the controversy are described here. The imperforate hymen occurred on the same side as the ureteric anomaly, indicating that the combined anomaly is derived from a deficit in a common denominator, the ipsilateral wolffian duct. The migration of the wolffian duct stopped short of the urogenital sinus, affected the development of the ureteric bud, and led to defective canalization of the vaginal plate and the imperforate hymen. By inference, normal hymen formation is also mediated by the wolffian duct and is derived from the vaginal bulbs of urogenital sinus origin externally and the müllerian ducts internally; the vagina is also of müllerian origin. Once the normal hymen perforates, there may be intermingling of the sinus and ductal epithelia.

Anomalies of the vagina and hymen when combined with ureteric defects may provide clues as to their origins. These two case histories describe the features of patients who had haematocolpos in one vagina of a double müllerian system. The ipsilateral anomalies of the ureter indicate that a faulty wolffian duct was instrumental in the subsequent malformation of the genital system. In combination with other known features of ectopic ureters, the anomalies described support the concept that in normal subjects the lower third of the vagina is müllerian and the hymen is derived from müllerian duct internally and urogenital sinus (vaginal bulbs) externally.

Case reports

Case 1

P.C., aged 13 years, complained of lower abdominal pain and dysuria for one week followed by the passage of a large amount of blood. At that time, examination of the introitus revealed a recent mini-perforation and a bluish bulge of the right hymen to the side of the hymen of the left vagina, with bloody discharge coming from it. A tender abdominal mass was palpable in the right iliac fossa. On rectal examination, a tense mass of banana shape, bulging into the anterior rectal wall, was palpated. An intravenous pyelogram revealed a hypertrophic but normal left kidney and no evidence of a right kidney.

Four days later, a patent left hymen and a stenotic orifice to the right of the rim of the left hymen were observed. Colposcopy through this opening revealed a right-sided vagina, cervix and uterus, and a septum between the two vaginas. Cystoscopy revealed a normal left ureteric orifice and an absent right ureteric orifice. On vaginoscopy a small orifice on the anterolateral wall of the right vagina was seen, near the recently perforated hymen, leading to a ureter and right-sided pelvic kidney. The vaginal septum was divided and one week later the right kidney and ureter were removed, following which the patient made an uneventful recovery. The kidney was dysplastic, measuring 1.5 × 0.8 cm (Fig. 5.1). The ureter showed muscle hypertrophy and fibrosis. The diagnoses included haematometrocolpos, imperforate hymen with recent perforation, and the ectopic ureter issuing into the dilated vagina.

Case 2

N.S., aged 15 years, had treatment in the newborn period for cloacal anomaly with a rectocloacal fistula, for which a temporary colostomy and later a rectal pull-through procedure were performed. Endoscopy at this early period revealed the urethral orifice on the anterior wall, the vaginal orifice on the apex and the rectal fistula on the posterior wall of the cloacal canal (Fig. 5.2a, b). In recent years, anorectal continence was maintained with the help of enemas. The right kidney and ureter were absent and the left upper tract was normal.

At puberty, the patient had increasing abdominal pain for five days. An X-ray of the abdomen showed an abdominal mass in the region of the right kidney, displacing the bowel forward and to the left.

Bimanual vaginal examination revealed a large pelvic and abdominal mass that displaced the left vagina towards the left. An ultrasound study of the abdomen revealed a 10-cm cystic mass posterior to the bladder with fluid levels.

Laparotomy revealed a normal right ovary that was hidden by a very dilated, blood filled, and completely sealed right fallopian tube. The right-sided, over distended uterus lay in the midline and to the right (Fig. 5.2c). The right uterus was opened, and a complete septum between the right and left uteri was displayed. A cruciate incision was made in the septum and the margins were sutured. The right tube was removed and the distal end ligated.

*Reproduced in part, with permission of Springer-Verlag Publications, from Luthra, M. and Stephens, F.D. (1988), Embryogenesis of the hymen and caudal end of the vagina deduced from uterovaginal anomalies. Pediatr. Surg. Int. 3: 422–5.

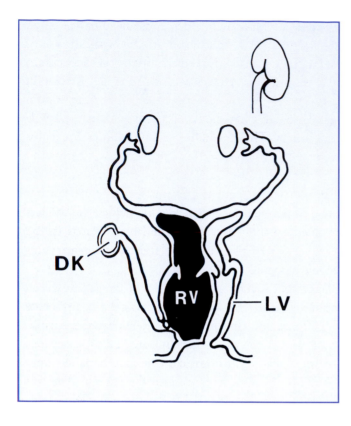

Fig. 5.1 *Case 1. Double vagina with right hydrometrocolpos and vaginal ectopic ureter (LV, left vagina; RV, right vagina; DK, dysplastic kidney) (Reprinted with permission from Luthra, M. and Stephens, F.D. (1988) Embryogenesis of the hymen and caudal end of the vagina deduced from uterovaginal anomalies. Pediatr. Surg. Int. 3: 422–5, Fig. 1.)*

The ovary was preserved. The left vagina and uterus were not enlarged but the left fallopian tube was distended. A cyst was present on the left ovary.

Both patients developed haematometrocolpos in the right component of a double vagina and uterus and abnormal ipsilateral upper urinary tracts. Case 1 had a bicornuate uterus and a dysplastic right pelvic kidney with its ureter issuing via Gartner's duct into the right vagina close to the imperforate hymen. Case 2 had a uterus didelphys, a short right vagina with imperforate hymen at the point of penetration of the cloacal canal, and agenesis of the right kidney and ureter.

The combination of unilateral müllerian and renal anomalies as in Case 1 is included in the Mayer–Rokitansky syndrome (Tarry *et al.*, 1986). The

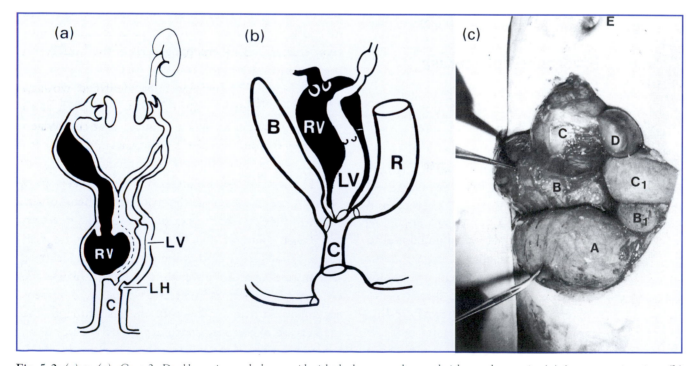

Fig. 5.2 *(a) to (c). Case 2. Double vagina and cloaca with right hydrometrocolpos and right renal agenesis. (a) Anteroposterior view. (b) Lateral view (LV, left vagina; RV, right hydrometrocolpos; LH, left hymen; C, cloaca; B, bladder; R, rectum). (c) Photograph of genital organs displayed at laparotomy. A, right haematocolpos; B, right haematometra; C, right hydrosalpinx; D, cyst of ovary; C₁, left fallopian tube; B₁, normal uterus; E, umbilicus.(Reprinted with permission from Luthra, M. and Stephens, F.D. (1988) Embryogenesis of the hymen and caudal end of the vagina deduced from uterovaginal anomalies. Pediatr. Surg. Int. 3: 422–5, Fig. 2.)*

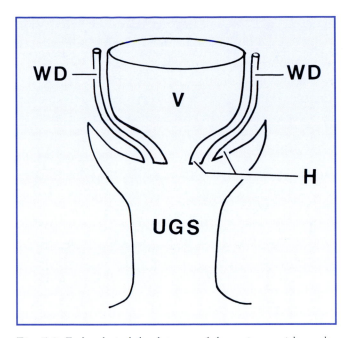

Fig. 5.3 *Embryological development of the vagina at eight weeks, showing wolffian ducts issuing between layers of hymen into urogenital sinus. V, vagina; WD, wolffian duct; UGS, urogenital sinus; H, hymen. (After Frazer, J.E. (1931), A Manual of Embryology. London, Baillière, Tindall and Cox, Fig. 266, p. 438.)*

combination is not uncommon with cloacal defects, though not included in the syndrome.

Normal embryogenesis of uterus, vagina and hymen

At six weeks' gestation the wolffian duct, which traverses the abdomen and pelvis, has entered the lower urinary tract of the fully divided cloaca and given rise to the trigone and ureteric bud. At six weeks, the coelomic epithelium dorsal and lateral to the developing gonad invaginates longitudinally to form a furrow, the lips of which meet to convert the furrow into the müllerian duct (fallopian tube). This tube first lies lateral and dorsal to the wolffian duct and its caudal, solid end, actively migrates and elongates alongside the wolffian duct in intimate contact with its basement membrane. It turns medially at the caudal end of the mesonephros, crossing ventral to the wolffian duct and meets its opposite member in the midline. The two solid, blunt ends of the müllerian ducts then migrate caudally side by side, canalizing and fusing as they go, to penetrate the wall of the urogenital sinus at the eighth week of gestation (Fig. 5.3).

Each müllerian duct is guided by the respective wolffian duct, migrates and develops independently of

the other, and usually one descends ahead of the other. The two müllerian ducts penetrate the posterior wall of the urogenital sinus between the orifices of the wolffian ducts on a mound called 'Müller's tubercle'. Two solid epithelial evaginations (sinovaginal bulbs) grow from the tubercle to meet the two solid tips of the fused müllerian ducts. This epithelial proliferation of the bulbs and the caudal ends of the müllerian ducts forms the solid vaginal plate. The vaginal plate and adjoining müllerian ducts elongate, canalize, and migrate from pelvic to perineal locations. Having guided the müllerian ducts to their destination and participated in the development of the vaginal plate, the wolffian ducts become atrophic.

Felix (1912) and Frazer (1931) considered that canalization occurred in the bulbar and vaginal components of the plate and that the hymen demarcated the junction between the müllerian and urogenital structures. Koff (1933) using histological evidence obtained from embryos and fetuses, claimed that the vaginal plate was formed mainly from vaginal bulbs, that the plate canalized predominantly in a caudocranial direction giving rise to the hymen, and that the hymen and caudal one-fifth of the vagina were formed from the plate and were therefore of urogenital sinus origin. Hence, the controversy concerning the morphogenesis of the hymen and vagina continued.

Witschi (1977) histologically identified wolffian duct structures in the walls of the vaginal plate down to the urogenital sinus. He claimed that the hymen was formed from sinus and müllerian epithelia with lateral contributions from the wolffian ducts. Frazer (1931) observed the termination of the wolffian ducts between the two layers of the hymen. Stephens' observations from a postmortem examination of a newborn baby with bilateral double ureters support the dual origin of the hymen and the müllerian contribution to the entire length of the vagina (Stephens, 1983d). The two ectopic upper pole ureters described by Stephens accompanied the lower pole ureters through the ureterovesical hiatuses, continued caudally beyond the trigonal orifices of these ureters, and remained submucosal along the trigone, urethra and urethrovaginal bridge; one issued to the exterior on the bridge but the other joined the remnant of the wolffian duct contiguous with the hymen. These observations support the findings of Witschi, firstly, that the hymen marked the junction of the canalized vaginal bulbs of the urogenital sinus and müllerian ducts at the introitus, and secondly, that the wolffian duct itself guides and mediates the caudal migration of the vaginal plate from pelvis to perineum.

Correlation of embryologic concepts with congenital defects of the vagina and urinary organs

The non-duplicated ectopic ureter of Case 1 issued in the distal end of the right-sided vagina, presumably via Gartner's duct, indicating that perhaps the wolffian duct and its attached ectopic ureter did not quite reach the urogenital sinus, thus impairing the influence of the duct on the development of the vaginal plate. The müllerian and sinus components of the plate both canalized incompletely, creating a thick, imperforate hymen. The müllerian component of the plate partially canalized and incorporated the lumen of the wolffian duct with its attached ureter.

Migration of the right müllerian duct of Case 2 was arrested close to, but not at, the cloacal canal owing to a defect of the right wolffian duct, as indicated by agenesis of the ipsilateral kidney. The left müllerian duct, accompanied by a normal wolffian duct and ureter, made contact with the vaginal bulbs forming the patent hymen. Absence of the right kidney and ureter indicates that the terminus of the right wolffian duct was defective, supporting the notion that the müllerian duct depends on the wolffian duct for its migration and contact and interaction with the ipsilateral vaginal bulb to form the hymen. Both müllerian ducts were barred from descent from pelvis to perineum owing to the lack of formation of the urorectal septum and persistence of the cloacal canal.

The two vaginal anomalies with their upper urinary tract defects support the concept of Witschi that the vagina is formed from the müllerian ducts though dependent on, and mediated by, the wolffian ducts.

Since the vaginal plate is derived from the solid ends of the müllerian ducts co-apting the solid vaginal bulbs, canalization may under abnormal conditions take place more from the sinus than from the vaginal components. The hymen may then be inside the introitus. If the müllerian duct is absent, the solid epithelial invagination of the sinovaginal bulbs induced by the wolffian duct may

elongate and, when canalized, create a blind, short vagina as in the testicular feminizing syndrome. An abnormally long vaginal plate in the presence of a normal wolffian duct may permit the formation of a long, canalized sinovaginal bulb that co-apts the müllerian duct more cranially than normal, creating an internal hymen, a septum, or a stenosis.

Witschi (1977) depicted traces of wolffian epithelium on the caudal part of the normal vaginal plate that he considered to be composed of müllerian and wolffian structures. With canalization of the plate, the hymen is formed of müllerian ducts cranially, urogenital sinus caudally and wolffian ducts laterally. With canalization of the normal plate and perforation of the normal hymen, sinus epithelium may subsequently intermingle with epithelium of the müllerian ducts and vice versa.

Unilateral renal and ureteric agenesis may be caused by defective bud formation from an otherwise normal wolffian duct. In this instance, the müllerian system may develop normally. If, however, the distal end of the wolffian duct is abnormal, the bud and vaginal plate may be affected. The vaginal plate may be defective, leading to anomalies of the distal one-third of the vagina. Under these circumstances the vaginal plate may fail to migrate or canalize, creating a persistent urogenital sinus anomaly with or without hydrocolpos (an anomaly referred to by McKusick et al., 1946, as 'transverse vaginal septum') or the plate may migrate towards or to the vestibule, but the hymen may remain imperforate. Case 1 supports this idea in that the accompanying ectopic vaginal ureter issuing near the imperforate hymen indicates some defect in the terminal wolffian duct that impaired the canalization of the vaginal plate.

In some patients, the kidney is normally developed yet major parts of the vagina and uterus or fallopian tubes are missing. In such instances, it is presumed that the normal process of disintegration of the mesonephric duct began prematurely but after the ureteric bud had developed and prior to the descent of the müllerian duct to the urogenital sinus. Under these circumstances, the müllerian deficiencies would correspond with the degree of caudal atrophy of the wolffian duct.

The hymen, therefore, is the product of the union of the müllerian duct and urogenital sinus epithelia, together with the transient presence laterally of wolffian duct epitheliam.

Intrinsic anomalies of the urethra

II

The male urethra

6

The pelvic urethra, common to male and female anatomy, extends from the internal urinary meatus of the bladder to the perineum and exhibits many variations in shape and size. These shapes are demonstrable by voiding cystourethrography in children, and by examination of postmortem specimens. Some shapes can be correlated with the intrinsic muscle of the urethra, while others may result from minor or major variations of development. Occult intrinsic abnormalities predominate in the male urethra, sometimes causing urinary obstruction, haematuria or dysuria.

In the female child, normal variants of shape are commonly revealed radiographically, but intrinsic anomalies of the urethra are rare. Both the male and female urethras exhibit misplaced ureters and many cloacal abnormalities, which are described in other chapters.

The anterior urethra in the male exhibits numerous intrinsic defects arising in glands and ducts in its walls and in the corpus spongiosum and corpora cavernosa. Hypo- and epispadias, anourethral and intersex forms are excluded from this chapter.

The advent of voiding cystourethrography (Higgins *et al.*, 1951) in the last 30 years has exposed many variants of normal and abnormal urethras, and it is only recently that the true clinical significance of many of these radiological features has been resolved. Many of these features, which occur commonly in children, can be explained as minor aberrations of normal embryology. The more uncommon but standard malformations are interpreted as major deviations of embryology, for which theories of abnormal development are proposed.

Symptoms pertaining to enuresis, urinary infection and obstruction have been the causes of investigation of the urinary tract in most children with intrinsic lesions of the urethra. Voiding cystourethrography (VCU), excretory urography by intravenous pyelography (IVP), urodynamic studies, endoscopy, and surgical exploration were used to identify or exclude the lesion in the urethra. Postmortem specimens of many intrinsic urethral abnormalities obtained from cadavers have been studied anatomically and histologically in order to provide objective data and aid the interpretations of the clinical and radiological observations.

Dynamic urethrography

The child or infant is placed in the supine position on the X-ray table. Non-toxic, non-irritating iodinated contrast medium, Renografin 30, diluted with saline or water to 15 per cent (anion diatrizoate), is introduced through a small calibre catheter. The medium is run in under gravity pressure until the viscus is full, or until the urge to micturate becomes intense. The catheter is then removed, and cystograms are obtained during fluoroscopy. In children who can start and stop micturition as required, anteroposterior, oblique and lateral projections of the urethra can usually be obtained. Within 20 seconds of the completion of voiding, fluoroscopy (or film) will demonstrate the presence or absence of residual content. Further films to detect ureteric emptying may be desired to estimate emptying times if vesicoureteral reflux has occurred. Videotaping of the voidance, or multiple low-radiation small films, may be substituted for the standard films.

Infants void spontaneously when the bladder is filled to capacity. Micturition time is so short that only one voiding film may be obtained, though if the bladder is enlarged by obstruction, the duration of voiding may be prolonged.

Occasionally, voiding may be possible only in the erect posture, in which event satisfactory films may be obtained. In some medical centres, the standing or sitting positions are used in routine dynamic urethrography. Micturition is usually successfully achieved in the supine position, which is preferred because it is convenient for catheterization, observation and fluoroscopy.

If cooperation is not forthcoming, the physician may resort to manual expression of the contrast solution from the bladder with the patient anaesthetized, but then the urethral filling is often imperfect, and the interpretation is sometimes less reliable.

When the bladder is chronically enlarged, and retention with overflow has occurred, it is a simple procedure to aspirate some urine and replace it with an equal quantity of Renografin 60 solution through a suprapubic needle under local anaesthesia. The Renografin dilutes in the urine of the bladder and the method avoids the risks of urinary infection from the catheter.

Often, a single film of the urethra, taken during micturition, is enough to disprove the presence of an anomaly. Sometimes, such a significant film can be obtained during the IVP series if the radiopacity of the bladder content is sufficient to demonstrate the urethra on voiding.

In boys, the true anteroposterior view causes superimposing of the wide column of iodide solution in the bulbous urethra on that of the membranous urethra, thus obscuring the detail in both segments (Fig. 6.1). A near anteroposterior position may be obtained by packing a small, folded hand-towel under one buttock, in order to tilt the pelvis and throw the bulbous urethra clear of the posterior urethra. The particular advantage of this view in the male is that it shows well the membranous portion of the urethra, the verumontanum, and the inferior crest and its terminal fins, whereas the oblique views show the bladder neck and lateral walls of the bladder more clearly.

The VCU is generally preferred to the retrograde injection urethrogram for demonstrating the posterior and anterior urethra. The anterior urethra is well demonstrated by injection techniques, but the procedure is more uncomfortable for the patient, more difficult to perform in young children, and does not show the features of the posterior urethra.

Absence of residual opaque medium immediately after micturition is a reliable guide to emptying efficiency, but the presence of residual volumes, especially after intermittent arrested micturition in the supine position, is not necessarily significant. In delayed films obtained from patients who exhibit primary vesicoureteral reflux or diverticula, the appearance of residual urine under these circumstances is usually false, the urine having returned into the bladder after micturition (Stephens, 1954).

Correlation of normal urethrographic criteria with normal anatomical features

Studies of both the cystourethrograms and the anatomy of the normal sphincters have helped to explain the

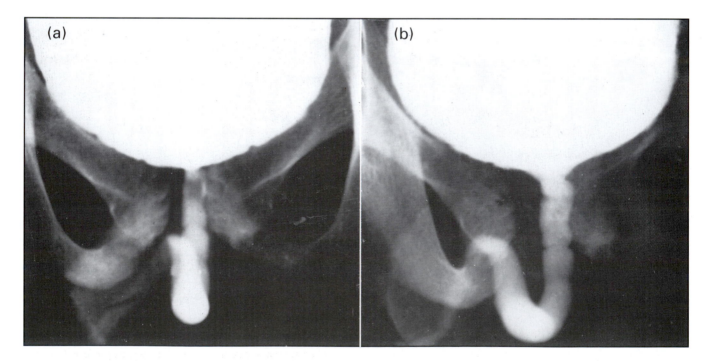

Fig. 6.1 *R.H., aged $8\frac{1}{2}$ years. (**a**) Normal urethrogram showing masking of membranous by the bulbous urethra in the true anteroposterior position. (**b**) The appearance in the slight oblique. (Reprinted, by permission, from Stephens, F.D. (1963), Congenital Malformations of the Rectum, Anus and Genito-Urinary Tracts. Edinburgh, Livingstone, Fig. 112, p. 212.)*

changes observed during micturition of normal and abnormal children and have provided explanations of some of the controversial issues posed by dynamic urethrography. Of particular interest are the variations of the shape, internal contours, and calibre of the normal bladder neck and urethra, the extent of the external voluntary sphincter compared with the descriptions of the postpubertal urethra, the 'milk-back' phenomenon and urethral peristalsis.

The normal bladder is finely crinkled during micturition, and the internal meatus adjusts to a diameter proportionate to the effort exerted by the bladder musculature (Fig. 6.2).

The posterior urethra, between the bladder outlet and the bulb, shows a cylindrical column of opaque fluid, narrowing slightly anteriorly and posteriorly at the site of the perineal membrane. The cylinder bulges slightly in the prostatic urethra. At the midpoint of the posterior urethra, or slightly above it, the verumontanum produces a small, oval 'filling defect' on the posterior wall. Below this, in the membranous urethra, the inferior urethral crest is sometimes visible as a midline longitudinal filling defect. Sometimes, the terminal fins of the crest are seen diverging caudally to either side (Fig. 6.3).

The bulbous urethra, larger in calibre, turns anteriorly at right angles to the posterior urethra below the perineal membrane. The bulb extends to the site of attachment of the suspensory ligament and is approximately as long as the child's penile urethra.

The penile urethra extends from the suspensory ligament to the external meatus. Its diameter is narrower in the proximal portion. Inside the external meatus is the local dilatation of the fossa navicularis. The diameter of the normal external orifice during micturition is almost equal to that of the local dilatation just proximal to it (Fig. 6.3).

The radiopaque column, demonstrable in the posterior urethra, can be obliterated in two zones by voluntary effort. Correlation of the anatomical studies described below with the radiographic interpretations shows these zones to correspond to the various sphincters of the urethra.

The highest level of occlusion is the internal urethral meatus (Fig. 6.4). At this site, the iodide column of the urethra is entirely eliminated from view by contraction of the internal sphincter, and the smooth, even contour of the bladder base is clearly defined in the cystogram. Between this and the second level, the

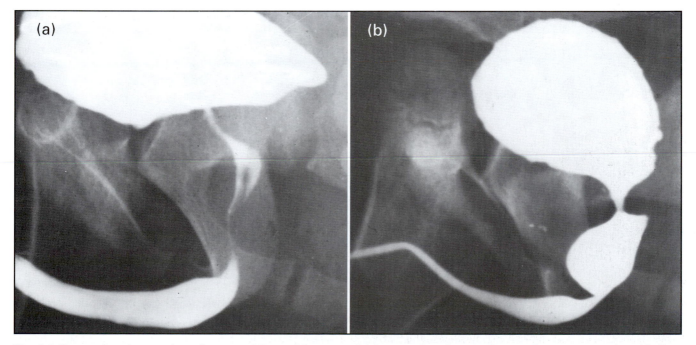

Fig. 6.2 *Retrograde and antegrade urethrograms. J.P., aged four years. (**a**) Injection through external meatus demonstrates penile and bulbous urethra. (**b**) Voiding of opaque medium distends whole urethra, demonstrating site of obstruction at junction of membranous urethra and bulb, with dilatation of posterior urethra and incomplete distension of anterior urethra. (Reprinted, by permission, from Stephens, F.D. (1983), Congenital Malformations of the Urinary Tract, New York, Praeger, Fig. 4.2, p. 87.)*

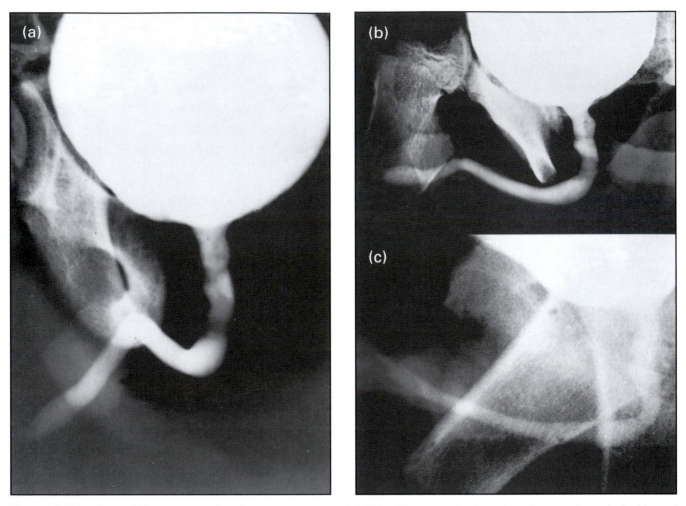

Fig. 6.3 *P.T., male, aged 12 years—normal voiding cystourethrogram. (**a**) Slight oblique view showing to best advantage the urethral calibre and the detail in the membranous urethra. (**b**) Full right oblique view which shows the bladder neck and anterior urethra most clearly. (**c**) Lateral view which demonstrates the posterior margin of the bladder neck. (Reprinted, by permission, from Stephens, F.D. (1963), Congenital Malformations of the Rectum, Anus and Genito-Urinary Tracts. Edinburgh, Livingstone, Fig. 113, p. 213.)*

urethra is occluded by the internal involuntary sphincter.

The second level lies near the verumontanum (Fig. 6.4). The obliteration of the zone of the urethra below this level is demonstrable by instantaneous radiography at the moment of voluntary arrest of micturition (Fig. 6.5). The upper portion of the iodide column in this zone becomes thinned in density and occlusion is complete caudally. This gradual occlusion in the male contrasts with the sudden, complete elimination of the column in the female (see Fig. 10.3). Presumably, prostatic tissue in the posterior and lateral walls of the urethra in the male renders the external sphincter less efficient at its upper limit; the lower limit of this zone is the upper surface of the perineal membrane, the level of

which is sharply defined by the contrast medium still remaining in the bulbous urethra (Figs 6.4 and 6.5). The greater strength of the external sphincter at the lower level ensures the occurrence of the 'milk-back' phenomenon—reverse flow of urine into the bladder at the time of sudden arrest of micturition.

A third level of occlusion in the male lies at the caudal surface of the perineal membrane and corresponds to the cranial limits of the bulbocavernosus muscle. The zone of occlusion extends distally from this point to approximately the region of the suspensory ligament. The urethra above retains its normal dimensions, but is cut off sharply at this level. Distally the narrow column of contrast fluid indicates collapse of the lumen of the penile urethra (Fig. 6.6).

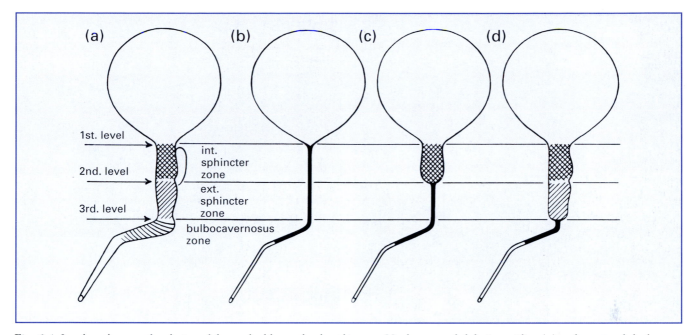

Fig. 6.4 *Levels and zones of occlusion of the urethral lumen by the sphincters. Urethra expanded during voiding (**a**) and unexpanded when not voiding (**b**); (**c**) shows internal sphincter zone expanded to the second level when the external sphincter is voluntarily contracted during voiding and (**d**) shows the internal and external sphincter zones expanded but the lumen is constricted by the voluntary action of the bulbocavernosus muscle.* (Reprinted, by permission, from Stephens, F.D. (1963), Congenital Malformations of the Rectum, Anus and Genito-Urinary Tracts. *Edinburgh, Livingstone, Fig. 114, p. 214.)*

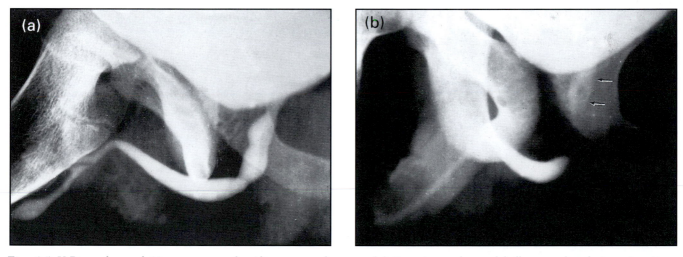

Fig. 6.5 *K.B., male, aged 11 years—normal voiding cystourethrogram. (**a**) Posterior urethra and bulbous urethra during micturition. (**b**) At the earliest moment of arrest of stream by external voluntary sphincter contraction, showing the prostatic urethra above (arrows) partially occluded and bulbous urethra full of opaque medium below the contracted segment.* (Reprinted, by permission, from Stephens, F.D. (1963), Congenital Malformations of the Rectum, Anus and Genito-Urinary Tracts. *Edinburgh, Livingstone, Fig. 115, p. 214.)*

Unusual configurations are sometimes discovered in the course of examination of boys with enuresis, dysuria, infection, haematuria, reflux, vesical diverticula or hypospadias, and in some, an upper-tract malformation may be found to coexist. Most of the urethras exhibiting such shapes do not cause a significant increase in the urethral resistance to flow of urine (Whitaker *et al.*, 1969; see Fig. 6.7).

The normal posterior urethra as displayed by VCU may dilate or contract from time to time according to the activity and moderating effects of the voluntary or

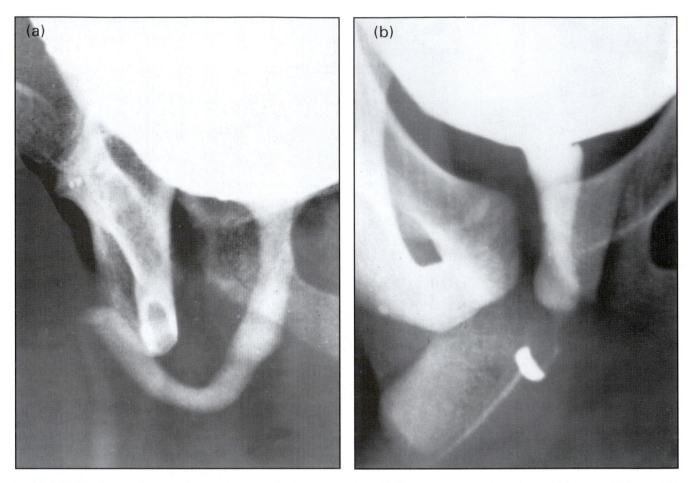

Fig. 6.6 *Voiding cystourethrogram showing the effect of sudden contraction of bulbocavernosus muscle on the urethral lumen. B.M., aged 12 years. (a) Free voidance. (b) The lumen occluded by the action of the bulbocavernosus muscle. Opaque medium is present in the collapsed urethra distal to bulbocavernosus and in the posterior urethra.* (Reprinted, by permission, from Stephens, F.D. (1963), Congenital Malformations of the Rectum, Anus and Genito-Urinary Tracts. *Edinburgh, Livingstone, Fig. 116, p. 215.*)

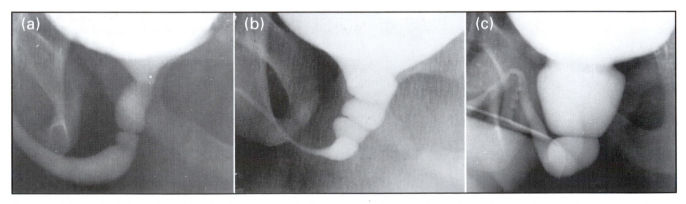

Fig. 6.7 *(a) Urethral rings. (b) Kinks. (c) Ectasia. VCU of patients showing non-obstructive variants of the posterior urethra and bulb.* (Reprinted, by permission, from Stephens, F.D. (1983), Congenital Malformations of the Urinary Tract, *New York, Praeger, Fig. 4.7, p. 90.*)

involuntary muscles of its walls, or the shape may be fixed and irregular.

Change of shape of the urethra during voiding due to changes in pressure and voluntary muscle action is not abnormal, but uncoordinated muscular activity may give rise to stop–start micturition, intermittent closure of the external and overexpansion of the internal sphincter zones typical of the dyssynergia syndrome.

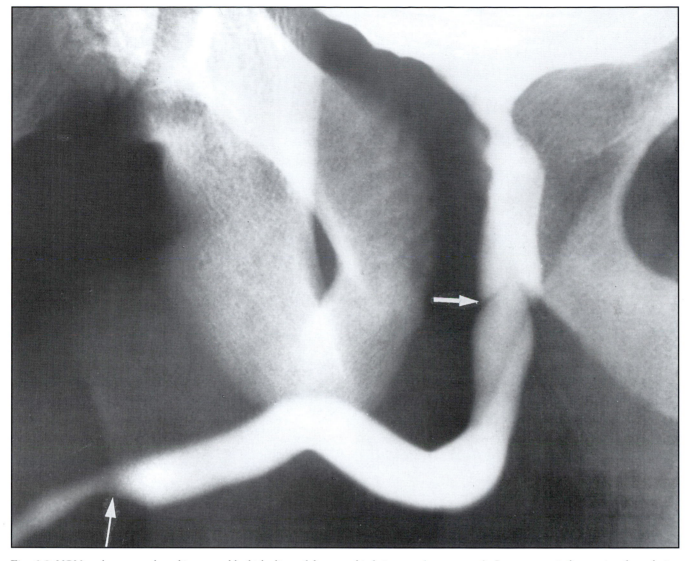

Fig. 6.8 *VCU to show normal marking caused by high plicae of the normal inferior crest (upper arrow). Lower arrow indicates site of angulation and pseudoconstriction caused by urinol. (Reprinted, by permission, from Stephens, F.D. (1983), Congenital Malformations of the Urinary Tract, New York, Praeger, Fig. 4.8, p. 91.)*

Fixed irregularities take the form of shallow-filling defects in the membranous urethra or sharp infolding of the anterior wall with dilatation of the urethra above it. Not infrequently, the membranous urethra exhibits one, two, or three ring-like indentations. Sometimes the prostatic urethra or the whole of the pelvic urethra and bulbous urethra, with or without these indentations, is oversized; some indentations, with time, undergo corrective modelling (Fig. 6.7). Oblique linear-filling defects, arising from each side of the verumontanum and coursing distally in the lateral walls without dilatation of the urethra cranially, are caused by normal lateral components of the inferior crest (Fig. 6.8). Infolding or kinking of the anterior wall of the urethra, usually accompanied by moderate dilatation of the prostatic urethra and sometimes the membranous and bulbous urethra, are examples of variants of shape and dimension (Fig. 6.9). An anterior indentation of the urethral lumen at the junction of membranous and bulbous urethra is attributed to the constricting action of the nuda muscle, a semidetached bundle of muscle fibres on the cranial aspect of the bulbocavernosus (Kjellberg, et al., 1957).

Embryological explanation of unusual shapes and indentations of the posterior urethra

General enlargement of the whole urethra may result from partitioning of an abnormally large cloaca or

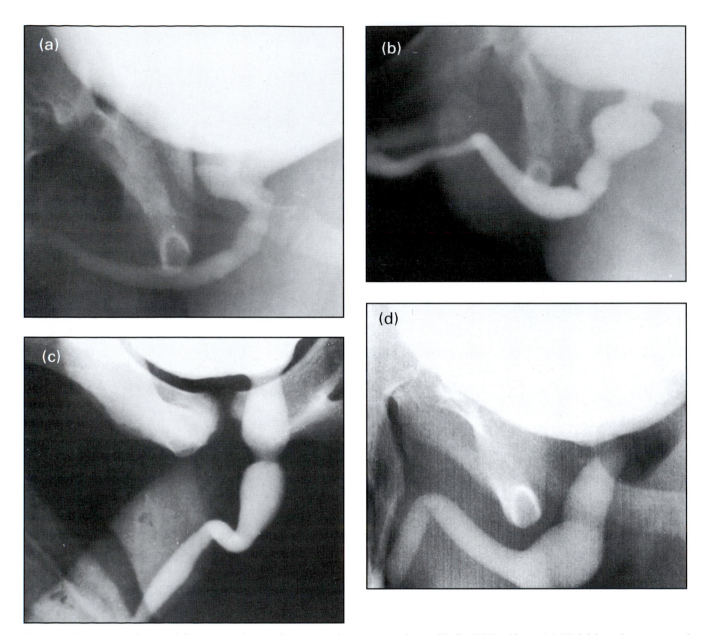

Fig. 6.9 *Variations in shape and dimensions of internal meatus and posterior urethra and bulb. VCU of boys.* (***a***) *With bilateral vesicoureteral reflux.* (***b***) *Right megaureter without reflux.* (***c***) *Coronal hypospadias without stenosis.* (***d***) *Enuresis. (Reprinted, by permission, from Stephens, F.D. (1983), Congenital Malformations of the Urinary Tract, New York, Praeger, Fig. 4.9, p. 92.)*

unequal partitioning of a normal cloaca (Fig. 6.10). Focal enlargement of the prostatic urethra may arise from excessive expansion and absorption of the wolffian ducts into the urinary tract. Focal enlargement of the bulbous urethra may be explained by congenital ectasia of the pars phallica of the urogenital sinus. Angulations of the urethra at the bladder neck (Fig. 6.10) and kinks in the anterior wall can be explained on the basis of angulation of the cloaca due to excessive ventral rotation of the hind end of the embryo to unusual alignment

of Tourneaux's fold with Rathke's plicae that partition the cloaca (Fig. 6.10). Circumferential indentations, single, double or triple in the zone of the membranous urethra, may demarcate irregular junctions of Rathke's plicae or persisting traces of the unabsorbed urogenital membrane (Fig. 6.10). This explanation presupposes that the membrane was thick owing to multilayering of the cells of its endo- and ectodermal components (Frazer, 1931c) or interposition of mesoderm between the two.

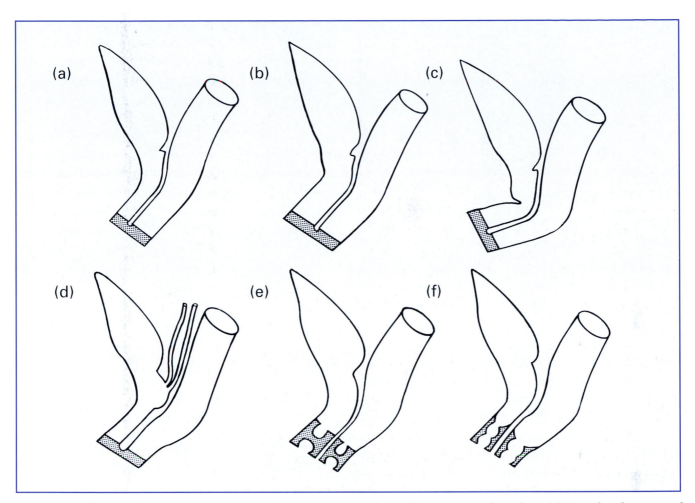

Fig. 6.10 *Possible embryological explanations of unusual dimensions, shapes and rings of the posterior urethra in boys. (**a**) Normal urethra at time of partition of cloaca (16-mm crown–rump length). (**b**) Dilated urethra due to posterior plane of urorectal septum. (**c**) Anterior flexion crease in urethral wall due to excessive rotation of the tail fold of the embryo. (**d**) Dilated prostatic urethra due to extreme expansion and incorporation of common excretory ducts into the urethra. (**e**), (**f**) Irregular penetration of a thick cloacal membrane leaving inelastic circumferential rings in the membranous urethra. (Reprinted, by permission, from Stephens, F.D. (1983), Congenital Malformations of the Urinary Tract, New York, Praeger, Fig. 4.10, p. 93.)*

Morphology of the sphincters of the urethra

Because voluntary contraction of the external sphincter results in the obliteration of so great a length of the urethral lumen, a microanatomical study was made to define the extent of the external sphincter and the zone occupied by the internal sphincter in children.

In postmortem specimens from three male subjects, the urethras were microscopically examined with regard to their normal relationships in the bony pelvis. Serial sections of 15-μm thickness were cut, and every tenth section was stained and examined.

It was found that the external voluntary sphincter conformed closely to the description by Wood Jones (1902), who emphasized the long cylindrical configuration of the voluntary musculature of the urethra in both sexes, rather than the character of a short band in the lower urethra in adults as described in *Gray's Anatomy* (1980).

Internal involuntary sphincter

The internal urethral meatus was surrounded by thicker smooth muscle to form the internal sphincter, which occupied less than the upper one-quarter of the posterior urethra in the male (Fig. 6.11). The internal sphincter lay chiefly cranial to the prostate, but the muscular tissue incorporated in the gland may exercise some sphincteric action.

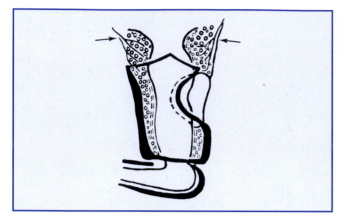

Fig. 6.11 *Diagram of muscles of bladder neck and urethra showing extent of external voluntary sphincter (heavy black), bulbocavernosus around bulb, internal involuntary sphincter around bladder neck (circles) with integrating longitudinal coat (arrows) and two layers of smooth muscle around the urethra (circles and coupled lines).* (Reprinted, by permission, from Stephens, F.D. (1983), Congenital Malformations of the Urinary Tract, *New York, Praeger, Fig. 4.11, p. 93.)*

External voluntary sphincter

In the male, a little more than the lower three-quarters of the posterior urethra was clothed by the external sphincter (Fig. 6.11). This voluntary sphincter was a strong layer of striated muscle, arranged obliquely for the most part, rising highest on the lateral and posterior aspects, and intermingling with the lower and outer fibres of the internal sphincter. The fibres passed caudally and anteriorly to meet those from the opposite side. The circular fibres were thinnest posteriorly above the prostate; they gained direct attachment to the sides of the gland in the middle of the urethra, and formed a strong circular muscle in the lower urethra above the triangular ligament.

Posteriorly in the membranous urethra, the voluntary muscle exhibited a central tendinous raphe somewhat similar to the linea alba of the abdominal wall.

Urethrographic studies indicated clearly that the external sphincter came first into action in voluntary arrest of micturition (Figs 6.5 and 10.3). This observation is in accord with that of Denny-Brown and Robertson (1933).

Smooth muscle of the urethra in the external sphincter zone

Inside the voluntary muscle coat were two layers of smooth muscle, an inner longitudinal and an outer circular. The outermost fibres of the circular layer were intimately related to the innermost voluntary fibres, and the thickness of the involuntary muscle approximately equalled that of the voluntary coat. The marginal muscle bundles contained a mixture of both smooth and voluntary fibres. The crossover of two types of muscle cells within the same bundle on the boundary line is unique to the urethra, and presumably has significance in coordination of voluntary-muscle activity with the smooth-muscle peristalsis. The function of these smooth-muscle coats is presumably peristaltic or detrusor; so regarded, they furnish an explanation of the undulating outlines observed on VCU and account for extrusion of the last drops of urine at the end of voiding.

Bulbocavernosus muscle

The fibres of this muscle encircled the posterior part of the bulb, arising posteriorly from the central point of the perineum, and more anteriorly diverging from the raphe along the caudal surface of the bulbous urethra to insert into the strong aponeurosis of the corpus cavernosum urethrae. Contraction of the bulbocavernosus muscle compresses the bulbous urethra and stops the flow of urine from the level of the perineal membrane. It can act as an accessory voluntary sphincter (Fig. 6.6).

The inferior crest of the urethra

Because valves of the urethra in children appear to be anomalies of the inferior part of the urethral crest, a special study was made of the normal crest in 30 specimens from male cadavers ranging in age from newborn to nine years (Fig. 6.12).

The verumontanum was situated on the posterior wall approximately at the midpoint of the posterior urethra or slightly above. The inferior crest arose as a midline continuation of the lower end of the verumontanum down the back of the membranous urethra.

In 18 specimens, the crest was a straight, tapering ridge that terminated by dividing into two or four fins, several millimetres above the spongy tissue of the bulb. These fins diverged laterally and distally in the membranous urethra to disappear at the level of the perineal membrane. In five specimens, the appearance was similar to that described, but a fine, central tapering ridge was continued toward the bulb beyond the diverging fins. In four specimens, the crest terminated without

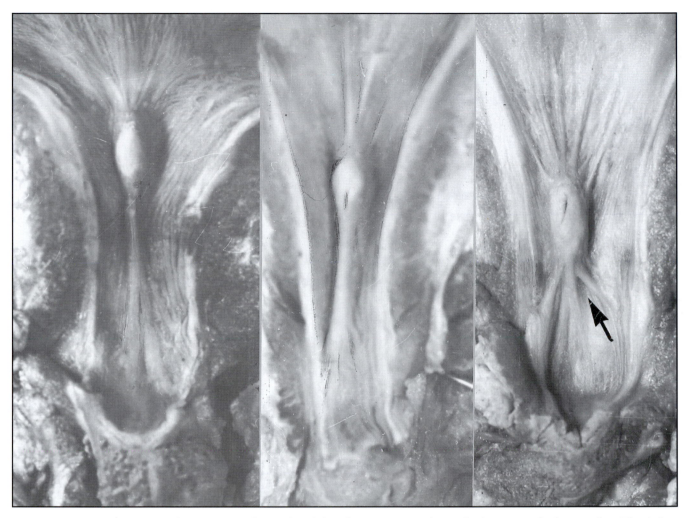

Fig. 6.12 *Necropsy specimens of the posterior urethras of three babies showing variants of normal inferior crests dividing into fins. The urethras are divided longitudinally down the anterior wall from bladder to bulb. Left. Thin crest dividing into two fins in mid-membranous urethra. Centre. Thicker and longer crest with several terminal fins. Right. Short inferior crest dividing high in membranous urethra, and two higher fins joining verumontanum directly (arrow). Note also variable patterns of the colliculi urethrae cranial to the verumontanum. (Reprinted, by permission, from Stephens, F.D. (1983), Congenital Malformations of the Urinary Tract, New York, Praeger, Fig. 4.12, p. 94.)*

dividing at the region of the perineal membrane. In two, the central ridge was short and tapered rapidly to disappear on the posterior wall, but two additional well-marked right- and left-side fins, meeting at the point of origin of the central ridge on the verumontanum, were present (Fig. 6.12). One further specimen showed only a doubtful left-sided terminal fin.

In some of the specimens examined, single or multiple very fine, oblique, mucosal ridges could be seen converging in a cranial direction on one or both sides of the central crest.

In all the normal specimens, the central crest was present, even though in some it was shorter than usual.

The mode of development of the external genitalia in the male has been controversial, especially in the region of the glans and prepuce. Recent thorough histological studies of Glenister (1954, 1956) and Altemus and Hutchins (1991) of fetal specimens are in close agreement on the embryogenesis of the normal urethra from the bulb to the external meatus. In this chapter the clinical features of hypospadias associated with descended testes are correlated with stages in morphogenesis of the external genitalia. In particular, the roles of the urethral plate and outer genital folds are emphasized regarding abnormal location of the orifice, the chordee and the preputial defects.

In some instances, the pathogenesis of the abnormality is known or strongly suspected. Genetic errors in enzyme formation leading to testosterone or dihydrotestosterone deficiency, a defect in the androgen receptor (incomplete androgen resistance) or testicular dysplasia can cause hypospadias in association with descended testes. However, in the majority of patients with hypospadias and scrotal testes, no such anomaly is recognizable. In some instances abnormal external forces may deform the otherwise normally developing genitalia accounting for some irregular forms of hypospadias. Intersex states and hypospadias associated with congenital rectourinary fistulas are not included here, but are discussed in Chapter 38.

Material and methods

In order that the embryogenesis of hypospadias could be deduced from the clinical appearances of the different forms of and markings of hypospadias genitalia, the features of 45 such patients were meticulously recorded diagrammatically. One extra report of a patient with a photograph was available as the sole representative of the perineal group of hypospadias by courtesy of Professor John Hutson. Special note was made of the site of the orifice, the ramifications of the penile raphe and its bifurcating branches, chordee, preputial and rotational defects and congenital curvature. On the basis of these data, correlations were observed between the known normal embryogenesis and that of hypospadias.

The anomalies were arranged in five groups depending on the position of the ectopic orifice. The terms used to signify the five groups together with the number of patients studied are as follows: perineal, one patient; clitoral, six; penile, ten (with subgroups: proximal, two; mid-penile, three; distal penile, five); coronal, six; and glandar, 23 (with subgroups: navicular, six; mid-glans, 11; subapical, six patients).

In the descriptions of the hypospadiac prepuce that follow, the term 'dog-ear' (Williams, 1952), is used frequently to describe the skin tuft on each side demarcating the angle between the border of the ventral wedge defect and the lip of the dorsal penile skin fringe (Fig. 7.1). The tuft has also been described as a cutaneous whorl (Williams, 1952) and a knuckle (Devine and Horton, 1973).

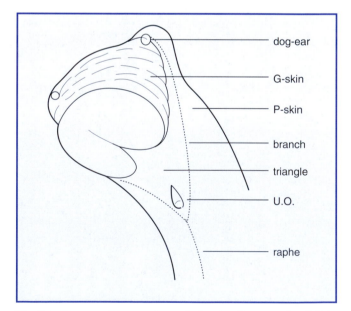

Fig. 7.1 *Features of hypospadias with chordee. Ectopic orifice (UO), triangle between branches of raphe and glans; penile skin of outer genital folds (P-skin); inner skin of prepuce (G-skin) and the two skin tufts (dog-ears of prepuce).*

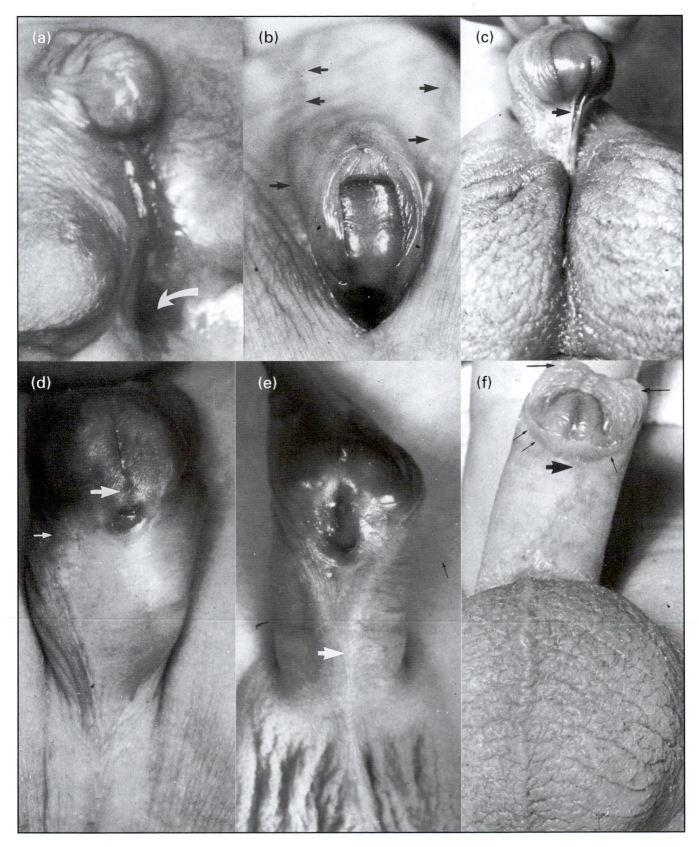

Fig. 7.2 (continued)

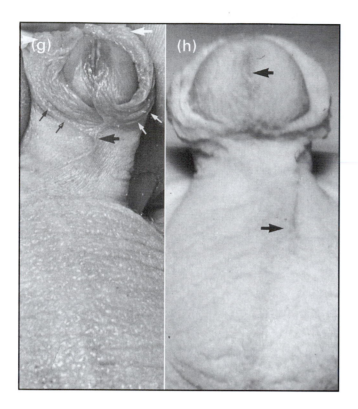

Fig. 7.2 *Hypospadias grouped according to ectopic orifice positions. (**a**) Perineal orifice (arrow). (**b**) Mid-scrotal orifice, clitoral conformation; branches of scrotal raphe track between body of penis and scrotum (arrows). (**c**) Proximal penile orifice, plate gutter between orifice and navicular groove (arrow). (**d**) Distal penile orifice separated by dry skin from coronal sulcus (top arrow); note deviated penile raphe (small arrow). (**e**) Coronal orifice confluent with navicular groove; mid-penile bifurcation of penile raphe (arrow); extended triangle. (**f**) Glandar navicular orifice at base of glans, rudimentary frenulum, irregular penile raphe bifurcating at corona (large arrow); branches and mini-triangle (small arrows); dog-ears (top arrow). (**g**) Mid-glandar orifice in fornix of navicular groove (arrow); rudimentary left-sided frenular leaflet, zigzag raphe with distal penile bifurcation (large arrow); branches (small arrows); dog-ears (large white arrows). (**h**) Subapical glandar orifice on ventral aspect of summit of glans (arrow); absent frenulum; proximal bifurcation of penile raphe (lower arrow); extended triangle; chordee.*

Results

Perineal ectopic orifice

The site of the anterior urethra was represented only by a long rudimentary midline wet red ridge that extended from the roof of the perineal orifice to the navicular groove on the glans (Fig. 7.2a). The penis, prepuce and glans and chordee were similar to those of the 'clitoral' group but the scrotal sacs containing the testes were completely separated by the deeply set rudiment of the urethra. The description of the raphe and its branches was not available.

Clitoral ectopic orifice

The urethral orifice was mid-scrotal and the body of the penis was folded at the region of the suspensory ligament upon itself in the manner of a clitoris and lay half buried between the halves of the upper scrotum (Fig. 7.2b). The glans lay close to the ectopic orifice or was tethered by a wet narrow gutter. In five of the six patients, the navicular groove was sagittal and in one the glans was rotated 20° towards the right. The preputial hood was oval, the dorsal fringe being retracted, the frenulum was lacking and the sides of the hood were attached both to the glans and upper scrotum. The scrotal raphe was central and bifurcated at the ectopic orifice. The branches of the raphe tracked longitudinally on each side between the dorsal skin of the penile shaft and scrotum (Fig. 7.2b). In this type of hypospadias there were no dog-ears on the prepuce.

Penile ectopic orifice

The ectopic orifice was located proximally in two patients (Fig. 7.2c), mid-penis in three (Fig. 7.3c) and distal in five (Fig. 7.2d). Chordee of mild-to-severe grade involving glans and body of penis occurred in all patients and the frenulum was lacking. The prepuce was arranged as a hood with two 'dog-ears' which were symmetric and lateral in eight and diagonally located in two. None exhibited penoglandar torsion. The 'dog-ears' lay at the angular junction of the central skin fold and the terminal fringe on the dorsolateral aspect of the split prepuce (Williams, 1952). The inner skin of the prepuce converged on the sides of the navicular groove and was devoid of frenulum. The penile raphe in nine bifurcated at or short of the orifice and the branches tracked anteriorly in symmetrical lines to end on the preputial dog-ears. The triangle on the shaft between the branches of the raphe distal to the orifice was covered by thin epidermis and in those patients in whom the bifurcation occurred short of the orifice, the urethra in this extended triangle lacked mobility beneath the delicate overlying skin. Occasional wet midline pits occurring between the ectopic orifice and the navicular groove denoted orifices of exposed Littré's glands. In some patients a narrow wet gutter extended from the ectopic orifice into the navicular groove. In two patients in whom the chordee was most marked the protruding arched shaft and glans were webbed to the underlying body of the penis (Fig. 7.2c).

Coronal ectopic orifice

The urethra issued very superficially into an oval coronal pit which verged on the posterior end of the navicular groove (Fig. 7.2e). The pit and the groove formed an hourglass shape with a transverse ridge between. The glans was tilted ventrally in five of the six patients, the frenulum was lacking and the prepuce formed a hood, the dog-ears of which were lateral and symmetrical in five, and diagonal in the patient with glans rotation. The raphe was central in three and deviated to one side in three. In two, apposing edges of the central raphe were separated by a shallow groove along the length of the penis. Though the ectopic orifice was coronal in location, the raphe bifurcated at the corona in only one and on the penile shaft in five (Fig. 7.2e). The branches tracked to the preputial dog-ears. The corpora cavernosa adjoining the corona were slightly curved ventrally.

Glandar ectopic orifice

This group of 23 patients is divided into three subgroups according to the location of the urethral orifice, navicular, mid-glans and subapical or distal glans.

Navicular orifice

In this subgroup (five), the orifice entered the posterior fornix of the navicular groove on the base of the glans and appeared small in calibre. The wings of the preputial hood encroached toward the midline and in two actually joined together to form a low transverse ridge or rudimentary frenulum (Fig. 7.2f). The frenulum was absent in three. The branchings of the penile raphe tracked from a ventral point of bifurcation just posterior to the ectopic orifice around the prepuce to the dog-ears

of the hood. Chordee was absent in two, and the glans was tilted ventrally in two and to the right in one.

Mid-glans orifice

The urethra in 11 cases was buried in the proximal glans and issued into the fornix of the foreshortened navicular groove about mid-way between the base and tip of the glans (Fig. 7.2g). The frenulum was absent in six, present but malformed in two and rudimentary in three. The raphe bifurcated on the distal penile shaft in six and more proximally in five. In one of these, the bifurcation was penoscrotal and accompanied by severe glandar chordee (Fig. 7.4). The branches of the raphe tracked to the dog-ears which were symmetrically located in eight and diagonal in three with penoglandar torsion. Chordee was absent in five, glandar in five and severe in one. Torsion of the glans to the left occurred in four.

Subapical orifice

In six cases, the urethra opened by a small orifice into the fornix of the much diminished navicular groove which lay on the ventral aspect of the summit of the glans (Fig. 7.2h). The proximal part of the glans overlying the glandar urethra was normal in appearance. In these patients the dog-ears of the prepuce were set laterally and diagonally in three exhibiting torsion of the glans. In three, the wings of the prepuce met in the midline at the corona and in three they united to form a false prepuce developed from skin derived from the glans (G-skin). The glans was rotated to the left in three. In four of these patients, the raphe bifurcated at the corona without chordee and in two bifurcation was penile with chordee.

Normal embryology of external genitalia

The development of the phallus begins by the coalescence of bilateral cloacal tubercles at the anterior end of the pars phallica of the urogenital sinus. These tubercles merge in the midline forming a prominent genital tubercle anterior to cloaca (Felix, 1912) (Fig. 7.3a). On the ventral aspect of this tubercle the cylindrical phallus projects and grows forward carrying with it a prolongation of the urogenital sinus known as the urethral

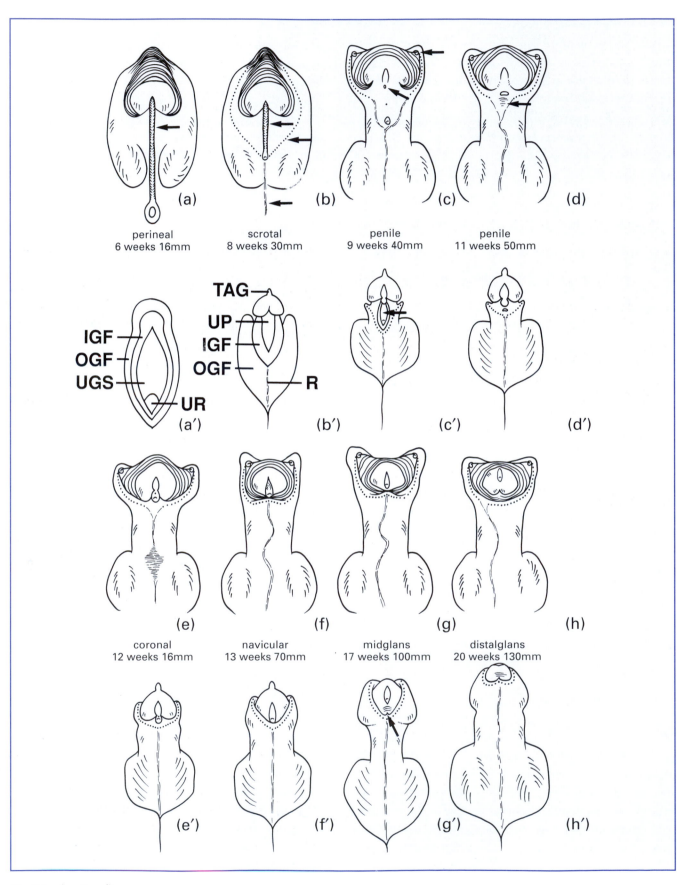

Fig. 7.3 (*continued*)

Fig. 7.3 *Diagrams of clinical forms of hypospadias and corresponding embryological stages of development of the urethra with approximate gestational times of occurrence and corresponding crown–rump lengths.* (**a**) *Perineal, rudimentary urethral plate (arrow); separated scrota.* (**a'**) *Roof of urogenital sinus remains uncanalized (IGF, OGF = inner and outer genital folds; UGS = urogenital sinus; UR = urethral orifice).* (**b**) *Scrotal orifice of clitoral hypospadias; perineal raphe (lowest arrow); bifurcation at orifice and branches (middle arrow); and rudimentary plate (top arrow).* (**b'**) *Roof of UGS partly canalized; partly uncanalized urethral plate (UP), scrotal raphe (R) and epithelial glandar tag (TAG).* (**c**) *Mid-penile orifice. Orifice of Littre gland (arrow); dog-ear (top arrow).* (**c'**) *Uncanalized plate in urethral groove (arrow); prepuce begins.* (**d**) *Distal penile orifice, raphe bifurcation mid-penile; posterior extended triangle (arrow).* (**d'**) *Urethral plate uncanalized anterior to orifice.* (**e**) *Coronal orifice confluent with navicular groove; prepuce deficient ventrally.* (**e'**) *Branches of raphe extending to dorsal fringe of prepuce; primitive ostium open.* (**f**) *Glandar navicular orifice projected onto base of glans; inner and outer layers of prepuce converge on posterior lip of orifice.* (**f'**) *Ventral component of prepuce developing; coronal orifice closes.* (**g**) *Mid-glandar orifice with lip rudimentary frenulum (arrow).* (**g'**) *Normal frenular attachments to glans (arrow).* (**h**) *Subapical distal glandar orifice mildly stenotic; deviated penile raphe; false prepuce formed chiefly from G-skin; skewed mini-triangle.* (**h'**) *Normal orifice on summit; prepuce, frenulum and raphe normal.*

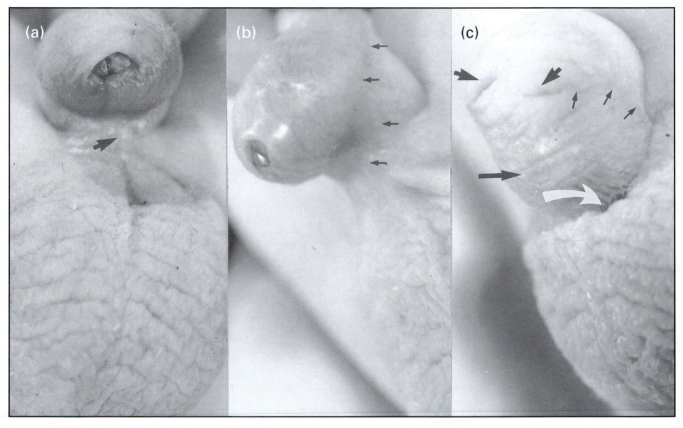

Fig. 7.4 *Chordee without hypospadias (cryptohypospadias).* (**a**) *Phimotic prepuce partly retracted exposing small meatus on glans; bifurcation of raphe (arrow).* (**b**) *Glans and shaft acutely angulated and false prepuce formed from everted G-skin; and left branch tracks to the dog-ear (small arrows).* (**c**) *Left branch of raphe ending on pit in left dog-ear (truncated arrow); left branch of raphe (small arrows); G-skin of false prepuce (lowest black arrow); and phimotic orifice hidden (white arrow).*

groove (Fig. 7.3c). The remaining basal crescentic part of the cloacal tubercle initially contributes the mesenchyme and dorsal skin cover of the phallus and laterally the inner and outer urogenital folds which wrap around the shaft and border the urogenital sinus and urethral groove. After the breakdown of the urogenital membrane, the sinus roof which forms the urethral plate is exposed (Fig. 7.3a'). As the genital tubercle grows, it carries with it the endodermal urethral plate to the tip of the glans. The epithelium of this plate proliferates to form a deep lamella that hollows out to form a gutter. This gutter tubularizes progressively from behind forwards by the meeting of its endodermal edges. This process is followed concomitantly by the meeting in the midline of the inner genital folds reinforced by the meeting of the outer folds. The plate in the cloacal sinus becomes the non-pendulous urethra; in the urethral groove, the plate forms the pendulous urethra up to the coronal sulcus.

The urethra of the glans is formed differently in its proximal and distal parts (Glenister, 1954, 1956). The urethral plate extends to the tip of the glans underlying a tag of surface epithelium and contributes to the formation of the proximal part of the glandar urethra. The inner genital folds combined with the preputial folds from each side close over the primitive ostium in the coronal sulcus projecting the orifice onto the base of the glans and creating the frenulum with its midline attachment to the glans (Fig. 7.3f', g'). The urethra distal to the frenulum becomes buried in the glans by the elevation of two parasagittal folds of surface epithelium which form a gutter in continuity with the more proximal urethra. This terminal glandar gutter is then bridged by proliferating glans epithelium which projects the orifice to the apex of the glans (Fig. 7.3h'). Here the roof of the urethra is in contact with a solid epithelial ingrowth underlying the surface tag in the centre of the glans. This epithelial ingrowth canalizes, the contacting walls disintegrate and the lumens of the terminal urethra and canalized ingrowth become one. By this union, the urethra is expanded to form the fossa navicularis and its orifice becomes a bigger sagittal meatus. The spongy tissue of the glans invests the urethra of the glans, rounding the ventral quadrant and tipping the meatus further dorsally.

Prepuce

The prepuce begins to form as a solid lamella of epithelial cells that dips into the floor of the coronal groove. Epithelial proliferation and desquamation causes a split in the lamella and raises a fold of skin which advances as a sleeve that covers the dorsum and sides of the glans. This sleeve has an inner layer of hairless skin derived from the glans (G-skin), an outer layer formed from the skin of the dorsum and outer genital folds (P-skin), with mesenchymal tissue between and a leading dorsal fringe. On the ventrum the prepuce formation is at first delayed by the presence of the primitive ostium in the coronal sulcus. The deficiency is at first wedge-shaped until the lamellas on each side unite with each other and with the inner genital folds at the apex of the wedge. This union occurs concurrently with the formation of the

floor of the proximal glandar urethra, the frenulum derived from G-skin and the preputial raphe from P-skin. Transient dog-ears situated at the distal corners of the wedge may be normal features that disappear on completion of the union of the two sides of the prepuce.

The raphe and scrotum

The right- and left-scrotal swellings arise in the outer genital folds. They enlarge to the sides of the non-pendulous phallus and merge to form a midline raphe and septate scrotum. The fusion of the outer genital folds over the urethral groove on the shaft creates a midline ridge in continuity with the scrotal raphe. With the union of the edges of the sleeve, the P-skin raphe advances along the outside of the prepuce and meets the inside G-skin raphe at the end of the prepuce.

Curvature of the penis

Kaplan and Lamm (1975) found three grades of ventral curvature of the shaft and glans in their study of the development of the penis in normal fetuses and concluded that moderate or marked ventral curvature was a natural phenomenon. The curvature involved all layers, was transitory and persisted well into the third trimester before gradual straightening occurred. No specimen exhibited fibrosis or fibrous chords.

Morphogenesis of hypospadias

The precise external features noted on the genital organs of hypospadiac patients indicate the underlying defective steps in their embryogenesis. These features include the ectopic position of the urethral orifice, the irregular penile raphe, the hooded prepuce and its dog-ears and the chordee structures.

Ectopic orifice

The anterior urethra is formed from three parts, the urogenital sinus, the urethral groove on the penis and the glans. The urogenital sinus defects lead to urethral orifices located on the non-pendulous phallus, the urethral groove defects lead to ectopic orifices on the pendulous part of the phallus and the glans evokes its own urethral faults. Most ectopic orifices were located near the corona and on the glans suggesting that the urethral plate is liable to become spent functionally in the part that elongates the most. Anterior to the ectopic orifice the plate on the shaft and glans lacks ability to form a urethra.

The urethral plate in the roof of the pars phallica of the urogenital sinus may lack the ability to canalize its deep lamella resulting in a perineal or scrotal ectopic orifice and a midline rudimentary plate in the form of a ridge or band between the orifice and glans. The plate prevents the inner and outer genital folds from advancing toward the midline. Hence the scrota are separated in the perineal group and partly cleft in the clitoral group (Fig. 7.3a, b).

An open midline ridge or gutter or pin-point duct orifices of presumed Littré's glands between the penile ectopic orifice and the glans in some patients indicate the persistence of the plate that failed to mature in its development (Figs 7.2c and 7.3c). The relative shortness of this spent plate suggests that it failed to elongate adequately with the corporal bodies.

The orifice of coronal hypospadias represents the persistence of the primitive ostium. Lack of coordinated development of the plate, inner genital folds and the preputial folds fails to project the urethra onto the glans (Fig. 7.3e, f).

The role of the plate on the glans is to stimulate surface epithelium to form the distal glandar urethra and the terminal solid epithelial ingrowth that on canalization augments the calibre of the meatus and fossa navicularis (Glenister, 1954). Lack of this stimulus results in a near terminal small orifice of the subapical hypospadias.

The irregular penile raphe

Normally the raphe is a midline ridge in the skin extending from the anus to the end of the prepuce demarcating the line of union of the outer genital folds from each side. These folds lag in their migration towards the midline more so distally than proximally in hypospadiac anomalies and the medial limits can be identified by the linear markings of the raphe and its branches. Sometimes the fold of one side overruns the midline to unite eccentrically with its opposite counterpart or some dovetailing is apparent by the zigzag course of the raphe. The raphe bifurcates at, or posterior to, the ectopic orifice, each branch tracking to the dog-ears on the prepuce indicating that the outer genital folds play a major part in the hypospadiac anomaly. These folds contain the mesenchyme that forms the dartos fascia

and subcutaneous tissue which are lacking in the triangle on the shaft between the branches of the raphe. This area is covered only by epidermis of the inner genital folds which clings to Buck's fascia anterior to the ectopic orifice. If the fork in the raphe is some distance posterior to the orifice, the urethra between the branches runs a superficial course beneath this thin epidermis.

The plate and the undifferentiated mesenchyme of the inner genital folds beyond the ectopic orifice in the triangle between the branches of the raphe have been identified as fascial bands, disorganized smooth muscle and remnants of spongy tissue in this area by Devine and Horton (1973), Avellan and Knutsson (1980) and by Page (1981).

Hooded prepuce, dog-ears and frenulum

The prepuce is an add-on sleeve with a dorsal and side fringes partly covering the glans. The sleeve based on the corona is derived externally from outer genital folds (P-skin) and internally from the glans epidermis (G-skin). At first, it has a ventral wedge-shaped deficiency owing to the tardy tubularization of the coronal urethra that precedes the development of the frenulum. When the urethral plate is functionally deficient as with hypospadias, the wedge deficiency persists and the frenulum does not develop. At the angle between the dorsal fringe and the lateral preputial borders of the wedge, lie the right and left dog-ears. The branches of the bifurcated raphe wind around the distal shaft onto the prepuce to end on the dog-ears. The dog-ears represent in the normal prepuce the most distal ventral points of union of the skin of the genital folds. The branches of the raphe on the prepuce mark the lines of separation of the P-skin derived from outer genital folds and the G-skin of the glans. The G-skin forms the concentric corrugations that converge ventrally on the opened out lateral corners of the navicular groove. When the ectopic orifice is glandar in location the wings of the navicular groove become closer and the attached converging G-skin folds then may meet in the midline or alternatively they may unite to form a shelf or even a complete false prepuce entirely from redundant G-skin (Figs 7.3f, g and 7.4). Then the medial limits of the outer folds are demarcated by the branches of the raphe tracking around the corona to the dog-ears.

The hood was slightly different in clitoral and perineal hypospadias. The outer genital folds were barred from their role in the formation of the pendulous urethra by the acutely flexed and buried shaft. This resulted in their union with the dorsal skin of the penis along the lines demarcated by the branches of the raphe which bypassed the prepuce and ran between the dorsal skin and the upper scrotum (Fig. 7.2B). There were no dog-ears on the prepuce in these patients.

Chordee

Chordee occurred in all hypospadiac subjects in the clitoral group, 15 of 16 of those of the combined penile and coronal groups and 11 of 22 of the glandar group.

The perineal and clitoral groups of hypospadiac patients presumably developed along female lines possibly because of testicular dysplasia of some degree. This would account for the hairpin bend of the corpora cavernosa. The phallus, instead of growing forward, turned posteriorly upon itself and remained half buried between the genital folds, thus resembling a clitoris. Alternatively, the defective urethral plate failed to elongate and prevented the corporal bodies from straightening at a very early stage.

Penile chordee occurred when outward growth of the phallus has begun. The spent plate fails to elongate in relation to the continued growth of the corpora cavernosa. In the more severe penile chordee anomaly, the short rudimentary plate tethers the glans to the ectopic orifice and a thin web of penile skin spans the concavity of the arched corpora cavernosa (Fig. 7.2c).

Bifurcation of the raphe on the shaft indicated that the triangle on the shaft between the branches is bereft of the layer of skin, subcutaneous tissue and dartos fascia that is normally carried in by the outer genital folds. The inner genital folds which normally form the corpus spongiosum are also defective. The resulting disorganization of the structures and fibrosis in this triangle lead to various grades of penile chordee. The same factors operate in the extended triangle when the raphe bifurcates some distance proximal to the orifice. The urethral wall between the fork and the orifice may be deficient in its spongiosa. The skin tethering and fibrosis are dominant features of chordee.

Glandar chordee may also result from a spent terminal plate as suggested by Rowsell and Morgan (1987) who showed histologically the epithelial strut joining the ectopic orifice to the bent glans. The glandar tilt and minimal penoglandar chordee may in some patients be the result of skin shortage in the mini-triangle or in others from arrest of the natural developmental process of straightening of the fetal phallus (Kaplan and Lamm, 1975).

Torsion of the glans in hypospadias patients

In nine of 28 glandar plus coronal hypospadiac patients, and in one each of the penile and clitoral types the glans was rotated on the shaft. The raphe was central or leaned to the opposite side before bifurcating. The short branch of the raphe tracked to the adjacent dog-ear and the other turned acutely crossing the midline behind the ectopic orifice to reach the diagonally located contralateral dog-ear. The deviated raphe and skewed triangle indicate that asymmetric coverage of skin and dartos fascia by the outer genital fold was halted on one side tipping up the glans towards the opposite side. Avellan and Knutsson (1980) identified a fibrous band tethering the glans beneath this deviated raphe on the distal penile shaft.

Chordee without hypospadias

When the urethral orifice is located on the ventral surface of the glans and the penis exhibits curvature and a cleft prepuce, the condition is classified as 'glandar hypospadias'. If, however, the prepuce covers the glans circumferentially the condition fulfils the criteria of 'chordee without hypospadias' (Fig. 7.4). In this latter condition, however, the prepuce is usually malformed in that: (1) the penile raphe bifurcates at the corona or on the distal penile shaft and the branches wind around the prepuce to dog-ears situated on the dorsum of the corona; (2) the prepuce is formed from typically corrugated and sometimes pigmented G-skin; and (3) the pale penile skin of the outer genital folds is lateral to the raphe and dorsally may intrude onto the prepuce between the dog-ears. These are the features of the false prepuce described earlier for hypospadias. In addition, the urethral orifice is usually smaller than normal and situated in a subapical or rarely an apical position.

In this condition, the spent distal glandar section of the urethral plate may account for the ectopic location and the small meatus. Arrest of migration of the P-skin of the outer genital folds results in the formation of the false prepuce entirely from G-skin. The chordee results from the skin, dartos and spongiosa defects in the mini-triangle on the shaft. The inner genital folds were defective in that the mesenchyme of the spongiosa failed to develop in this triangle area (Devine and Horton, 1973). The terms 'cryptohypospadias', used by Avellan and Knutsson (1980), or 'distal glandar hypospadias' are more in accord with the authors' concepts of the embryology of this condition which is included in the subgroup of glandar hypospadias.

Coronal hypospadias with intact prepuce without chordee

This is an unusual anomaly. The P-skin of the prepuce may appear completely normal externally including the central raphe and absence of dog-ears. When the glans

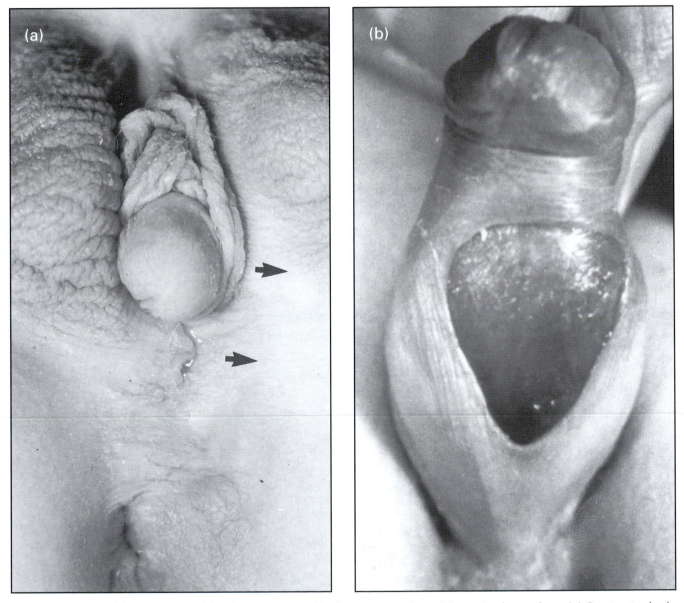

Fig. 7.5 *Anomalies of the genitalia, possibly deformations, caused by foot pressure at six weeks' gestational age or later. (**a**) Compression by the foot on the dorsum of the penis and adjoining scrotum creating ventral penile angulation and rotation and hypospadias (arrows indicate scar of healed pressure sore). (**b**) Ventral compression causing widening of penile shaft and wide defect of the floor of the urethra. Note urethra patent beyond the cleft to the meatus on the glans.*

is fully exposed the primitive coronal ostium which is usually large, is revealed (Duckett and Keating, 1985; Hatch *et al.*, 1989; Attalla, 1991). The prepuce forms normally except that the frenular attachment to the glans is missing and the G-skin unites in the midline proximal to the lip of the megameatus to complete the inner skin of the prepuce. Chordee is usually absent. This anomaly is due to a defect of the urethral plate beyond the corona. In other examples of this anomaly, the glans may be covered by a false prepuce developed entirely from G-skin. The limits of the P-skin formed from outer genital folds are indicated by the penile raphe which stops short and bifurcates at the distal end of the shaft or part way along the prepuce. Each branch of the bifurcated raphe then tracks to the ipsilateral coronal dog-ear marking the limits of encroachment of the P-skin on the false prepuce. Here the spent plate plus the defective outer genital folds lead to the combination of the coronal megameatus and false prepuce.

Deformation of the external genitalia

Ben-Ari *et al.* (1985) found minor anomalies of the penis in their prospective study of all neonates admitted to hospital, totalling 274 babies. Three patients had major hypospadiac defects and were excluded from the analysis. They found that the spontaneous direction of the non-erectile penile shaft was off-centre in 23.2 per cent and the prepuce did not cover the glans in 10 per cent. The direction of the meatus was off-centre in 2.2 per cent and in these subjects the penile raphe was deviated ipsilaterally. Deviations of the raphe but with central meatus occurred in 9.3 per cent, split raphe in 1.8 per cent and zigzag raphe in 7 per cent. In all these subjects, the aberrations were not of clinical significance.

In the patients with hypospadias described here, all these aberrations formed part or parts of the major defect (Cook and Stephens, 1988). Between six and eight weeks' gestational age of the fetus when the hip and knee joints mobilize, the feet come to lie over and may press on the developing external genitalia (Cook and Stephens, 1988). Temporary leakage of amniotic fluid at this stage may cause the amniotic membrane to shrink transiently on these soft-growing and protruding structures creating minor or major permanent mutual deformations of the genitalia and of foot or toes. In particular, the same minor anomalies described by Ben-Ari *et al.* and some forms of hypospadias may be caused by this gentle or severe transient compression, e.g. deviations of the raphe, rotation of the glans, pressure sore or scar or ventral urethral fistula and some hypospadiac and scrotal defects (Fig. 7.5). The deformations of the foot associated with hypospadias are minor or major talipes or overlapping or irregular toes. Early amniotic rupture syndrome should be suspected if genital and foot anomalies occur together (see Chapter 36). Such deformations resulting from compression are unlikely to occur in future members of the family because they are non-genetic and hence the recognition of this association is important in counselling of parents of afflicted children.

Congenital intrinsic lesions of the posterior urethra

The particular radiographic features of congenital urethral anomalies, as observed by the method of voiding cystourethrography, are sufficiently characteristic of each type to be diagnostic in most instances. Whenever possible, the results of morphological and embryological studies in addition to the clinical features of the anomaly are described.

Posterior urethral valves

Young *et al.* (1919) proposed a classification designed to include all types of congenital urethral valves. The authors named described three types. In Type 1, the valve consists of oblique posteroanterior mucosal folds, directed distally from the verumontanum or inferior urethral crest.

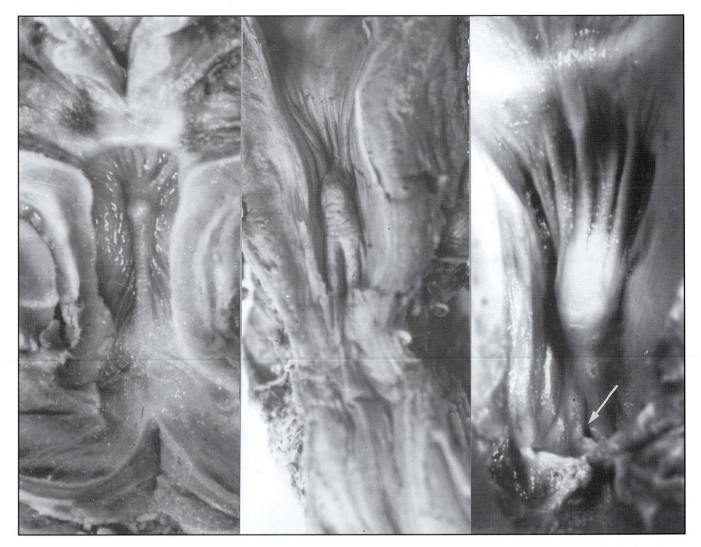

Fig. 8.1 *Normal and abnormal inferior crest of Type 1 valves. Left. Hypertrophic posterior urethra resulting from anterior urethral valve showing normal inferior crest. Centre and right. Posterior urethra and bifurcated short and medium length inferior crest with thick fins incised anteriorly (centre) but in continuity (right). Note the sagittal slit-like lumen between the fins (arrow). (Right photograph reprinted, by permission, from Stephens, F.D. (1963), Congenital Malformations of the Rectum, Anus and Genito-Urinary Tracts. Edinburgh, Livingstone, Fig. 121, p. 220.)*

Type 2 depends for its valve action on posteroanterior folds, which diverge from the verumontanum upwards toward the internal urethral orifice. Type 3 appears as a disk-shaped membrane or mucosal stricture.

In the experience of Young and his co-workers of these variants, Type 1 occurred most and Type 2 least frequently.

Type 1 valves

Type 1 congenital urethral valves occur almost exclusively in males. They are located in the segment of the urethra lying between the verumontanum and the perineal membrane. They are intimately related to the diverging fins of the inferior portion of the urethral crest. Of 19 postmortem specimens investigated, the fins arose from the inferior extremity of a crest of approximately normal length in three cases (Fig. 8.1), in nine from a crest of medium length, and in seven, the fins merely met in the midline at the verumontanum or joined the inferolateral aspects of the verumontanum.

The fins were firm, unyielding structures that diverged from the midline posteriorly, and traversed the lateral walls to meet in the midline anteriorly at a more caudal level (Fig. 8.2). Their tautness drew the mucosa of the lateral walls into two valve cusps, the selvaged edges of which lay contiguous in the sagittal plane, somewhat like vocal cords. Their inflexibility contrasted with the expansile urethral walls above, which dilated, hypertrophied, and ballooned laterally and anteriorly during micturition.

The craniocaudal slitlike urethral lumen between the fins was characteristic of Type 1 valves. The slit was narrowed in side-to-side dimensions, and varied in anteroposterior measurement from approximately 0.3 cm to more than 1 cm. The walls of the urethra, caudal to the valves, were not abnormally thickened.

In Type 1 valves, the obstructive effect of the folds is valvular, but in some, a true constriction of the lumen in both lateral and anteroposterior diameters is superimposed.

Secondary dilatation and hypertrophy of the urinary tract occurred above the valves (Fig. 8.2). Some degree of renal damage had occurred from back-pressure effects in most cases, and in some, hypoplasia and dysplasia of the kidneys and ureters were accompanying features.

The following differences between the conformation of the normal inferior urethral crest and its terminal

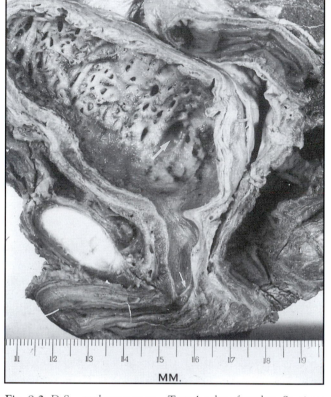

Fig. 8.2 *D.S., aged seven years—Type 1 valve of urethra. Specimen of bladder and urethra showing right valve (small white arrow) and hypertrophy of bladder and urethra. Note mouths of multiple saccules; large white arrow indicates mouth of the one and only diverticulum— no vesicoureteral reflux. (Reprinted, by permission, from Stephens, F.D. (1983), Congenital Malformations of the Urinary Tract, New York, Praeger, Fig. 5.2, p. 108.)*

fins, and that which results in valves of the urethra, were noted:

1. The verumontanum, the crest, and the fins were all larger and tougher than normal.
2. In the great majority, the inferior crest was abnormally short or absent. In only two out of 30 normals was the crest short, and in none was it absent.
3. In valves, the fins were thick, unbroken, mucosal structures that swept around and across the lumen to join together anterior to the urethral channel; they contrasted with the brief, delicate, tapering ridges of the normal fins.
4. Caudal to the point of deviation of the fins to form valves, the crest was invariably absent.

It would appear, from the study of the specimens indicated, that valves in most cases represented more than hypertrophy of normal folds of the urethra. The fins were actually extended anteriorly to encircle the urethral lumen, and the bifurcation of the fins occurred commonly at a high level at the expense of the inferior urethral crest.

From the above descriptions, it appears that Type 1 valves are malformations of the inferior urethral crest. The normal inferior crest is considered by the author (76) to be a bilateral structure formed by the ends of the wolffian ducts, which are initially solid, but soon canalize and issue into the cloaca close to one another near the anterior end of the cloacal membrane in the 4.2-mm embryo (Keibel and Mall, 1912b). At this stage, the urorectal septum is dividing the cloaca, and the orifice of the duct is undergoing a change from anterior-to-posterior and from caudal-to-cranial locations in the cloaca (Fig. 8.3). The shift of each orifice may take place by the disappearance of the apposing epithelial walls of the ducts and cloaca as far cranially as the site of the future verumontanum. Ridges on the side and posterior walls of the urethra represent vestiges of the duct left by the receding orifice. They converge from each side on the posterior wall of the urethra forming the inferior crest, which blends with the verumontanum (Müller's tubercle). Cranial to Müller's tubercle, the process of absorption of the wolffian ducts and ureters into the upper urethra and bladder base continues, forming the trigone.

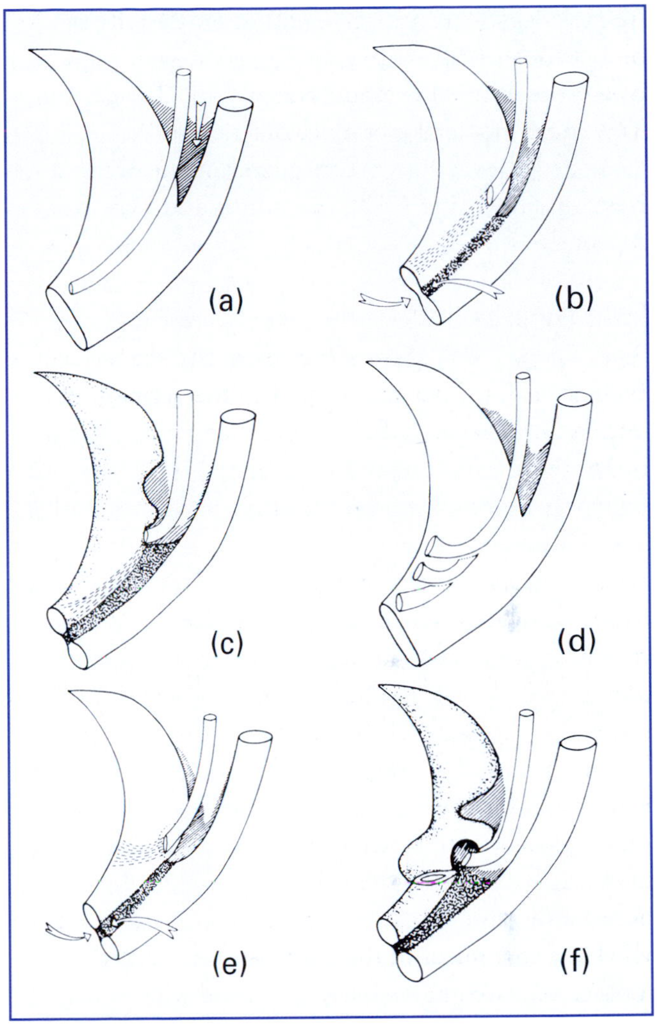

The embryological significance of the snail-track vestiges of the receding wolffian ducts is suggested by the lack of these structures in a male baby who died at birth from congenital absence of the kidneys and all structures derived from wolffian and müllerian ducts, namely ureters, vasa deferentia, vesicles and the utriculus masculinus. The urethra was of normal calibre, and the verumontanum was slightly more elongated than normal. The inferior crest was deficient and there were no fin-like folds radiating from any part of the midline of the urethra below the verumontanum. The superior crest and trigonal thickenings were absent and the bladder was very small. This specimen provides evidence that supports the contention that the snail tracks are the vestiges of the distal extremities of the wolffian ducts.

Type 1 valves result from errors of formation of the fins and crest and so relate to defective integration of

Fig. 8.3 *Embryology of Type 1 valves. (**a–c**) Development of the normal inferior crest. Migration of the orifice of the wolffian duct, from its anterolateral position in the internal cloaca close to the anterior part of the cloacal membrane, to the site of the verumontanum on the posterior wall of the urinary tract occurs synchronously with partition of the cloaca: dots denote the pathway of migration on the urethral wall taken by the receding orifice of the duct. These pathways on each side are swept posteriorly in the lateral ingrowths into the cloaca (Rathke's plicae), which form the urorectal septum caudal to the verumontanum. These pathways are presumed to be represented by epithelial ridges that remain as the terminal fins and normal inferior crest, which is thus a bilateral midline structure spanning the membranous urethra to the verumontanum. (**d–f**) Abnormal anterior positions of the wolffian duct orifices and abnormal migration of the terminal ends of the wolffian ducts creating oblique but circumferential 'valve' structures, leading posteriorly to the verumontanum. (**d**) The abnormally located right and left orifices are presumed to lie contiguous on the anterior wall of the cloaca and as they retract symmetrically to the verumontanum, the vestiges of the wolffian ducts remain as oblique abnormally hypertrophic ridges in the side walls of the membranous urethra. The inferior crest caudal to the point of junction of these ridges which comprise the 'valve' is absent. (Reprinted, by permission, from Kaplan, G.W. (1976), in Clinical Pediatric Urology, P.P. Kelalis and L.R. King (eds). Philadelphia, Saunders, Vol. 1, Fig. 10G-5, p. 305.)*

the wolffian ducts into the urethra. The duct orifices are presumably at first misplaced, being located on the anterior instead of the anterolateral walls of the cloaca (Fig. 8.3). The orifices may be contiguous and issue at or somewhat cranial to the cloacal membrane. Contact between the walls of the orifices in the extreme anterior location may lead to an anterior web formation in the urethra. With relocation of the orifices from these sites, the snail-like vestiges of the ducts form circumferential but oblique 'cusps', like vocal cords, which meet on the posterior wall to form a short crest or converge directly on the verumontanum (Fig. 8.1). The thick nature of some of the 'cusps' may be due to deficient integration of the initially solid ends of the ducts into the walls of the urethra.

Tolmatschew (1870) believed that valves result from simple hypertrophy of the normal folds of the urethra. In the majority of the patients, the folds, as enumerated above, are not only thickened but are abnormal in other aspects.

Lowsley (1914) considered that the valve-like malformations he described were related to defects in development of the wolffian and müllerian ducts. His explanation was based on histological study of the normal and abnormal urethra. In the normal, he found that the ducts in question entered the urethra at the verumontanum, ensheathed in connective tissue,

which disappeared on the urethral floor below the entry of the ducts. In Lowsley's specimen, this connective tissue persisted beyond the verumontanum, gaining attachment to the walls of the urethra in such a fashion as to obstruct the lumen. This author's observations and embryological theory are partly complementary.

The interpretation of voiding cystourethrography in valvular obstruction

Most patients are now investigated by dynamic radiography in the manner described earlier in this chapter, and by Jorup and Kjellberg (1948).

The water-soluble contrast solution, forced by natural effort of micturition into the posterior urethra, sometimes dilates this structure to two or three times its normal diameter. The internal urethral meatus opens proportionately to the natural muscular effort. The contrast medium in the dilated posterior urethra above the valves undermines the partly open internal urinary meatus, billows out the anterior wall, and balloons the lateral walls around and in front of the linear filling defects, which represent the cusps of the valves. Posteriorly, the wall, reinforced by fibromuscular and glandular tissue of the prostate gland, remains flattened except for the central enlarged verumontanum, which appears as a filling defect at approximately the middle,

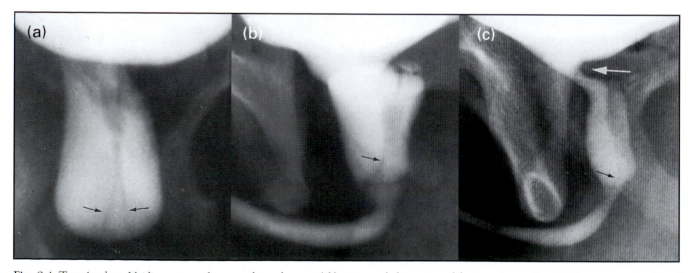

Fig. 8.4 *Type 1 valves. Voiding cystourethrogram shows degrees of dilatation and obstruction of the posterior urethra.* (**a**) *Anteroposterior view of filling defects of the valve cusps of W.H.* (**b**) *Oblique view of cusps of J.C.* (**c**) *Oblique view of cusps and only mild obstruction and dilation of posterior urethra. Note also the harmless accentuation of the posterior lip of the internal urinary meatus (white arrow; cusps indicated by black arrows).* ((**a**) *reprinted, by permission, from Stephens, F.D. (1963),* Congenital Malformations of the Rectum, Anus and Genito-Urinary Tracts. *Edinburgh, Livingstone, Fig. 124, p. 224.)*

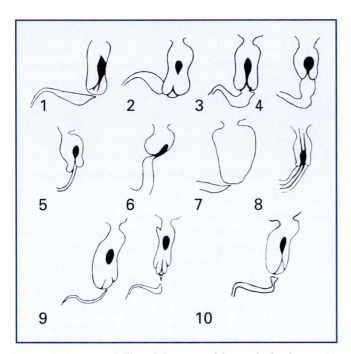

Fig. 8.5 *Tracings of filling defects caused by urethral valves in 10 different urethrograms showing variations in X-ray patterns. (Reprinted, by permission, from Stephens, F.D. (1963), Congenital Malformations of the Rectum, Anus and Genito-Urinary Tracts. Edinburgh, Livingstone, Fig. 125, p. 225.)*

or a little to the cranial side of the central point of the prostatic urethra. Occasionally, reflux of the solution displays the lumens of the ejaculatory ducts or utriculus masculinus.

The linear filling defects of the medial margins of the valves are visible, sometimes very faintly, in part or whole of their respective courses (Fig. 8.4). The course on each side is caudal downward and anterior, diverging from the filling defect of the verumontanum or from the short posterior crest and converging near the anterior wall. The smooth, lower, rounded contour of the dilated urethra may be notched in one or two places by the filling defects of the valve margins (Fig. 8.5). The lumen of the posterior urethra below the level of the valves is collapsed and shows as a narrow column of iodide; whether the whole or part of the membranous urethra was so delineated is determined by the level of the valves. The bulbar and penile urethral segments diminish in calibre in proportion to the degree of obstruction above. The rounded lower margin of the enlarged, distended urethra lying cranial to the fine streak of contrast medium representing the collapsed lumen of the

membranous urethra confirms the presence of obstruction and faint filling defects caused by the large verumontanum and the thick cusps usually determines the diagnosis of Type 1 valves.

Young and Davis (1926) described under Type 1 an example of a univalve; that is, a lateral, thick, unilateral cusp. A voiding cystourethrogram of one patient studied showed a well-marked filling defect of a predominant right-sided cusp and only a faint defect demarcating a normal lateral fin on the left side (Fig. 8.6). The right cusp was resected endoscopically with complete relief of the obstruction.

The bladder, ureters, and kidneys with urethral obstruction

Upper urinary-tract dilatation, sacculation of the bladder, tortuosity of the ureters, hydronephrosis of varying degrees of renal atrophy or hypodysplasia are usually present; vesicoureteric reflux is demonstrated in approximately one-third of the patients, and in some, an associated vesical diverticulum, into which the reflux ureter opens, coexists.

The bladder neck or collar of muscle that surrounds the internal urethral meatus in patients exhibiting valves of the urethra, or for that matter any obstruction in the urethra caudal to it, is hypertrophic and even more prominent than normal (Fig. 8.4c). It is a temptation to regard this structure as a contributor to the main obstruction, which has been proved to lie at a lower level. But in none of the patients has it been proved that the bladder neck ever caused obstruction or impaired the flow of urine subsequent to adequate treatment of the valves. The temptation to resect this structure should be rigorously resisted.

Type 2 valves

Young et al. (1919) described the Type 2 valve: 'A ridge ... passes upwards from the verumontanum and divides into two valve-like folds which attach to the urethra just outside the urethral sphincter.' The normal superior crest and the diverging mucosal plications conform to this description and become conspicuous, multiple and exaggerated in the dilated urethras of patients with Types 1 and 3 valves (Fig. 8.1, right). The Type 2 valve has not been generally accepted as an obstructing entity.

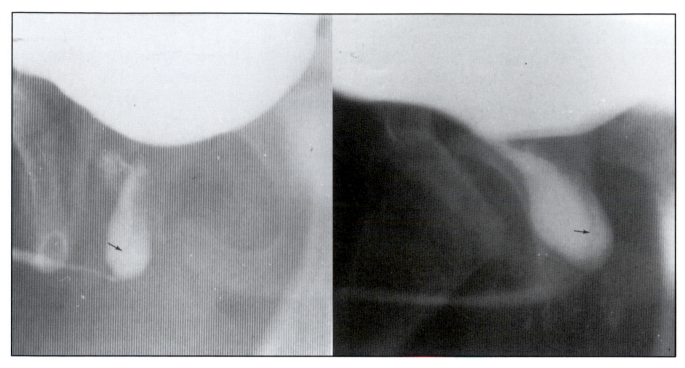

Fig. 8.6 *Type 1 univalve. Voiding cystourethrogram demonstrating filling defect of one cusp only (black arrow) in different oblique views. Note collapsed bulbous urethra distal to the obstruction. (Reprinted, by permission, from Stephens, F.D. (1983),* Congenital Malformations of the Urinary Tract, *New York, Praeger, Fig. 5.6, p. 111.)*

Type 3 valve: mucosal stricture or diaphragm
Necropsy specimens of Type 3 valves

Six specimens were studied from male infants in whom the obstruction lay in the region of the junction of membranous urethra and bulb. In three, the obstruction was a circumferential mucosal narrowing to a pinpoint calibre (Fig. 8.7). In three other specimens, the urethra was partially occluded by a diaphanous diaphragm set transversely across the lumen. In one, there were two orifices in the diaphragm. In another specimen, the diaphragm was formed by a flat septum posteriorly and a nipple-like prolongation anteriorly (Fig. 8.8). The orifice lay in the sagittal plane on the posterior aspect of the nipple. Both the septal part and the nipple, which no doubt ballooned with each effort of micturition, impeded the flow of urine. In all six, secondary hypertrophy and dilatation were seen in the urinary tract above the obstruction and normal urethra below; in three, the urethra was angulated a short distance caudal to the entry of the utriculus masculinus.

The appearance of the verumontanum and inferior crest differed from that described in the Type 1 valve anomalies. In none was there any evidence of hypertrophy of the verumontanum or crest or fins. In one example of mucosal stricture, the verumontanum was represented by a depression in the posterior urethral wall into which opened the ejaculatory ducts, side by side. Emerging from the pit was a fine central crest, which faded out at a point just proximal to the site of the stricture. In the two other examples of mucosal stricture, the verumontanum was normal in size, and the central crest was of the calibre of fine cotton, terminating proximal to the obstruction or dividing into two fins that terminated on the diaphragm (Fig. 8.7).

In three specimens of the urethral diaphragm, the slender crest terminated at a point proximal to the diaphragm by dividing into two fine fins, which bordered the edges of the posteriorly situated small orifice of the membrane (Fig. 8.8).

In three specimens of the Type 3 group, including one example of the diaphragm, the ducts of Cowper's glands could be traced distal to the obstruction.

Strictures or stenoses of congenital origin occur commonly at the site of the bulbomembranous junction (Lowsley and Kirwin, 1944). Bazy (1903) described a clinical case of valve-like obstruction in this region, which he attributed to the persistence in part of the urogenital membrane. Young and Davis (1926) considered

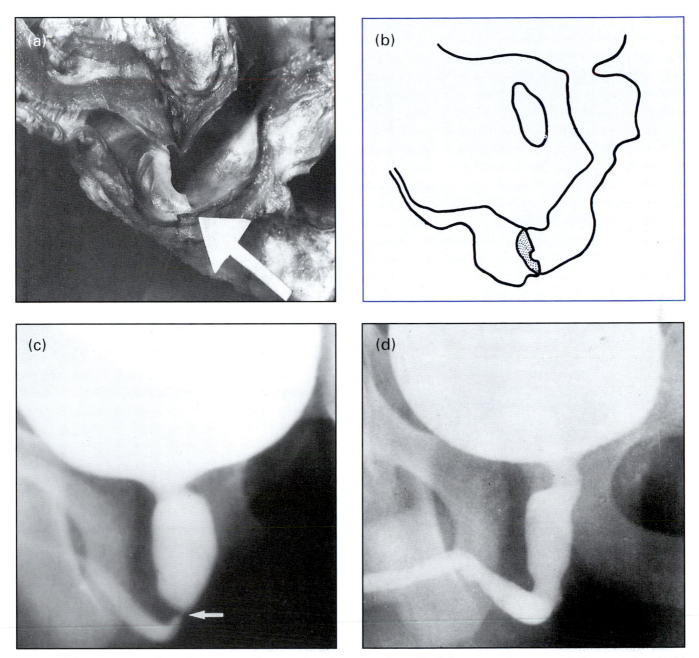

Fig. 8.7 (**a**) *Transverse membrane shown in sagittal section of membranous urethra and bulb (autopsy specimen, arrow indicates membrane).* (**b**) *Drawing of membrane and whole length of urethra.* (**c**) *R.D., aged three years—voiding cystourethrogram showing filling defect of obstruction by Type 3 valve.* (**d**) *Absence of obstruction after two urethral dilatations.* ((**a**),(**c**),(**d**) *reprinted, by permission, from Stephens, F.D. (1963), Congenital Malformations of the Rectum, Anus and Genito-Urinary Tracts. Edinburgh, Livingstone, Figs 126A, 127A,B, pp. 226, 228.* (**b**) *reprinted, by permission, from Field, P.L. and Stephens F.D. (1974), Congenital urethral membranes causing urethral obstruction.* J. Urol. 111: 250, Fig. 1B.)

that Bazy's suggestion was probably the explanation of mucosal stricture at this site.

The preceding six examples of Young's Type 3 lend support to this embryological explanation, as all are unassociated with abnormalities of the inferior crest, and doubts still exist as to the exact site of the urogeni-

tal membrane relative to the uroanatomy of the fully developed fetus (Currarino and Stephens, 1981).

Voiding cystourethrography was not performed during life in any of the six children who provided specimens of mucosal membrane, but at the necropsies of two of them, the bladder and urethra were distended to capac-

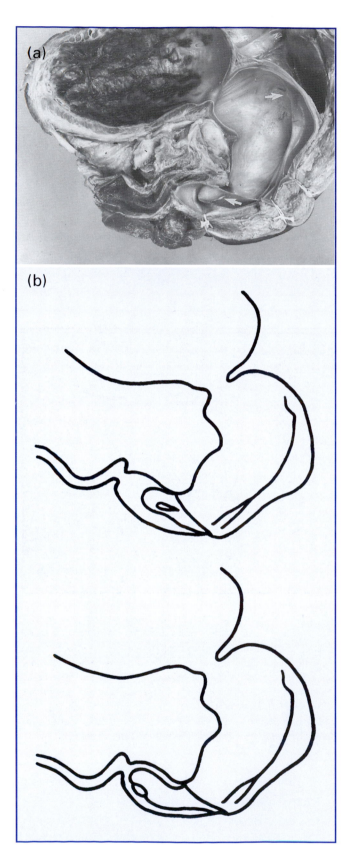

Fig. 8.8 *Wind sock membrane. (**a**) Obstructing membrane attached in membranous urethra and ballooned like wind sock into expanded bulbous urethra—orifice is subterminal (distal arrow); note very small verumontanum (rostral arrow) and elevated Kiel of inferior crest drawings in (**b**), indicate filling of wind sock at autopsy and presumed filling during micturition. Note the dilatation of the urethra due to bougienage by the membrane. ((**a**) reprinted, by permission, from Stephens, F.D. (1963),* Congenital Malformations of the Rectum, Anus and Genito-Urinary Tracts. *Edinburgh, Livingstone, Fig. 126C, p. 226. (**b**) reprinted, by permission, from Field, P.L. and Stephens, F.D. (1974), Congenital urethral membranes causing urethral obstruction.* J. Urol. *111: 250, Fig. 2B,C.)*

ity with radiopaque solution. Radiographs demonstrated the narrowing of the stricture, the proximal dilatation and the pronounced angulation of the urethra below the entry of the ejaculatory ducts.

The origin of the Type 3 obstruction lesion near the bulbomembranous junction may be difficult to determine. The features typical of a membrane or stricture are that the constriction or attachments of the membrane are transverse to the axis of the urethra, the fins and inferior crest are very fine and not involved and the verumontanum is not hypertrophied. In contrast, the Type 1 valve is obliquely oriented in the axis of the urethra and is made up of thick fins of the bifurcated inferior crest and the verumontanum is large.

These criteria are more likely to be determined accurately in the postmortem specimen and the issue may be regarded, therefore, as of academic interest only. The simple membrane and stricture of the Type 3 valve, however, are sometimes amenable to treatment by simple dilatation. The Type 1 valve deformity shows little, if any, permanent improvement by similar treatment.

Type 3 valves observed in patients

In an analysis of 111 cases of valves of the urethra, Cass and Stephens (1975) found 23 (21 per cent) examples of Type 3 valves compared with 87 (79 per cent) of Type 1 valves. Most conformed to the above description with variation in the level of circumferential attachment to the membranous urethra, the area of the membrane, the site and size of the orifice in the membrane, and the extent of the dilatation above and below the membrane.

Voiding cystourethrography together with excretory pyelography, were usually the first radiological examinations undertaken prior to endoscopy. The urethral configurations showed many variations and some resembled Type 1 valve appearances already described; others exhibited gross dilatation of the urethra proximal to the obstructing agent with filling defect at the site, while yet others were confounding. After repeat voiding cystourethrography with standard-sized spot films and correlation of endoscopic findings, it was possible to piece together the filling defects and the urethral anatomy and recognize the obstructing agent. Urethral dilatation, involving the whole of the posterior urethra down to the perineal membrane, or even below it, together with absence of the oblique filling defects so typical of Type 1 valves, are two characteristics of Type 3 valves. The wind-sock variety of membrane, however, has its own array of radiographic filling defects.

If the attachment were close to the verumontanum and the cross-sectional area large, the membrane was baggy and bulged distally during voiding, dilating by bougienage effect the membranous urethra distal to it (Fig. 8.9). In two babies, the membranes were noted to be elongated in the form of a sock, attached circumferentially high in the membranous urethra, with the foot of the sock floating distally in the stream of urine. The perforations in the 'socks' were subterminal and large or small; in one, the sock was long and smooth and in one, the 'toes' were much expanded. The voiding cystourethrography shows the faint filling defects of these elongated membranes, which billow in the stream like 'wind socks'. It shows also the smooth, rounded end of

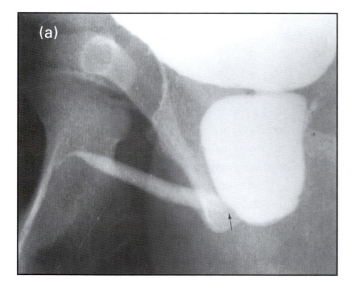

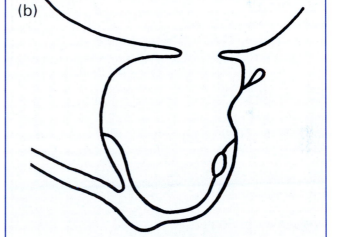

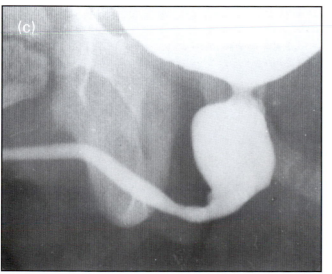

Fig. 8.9 (a) Voiding cystourethrogram shows filling defect (arrow) across bulbous urethra, with proximal dilatation. (b) Overlay drawing depicting the position of the membrane present but not visible in (a). (c) Voiding cystourethrogram after resection of membrane showing uninterrupted lumen. ((a),(b) reprinted, by permission, from Field, P.L. and Stephens, F.D. (1974), Congenital urethral membranes causing urethral obstruction. J. Urol. 111: 250, Fig. 3A, B. Fig. 5.9c Reprinted, by permission, from Stephens, F.D. (1983), Congenital Malformations of the Urinary Tract, New York, Praeger, p. 114.)

the sock or the 'toes' of the multiloculated sock lying in and plugging the bulbous urethra (Figs 8.10 and 8.11). Endoscopically, the view is less confusing if the nature of the lesion is first discerned by radiography. The orifice in the membrane may be found by distending and searching the urethral lumen distal to the sock. The miniature endoscope can then be directed through the orifice in the membrane to view the verumontanum and internal urinary meatus. The membrane may be inverted by the irrigating water pressure bringing the eccentric orifice more readily into view (Fig. 8.10).

The membranes in these two babies were thin and translucent and readily fulgurated with the loop of the resectoscope. If, after endoscopic examination, the diagnosis is unsolved, a retropubic cystourethrotomy will provide clearer evidence as to the cause of the obstruction and better access for direct excision of the membrane.

Embryology of Type 3 valve

Bazy (1903) ascribed a clinical example of valve-like obstruction in the region of the junction of the posterior and anterior urethra to persistence in part of the urogenital membrane. This explanation is readily acceptable for the simple diaphragm (Fig. 8.7) and the simple stricture at this level, and also for complete imperforate thin or thick diaphragms or long strictures that lie

between the membranous and bulbous parts of the urethra. The persistence of the urogenital membrane may also explain the variants described by Field and Stephens (1974) (Figs 8.9–8.11).

The urogenital membrane is the anterior portion of the cloacal membrane, which is divided by the urorectal septum, the posterior portion of the cloacal membrane being the anal membrane. Almost immediately after the partitioning of the cloaca is completed at the 16-mm stage of embryonic development, the urogenital membrane disappears, leaving little or no trace of its former presence.

The cloacal membrane forms under normal circumstances from the close apposition of the endoderm of the expanded hindgut with the ectoderm of the hind end of the embryo. It is a membrane composed of two layers of epithelium with little, if any, mesoderm between. The urogenital membrane, like the anal membrane, is indented from inside and outside and perforates (Frazer, 1931c). If the membrane persists circumferentially, it may account for minor constrictions visible on voiding cystourethrography in some children, or if the greater part remains, a ring stricture or diaphanous membrane constricts the lumen (Fig. 8.12).

If the cloacal membrane were thick, owing to the presence of mesoderm between the layers, the cloacal membrane would become an impenetrable barrier or

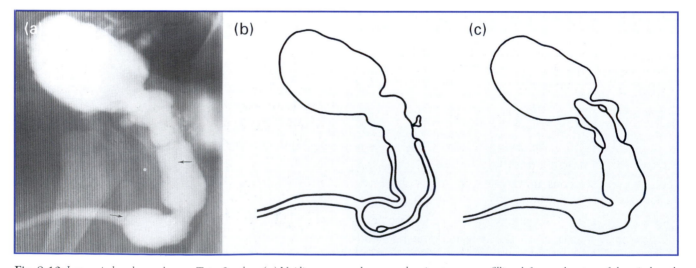

Fig. 8.10 *Long wind sock membrane, Type 3 valve. (a) Voiding cystourethrogram showing transverse filling defect at the apex of the wind stock membrane (distal arrow). Longitudinal linear filling defects in posterior urethra represent walls of membrane (rostral arrow). (b) Overlay diagram shows extent of membrane; inversion of the membrane as seen endoscopically during filling of urethra caudal to membrane. (Reprinted, by permission, from Field, P.L. and Stephens, F.D. (1974), Congenital urethral membranes causing urethral obstruction. J. Urol. 111: 250, Fig. 4.)*

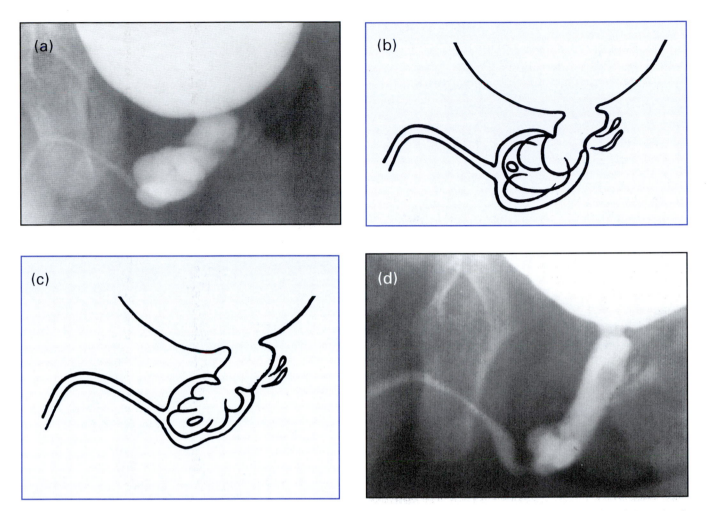

Fig. 8.11 *Multiloculated wind sock membrane. Type 3 valve. (**a**) Preoperative voiding cystourethrogram shows overlapping filling defects of multiloculated membrane. (**b**) Overlay diagrams of filling defects and loculi. (**c**) Interpretation of membrane as seen endoscopically. (**d**) Postoperative voiding cystourethrogram after resection of central obstructing loculus. (Reprinted, by permission, from Field, P.L. and Stephens, F.D. (1974), Congenital urethral membranes causing urethral obstruction. J. Urol. 111: 250, Fig. 5.)*

undergo partial or even complete perforation by longer and complex indents from inside and outside creating a varied array of membranes or stenoses (Figs 8.10–8.12) or just minor variations of shape in the membranous or bulbous urethra (see Fig. 6.7).

Two specimens from babies born with complete obstruction exhibited a thick barrier between the membranous and bulbous urethra. Presumably, mesoderm migrated between epithelial layers of the cloacal membrane, separating the membranous urethra from bulb (Fig. 8.13). A hint as to the depth of the barrier is obtained from a third specimen and urethrogram demonstrating a long stricture shown in Fig. 8.14. The thick urogenital membrane is canalized by an endodermal pit represented by the beak in the membranous

urethra and by a caudal pit, which meets it and forms the narrow segment (Fig. 8.14b).

Voiding cystourethrography, urethroscopy and the specimens serve to identify the various membranes, the origins of which may be explained on the basis of irregular canalizations of the urogenital membrane (Fig. 8.15).

Type 4 valves

Another abnormality distinct from Types 1, 2 and 3 sometimes gives rise to valvular obstruction that is usually partial, but on rare occasions is complete, even though the lumen is not abnormally small. This abnormality is a deep infold of the anterior and anterolateral walls that override the lumen of the membranous urethra. Unlike the valves described by Young, the

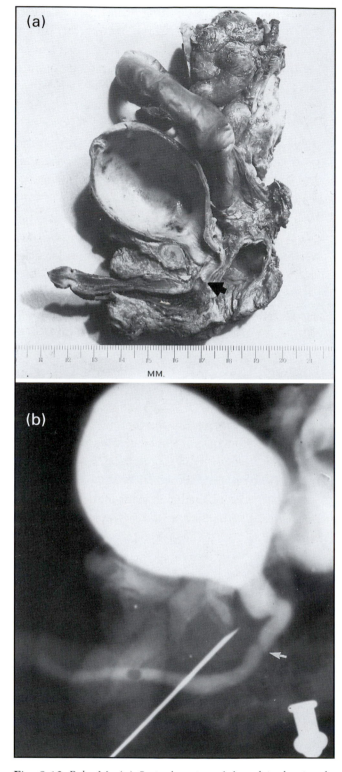

Fig. 8.12 *Baby M. (**a**) Sagittal section of the pelvis showing the urinary tract and rectum. The arrow marks the obstructing stricture which is also shown on voiding cystourethrography (**b**) as a transverse filling defect (arrow). ((**a**) reprinted, by permission, from Stephens, F.D. (1963), Congenital Malformations of the Rectum, Anus and Genito-Urinary Tracts. Edinburgh, Livingstone, Fig. 126B, p. 226. (**b**) Reprinted, by permission, from Stephens, F.D. (1983), Congenital Malformations of the Urinary Tract, New York, Praeger, Fig. 5.12B, p. 117.)*

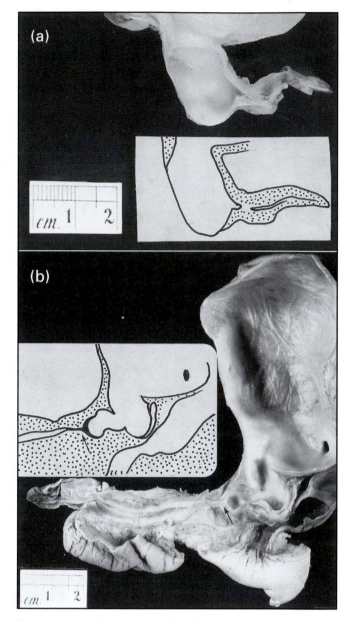

Fig. 8.13 *Imperforate urogenital membrane. (**a**) Baby D.A.—specimens of urethra and overlay drawing to show the site of occlusion at junction of membranous urethra and bulb, and dilation of the posterior urethra and bladder. (**b**) Baby R.—specimen of bladder and urethra and overlay drawing of urethra showing point of occlusion (arrows) with irregular dilatation of the posterior urethra and bladder (inset). (Reprinted, by permission, from Stephens, F.D. (1983), Congenital Malformations of the Urinary Tract, New York, Praeger, Fig. 5.13, p. 118.)*

obstructing agent is formed in the anterior instead of the posterior wall and lies below the level of, and is unrelated to, the verumontanum or inferior crest of the urethra. The lumen of the urethra at the point of obstruction is a coronal slit, is non-stenotic, and is bordered anteriorly by a sharp, sickle-shaped mucosal apron. This type is called the Type 4 urethral valve (Fig. 8.17).

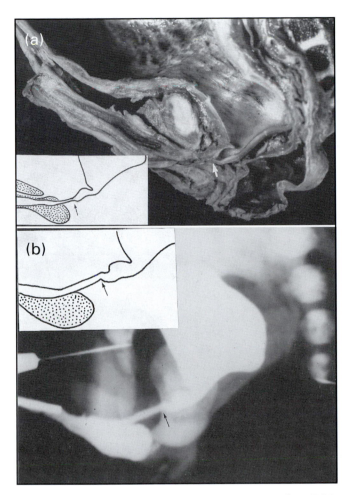

Fig. 8.14 *Urogenital membrane stenosis in Baby R.M. (a) Stenoses of urethra at junction of membranous urethra and bulb (arrow) and beaking above it indicating irregular penetration of urogenital membrane. (b) Retrograde urethrogram showing patency, stenosis (arrow) and beaking. Note opaque medium in bulbospongiosum. Insets are explanatory tracings. (Reprinted, by permission, from Stephens, F.D. (1983), Congenital Malformations of the Urinary Tract, New York, Praeger, Fig. 5.14, p. 119.)*

1. Membranous urethra exiting from the prostatic urethra along the anterior wall with: (a) normal calibre, five examples; (b) narrow calibre, four examples; (c) high 'take-off', two examples partly resembling Type 4 valves.
2. Modified Young's Type 1 valve. One full-term baby and two fetuses (identical twins aborted at 18 weeks' gestational age) exhibited a short anterior nipple-like diverticulum of the dilated prostatic urethra directed distally overlying and compressing the narrow calibre eccentrically exiting membranous urethra.
3. Modified Young's Type 3 lesion; five specimens. The prostatic and membranous urethral segments were widely dilated. In the region of the perineal membrane, four exhibited an abrupt narrowing of the exiting urethra, and in the fifth specimen, the lumen was totally occluded (Fig. 8.17). In two specimens, the urethra has been transected and the distal part was not examined.

Urethras with profiles (2) and (3) were undoubtedly severely obstructive and with profiles (1b, c) were likely to be mechanically obstructive (Fig. 8.17b). Profile (1a) specimens may not be obstructive and may resemble the urethral profile of some surviving prune belly syndrome patients (Stephens, 1983).

The dilated prostatic urethra in many of the prune belly patients exhibits a preponderance of expansion posteriorly with the ejaculatory ducts issuing into a shallow crater in the deepest part. It is likely that the seminal vesicles are abnormal, especially the distal end of the duct which over expands and extrophies into the prostatic urethra (Fig. 8.16 and Chapter 37). This overexpansion creates the posterior expanded pocket of the prostatic urethra, and alters the alignment of the prostatic and membranous segments. In so doing, the anterior and anterolateral walls infold, form a shelf across the lumen and angulate the urethra. This same abnormal embryological sequence may apply, though in lesser degree, to non-prune belly patients who exhibit the dilated prostatic urethra.

The prostatic and membranous urethral profiles in prune belly syndrome specimens

In this study of 21 postmortem specimens (Stephens and Gupta, 1994), the profiles of the pelvic urethra were examined in some by cystourethrography and in 19 by dissection.

The posterior, caudal and side walls of the prostatic segment were extremely dilated in all specimens. Three different profiles of the membranous urethra were identified (Fig. 8.16).

Bulbar urethral strictures*

Strictures of the bulbar urethra in boys are not uncommon and in most cases are due to surgery on the urethra,

---

*Reproduced in part, with permission, of the Williams and Wilkins Co., from Currarino, G. and Stephens, F.D. (1981), An uncommon type of bulbar urethral stricture sometimes familial, of unknown cause: congenital versus acquired. J. Urol. 126: 658–62.

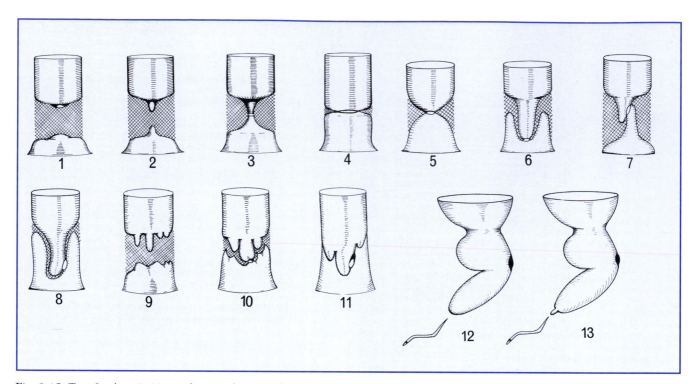

Fig. 8.15 *Type 3 valves. 1–11: canalization of urogenital membrane. 1, 2, 3 and 4 show the normal canalization of the urogenital membrane; 4, normal slight constriction at the level of the perineal membrane; 5, stricture formation; 6, canalization, chiefly by central downgrowth and some circumferential ingrowth of the membrane creating a bulging membrane with central stenotic small orifice; 7, 8, side opening creating the valvular wind sock membrane; 9, 10, 11, the multiple downgrowth with corresponding ingrowth creating the compound wind sock; 12, 13, variations of imperforate urogenital membrane as seen in specimens of newborn babies. (Reprinted, by permission, from Kaplan, G.W. (1976), in Clinical Pediatric Urology, P.P. Kelalis and L.R. King (eds). Philadelphia, Saunders, Vol. 1, Fig. 10G.6, p. 305.)*

urethral instrumentation, external trauma or infection (Devereux and Williams, 1972). The urethral features of six children with a short stricture of the bulbar urethra without an apparent cause are described here. A similar stricture, interpreted as congenital in origin, has been described in the literature in a few patients (Amsler, 1961; Viville *et al.*, 1971; Rao, 1975; Michon, 1978; Redman and Fraiser, 1979). The various possibilities concerning the aetiology of the lesion are considered.

Between 1969 and 1977, six white boys were clinically evaluated at Children's Medical Center, Dallas, Texas, because of voiding problems due to a short stricture of the bulbar urethra without preceding trauma to the perineum, urethral instrumentation or urinary tract infections (Table 8.1). No family history of the same disorder was recorded in any of the children. The presenting symptoms, treatment and results are outlined. The stricture was demonstrated by voiding and retrograde urethrography but in some instances the retrograde study outlined the actual length of the stricture more accurately. The retrograde urethrograms of these six

patients are shown in Fig. 8.18. The cystourethrograms were normal except for vesicoureteral reflux in Cases 5 and 6. The excretory urograms demonstrated normal upper urinary tracts in all six patients. Urethroscopy confirmed the presence of a short stricture in the bulbar urethra without any other urethral abnormalities proximally or distally. In two patients, the stricture was described as a thin iris membrane. Cystoscopy revealed trabeculations of the bladder in Cases 4 and 6 and slight patulous ureteral orifices in Cases 5 and 6. The blood urea-nitrogen, urinalysis and routine urine cultures were normal except for traces of haemoglobin and a few red blood cells in the urine of Cases 4 and 6.

Possible cause of stricture
Acquired lesion
Trauma. Injury to the urethra is the most common cause of urethral stricture, especially in children, and in some cases it is iatrogenic (from urethral surgery, endoscopic procedures and urethral catheterizations, especially long-term catheter drainage) (Devereux and

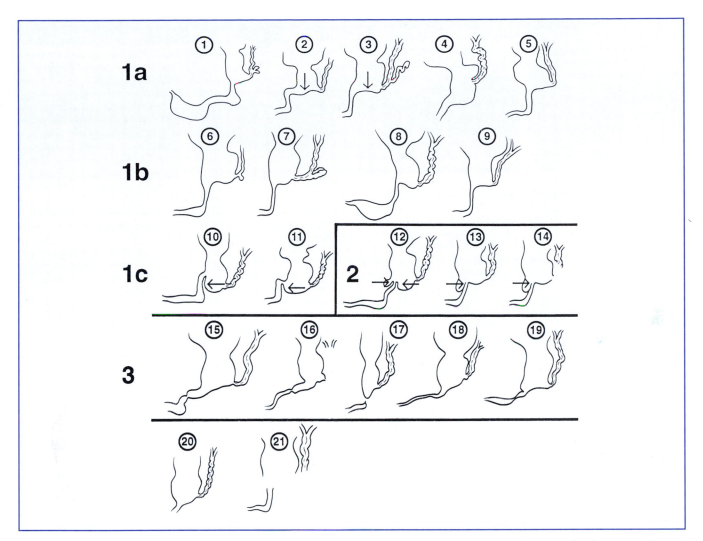

Fig. 8.16 *Prune belly syndrome; profiles of urethra and seminal ducts and vesicles. 1a,b,c, membranous urethra normal and narrow calibre and 'high take-off'; 2, modified Young's valve, type 1; 3, modified Young's valve type 3; unclassified #20 and #21. Arrows indicate valve or potential activation of valve. Banding of seminal ducts 19, and not known #6 and #16; urachal fistula, #5, #19, and #21; scaphoid megalourethra, #1 and #8; identical twin fetuses #13 and #14; seminal vesicle present #7, rudimentary #1, #3 and #6, not known #14, #16 and #21, absent in remainder. (Reprinted, with permission, after Stephens, F.D. and Gupta, D. (1994), Pathogenesis of prune belly syndrome. J. Urol. 152: 2328–31 Fig. 1.)*

Williams, 1972). Less frequently, the urethra is traumatized by a fall astride a sharp edge, such as a bicycle bar, a direct blow to the perineum, a penetrating injury or pelvic fractures. Traumatic strictures may occur anywhere in the urethra but they are particularly frequent in the bulbar area where they may be short. A negative history makes the possibility of trauma an unlikely cause but does not exclude it entirely, since trauma, possibly of a minor nature, could have been forgotten.

Infections. Urethritis due to *Neisseria gonorrhoea* is the best known type of infection that can cause strictures in the urethra. The strictures predominate in the bulbar urethra, presumably because of a predominance of mucous glands in that area (Singh and Blandy, 1976).

They may be as discrete as those described in this report but they are rarely single and the rest of the urethra usually shows some additional abnormalities. Other venereally transmitted urethritis, possibly caused by *Chlamydia trachomatis*, can apparently cause strictures of the bulbar urethra (Dunlop, 1961). It is assumed that strictures also can be produced by other primary non-venereal infections due to bacteria or other agents, including viruses, but this is not well documented. A form of 'non-specific' urethritis, for which no agent could be isolated, was described by Williams and Mikhael (1971) in 17 boys 5–15 years old. Blood-stained discharge, urethral bleeding apart from micturition and haematuria were reported in 14 of these

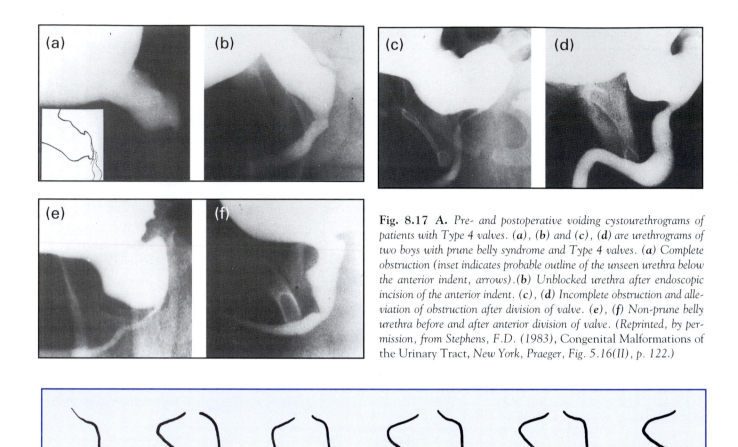

Fig. 8.17 A. *Pre- and postoperative voiding cystourethrograms of patients with Type 4 valves. (a), (b) and (c), (d) are urethrograms of two boys with prune belly syndrome and Type 4 valves. (a) Complete obstruction (inset indicates probable outline of the unseen urethra below the anterior indent, arrows). (b) Unblocked urethra after endoscopic incision of the anterior indent. (c), (d) Incomplete obstruction and alleviation of obstruction after division of valve. (e), (f) Non-prune belly urethra before and after anterior division of valve. (Reprinted, by permission, from Stephens, F.D. (1983), Congenital Malformations of the Urinary Tract, New York, Praeger, Fig. 5.16(II), p. 122.)*

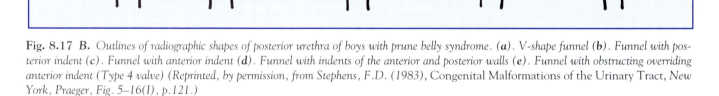

Fig. 8.17 B. *Outlines of radiographic shapes of posterior urethra of boys with prune belly syndrome. (a). V-shape funnel (b). Funnel with posterior indent (c). Funnel with anterior indent (d). Funnel with indents of the anterior and posterior walls (e). Funnel with obstructing overriding anterior indent (Type 4 valve) (Reprinted, by permission, from Stephens, F.D. (1983), Congenital Malformations of the Urinary Tract, New York, Praeger, Fig. 5–16(I), p.121.)*

patients and dysuria, enuresis and diurnal frequency in five. At urethroscopy an inflammatory process was observed in the bulbar urethra in 11 cases and in the posterior urethra in six. A bulbar urethral stricture developed in two patients, which was diagnosed by endoscopy. Although previous venereal urethritis, possibly mild or subclinical, cannot be excluded in some older individuals, this is not a consideration in children. However, the possibility exists that this stricture might have resulted from some other type of urethritis, particularly the disorder reported by Williams and Mikhael

(1971), but this cannot be confirmed on the basis of available evidence.

Abnormality of Cowper's ducts. This is added to the list of possible causes of urethral stricture in view of the fact that the location of the lesion corresponded quite well to the openings of these ducts. Two examples of opacified Cowper's ducts were observed as an incidental finding on routine voiding urethrograms (Fig. 8.19A, B). Possibly related to these ducts is another finding occasionally seen on voiding urethrograms, which consists of a small rounded filling defect or mound in the floor of

Table 8.1 *Clinical data on six patients with bulbar urethral strictures*

Case No.	Age at diagnosis (years)	Initial symptoms	Initial treatment and course	Definitive treatment	Follow-up
1 (Fig. 8.18a)	8	Acute urinary retention	Urethral dilations with some improvement initially, second episode of urinary retention at 10 years followed by poor urinary stream	Patch graft urethroplasty at 11 years	Normal voiding cystourethrogram and retrograde urethrogram, no symptoms at 4 months
2 (Fig. 8.18b)	9	Acute urinary retention	Urethral dilations with some improvement initially, second episode of urinary retention at $9\frac{1}{2}$ years	Patch graft urethroplasty at $9\frac{1}{2}$ years	Normal voiding cystourethrogram and retrograde urethrogram, no symptoms at 1 year
3 (Fig. 8.18c)	$11\frac{1}{2}$	Weak urinary stream for 1–2 weeks	Urethral dilations with improvement	Patch graft urethroplasty at 12 years	Lost to follow-up
4 (Fig. 8.18d)	12	Bed wetting for 2–3 years	Urethral dilations, development of a short false passage that healed promptly		Normal voiding cystourethrogram and retrograde urethrogram, bed wetting continues at 7 months
5 (Fig. 8.18e)	13	Enuresis and blood stained sheets at night for 3 weeks	Urethral dilations with gradual improvement		Normal voiding cystourethrogram and retrograde urethrogram, no symptoms at 4 years
6 (Fig. 8.18f)	13	Dysuria, frequent urination and occasional terminal haematuria for 1–2 months	Urethral dilations with marked improvement at time of discharge from hospital		Lost to follow-up

Source: Currarino, G. and Stephens, F.D. (1981), An uncommon type of bulbar urethral stricture, sometimes familial, of unknown cause: congenital versus acquired. *J. Urol.* 126: 658. Published with permission of the Williams and Wilkins Co.

the bulbar urethra. Five instances have been reported by Moskowitz and associates (1976), and we have two cases, including a one-day-old newborn (Currarino and Stephens, 1981) (Fig. 8.19C, D). At urethroscopy the lesions appear cystic and they are found to be filled with clear, sometimes blood-tinged fluid upon unroofing. They are believed to represent obstructed Cowper's ducts but whether this is true for all cases is not certain. In one case reported by Moskowitz and associates, a voiding urethrogram after fulguration of the cyst showed reflux into a Cowper's duct at the same level, suggesting that the cyst very likely originated from this structure (Moskowitz *et al.*, 1976). These observations raise the possibility that the stricture might have originated from an abnormality of these ducts, perhaps on the basis of infection or from rupture of one of the urethral cysts.

Congenital anomaly

Several patients have been reported in whom a bulbar urethral stricture, similar to that described in this series, was interpreted as being congenital in origin because of the negative history of trauma or infection, the occasional familial occurrence of the lesion and the appearance of the stenosis, which was sometimes described as a delicate membrane without local fibrosis. Amsler (1961), reported on three patients, 26, 29 and 25 years old, respectively. The first patient had an episode of acute urinary retention when he was five years old and problems with urination thereafter, the second had difficulties with urination for many years and the third had had some dysuria and a weak urinary stream since early life. The urethrogram of the second patient also showed reflux of contrast material into a cavity that

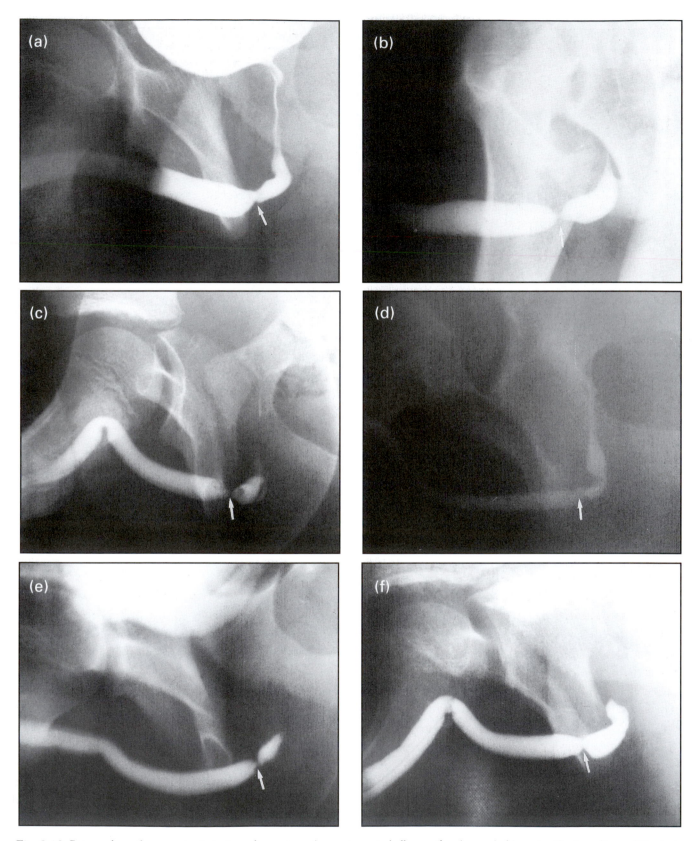

Fig. 8.18 *Retrograde urethrograms in six patients demonstrate short stricture in bulbar urethra (arrows). Note opacification of part of Cowper's duct. (Reprinted, with permission, from Currarino, G. and Stephens, F.D. (1981), An uncommon type of bulbar urethral stricture, sometimes familial, of unknown cause: congenital versus acquired. J. Urol. 126: 658–62, Fig. 1.)*

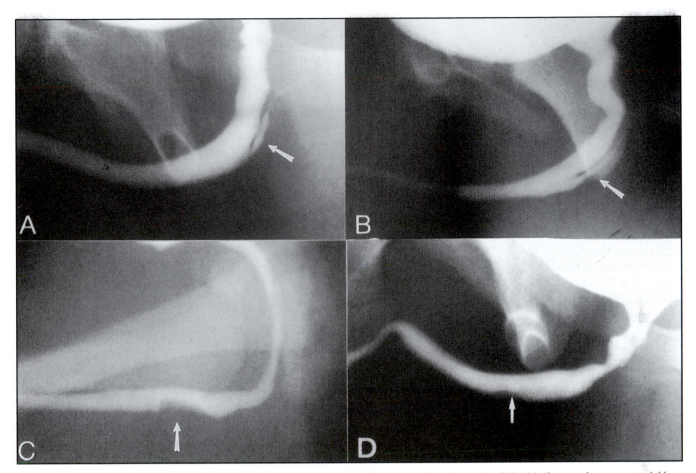

Fig. 8.19 A,B. *Voiding urethrograms in two children show opacification of Cowper's ducts (arrows).* **C,D**. *Voiding urethrograms in children reveal filling defect in ventral surface of bulbar urethra believed to represent obstructed Cowper's duct (arrows). Urethrogram* **C** *was done in one-day-old newborn investigated because of 'imperforate anus'. (Reprinted, with permission, from Currarino, G. and Stephens, F.D. (1981), An uncommon type of bulbar urethral stricture, sometimes familial, of unknown cause: congenital versus acquired. J. Urol. 126: 658–62, Fig. 2.)*

probably represented a dilated Cowper's duct. Viville and associates (1971) reported two cases, including a 26-year-old man who had had problems with urination since early life, with a more recent development of dysuria and weak urinary stream. The retrograde urethrogram showed a membrane-like stenosis of the bulbar urethra together with opacification of a Cowper's duct. The second patient was a 34-year-old man with a long-standing history of dysuria, occasional haematuria and a weak urinary stream for as long as he could remember. Rao (1975) reported on three patients, 20, 18 and 21 years old, respectively. The symptoms were difficulty in passing urine in the first patient, difficulties in passing urine for some time and an episode of urinary retention in the second, and a long history of weak urinary stream and enuresis for two years in the third. Michon (1978) described a similar bulbar urethral stricture in a 42-year-

old man and his 28-year-old son, and a 'double juxtabulbar' stricture in another son aged 23 years. Their symptoms were dysuria and a weak urinary stream in the father, two recent episodes of urinary retention and a weak stream in the first son and severe dysuria in the second son. Redman and Fraiser (1979) reported on two brothers, including a 7-year-old boy who presented with urinary retention and a history of haematuria on three occasions, and his 13-year-old brother, who had had some haematuria when he was 12 years old.

There is no definite evidence that the stricture described in these patients was truly congenital. Its occurrence in a father and his two sons (Michon, 1978) and in two brothers (Redman and Fraiser, 1979) is suggestive but not conclusive. More convincing evidence would be the observation of a similar lesion in newborns or infants.

A possible embryogenesis of bulbar urethral stricture

The local stricture or diaphragm was located in the bulbar urethra close to the point of entry of Cowper's ducts and also close to the entry of a rare type of recto-bulbar fistula (Fig. 8.20) (Currarino et al., 1978). This trio of anomalies at this site favours an embryological explanation. One of us (F.D.S.) has studied one specimen with a long stenosis and two with complete obstructions of the urethra in three newborns who died within hours after birth. The most distal part of the stenosis or occlusion reached into the bulb and the most proximal extended into the membranous urethra.

Congenital membranes or strictures in the region of the membranous urethra and adjoining bulb may be derived from the urogenital membrane. Normally, this membrane consists of two cell layers and breaks down at the 16-mm stage when the urorectal septum completes the partitioning of the cloaca. However, this membrane may be thick, consisting of many layers of ectodermal or endodermal cells, or because mesodermal cells may grow between the layers. The membrane then is canalized by ectodermal and endodermal pits that meet and create the lumen through the membrane. The 'pitting' may be complete, leaving no trace of the membrane, or it may be incomplete. When incomplete a peripheral ring, stricture or diaphanous membrane may

remain, or an occluding bar of tissue may separate the prostatic urethra from the bulbar urethra. The level of attachment of the membrane to the urethra or the extent of the bar depends on the manner of pitting and the depth of each pit contributing to the canalization. If the ectodermal pitting predominates the attachment of the membrane will be high and if endodermal, the attachment will be low (Fig. 8.21) (Field and Stephens, 1974).

The level of the original urogenital membrane in the urethra of a full-term neonate is obscure and embryologists are non-committal in this respect, although the level of the anal membrane is clear and denoted by the abrupt change from rectal mucosa to skin on the anal valves.

At the 16-mm stage, the urogenital sinus in its distal segment reaches, expands and elongates in the sagittal plane to form the so-called pars phallica, which contributes to the formation of the anterior urethra (Fig. 8.22a). At the same time, the perineal mound builds up in the depths of the external cloaca, separating and elongating the once co-apting walls of the urethra and anus (Fig. 8.22b–d). These combined processes broaden the original zone of the urogenital membrane (Fig. 8.22e). Urethral strictures, membranes and occlusions in the adjoining parts of the membranous and bulbar urethra may be the vestiges of the urogenital

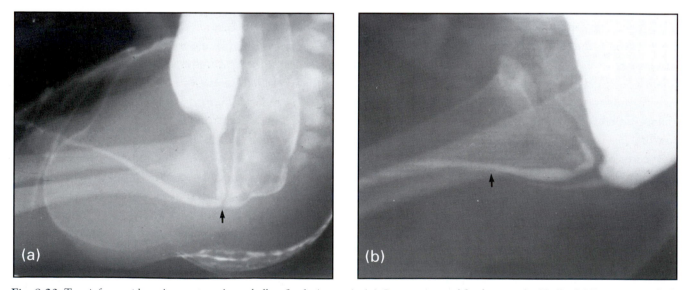

Fig. 8.20 *Two infants with anal agenesis and rectobulbar fistula (arrows). (a) Common type of fistula to urethral bulb. (b) Rare type in which fistula is thin and long, terminating much more distally in ventral surface of bulbar urethra. (Reprinted, with permission, from Currarino, G., Votteler, T.P. and Kirks, D.R. (1978), Anal agenesis with rectobulbar fistula. Radiology 126: 457.)*

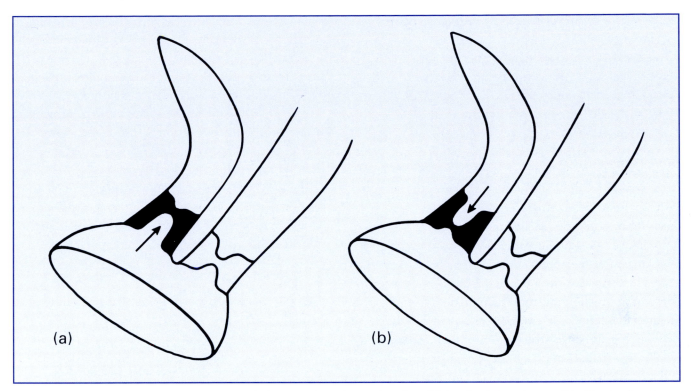

Fig. 8.21 *Diagram shows manner of breakdown of thick urogenital membrane of ectodermal (**a**) and endodermal pitting (**b**). (Reprinted, with permission, from Currarino, G. and Stephens, F.D. (1981), An uncommon type of bulbar urethral stricture, sometimes familial, of unknown cause: congenital versus acquired. J. Urol. 126: 658–62, Fig. 4.)*

membrane and denote the zone in which they are located.

The ducts of Cowper's glands originate deep in the pars phallica approximately two weeks after the urogenital membrane has disappeared and during the phase of elongation of the sinus. This elongation, which also incorporates the ducts, is brought about in part by extension of the urorectal septum into the external cloaca, forming the normal perineal mound (Fig. 8.22), which widely separates the anal canal from the urethra. Subsequently, the mound and the pars phallica are covered over to form the perineum and bulbous urethra, respectively, by the inner genital folds, which carry Cowper's ducts with them to the floor of the bulbar urethra.

With agenesis of the perineal mound, the anal canal and urogenital sinus orifices remain co-apted and both are enveloped by the genital folds, thus forming a rectobulbar fistula. The folds carry Cowper's ducts to the floor of the bulb beyond the origin of the fistula (Kitchen, 1971). With hypogenesis of the mound, the anal canal and sinus are separated by a thin wedge of perineal mound that intervenes between the enveloping folds and projects the tenuous fistula into the floor of the bulb to a point to, or beyond, the orifices of the two ducts of Cowper (Kitchen and Stephens, 1971). Two necropsy specimens exhibited this anatomy.

The original zone of the urogenital membrane may be much broadened by growth of the inner genital folds and perineal mound, and is delimited probably distally by the orifices of Cowper's ducts. These ducts also denote the distal limit of the contribution of the normal perineal mound to the bulbar urethra and the orifice of the rare tenuous rectobulbar fistula. Strictures and membranes occurring in the membranous urethra and bulb are possibly vestiges of an abnormally thick and partly broken down urogenital membrane. It is possible that the strictures exemplified in Cases 1 to 6 are vestiges of the urogenital membrane.

The findings in these cases and those reported to the literature do not provide a clear-cut answer as to the cause of this uncommon type of stricture. Trauma is possible but unlikely. The possibility of a form of urethritis, particularly at the level of the Cowper's ducts,

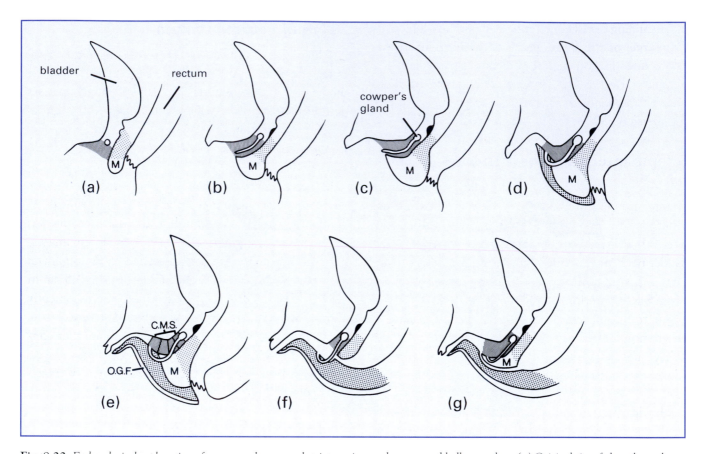

Fig. 8.22 *Embryological explanation of some membranes and strictures in membranous and bulbar urethra.* (**a**) *Original site of cloacal membrane and Cowper's gland.* (**b**), (**c**) *Broadening of membrane zone (shading in urethra) and lengthening of Cowper's duct with growth of perineal mound (M).* (**d**) *Envelopment of bulbar urethra and perineal mound by inner genital folds (heavy dotted area) carrying Cowper's ducts with them.* (**e**) *Outer genital folds (OGF) merge over inner genital folds forming raphe; levels of membranes and strictures (CMS) occurring in membranous and bulbar urethra.* (**f**) *Rectobulbar fistula caused by agenesis of perineal mound.* (**g**) *Rectobulbar fistula with hypogenesis of perineal mound; fistula and zone of broadened cloacal membrane projected anteriorly by thin mound and covered by inner genital folds.* *(Reprinted, with permission, from Currarino, G. and Stephens, F.D. (1981), An uncommon type of bulbar urethral stricture, sometimes familial, of unknown cause: congenital versus acquired. J. Urol. 126: 658–62, Fig. 5.)*

is appealing but cannot be proved. The theory of a congenital anomaly is supported by case reports of familial incidence.

One other diaphenous diaphragm with small central perforation has been identified endoscopically in the bulbar urethra of a neonate by one of us (F.D.S.). Therefore, it is suggested that until more evidence becomes available this type of localized stricture should be recorded as developmental in origin.

Marion's disease of congenital origin

The term 'neuromuscular incoordination of the bladder neck' is used as descriptive of the situation in which obstruction occurs in the region of the internal sphinc-

ter, without obvious anatomical or neurological cause. Marion (1933) described congenital and acquired types of this disease of the bladder neck. In his view, the congenital form was due either to muscular hypertrophy, comparable to congenital hypertrophy of the pylorus, or to absence or deficiency of the plexiform dilator fibres of the bladder neck.

In Marion's disease, the bladder and upper urinary tract show all the typical effects that ensue on obstruction. The internal sphincter shares in the hypertrophy, but the urethra is otherwise normal in appearance.

The congenital form of this disease is a very rare entity. The diagnosis seems to be made seldom nowadays, possibly because of the greater accuracy in distinguishing other causes of urethral obstruction. The better understanding of vesicoureteral reflux, urinary infection, dyssynergia of the sphincters, and occult neuropathic lesions affecting the spinal cord may also explain the extreme rarity of the congenital form of Marion's disease. The acquired form is likewise a very rare and ill-understood entity.

Ectopic internal urinary meatus

Studies of lateral views of the bladder neck during voiding cystourethrography reveal that the internal urinary meatus may be located centrally in the bladder base with well-marked lips anterior and posterior to the bladder neck, or it may hug the back of the pubis with a relatively long posterior lip or lie posteriorly with an exaggerated anterior lip. The positioning does not appear to be important in the normal functioning of continence in children. However, in one male baby, the internal meatus was located on the anterior wall of the bladder cranial to the pubis symphysis, and the long posterior lip formed a flap valve obstruction (Fig. 8.23). The bladder was extremely large, and urine overflowed drop by drop from the urethra. After extensive resection of the posterior bladder neck and partial cystectomy, the patient learned to void and became continent and has made good progress for at least 15 years.

Polyp of verumontanum

A tally of the published case reports of congenital polyps of the prostatic urethra was made by Downs (1970). He analysed 28 case reports including five of the six described herein. The polyps were composed of fibrous tissue, but with the addition in some of smooth muscle, small cysts, or neural tissue covered by transitional epithelium.

In six children between the ages of three and six years, a pedunculated polyp partially and intermittently obstructed the posterior urethra. In two, bleeding was also a presenting symptom. The polyps, approximately 1 cm in diameter, were each attached to the region of the verumontanum by a stout stalk measuring 1.5 cm in length. Two of the polyps examined microscopically were observed to consist of vascular connective tissue covered with transitional epithelium, and another consisted of a mass of small cysts lined by one or more layers of cuboidal epithelium within an encasement of transitional epithelium.

Voiding cystourethrography

Cystography revealed a rounded 'filling defect', due to the presence of the polyp, in the base of the bladder adjacent to the bladder neck. On micturition, the polyp

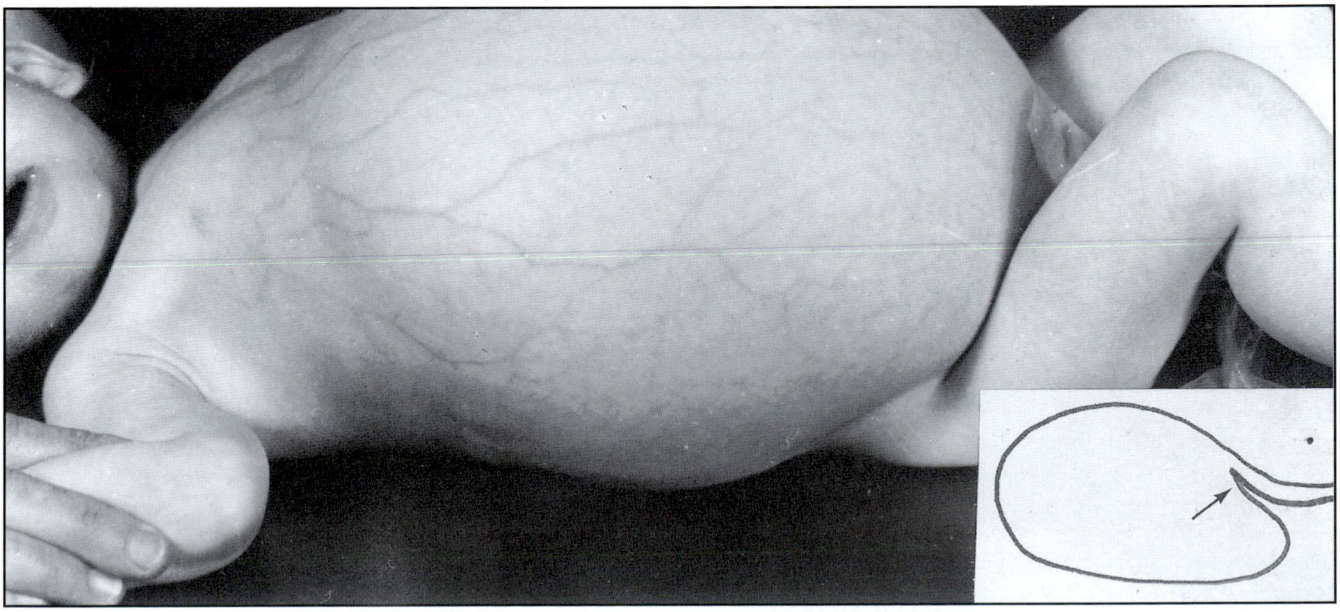

Fig. 8.23 Anterior locus of internal meatus. Male baby P.C., aged four months—gross distension of bladder occupying abdominal cavity. Obstruction at internal urinary meatus due to high insertion of urethra into anterior wall of bladder and flap valve effect of posterior lip of internal sphincter (inset, arrow). (Reprinted, by permission, from Stephens, F.D. (1983), Congenital Malformations of the Urinary Tract, New York, Praeger, Fig. 5.17, p. 123.)

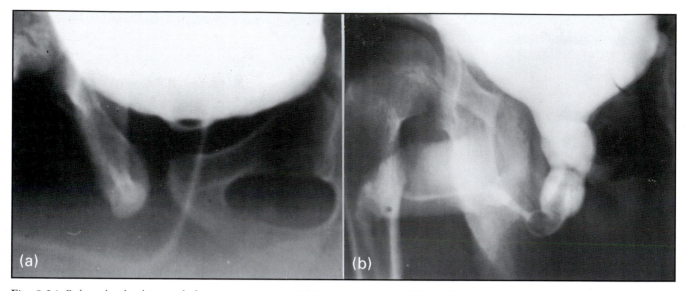

Fig. 8.24 *Pedunculated polyp attached at verumontanum. (**a**) Cystogram showing filling defect of polyp in lumen of bladder at the internal urinary meatus. (**b**) Voiding cystourethrogram showing filling defects of another polyp and its stalk in bulb and membranous urethra. The urethra in the bulb is partially obstructed by the polyp. ((**a**) reprinted, by permission, from Stephens, F.D. (1963),* Congenital Malformations of the Rectum, Anus and Genito-Urinary Tracts. *Edinburgh, Livingstone, Fig. 129A, p. 232.)*

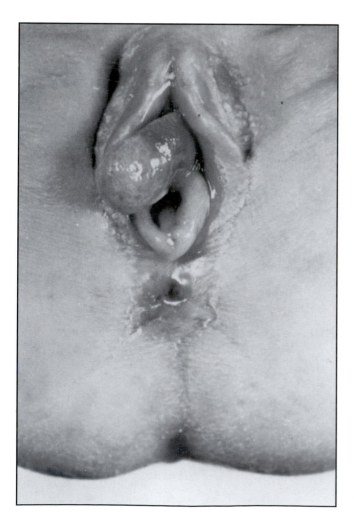

Fig. 8.25 (left) *Polyp in female urethra. Baby D.B.—neonate with spina bifida occulta, paretic bladder and myomatous urethral polyp suspended by a pedicle from the posterior wall of the distal urethra. (Reprinted, by permission, from Stephens, F.D. (1983),* Congenital Malformations of the Urinary Tract, *New York, Praeger, Fig. 5.19, p. 124.)*

on its stalk, fixed at the verumontanum, turned down and wedged itself in the lower membranous urethra and bulb (Fig. 8.24).

The posterior urethra and upper urinary tract were only very slightly dilated. The kidneys showed no evidence of damage due to back pressure. The urethra below the wedged polyp was normal in calibre. Voiding cystourethrography subsequent to removal of the polyp and stalk revealed a urethra of normal calibre and contour in all the children. Apart from these polyps, pedunculated as described, arising from the verumontanum and probably of congenital origin, no instance of obstruction to the urinary flow by an enlarged verumontanum *per se* was observed by means of voiding cystourethrography.

The polyps can be removed either endoscopically by division of the base of the stalk with the cutting loop in boys whose urethra admits an 18F sheath, or in babies by suprapubic cystostomy, transfixion and ligation, and division of the stalk near its attachment to verumontanum.

A urethral polyp similar to that already described was observed in a newborn female baby (Fig. 8.25). It consisted of fibrous tissue covered by transitional epithelium. The stalk was attached to the caudal end of the urethra and the polyp prolapsed into the vestibule. The similarity of the polyps of the male and female urethra suggests a common embryology.

Embryology of urethral polyp

The pedunculated polyp arising in the site of the verumontanum in the male may be a development malformation of Müller's tubercle. This tubercle is formed by the müllerian ducts, which penetrate into the urogenital sinus between the orifices of the wolffian ducts. The epithelia of the sinus and ducts undergo active proliferation, forming a mound with sinus and a solid cord of cells, which later canalizes. In the male, further development of the müllerian structures is arrested, and the Müller's tubercle shrinks and remains as the verumontanum, into which open centrally the vestigial prostatic utricle and laterally each wolffian duct (vas deferens). In the female, the tubercle is replaced by the widened vaginal orifice and hymen, which 'migrate' caudally from pelvis to perineum. Concurrently with this relative shift, the pelvic urethra elongates, and the urogenital sinus folds outward to become the vestibule. The polyp in the male and female may represent persistence of Müller's tubercle, either whole or in part, and the stalk is composed of drawn-out urogenital sinus epithelium together with a central core of fibrous tissue and blood vessels. The polyp is a hamartoma comprising glands, cysts, muscle or neurovascular tissue arising in the prostatic part of the urethra.

Another explanation for polyp formation may be found in the developmental processes of the urorectal

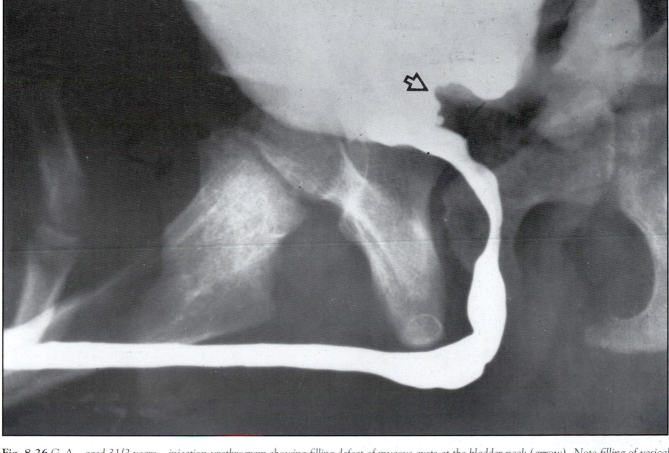

Fig. 8.26 G.A., aged 31/2 years—injection urethrogram showing filling defect of mucous cysts at the bladder neck (arrow). Note filling of vesical diverticulum. (Reprinted, by permission, from Stephens, F.D. (1983), Congenital Malformations of the Urinary Tract, New York, Praeger, Fig. 5.20, p. 125.)

septum. The polyp occurs at the meeting point of Tourneux's fold and Rathke's plicae which divide the cloaca into urinary and rectal components. At such a site, proliferation and sequestration of the cloacal epithelium may occur with polyp formation in the urethra at the level of the verumontanum or on the anterior wall of the rectum. Stalk formation may be caused by traction exerted by peristaltic propulsion of the polyp.

Cysts of the bladder neck

A large cyst caused obstruction at the bladder neck in one male child. The symptoms of obstruction were insidious, and overflow incontinence was noted at two years of age. At the age of $3\frac{1}{2}$ years, voiding cystourethrography was performed. This showed a large 'filling defect' in the trigone region, bulging into the bladder and partially occluding its outlet. A large vesical diverticulum was also apparent (Fig. 8.26).

Subsequent to surgical marsupialization of the cyst into the bladder, voiding cystourethrograms displayed a free urethral outlet, very small outpouching of the trigone at the site of marsupialization, and persistence of the vesical diverticulum, which was later excised. Williams (1958a) reported a similar example of a cyst blocking the bladder outlet in a female baby. This cyst measured approximately 2.5 cm in diameter. It contained pus. The roof of the cyst exhibited several small satellite cysts on its surface. Histological examination revealed that these cysts were lined by transitional epithelium, and that there was evidence of inflammation in their walls.

Diverticula of the anterior urethra

Dilatations of the anterior urethra are found in two forms: the saccular, arising from the floor of the urethra (Campbell, 1951a); and the diffuse megalourethra which occurs as either a scaphoid or fusiform deformity.

Saccular diverticula

Most of the saccular diverticula obstruct the flow of urine as evidenced by weak stream and straining; in large diverticula, a tense, localized swelling appears synchronously at the corresponding site along the urethra in the perineum or penis. They occur more often in the proximal half of the penile urethra (Fig. 9.1) and the distal half of the bulbous urethra, in contrast with the megaduct of Cowper, which lies in the proximal half of the bulbous urethra.

The opening of the orifice of the diverticulum into the urethra may be narrow and circular or wide and long, and the body of the diverticulum may be round or sausage-shaped. A round, pendulous diverticulum (Fig. 9.2) resulting from a focal defect of the corpus spongiosum lies within the tunica albuginea and, when

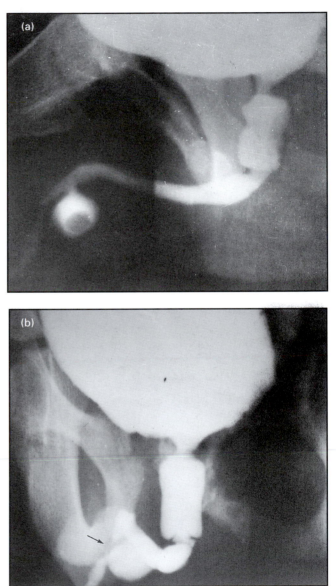

(a)

(b)

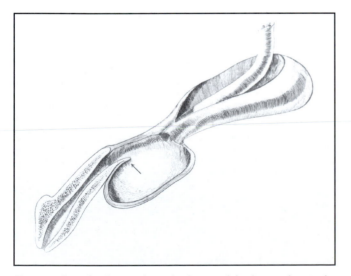

Fig. 9.1 *Saccular diverticulum. At the site of the diverticulum in the penile urethra, the corpus spongiosum is deficient; more proximally it is absent from the roof and sides of the bulbous urethra. The arrow indicates the site of the 'gate' action (the corpora cavernosa are not shown). (Reprinted, by permission, from Dorairajan, T. (1963), Defects of spongy tissue and congenital diverticula of the penile urethra. Aust. N.Z. J. Surg. 32: 219, Fig. 1.)*

Fig. 9.2 *Saccular diverticulum. M.S., aged four years—voiding cystourethrogram showing saccular diverticulum of the penile urethra with narrow neck, non-obstructive when filling (a) but impairing the flow (arrow) when full (b). Note air bubble in diverticulum and Type 1 valves of posterior urethra. (Reprinted, by permission, from Smith, E.D. (1980), Malformations of the bladder and urethra, and hypospadias, in Pediatric Surgery, T.M. Holder and K.W. Ashcraft (eds). Philadelphia, Saunders, Fig. 58.14, p. 769.)*

tense, compresses the urethral lumen. The elongated diverticulum with a long orifice opening into the urethra results from a more widespread defect of spongy tissue. It also distends within the fibrous tunica and obstructs the urethral lumen. The thin common wall between the distal penile urethra and distal pouch of the diverticulum forms a flap valve or 'gate', obstructing urine flow (Fig. 9.1).

Voiding cystourethrography displays the sacculation of the penile urethra. The radiopaque medium flows freely into the saccule demonstrating a rounded or oval shape which may be small or large. The urethra distal to the diverticulum is not stenotic but appears collapsed. A linear-filling defect between the opaque medium in the urethra and diverticulum proximal to the orifice indicates the length of the common wall shared by both structures and characterizes the diverticulum (Fig. 9.3).

Histological studies of one specimen revealed that the saccule was lined by transitional epithelium and indicated that the spongy tissue of the urethra was rudimentary and that it displayed an abnormally large amount of fibrous tissue. This spongy layer was spread very thinly over the whole wall of the diverticulum and the roof of the urethra corresponding with the length of the diverticulum, which lay in the proximal half of the pendulous urethra (Fig. 9.1).

Examination of the spongy tissue proximal to the diverticulum showed a gradual thinning from the bulb toward the diverticulum. Furthermore, the corpus spongiosum was also incomplete on the roof and sides of the bulbous urethra (Dorairajan, 1963).

These observations indicate that a diverticulum represents the local manifestation of a more widespread developmental derangement of the corpus spongiosum. The defect is more severe and apparent in the floor, side walls and roof of the urethra at the site of the diverticulum, but an occult defect of the spongy tissue around the side walls and roof of the urethra, proximal to the diverticulum, coexists (Fig. 9.1).

Embryogenesis of saccular diverticula

The spongy tissue is normally formed from the inner genital folds, which grow together from either side of the urogenital sinus to meet in the midline, covering-in the male urethra from behind forward. The vascular sponges in the mesenchyme within the folds also meet first posteriorly to form the bulb of the urethra. This vascular spongework then envelops the urethra on all sides and extends throughout the length of the bulbous and penile urethra and is encased within the tunica albuginea of the corpus spongiosum.

Incomplete migration of the spongy tissue and rudimentary development of its vascular network account for the defective closure of the bulbous urethra. Local deficiency of the spongework accounts for pocket-like out-pouchings of urethral epithelium within the limits of the tunica albuginea and the proximal half of the pendulous urethra.

Surgical procedures

The obstructive mechanism is a gate action. The 'door' consists of the caudal common wall of urethra and

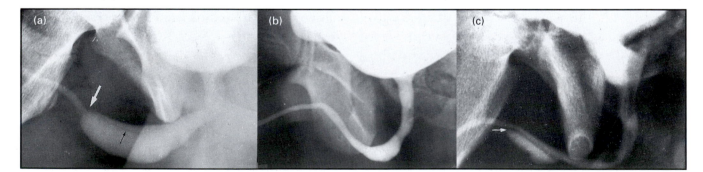

Fig. 9.3 *Large and small saccular diverticula in bulbous urethra.* (**a**) *J.C., aged 14 years—voiding cystourethrogram (VCU) showing compression of urethra (white arrow) by the distal part of the ballooned saccule. Black arrow indicates filling defect caused by the common wall of urethra and diverticulum.* (**b**) *VCU after open repair of urethra.* (**c**) *R.B., aged four years—VCU flap valve clearly shown as a filling defect between diverticulum and urethra (arrow). ((**a**), (**b**) reprinted, by permission, from Dorairajan, T. (1963), Defects of spongy tissue and congenital diverticula of the penile urethra. Aust. N.Z. J. Surg. 32: 219, Fig. 2A,B. (**c**) reprinted, by permission, from Stephens, F.D. (1963), Congenital Malformations of the Rectum, Anus and Genito-Urinary Tracts. Edinburgh, Livingstone, Fig. 132A, p. 235.)*

diverticulum. This door is hinged distally and shuts the urethral lumen when the pressure during voiding rises in the diverticulum.

Endoscopic division of the gate is adequate treatment for the small diverticulum (Fig. 9.3c), but excision of the redundant walls and the gate, together with reconstruction of the urethra, are necessary for the more extensive and capacious lesions (Fig. 9.3a). In babies with retention and urinary infection or uraemia, the diverticulum may be temporarily and expeditiously marsupialized to the skin.

Diffuse enlargement or megalourethra

This uncommon diffuse enlargement of the urethra affects a more extensive part of the penile urethra, which becomes ballooned during micturition, distorting the contour of the surrounding structures.

Two types of abnormality, depending on the extent of associated defects of formation of erectile tissue of the penis, are found. In one type, only the corpus spongiosum is affected; when the urethra fills with urine, its ventral wall balloons, while the dorsal wall is splinted to the corpora cavernosa. The dilated urethra assumes a scaphoid shape. In the second type, the erectile tissue is defective in the corpora cavernosa as well; the urethra, when full, distends circumferentially and becomes fusiform in appearance.

Scaphoid megalourethra: a defect of the corpus spongiosum

In scaphoid megalourethra (Fig. 9.4), the penis is elongated, and the skin redundant, being raised in circumferential folds; the glans is small and tilted dorsally; both corpora cavernosa can be palpated in their whole length on the dorsum of the penis. The spongy urethra, when empty, is impalpable within the baggy redundant skin of the ventral aspect of the penis. During voiding urethrography, the affected segment of the penile urethra expands as a sausage-shaped swelling, which becomes tense during the flow of urine and flaccid on cessation of micturition. The inlet and outlet are funnelled and there is no valvular obstruction (Fig. 9.5).

A bizarre array of anomalies, occurring in some children, are so similar and unusual that they may represent a syndrome of anomalies. These malformations include

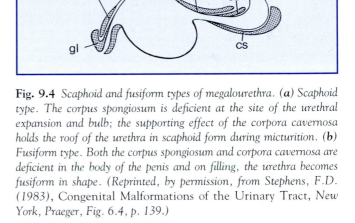

Fig. 9.4 *Scaphoid and fusiform types of megalourethra. (a) Scaphoid type. The corpus spongiosum is deficient at the site of the urethral expansion and bulb; the supporting effect of the corpora cavernosa holds the roof of the urethra in scaphoid form during micturition. (b) Fusiform type. Both the corpus spongiosum and corpora cavernosa are deficient in the body of the penis and on filling, the urethra becomes fusiform in shape. (Reprinted, by permission, from Stephens, F.D. (1983), Congenital Malformations of the Urinary Tract, New York, Praeger, Fig. 6.4, p. 139.)*

local dilatation of the prostatic urethra, megacystis, vesical diverticula, megaureters, vesicoureteral reflux and renal hypoplasia (Fig. 9.6).

Campbell (1951b) described one similar patient. Boissonnat and Duhamel (1962) reported case notes of a baby with prune belly deformities and scaphoid megalourethra. Johnston and Coimbra (1970) drew attention to the gradation from near-normal calibre to extreme dilatation of the penile urethra, and also the association, in one patient, of a wide, cutaneous fistula from the floor of the scaphoid urethra. These authors describe a patient with Down's syndrome who died and whose scaphoid megalourethra was examined histologically. It contained no erectile tissue in the whole circumference of the wall. The corpora cavernosa and glans exhibited histologically normal cavernous tissue.

The operation for scaphoid megalourethra described by Nesbitt (1955) diminishes the lumen and offers a satisfactory cosmetic result.

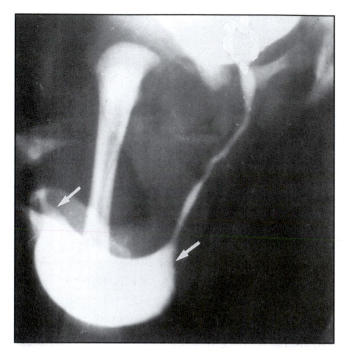

Fig. 9.5 *Voiding cystourethrogram of C.E. showing scaphoid expansion of the penile urethra (arrows indicate the funnel-shaped inlet and outlet). (Reprinted, by permission, from Dorairajan, T. (1963), Defects of spongy tissue and congenital diverticula of the penile urethra. Aust. N.Z. J. Surg. 32: 219, Fig. 4.)*

Fusiform megalourethra

One stillborn baby exhibited fusiform megalourethra (Fig. 9.7), which involved the corpus spongiosum and both corpora cavernosa. The penis was elongated, the skin was redundant, the glans was small and, in this instance, the shaft of the penis was flaccid because of focal absence of both the corpus spongiosum and corpora cavernosa in the vicinity of the suspensory ligament. This condition occurred in association with a congenital rectovesical fistula. It may also occur in patients exhibiting the 'forme fruste' of vesical exstrophy with skin-covered split symphysis and anterior abdominal wall.

Urethrography in the postmortem state demonstrated a wide fusiform expansion of the penile urethra; focal absence of the corpora cavernosa in addition to the corpus spongiosum accounted for the fusiform bulging of the urethra. There was no radiographic evidence of urethral obstruction.

The pathological anatomy and histological structure of the specimen from the stillborn infant exhibiting fusiform megalourethra are depicted in Fig. 9.7. There it

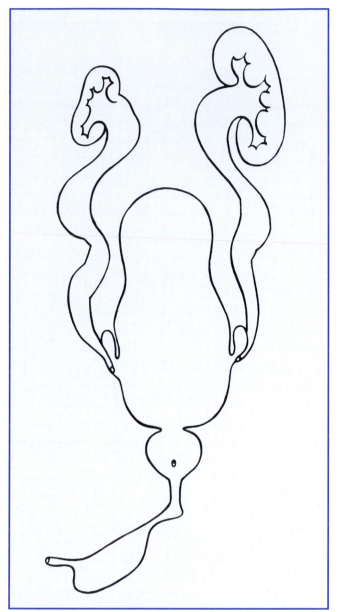

Fig. 9.6 *Scaphoid megalourethra; associated malformations of the urinary tract. Enlargement of the prostatic urethra, megacystis, vesical diverticula, megaureters and hypoplasia of the kidneys. (Reprinted, by permission, from Dorairajan, T. (1963), Defects of spongy tissue and congenital diverticula of the penile urethra. Aust. N.Z. J. Surg. 32: 219, Fig. 5.)*

is shown that the bulbous urethra lay in a gutter formed by the incomplete envelope of corpus spongiosum; that at the junction of bulb with penile urethra, the spongy tissue of the urethra terminated abruptly and reappeared in the glans; and that the defect of development of the erectile tissue affected the corpora cavernosa to a similar extent (Dorairajan, 1963).

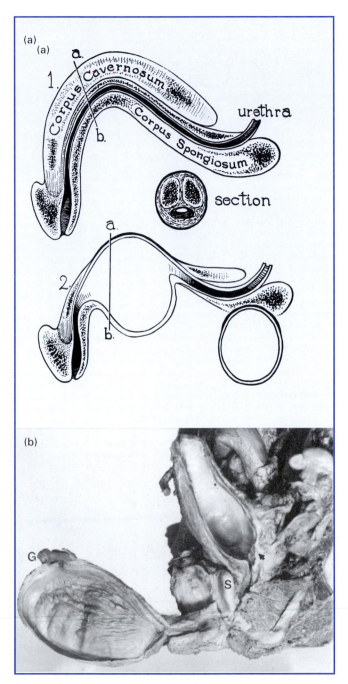

Fig. 9.7 *(a) Fusiform megalourethra. Compare the sagittal and cross-sections (insets) of the normal (1) with the abnormal (2) in which both corpora cavernosa and spongiosa are deficient in the expanded zone and defective in the zone of the bulbous urethra. (b) Specimen of fusiform megalourethra associated with rectovesical fistula. Note absence of corpus spongiosum and corpora cavernosa in penile urethra but presence of glans and some cavernous tissue (G = glans; S = symphysis; arrow shows fistula). (Reprinted, by permission, from Stephens, F.D. (1963), Congenital Malformations of the Rectum, Anus and Genito-Urinary Tracts. Edinburgh, Livingstone, Fig. 137, p. 238.)*

The histological studies showed that the structure of the spongy tissue of the bulb and glans penis was abnormal; the vascular network was overloaded with fibrous tissue. In the expanded urethra, the spongy tissue was absent, and the urethral epithelium lay upon the fibrous wall of the tunica albuginea.

It was possible to recognize, both clinically and radiographically, the obstructive effect of the saccular diverticulum. No such obstruction could be found in living patients with the diffuse megalourethra. However, distal obstruction was found in two aborted fetuses. In these two fetuses, the distal urethra of the glans was totally obstructed by an uncanalized epithelial plug associated with extreme ectasia of the pendulous urethra. A defect in the embryological sequence of events in the formation of the urethra of the glans may be one of the causes of megalourethra. The two fetuses were aborted because of major anomalies including megacystis detected by routine ultrasound examination during the pregnancies. Both fetuses were autopsied. The genitourinary and rectal organs were removed *in toto* and dissected microscopically with special attention to the pelvic, bulbar and penile urethra. The urethra of the glans was also cut in serial sections.

Case 1. Fusiform megalourethra

A male fetus, S.K., gestational age 14 weeks, weighing 62 g, was aborted because of gross dilatation of the bladder and prostatic urethra detected ultrasonographically. The amniotic fluid volume was small but within normal limits as assessed by ultrasonography. Multiple anomalies were found at autopsy, namely extreme total scoliosis, gastroschisis, high rectal atresia lacking rectourinary communication and urethral obstruction.

The urinary tract anomalies included partial obstruction in mid-pelvic urethra, possibly Type 1 valve, megacystis, bilateral intrarenal hydronephrosis and small kidneys with oligonephronia, dysplasia and intrarenal calcification. The ureters were straight and only slightly dilated and both exhibited vesicoureteral reflux when tested in the postmortem state.

The pendulous urethra was ectatic, full of fluid, incompressible and fusiform in shape (Fig. 9.8a). The bulbar urethra and urethra in the glans were not dilated. A small white solid tag was attached to the tip of the glans (Fig. 9.9).

On microscopy the walls of the megalourethra were found to be stretched around the distended lumen. The very thin corpus spongiosum was barely recognizable except for the presence of sparse sinusoidal capillaries. The mesenchymal precursor of the corpora cavernosa was present as a thin undivided arch thinnest in mid urethra and spread over the dorsal third of the circumference of the urethra (Fig. 9.10c). The epithelial lining was transitional in type and no glands were identified in the sections examined.

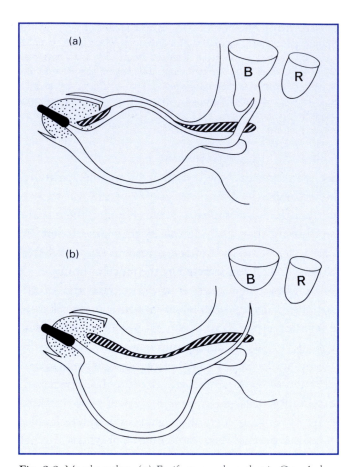

Fig. 9.8 *Megalourethra. (**a**) Fusiform megalourethra in Case 1 shows defective erectile tissue of corpora cavernosa (hatched area), epithelial tag and ingrowth blocking urethra of glans (black area), mid pelvic partial urethral obstruction and high rectal atresia. (**b**) Case 2 demonstrates scaphoid type with intact (although thinner) corpora cavernosa, similar epithelial plug in glans (black area), total occlusion of internal urinary meatus and high rectal atresia. B = bladder, R = rectum. (Reproduced, by permission, from Stephens, F.D. and Fortune, D. W. (1993), Pathogenesis of megalourethra. J. Urol. 149: 1512–16, Fig.1.)*

The bulbar and membranous urethra lying caudal to the mid-pelvic urethral obstruction was not dilated. The junction between the bulbar urethra and the megalourethra was abrupt.

At the level of the coronal sulcus, the junction was also abrupt, the urethra in the proximal glans being very narrow in calibre. Distally, it was occluded by a solid core of squamous epithelial cells extending to the site for the meatus and beyond the glans as a squamous epithelial tag. The deepest part of the core was partly calcified (Fig. 9.10a, b). The mucosa of the patent urethra of the proximal glans was autolysed. Erectile tissue of the glans surrounded the core of the squamous epithelium distal to the frenulum.

Case 2. Scaphoid megalourethra
A male fetus, C.T., gestational age 19 weeks, weighing 170 g was aborted because of gross megacystis and oligohydramnios detected ultrasonographically. The fetus was moderately macerated.

The anomalies included lumbar scoliosis, absence of three toes on left foot, anorectal atresia, atresia of the internal urinary

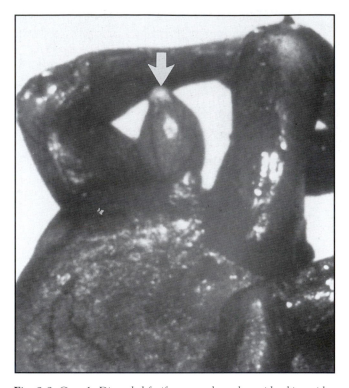

Fig. 9.9 *Case 1. Distended fusiform megalourethra with white epithelial tag on glans (arrow). (Reproduced, by permission, from Stephens, F.D. and Fortune, D.W. (1993), Pathogenesis of megalourethra. J. Urol. 149: 1512–16, Fig. 2.)*

meatus, gross megacystis, mildly dilated ureters, oligonephronic horseshoe kidneys and megalourethra of the scaphoid type (Fig. 9.8b). The ureters were slightly tortuous and only mildly dilated above normal dimensions. The scaphoid curve of the phallus was gentle and limited to the distal third.

The epithelium of the megalourethra was autolysed. Two slender paramedial thickenings in the undivided dorsal arch of mesenchyme representing immature corpora cavernosa were recognizable. The corpus spongiosum composed of undifferentiated mesenchyme was thick dorsal to the lumen, becoming thin on the ventral aspect. Sparse thin-walled sinusoids lying in the mesenchyme were present in the wall.

The bulbar urethra was attenuated but patent and the crura of the corpora cavernosa were identified. The bulbospongiosus and accompanying muscle were orientated around the urethra of the bulb.

The urethra in the glans was patent proximally, and distally was represented by a non-canalized partly calcified squamous epithelial core, part of which protruded as a tag from the tip of the glans (Fig. 9.11). The urethra in the proximal segment of the glans was narrow and contacted the solid core. Its epithelium had autolysed. The prepuce had formed around the glans. Erectile tissue of the glans surrounded the uncanalized segment of the urethra beyond the attachment of the frenulum.

In both fetuses, the distal urethra in the glans was totally blocked by an uncanalized squamous epithelial

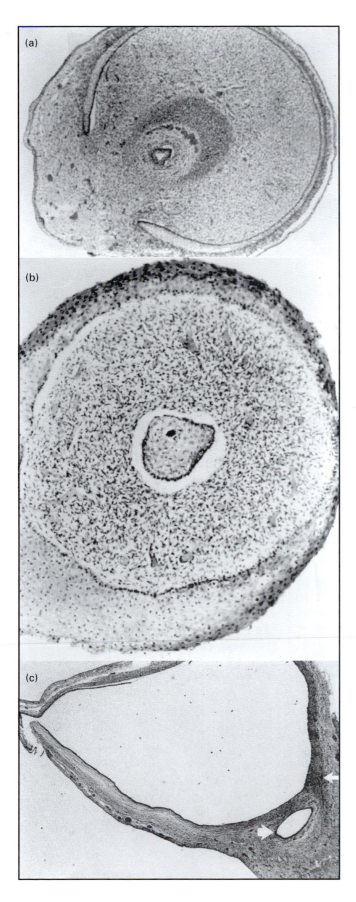

Fig. 9.10 *Case 1. (**a**) Small-calibre proximal urethra of the glans. (**b**) Uncanalized epithelial ingrowth with calcification (black speck) in distal urethra in transverse sections. Reduced from ×50. (**c**) Transverse section of proximal megalourethra shows wide lumen, compressed mesenchyme of corpora cavernosa (small arrow) and tapering urethra (large arrow) near bulb. Reduced from ×20. (Reproduced, by permission, from Stephens, F.D. and Fortune, D.W. (1993), Pathogenesis of megalourethra.* J. Urol. *149: 1512–16, Fig. 3.)*

core. In Case 1, the pelvic urethra was partially obstructed but in Case 2 the pelvic urethra was totally blocked. Fluid under tension accumulated in the megalourethra and may have been urine in Case 1, but in Case 2, the lumen was blocked at both ends, and the fluid may have been secreted by the mucosal lining.

Though the structure of the proximal and distal urethra of the glans was similar in both, and the degree of obstruction the same, the megalourethra in one was fusiform in type and in the other scaphoid.

Both fetuses exhibited anorectal agenesis and Case 2 had in addition atresia of the urethra at the internal urinary meatus.

The proximal urethra of the glans in both fetuses was a short narrow calibre segment intervening between the megalourethra and the uncanalized epithelial ingrowth.

The corpora cavernosa in both megalourethras were represented by an undivided arch of mesenchyme that was sparse in Case 1 and formed into two longitudinal but non-separated slight thickenings in Case 2.

In Case 1, of 14 weeks' gestational age, amniotic fluid volume was within normal limits. In the absence of an influx of urine to supplement fluid already formed from the amniotic membrane and in this fetus the peritoneal surface of the extraabdominal intestines, amniotic fluid remained near normal in volume. This state is well recognized by ultrasonologists, and if the pregnancy had not been terminated the volume would have been reduced gradually by absorption during the next several weeks and oligohydramnios would eventuate. This explains the presence of amniotic fluid in this fetus with total urinary tract obstruction (Bronshtein *et al.*, 1990).

The urinary tracts described in Cases 1 and 2 were totally obstructed, the kidneys were arrested in their development at a very early stage and the sparse ducts and nephrons exhibited back-pressure dilatations of the ampullae and Bowman's capsules. The pelvis, calyces and ureters were only slightly dilated in contrast with

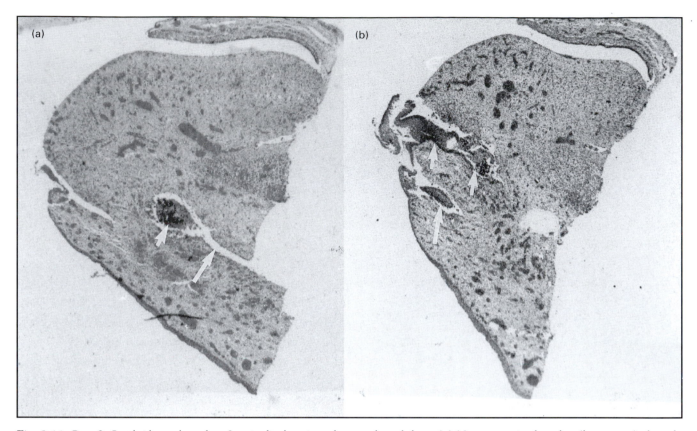

Fig. 9.11 *Case 2. Scaphoid megalourethra. Longitudinal sections show urethra of glans. (**a**) Narrow proximal urethra (long arrow) abuts the uncanalized epithelial ingrowth. (**b**) Parallel section shows solid epithelial ingrowth in distal segment (short arrows) and tag protruding from it. Long arrow indicates epithelium of glans adjoining frenulum. Reduced from ×20. (Reproduced, by permission, from Stephens, F.D. and Fortune, D.W. (1993), Pathogenesis of megalourethra. J. Urol. 149: 1512–16, Fig. 4.)*

the extreme dilatation of the bladder (Bronshtein *et al.*, 1990). This apparent discrepancy may be explained on the basis of early cessation of urine flow in the face of complete obstruction at this very early stage of development.

Embryogenesis of diffuse dilatations of the anterior urethra

The abnormalities of the spongy tissue described may be explained on the basis of defective development of the genital folds.

The penile and glandular urethra are normally formed by the phallic portion of the urogenital sinus. In the male, the urethral folds that form the margins of the urogenital sinus approach each other in the midline posteriorly and close in the sinus from behind forwards. This fusion of the folds extends to the coronary sulcus of the glans. The closing and embedding of the bulbous and penile segments of the urethra occur first at the back of

the bulb and extend from there to surround the urethra, advancing anteriorly as fusion of the urethral folds progresses. These folds carry with them the mesenchyme that forms the vascular erectile tissue. The urethral canal so formed issues in an ostium at the base of the glans.

An extensive circumferential defect of development of erectile tissue of the urethral folds leads to scaphoid dilatation of the penile urethra, which bulges ventrally and is splinted dorsally by the intact corpora cavernosa. When the defect includes both corpora cavernosa as well as the corpus spongiosum, the penis is floppy and the urethral dilatation becomes fusiform in shape during micturition. A further variant of urethral dilatation was reported in which the erectile tissue was absent from a segment of the corpus spongiosum and one of the two corpora cavernosa. Since each corpus cavernosum develops concurrently and independently from the corpus spongiosum, any combination of defects of these three structures may occur.

The degree of dilatation of the scaphoid urethral lumen varies from patient to patient being just above normal in some and gross in others (Johnston and Coimbra, 1970). Adamson and Burge (1990) reported the occurrence of urethral ectasia in a patient whose corpora cavernosa and spongiosa were fully developed and considered that this anomaly represents a third form of megalourethra. No cause has been found for the megalourethra, though speculation ranges through possible temporary distal urethral obstruction occurring in the fetus, to a mesenchymal defect affecting the genitourinary tracts or other parts of the body.

The two aborted fetus specimens described above raise the probability of distal penile obstruction as a cause, and direct attention to the glandular urethra.

Embryology of the glans

According to Glenister (1954, 1958) and Altemus and Hutchins (1991) the urethra of the glans forms in two parts, the proximal segment extending from the coronal sulcus to the frenulum and the distal segment from the frenulum to the summit of the glans. The proximal segment is a prolongation of the penile urethra formed from the urethral plate but overlaid by the frenulum and invested by corpus spongiosum. In the distal segment, surface epithelium of the glans forms two longitudinal folds distal to the frenulum that unite to tubularize in continuity with the proximal urethra, thus projecting the ostium to the epithelial tag at the summit of the glans. Under the tag, proliferating surface epithelium has formed a solid core abutting the end of the plate overlying the roof of the newly formed distal urethra. The core canalizes and its lumen gains continuity with that of the proximal and distal urethra by disintegration of the common wall. In so doing, the lumen becomes expanded into the fossa navicularis and the lacuna magna (Figs 9.12–9.14).

The spongy tissue of the glans migrates around the sides and floor of the distal segment rounding the ventral quadrant and tilting the glans and meatus upwards (Glenister, 1954; Williams, 1952).

In normal development of the glans, the proximal segment is formed by about 14 weeks' gestation and by 18 weeks' canalization of the core and union with the underlying urethra should be complete. The distal urethra in the two rare specimens described above was uncanalized at 14 weeks in Case 1 and at 19 weeks in Case 2. The process of canalization of the epithelial core had not even begun, indicating perhaps a possible late

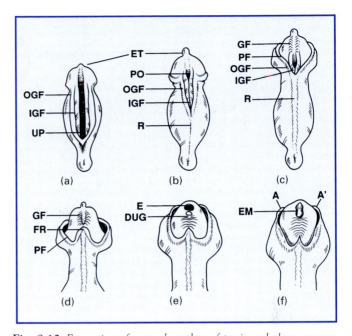

Fig. 9.12 *Formation of normal urethra of penis and glans as seen from ventral aspect.* (**a**) *Urethral plate (UP) extending from bulb to epithelial tag (ET) on tip of glans and flanked by inner (IGF) and outer (OGF) genital folds.* (**b**) *Progressive union of edges of urethral plate and inner genital folds from bulb to primitive ostium (PO) at base of glans to form urethra followed by union of outer genital folds (OGF) to form raphe (R).* (**c**) *Ostium projected onto proximal half of glans by similar process as shown in* (**b**), *and longitudinal folding of surface epithelium of glans (GF) in continuity with inner genital folds.* (**d**) *Preputial folds (PF) combine with outer and inner genital folds to form frenulum (FR) and floor of proximal urethra of glans.* (**e**) *Longitudinal folds of surface epithelium of glans (GF) unite to form the distal urethra of glans (DUG) projecting ostium to tip of glans contiguous with canalized epithelial core (E).* (**f**) *Apposing walls of ostium and canalized core disintegrate to form elliptical external meatus (EM). Prepuce is completed by union of preputial folds (not shown) from frenulum to points A to A', thus covering entire glans. Raphe traverses prepuce but stops at frenular attachment to glans. (Reproduced, by permission, from Stephens, F.D. and Fortune, D.W. (1993), Pathogenesis of megalourethra. J. Urol. 149: 1512–16, Fig. 5.)*

onset or as suggested by the calcification in the core, possible arrest of development. The narrow-calibre proximal urethra of the glans formed from the plate coapted the uncanalized epithelial core. The preputio-urethral folds had formed the frenulum on the proximal glans and had completely occluded the primitive ostium at the corona (Fig. 9.12). The distal urethra of the glans failed to form and the mesenchyme of the glans migrated around the uncanalized epithelial core. The urethral plate of the proximal segment abutting the solid epithelial core canalized but, lacking the enhancement in calibre created by coalescence with the distal segment, remained slender and became embedded deep

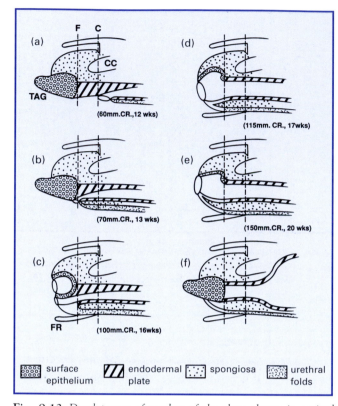

Fig. 9.13 *Development of urethra of the glans shown in sagittal section in normal (**a**) to (**e**) and abnormal (**f**) states. Proximal urethra of the glans lies between coronal (**c**) and frenular (**f**) lines, distal urethra between F line and tip of glans. F line denotes the site of the attachment of frenulum. Penile urethra lies to right of coronal line. CC, corpus cavernosum. (**a**) Urethral plate (hatched area) extends onto glans beyond primitive ostium to future site of attachment of frenulum to glans. (**b**) Urethral plate tubularizes in same manner as that of penile urethra, thus projecting primitive ostium distally from C to F lines. Note surface epithelial tag and core abutting plate. (**c**) Canalization of epithelial core. Glans folds united (white triangle) thus projecting ostium to tip. Spongy mesenchyme appears deep to outer genital folds. Prepuce and frenulum are formed by midline union of frenulopreputial folds (FR). (**d**) Common wall between canalized ingrowth and distal urethra of glans disintegrates creating a large meatus, fossa navicularis and lacuna magna. Spongy mesenchyme of glans migrates around distal urethra. (**e**) Further migration of spongiosa into floor of distal urethra of glans, rounding under quadrant and tipping meatus dorsally. (**f**) Urethra of the glans in megalourethral anomaly. Failure of canalization of epithelial core accompanied by arrest of formation of distal urethra, investment of core by erectile tissue, sealing of primitive ostium and excessive dilatation of penile urethra. Fetal crown–rump (CR) length and approximate fetal age are depicted beneath each diagram. (Reproduced, by permission, from Stephens, F.D. and Fortune, D.W. (1993), Pathogenesis of megalourethra. J. Urol. 149: 1512–16, Fig. 6.)*

in the glans. The penile megalourethra expanded because of the complete obstruction caused by the persisting epithelial core in both fetuses.

In patients with megalourethra who survive and in whom no obstruction can be found in the urethra of the glans, it is proposed that the proximal and distal urethra of the glans formed in the normal manner but canalization of the epithelial core was delayed creating, temporarily, a high degree of obstruction. The distal urethra of the glans eventually opened up but not before the pendulous urethra had become overdistended. Moderate delay may give rise to compression and arrest of formation of the relatively unsupported corpus spongiosum and to grades of scaphoid megalourethra. Maximum delay may lead to prolonged maximum distension of the pendulous urethra and hindrance, not only of the development of the corpus spongiosum urethrae, but also the corpora cavernosa within Buck's fascia. When both these structures are compressed, the formation of the erectile tissue in the pendulous urethra is arrested and the distended megalourethra appears fusiform in shape.

Associated anomalies

Shrom *et al.* (1981) reviewed 26 cases of megalourethra and noted that 21 exhibited the scaphoid and five the fusiform types. In four of the 21, the scaphoid megalourethra was an isolated anomaly and in two others the upper tracts were also dilated whereas in the fusiform group of five, none was an isolated anomaly and all had other urologic defects; two had 'imperforate anus' and four died. Of the 15 remaining scaphoid megalourethra patients, eight exhibited the prune belly syndrome, eight had ectasia of ureters and four were recorded as having other system defects.

Beasley *et al.* (1988) calibrated the anterior urethra of patients with prune belly syndrome and concluded that the anterior urethra was abnormally dilated. They postulated that a transient obstruction in the glans caused by delay in the normal embryologic union of the lumen of the ectodermal urethra of the glans with that of the penile urethra induced the ectasias of the prune belly syndrome.

Delay in canalization of the epithelial core of the glans may be the factor that leads to megalourethra either alone or in company with other developmental, though probably unrelated anomalies, such as reflux megaureters, prune belly syndrome and cloacal defects.

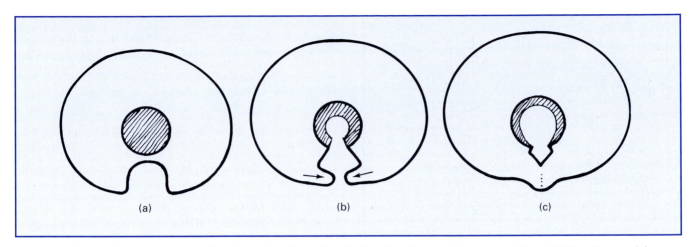

Fig. 9.14 *Schematic transverse section of developing glanular urethra. (**a**) Ectodermal ingrowth in centre of glans. (**b**) Canalization of the ectodermal ingrowth; genital folds and preputial folds beginning to fuse (arrows) to form the floor of the glanular urethra. (**c**) Glandular urethra completely formed. (Reprinted, by permission, from Sommer, J.T. and Stephens, F.D. (1980), Dorsal urethral diverticulum of the fossa navicularis: symptoms, diagnosis and treatment. J. Urol. 124: 94, Fig. 7.)*

The ducts of Cowper's (bulbourethral) glands

Cowper's glands are paired and lie posterolateral to the membranous urethra, caudal to the external urethral sphincter, cranial to the corpus spongiosum and bulbo-cavernosus muscles, and medial to the voluntary fibres of the pubourethralis muscle. The two ducts course medially and posteriorly from the glands between the cavernous tissue of the bulb and the urethral mucosa and run side by side to issue into the floor of the bulbous urethra. The orifices of the ducts normally issue together along the bulbous urethra. Ectasias are termed cysts of the ducts of Cowper's glands or Cowper syringoceles (Maizels *et al.*, 1983).

Anomalies of these ducts are discovered in the course of investigation of symptoms such as spotting of blood or postvoiding dribbling of urine or intermittent impairment of flow and discomfort during voiding.

Radiography of Cowper's duct

One or rarely both ducts may show reflux on voiding cystourethrography as a fine radiopaque line beneath the floor of the bulbous urethra or as an ectatic pear-shaped or bi- or triloculated duct leading to a narrow proximal tubular extension into the acini of the gland (Eding, 1953) (Figs 9.15 and 9.16). The large reflux orifice may be located anywhere in the floor of the posterior half of the bulbous urethra, and because the duct is in the submucosal layer, the apposing walls are thin and relatively avascular. The loculations may be due to developmental ectasia of the acini that lie in the walls of the main duct (Fig. 9.15). Less commonly, the orifice of the duct may be stenosed or occluded, in which event, the overexpanded duct encroaches on the lumen of the urethra (Fig. 9.16c).

Surgical procedures

The thin common wall between bulbous urethra and duct and its meatus is usually conspicuous endoscopically: the dysuria and haemorrhage are cured by resection of this common wall in the bulbous urethra.

The duct orifice, however, may lie more posteriorly at the back of the bulb. The orifice and common wall are not then precisely accessible to the endoscopist, and a perineal procedure is preferable as indicated in the following case report.

Case study

M.G., aged five years, complained of intermittent stoppages and difficulties with micturition over a period of six months. On one occasion, an attack of acute retention was relieved by catheter. Voiding cystourethrography demonstrated an ectatic duct resembling a diverticulum arising from the junction of the membranous urethra with the bulb. The lumen of the diverticulum lay parallel to the posterior wall of the bulbous and membranous urethra, terminating at the level of the verumontanum. During voiding, the diverticulum distended and compressed the urethra and remained full for at least 10 minutes after voiding (Fig. 9.17). Urethroscopy showed that the small orifice of the diverticulum was directed toward the perineum, and lay on the back of the bulbous urethra. Surgery was

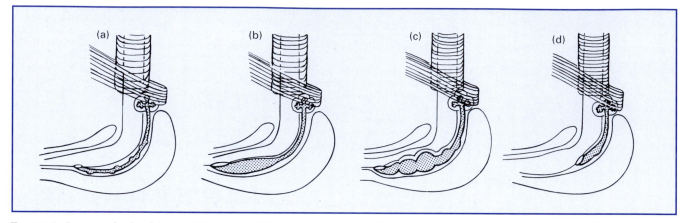

Fig. 9.15 *Cowper's gland and duct.* (*a*) *Normal gland lies cranial to the perineal membrane, caudal to the external sphincter and partly covered by the pubourethral muscle. The duct runs between the urethral epithelial layer and the corpus spongiosum. Note small glands opening into side of duct in its subepithelial course.* (*b*),(*c*). *Ectatic ducts, orifices and glands partly impinging on urethral lumen.* (*d*) *Abnormal entry site of duct into back of the bulb. (Reprinted, by permission, from Stephens, F.D. (1983), Congenital Malformations of the Urinary Tract, New York, Praeger, Fig. 6.8, p. 142.)*

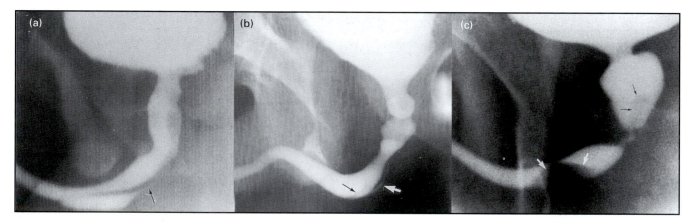

Fig. 9.16 *Cowper's duct ectasia.* (*a*) *R.D., aged two years—voiding cystourethrogram (VCU) showing opaque medium refluxing into the dilated duct which slightly compresses the bulbous urethra. More cranially, the duct (arrow) is minimally dilated indicated by arrow.* (*b*) *B.K.K.—VCU showing irregular lumen of posterior urethra (black arrow) reflux into the slightly ectatic ducts.* (*c*) *R.A.—stenosis of Cowper's duct with filling defect in dilated posterior urethra (black arrows) and in bulbar urethra caused by the distended enlarged duct (white arrows). (Reprinted, by permission, from Stephens, F.D. (1983), Congenital Malformations of the Urinary Tract, New York, Praeger, Fig. 6.9, p. 142.)*

performed through the perineum. The bulbous urethra was laid open, and the orifice of the diverticulum was identified. The diverticulum was found to lie in the submucosal plane of the membranous urethra. Simple diathermy excision of the thin septum that formed the wall common to urethra and diverticulum alleviated all symptoms (Fig. 9.17).

Embryogenesis of Cowper's duct cyst

Cowper's glands develop as solid paired epithelial buds growing from the urogenital sinus at the junction of the pelvic and perineal urethra. The glands come to lie above the perineal membrane. The ducts elongate with lengthening of the bulbous urethra, canalize and issue into the floor of the bulb to either side of the midline by very small orifices. At the cranial ends, mucus-secreting acini form in lobules, and small acini also arise at intervals along the course of the ducts (Fig. 9.15a). By faulty development, the duct and orifice may be diffusely ectatic, or the duct may exhibit irregular ectasia resulting from a combination of ectasia of the duct and the mucous glands in the wall, or the orifice of the duct may be stenosed or occluded.

The urethral glands and the valve of Guérin

Morgagni described the urethral glands (lacunae urethralis) in 1719. These glands in the penile and glandar urethra comprise the glands of Littré and the lacuna magna or 'valve' or sinus of Guérin.

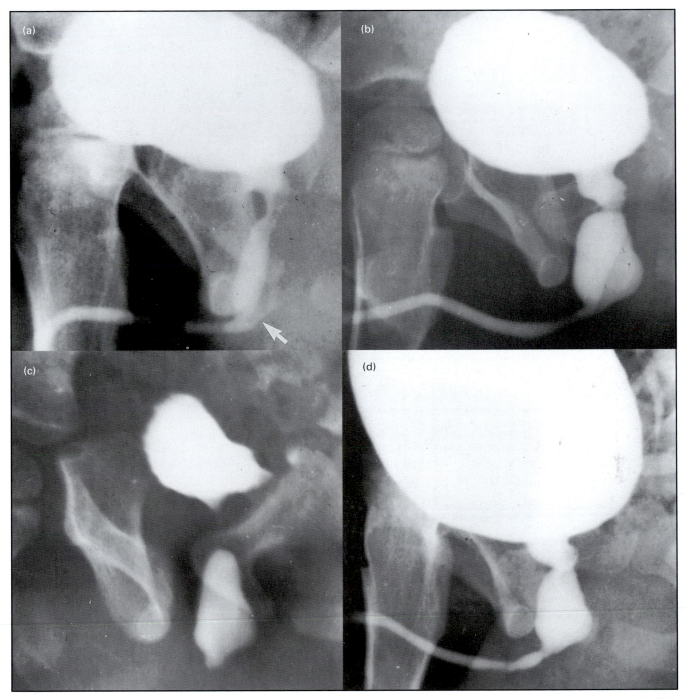

Fig. 9.17 *Voiding cystourethrograms showing reflux into an ectatic duct arising from the back of the bulb. (**a**) Cowper's duct (arrow). (**b**) Wide distension of the ectatic gland. (**c**) Residual content in the ectatic duct and gland and bladder after voiding. (**d**) Urethral lumen after marsupialization of the ectatic duct into the posterior urethra. (Reprinted, by permission, from Stephens, F.D. (1963),* Congenital Malformations of the Rectum, Anus and Genito-Urinary Tracts. *Edinburgh, Livingstone, Fig. 139, p. 241.)*

Littré's glands

Littré's glands are located chiefly in the bulbous and distal penile urethra. Multiple small puncta in the floor and side walls denote the orifices of the short ducts, which are directed cranially under the mucosa of the urethra. Most of the ducts drain short branching tubular glands. Ordinarily, these orifices are so small that they escape notice during endoscopic examinations, but occasionally, the orifice and duct are conspicuous because of their wide calibre. These ectatic ducts may be opacified during the voiding cystourethrography, appearing as a linear streak several millimetres long lying parallel to the wall of the urethra. Recurrent painless bleeding after micturition is the symptom that is presumably caused by overstretching by reflux of urine of the delicate duct wall, and that subsides after endoscopic resection of this common wall.

These ducts form as outgrowths from the urethral lining at about the ninth week of embryonic life at the time of fusion of the genital folds and tubularization of the anterior urethra. They do not penetrate the cavernous structures, but grow backwards parallel to the urethra. Developmental overgrowth of the duct may account for this occasional anomaly.

Lacuna magna

The lacuna magna or sinus of Guérin is a dorsal diverticulum in the roof of the fossa navicularis, and is present in approximately 30 per cent of boys as either a small pit or a sinus of up to 4–6-mm long. The sinus is directed cranially adjacent and parallel to the urethra, and is the only diverticulum of the anterior urethra arising from the roof. Guérin (1864) called it a valve because it sometimes impaired the retrograde passage of a sound but did not obstruct orthograde flow of urine.

Histological examinations of the lacuna magna obtained from postmortem specimens revealed a sinus lined by squamous epithelium in the depths of which were situated nests of mucous glands.

This diverticulum, however, may cause intermittent postvoid spotting of blood from the meatus, microhaematuria or frank haematuria, or sometimes discomfort or severe pain in the vicinity of the glans during voiding. The onset of symptoms in the children studied ranged from four to nine years in four children previously reported (Sommer and Stephens, 1980). The factors triggering the symptoms may be changes in the orientation of the orifice by growth resulting in a cusplike distal lip that directs urine flow into the diverticulum, causing overstretching of the walls of the sinus.

Voiding cystourethrography, undertaken for symptoms of haematuria or dysuria, may reveal the lacuna magna, which appears as a smooth, spherical radiopaque globule overlying the fossa navicularis (Figs 9.18 and 9.19).

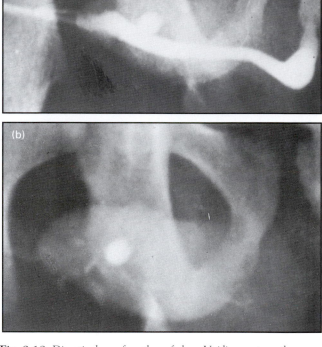

Fig. 9.18 *Diverticulum of urethra of glans. Voiding cystourethrogram showing expanded dorsal diverticulum with residual filling during (**a**) and after (**b**) voiding (symptom: painless postvoiding spotting of blood). (Reprinted, by permission, from Sommer, J.T. and Stephens, F.D. (1980), Dorsal urethral diverticulum of the fossa navicularis: symptoms, diagnosis and treatment. J. Urol. 124: 94, Fig. 4.)*

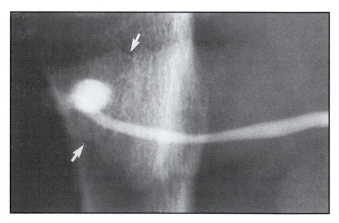

Fig. 9.19 *Diverticulum of the urethra of the glans. Voiding cystourethrogram showing rounded dorsal diverticula overlying urethral lumen: corona marked by arrows (symptom: pain in glans penis during voiding). (Reprinted, by permission, from Sommer, J.T. and Stephens, F.D. (1980), Dorsal urethral diverticulum of the fossa navicularis: symptoms, diagnosis and treatment. J. Urol. 124: 94, Fig. 2.)*

Errors of interpretation may occur if the urethrogram is carried out with the boy in the supine position because radiopaque droplets may hang under the corona

(Fig. 9.20), or be splashed on towels, or because the urethra of the glans lies beyond the limit of the film frame or is obscured in a dark corner of the film.

The lacuna magna may be probed or viewed endoscopically to confirm its presence. Probing can be carried out using Xylocaine jelly for local anaesthesia or general anaesthesia as a preliminary to endoscopy. A lacrimal probe or the eye end of a fine, straight needle passed along the roof of the fossa navicularis in the midline will arrest in the blind end of the diverticulum. By gradual withdrawal and ventral tilting, the probe can be disengaged from the diverticulum into the lumen of the urethra. In this way, it is possible to estimate the depth of the lacuna (Fig. 9.21a).

Surgical treatment

The proximity of the orifice of the lacuna magna to the meatus in the glans makes endoscopy tricky in small boys. The orifice is a transverse slit lying astride the roof of the fossa navicularis, and its interior cannot be inspected, though a ureteric catheter may be directed into it.

Transmeatal marsupialization of the diverticulum into the urethra by division of the common wall proved to be effective. One fine blade of a small pair of blunt-pointed scissors can be probed into the depths of the diverticulum and the other blade concurrently directed along the floor of the urethra. The common wall is then cut to complete the marsupialization (Fig. 9.21). Alternatively, the common wall may be divided by endoscopic fulguration. No serious bleeding occurs and the symptoms are usually eliminated.

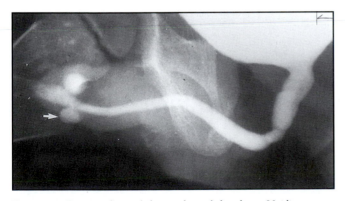

Fig. 9.20 *Diverticulum of the urethra of the glans. Voiding cysto-urethrogram showing the distended dorsal diverticulum and droplet hanging from the corona mimicking a ventral diverticulum (arrow). (Reprinted, by permission, from Stephens, F.D. (1983), Congenital Malformations of the Urinary Tract, New York, Praeger, Fig. 6.13, p. 145.)*

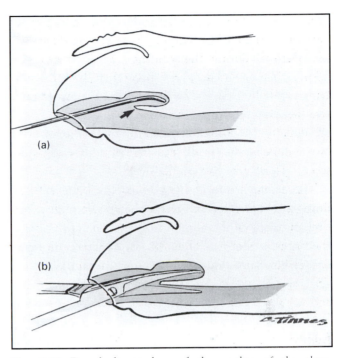

Fig. 9.21 *Dorsal diverticulum of the urethra of the glans. (a) Identification and measurement of depth of diverticulum by lacrimal probe. (b) Transmeatal marsupialization by division of the adjacent walls of the diverticulum and urethra with scissors. (Reprinted, by permission, from Sommer, J.T. and Stephens, F.D. (1980), Dorsal urethral diverticulum of the fossa navicularis: symptoms, diagnosis and treatment. J. Urol. 124: 94, Fig. 5.)*

Embryogenesis of the lacuna magna

The concepts of Glenister (1954, 1956) concerning the development of the glanular and penile urethra are supported by the anatomical and histological studies of the lacuna magna of Sommer and Stephens (1980) and Stephens and Fortune (1993).

The genital tubercle develops at the anterior end of the phallic part (urethral plate) of the urogenital sinus (Fig. 9.12a). When the tubercle elongates to form the body of the penis, the urethral plate also elongates, retaining its contact with the base of the glans (Fig. 9.12b). The urethral plate is then tubularized by the midline meeting from behind forward of the inner genital folds or edges of the plate to form, first, the bulbous and then the penile parts of the urethra to the base of the glans (Fig. 9.12c).

The outer ectodermal genital folds also meet in the midline from behind forward, merging into and over the uniting inner folds. The line of fusion is demarcated by the perineal and penile raphe. The outer folds, however, continue fusion beyond the base of the glans, prolong the tubularized urethra onto the undersurface of the glans, and join with the preputial folds to form the frenulum (Fig. 9.12d,e,f).

A solid ectodermal core develops in the centre of the glans, grows inward parallel with, but overlying, the roof of the new urethra on the underside of the glans, and becomes canalized (Fig. 9.12c,d). The contiguous walls of this ectodermal ingrowth and the urethra break down to establish urethral continuity (Fig. 9.12d,e,f). This natural 'anastomosis' coalesces the orifices of the sinus and glandar urethra and the lumens of both into one capacious orifice and fossa navicularis respectively (Figs 9.13 and 9.14).

Normally, curvilinear markings may remain in the fossa navicularis along the line of anastomosis. In some normal individuals, the anastomosis may be incomplete in the deepest part of the ectodermal sinus, giving rise to a small pit known as the 'lacuna magna'. If the sinus is abnormally long and the anastomosis incomplete, the lacuna may become a diverticulum and give rise to the symptoms and signs described here (Fig. 9.13).

Histological studies provide clues that support this embryology. The epithelium of the entire glandar urethra was squamous and extended proximally to the penile urethra which was lined by a transitional type of epithelium.

Congenital meatal stenosis

Congenital meatal stenosis may occur as a narrowing of the normally situated glanular orifice or in association with hypospadias.

Congenital stenosis of the normally located orifice is exceptionally rare, presumably because developmentally it is a compound of two orifices. In circumcised children, acquired stenosis of the orifice is common and follows meatal ulceration.

Hypospadiac meatal stenosis is not uncommon and occurs in the ectopic meatus, which may be concealed in the floor of the blind meatus, or exposed on the glans, corona or shaft of the penis (Fig. 9.22). Coronal or penile ectopic orifices may be accompanied by a blind sinus, the orifice of which lies slightly anterior, and the body of the sinus co-apts the roof of the urethra for a distance of approximately 2 cm. The sinus is made use of in the anterior meatotomy procedure described by Browne (1950) for enlarging the stenotic ectopic orifice.

Meatal stenosis causes prolonged, painless micturition, a fine-calibre jet and, in hypospadias, a deviated stream (Fig. 9.22). Catheter calibration of the meatus is the most accurate method of determining stenosis when in doubt. The normal calibre is 10F or larger (see Appendix 1, page 437).

Voiding cystourethrography shows the whole of the opacified urethra expanded to no more than maximal normal calibre even when the stenosis is severe.

In meatal stenosis associated with hypospadias, the calibre of the whole urethra is sometimes enlarged greatly and out of all proportion to the degree of narrowing. In fact, even where no narrowing exists at all, the calibre may be excessively large. The urethral dilatation is sometimes a developmental anomaly, an ectasia

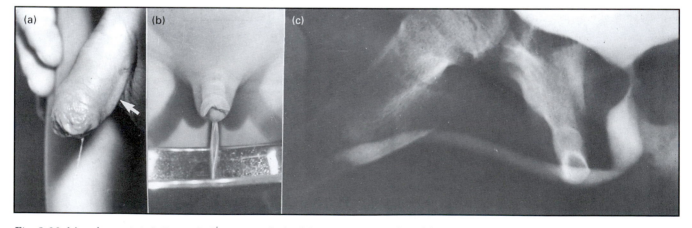

Fig. 9.22 *Meatal stenosis in L.P., aged $10\frac{1}{2}$ years, with glandular meatal hypospadias. (**a**) Extremely fine stream; note maximal distension of the urethra during voiding (arrow). (**b**) Wide stream after meatotomy. (**c**) Voiding cystourethrogram in same boy. Note general distension of the urethra proximal to the meatus. ((**a**) reprinted, by permission, from Stephens, F.D. (1963), Congenital Malformations of the Rectum, Anus and Genito-Urinary Tracts. Edinburgh, Livingstone, Fig. 142, p. 243.)*

associated with the hypospadias deformity and independent of obstruction.

Phimosis

The prepuce covers the glans and may be short or excessively long and exhibit congenital or acquired stenosis. Most developmental stenoses do not obstruct the stream but are regarded as being too narrow if the prepuce cannot be freely rolled back exposing the glans. Smegmaliths and balanitis may complicate the condition. Tight stenosis of a large prepuce causes urine to be dammed back and a swelling to appear during voiding (Fig. 9.23). The phimosis may be congenital or acquired either from constant wetting and infection as with some patients with neuropathic bladders or following faulty circumcision. The regular subpreputial irrigations with each voiding cleanses the glans and inhibits infection.

Congenital 'bladder neck' dysfunction

The preceding descriptions encompass a wide range of abnormalities that lead to an equally wide range of symptoms—those of infection, of uraemia or urethral blockage. But it is to be noted that idiopathic 'bladder neck' hypertrophy (Marion, 1933) and fibroelastosis (Bodian, 1957), previously considered to be common forms of obstruction in children, are now rarities. Features that incriminated the bladder neck in children in the 1950s and 1960s resulted from the introduction of routine voiding cystourethrography. The narrow internal meatus, sacculations in the bladder wall or diverticula, megacystis, presence of residual urine and vesicoureteral reflux were attributed to fibrosis, fibroelastosis or hypertrophy of the bladder neck. Now the bladder neck has been exonerated since it has come to

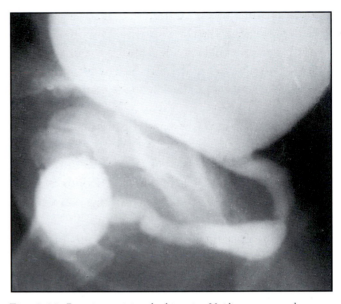

Fig. 9.23 *Postcircumcisional phimosis. Voiding cystourethrogram showing subpreputial collection of contrast medium and distended penile urethra. (Reprinted, by permission, from Stephens, F.D. (1983), Congenital Malformations of the Urinary Tract, New York, Praeger, Fig. 6.19, p. 149.)*

be realized that the calibre of the internal meatus is inconstant and unpredictable, rarely structurally abnormal, and not a cause of vesicoureteral reflux or megacystis–megaureter syndrome. Many of the symptoms such as dysuria, frequency of micturition, enuresis, stop–start micturition and urgency are related to so-called 'dyssynergia of the vesical detrusor and external sphincter of the urethra'. The symptomatology of the dyssynergia syndrome results from impairment, usually self-limiting, of the complex neuromuscular mechanisms of micturition, and furthermore, vesical diverticula in children once regarded as pathognomic of outlet obstruction often result from congenital flaws in the muscle meshwork of the bladder.

Congenital intrinsic lesions of the female urethra

The urethral image in the female as demonstrated radiographically during voiding is now familiar to the clinician, but the many configurations of the bladder neck, urethra and outlet are still confusing. The interpretation of the radiological features is helped by the correlation of the anatomy of the muscular sphincters that shape the urethra during the act of micturition and the current urodynamic and electromyographic studies of urethral function.

The technique of the radiographic procedure is similar in many respects to that already described for boys. The anteroposterior posture is, however, suited for demonstration of the lower two-thirds of the female urethra, and because of the overlap of the bladder lumen on the bladder neck, the oblique or lateral views demonstrate the upper one-third of the urethra more clearly (Fig. 10.1).

The bladder during voiding becomes crinkled, the internal meatus widens as the vesical detrusor contracts and the urethra exhibits many variations of shape (Fig. 10.2).

Most commonly, the urethra shows up as an almost cylindrical column with, sometimes, a gentle bulging of its upper and middle zones, which taper quite rapidly to a narrower calibre at the external orifice. In females, the terminal urethra is sagittally elongated, but rarely stenotic, and may be directed anteriorly (Fig. 10.1).

In some children, the force of the detrusor and the excessive relaxation of the sphincters combine to create an unusually wide lumen, thus mimicking the features of obstruction at or near the outlet (Fig. 10.1c).

In female children whose streams are very forceful, waves suggestive of peristaltic activity are sometimes seen on the anterior urethral outline (Fig. 10.1b).

During the course of micturition, the urethral shape may change from cylindrical to fusiform to arrowhead to conical or to wineglass, before the last, thin column of opaque medium is extruded by peristalsis from the urethra (Fig. 10.2). These shapes reflect the activity of the involuntary and voluntary muscles of the urethral walls and are all variants of normal.

In the female urethra, sudden cessation of micturition by voluntary effort occludes the longer and lower striated sphincter zone of the urethral column. The lowest part of this zone closes first, quickly followed by the remainder, with radiographically demonstrable retro-

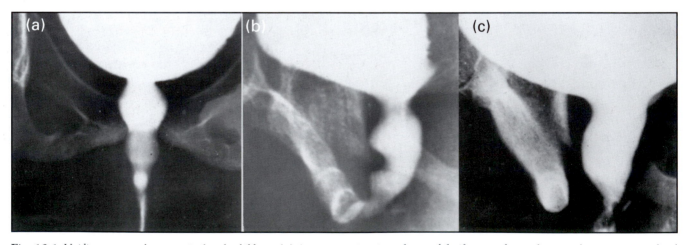

Fig. 10.1 *Voiding cystourethrograms in female children. (**a**) Anteroposterior view of normal fusiform urethra and narrow but not stenotic distal urethra. (**b**) Oblique view showing better view of bladder neck and wider sagittally oriented distal urethra. (**c**) Wide urethra of enuretic child with non-stenotic but radiographically narrow outlet. (Reprinted, by permission, from Stephens, F.D. (1963),* Congenital Malformations of the Rectum, Anus and Genito-Urinary Tracts. *Edinburgh, Livingstone, Figs 117 and 118, p. 216.)*

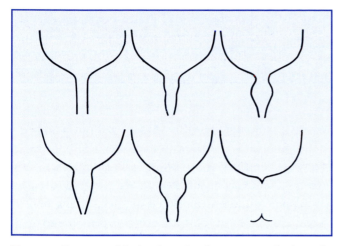

Fig. 10.2 *Diagrams of the female urethra depicting normal radiographic configurations with descriptive terms. Note also variations in the width of the bladder neck. The shapes may change from one to another in the same child during voidance. (Reprinted, by permission, from Stephens, F.D. (1983), Congenital Malformations of the Urinary Tract, New York, Praeger, Fig. 7.2, p. 155.)*

grade emptying of the opaque medium into the bladder. This is known as the 'milk-back phenomenon'. Sudden occlusion of this zone by the external sphincter precedes closure of the internal sphincter and a short, sharply cut-off cup-shaped segment of the urethra amounting to one-quarter or one-fifth remains momentarily filled in free communication with the bladder. Finally, this upper zone closes, leaving only the smooth outline of the bladder base (Fig. 10.3).

Sphincters of the female urethra

Specimens of the pelvic organs from newborn female subjects were prepared *en bloc* in paraffin and cut in serial sections of 15-μm thickness and studied microscopically.

The involuntary muscle was heaped around the internal meatus and the upper one-quarter of the urethra in mainly transverse orientation. In the lower three-quarters of the urethra, the involuntary muscle was disposed beneath the mucosa in two layers, an inner longitudinal and an outer circular and oblique, thus equipping the urethra for peristalsis (Fig. 10.4).

Surrounding the lower three-quarters of the urethra is the circularly arranged intrinsic voluntary muscle of the external sphincter. Some voluntary-muscle fibres can be identified in some urethras as high as the internal meatus.

The narrowest sites in the female urethra are at the perineal membrane where the urethra is fixed to this membrane, which is rigid and holds the otherwise distensible tube to a fixed circumference and diameter, and the external urethral orifice. The normal orifice of the urethra has been accurately calibrated (Immergut *et al.*, 1967; see also Appendix 1, page 438) and subsequent calibrations of other children with urinary infection or vesicoureteral reflux have been shown to be within the normal range for age (Immergut and Wahman, 1968).

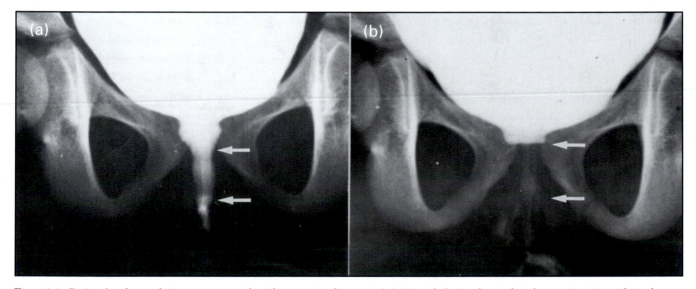

Fig. 10.3 *D.A., female, aged six years—normal voiding cystourethrogram.* (**a**) *Upper bulge in the urethra demarcating internal involuntary sphincter zone.* (**b**) *The zone of urethral lumen obliterated by contraction of voluntary external sphincter and the internal sphincter still open. Arrows indicate external sphincter zone. (Reprinted, by permission, from Stephens, F.D. (1963), Congenital Malformations of the Rectum, Anus and Genito-Urinary Tracts. Edinburgh, Livingstone, Fig. 119, p. 217.)*

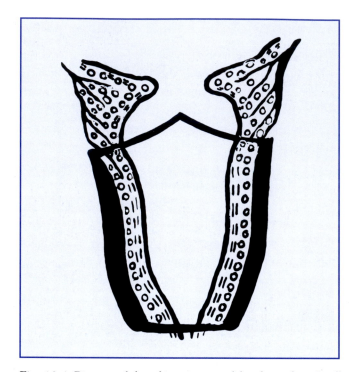

Fig. 10.4 *Diagram of the sphincter zones of female urethra. Small circles represent involuntary circular muscle of the internal sphincter and the outer circular muscle coat of the urethra. Coupled lines represent longitudinally oriented smooth muscle in the bladder and urethra. Black bands indicate extent of the external voluntary muscle sphincter.* (Reprinted, by permission, from Stephens, F.D. (1983), Congenital Malformations of the Urinary Tract, *New York, Praeger, Fig. 7.4, p. 156.*)

The external meatus is rarely, if ever, stenotic in young female children.

Urethral symptomology of female children

Symptoms such as dysuria, frequency, urgency or hesitancy of micturition, impulsive voiding, dribbling of urine or enuresis may accompany acute urinary-tract infections or arise from delays in maturation of the neural arcs and higher centres. These delays induce dyssynergia in the bladder sphincter and nocturnal or diurnal enuresis. The bladder neck was previously considered to be hypertrophic or exhibit fibroelastosis leading to impairment of micturition and surgical procedures such as resection of the bladder neck or Y–V plasty procedures were undertaken to reduce resistance to urine flow. However, these procedures have failed to gain the expected relief of symptoms and are now rarely indicated. 'Distal urethral stenosis' in female children was diagnosed by bougie-à-boule calibrations, the 'stenosis' lying either at the site of penetration of the urogenital membrane by the urethra or at the meatus, or both (Lyon and Smith, 1963). This narrow segment was regarded as a significant obstruction and a possible cause of stasis and infection. Subsequent calibration studies (Immergut and Wahman, 1968) of normal female urethras showed that calibrations of the urethras of children with recurrent urinary infection fall within the normal range for age. However, any sudden change in calibre converts laminar to turbulent flow, creating eddies that may carry meatal organisms into the bladder during voiding (Cox et al., 1968). Hence the wide urethra and the narrow normal calibre at the distal end may promote infection, which is further enhanced by the milk-back phenomenon observed radiographically in patients with dyssynergia of the sphincter muscles. The reasons for improvement of symptoms of the recurrence rate of infection derived from urethral dilatation in some patients may be due to improvement in the voiding patterns and not to the presence of an underlying congenital stenosis of the urethra.

Embryogenesis of the distal urethra

The urethra in females is unlikely to be anatomically stenotic because of the simplicity of its origins. When the internal cloaca is partitioned by the urorectal septum, the wolffian ducts then open into the anterior urinary compartment at the level of the verumontanum (Müller's tubercle), caudal to the bladder neck. These ducts demarcate the urethra cranial and the urogenital sinus caudal to their point of entry. The urethra elongates and undergoes local expansion resulting from absorption into its walls of the adjoining terminal segments of the wolffian ducts, and the urogenital sinus expands and exstrophies to form the vestibule in the vulva. The process of expansion of the urogenital sinus is enhanced by the arrival and rapid growth and expansion of the müllerian ducts, which migrate caudally from a pelvic to a perineal location. All these embryological events favour expansion or overexpansion of the female urethra in addition to normal growth. In some female children, the pelvic urethra is shown by voiding cystourethrography to be extremely wide. This widening might develop as a result of overexpansion and absorption of the terminal ends of the wolffian ducts into the urethra.

Skene's glands (paraurethral glands)

Skene's glands are single tubular glands that arise as multiple urethral epithelial outgrowths from the vesicourethral canal around the site of entry of the wolffian ducts at about the 11-week stage of development. They become prostatic ducts and glands in the male, but in the female, these ducts are farther apart and eventually come to be in the external urinary meatus between the meatus and hymen. In the newborn period, a blocked Skene's duct may form a large cyst, which partially extrudes into the vestibule compressing and deflecting the urethral meatus sideways. The cyst is sessile, one-third within and two-thirds outside the meatal margin, and is tense, yellow and thin-walled. It may resemble a bulging hymen associated with hydrometrocolpos, but lateral deflection of the meatus on the side of the cyst typifies the cyst (Fig. 10.5). A prolapsed ureterocele protrudes from the urethra, but is fleshy and protrudes through the meatus and usually retracts spontaneously.

Bartholin's gland

The major vestibular glands of Bartholin arise one on each side from the pars phallica of the urogenital sinus as solid epithelial buds at about the ninth week of development. At first, the buds issue into the sinus caudal to the site of the müllerian ducts but with progressive exstrophy of the pars phallica and pars pelvina of the sinus and the descent of the müllerian ducts (vagina and hymen), the Bartholin ducts open finally in the vestibule on either side of the hymen (see Fig. 1.8). The gland comes to lie lateral to the vaginal orifice against the ischiopubic ramus deep to the bulbospongiosus muscle and cavernous tissue. The gland is mucus secreting and has a central reservoir into which open tributaries that carry the mucus to it. The main duct, also

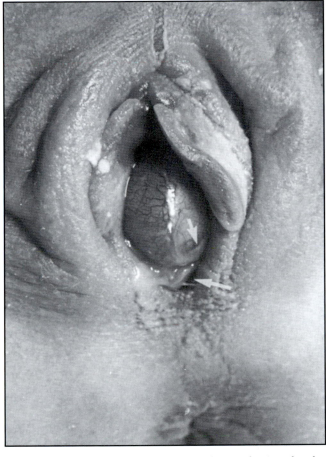

Fig. 10.5 *Skene's duct cyst. Vulva of newborn Baby A with right-sided cyst deflecting, flattening and protruding the external urethral orifice to the left (upper arrow) and vaginal introitus (lower arrow). (Reprinted, by permission, from Stephens, F.D. (1983), Congenital Malformations of the Urinary Tract, New York, Praeger, Fig. 7.5, p. 156.)*

lined by mucus-secreting epithelium, emerges from the reservoir and issues into the vestibule at the base of the external surface of the hymen on each side. This gland and duct rarely exhibit abnormalities during infancy or childhood. Cystic dilatation may arise from blockage of the main duct. Infections in this gland are rare before puberty.

The bladder

III

The routine use of micturition cystourethrography in paediatric urology in the last 30 years has made clinicians aware of many aspects of bladder function and anatomy that had not been fully considered hitherto. These include many normal variants of shape and size of the bladder and bladder neck, ureterovesical incompetence, hiatal hernias, sacculations, and small, large and multiple diverticula, all of which are better demonstrated during the act of voiding. The impact of the new radiographic data led to differences of opinion regarding the clinical significance of various shapes and sizes of the bladder, bladder neck and urethra and the aetiology of vesical diverticula, reflux, cystitis and enuresis. As the result of combined radiological, pathological, experimental and urodynamic studies, it has been found that the urotracts present many variations in contour and activity, which mimic abnormal patterns but have no long-term clinical significance. The embryogenesis of these variants, together with descriptions of the bladder and urethral musculature and the normal and abnormal structure of the ureterovesical hiatus, are included in this chapter.

Exstrophy of the bladder is excluded, and urorectogenital anomalies and the prune belly syndrome are described in Chapters 2 and 37, respectively.

Radiological anatomy

The bladder has labile walls that constitute the body or vertex, and a fundus, which is a firm, triangular muscular platform anchored directly to the pubis and indirectly through the urethra to the urogenital diaphragm. When empty, the vertex tilts ventrally, and the superior wall rests upon the inferior wall. With filling, the bladder becomes spherical, pear-shaped or conical, rising up into the lower abdomen upon the base. With the act of voiding, the vertex maintains a globular shape, diminishing in size until nearly empty, when the bladder base becomes tubular and similar in dimensions to the urethra. The ureters enter the posterolateral corners of the bladder base. The internal urinary meatus lies at the caudal and anterior apex of the trigone on the bladder base.

The lateral wall of the bladder may bulge on either or both sides giving the appearance of 'ears'. In the newborn period, the ears may be long enough to extend in a paraperitoneal plane into the inguinal canals. These ears result from temporary weakness in the lateral walls, which strengthen postnatally as more circular muscle bundles form in the hypoplastic areas.

In infants, the bladder is abdominal and the urethra pelvic, the internal meatus lying behind the upper surface of the symphysis pubis. In adults, the normal bladder is accommodated mainly in the relatively larger and deeper pelvis.

The position of the internal urinary meatus in infants is located close behind the symphysis pubis and exhibits a well-marked posterior lip during voiding. It may, however, lie further back, in which event, the anterior lip becomes equal to or greater than the posterior lip as shown by voiding cystourethrography (see Fig. 6.5). Very rarely, the internal meatus may be located high on the anterior bladder wall above the pubis, in which event, the posterior lip may be so long that it acts as a flap valve and fails to retract to open the meatus, causing severe obstruction to the bladder outlet (see Fig. 8.23).

Musculature

The arrangement of the detrusor muscles is more readily understood if the layers are described first in the empty bladder when the vertex has an upper and lower wall attached posteroinferiorly to the trigonal platform.

The circular muscle coat of the vertex is constructed in loose rungs made up from a circularly oriented meshwork of bundles of fibres. These rungs rest on the bladder base and rise up over the dome. Around the bladder base itself, the circular rungs are packed more tightly and diminish in circumference toward the internal urinary meatus.

The inner longitudinal coat is delicate, incomplete and, on the dome, intermingles with the circular rungs.

It is chiefly oriented over the superior and inferior walls and is weak laterally but reinforces and guards the medial end of the ureterovesical tunnel (Figs 11.1 and 11.2).

It is continued as a thin and incomplete layer through the internal meatus but reconstitutes into a definite inner longitudinal coat in middle and distal urethra, where it is in intimate contact with the outer circular smooth muscle coat. These two coats in the pelvic urethra, inner longitudinal and outer circular, equip the urethra with the function of peristalsis (see Figs 10.1 and 10.4).

The outer longitudinal layer is more robust, covering the posterior and anterior walls of the vertex. Superiorly, the muscle bundles cover and intermingle in a feltwork of fibres on the dome. Inferiorly, the muscle tendrils of the outer coat penetrate the circular muscle of the bladder neck; some of the fibre bundles of the posterior longitudinal coat traverse the bladder neck from back to front through and integrating into the circular muscle sphincter. The longitudinal muscle of the anterior wall gains strong anchorage to both the pubis through the

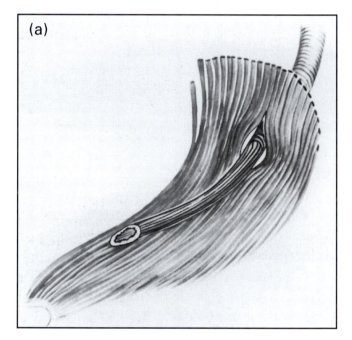

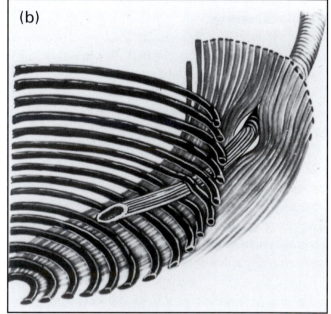

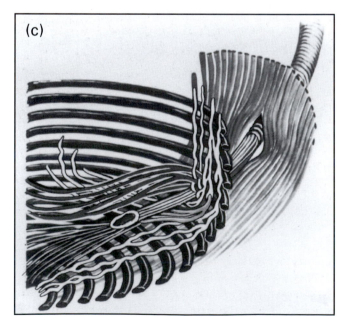

Fig. 11.1 *Normal ureterovesical hiatus. Entry of ureter through split in the posterior longitudinal muscle (**a**) and through circular muscle (**b**). (**c**) Inner longitudinal and some submucosal circular bundles interdigitating into roof and sides of the hiatus (thick white lines = longitudinal muscle). (Reprinted, with permission, from Stephens, F.D. (1978), The normal and abnormal ureterovesical hiatus: methods of correction of vesicoureteral reflux and paraureteral diverticula. J. Cont. Ed. Urol., Fig. 1.)*

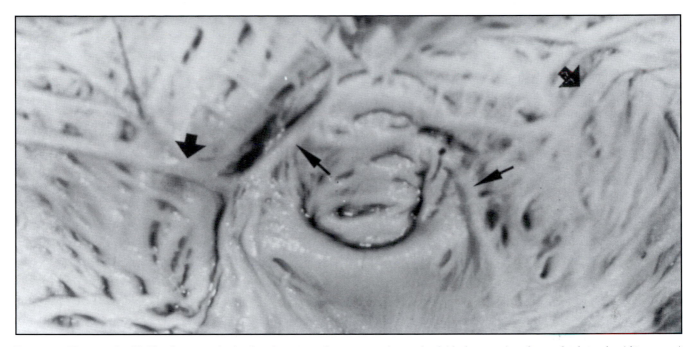

Fig. 11.2 *Hypertrophic bladder due to urethral valve obstruction showing inner longitudinal (thick arrows) and superficial circular (thin arrows) muscle bundles interdigitating around the hiatus. (Reprinted, with permission, from Stephens, F.D. (1978), The normal and abnormal ureterovesical hiatus: methods of correction of vesicoureteral reflux and paraureteral diverticula. J. Cont. Ed. Urol., Fig. 2.)*

pubourethral ligaments and the urethra through fasciculi that integrate into the internal sphincter and gain attachment to the sleeve of the external sphincter. This arrangement gives toeholds to the longitudinal coats, which draw the dome of the bladder toward the base and retract the walls of the internal urinary meatus during voiding. These coat-tails of the outer longitudinal muscle coat resemble the coat-tails of the outer longitudinal muscle of the rectum, which split up the internal and external sphincter muscles of the anus.

When the bladder fills, the walls stretch and the bladder becomes ovoid, the axis being directed anteriorly from the fundus to the umbilicus. The superior wall rises up and the lateral borders become rounded. The stretched lateral walls, especially near the base, are formed by the rungs of the circular muscle coat only. They are relatively weak in young children and are apt to exhibit bulges, saccules or diverticula, when the bladder is full and contracting (see Fig. 12.5e).

The ureters enter the bladder in the posterolateral corners between the fundus and vertex through the hiatus, which is bordered by all three muscle coats. Together with Waldeyer's fibromuscular sheath, they provide a watertight seal around the ureters and prevent the formation of saccules alongside the ureter in the muscular tunnel (Fig. 11.3). Having penetrated the

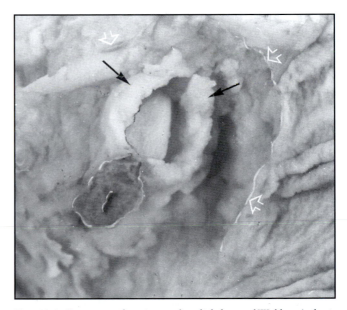

Fig. 11.3 *Dissection of specimen of medial sleeve of Waldeyer's fascia of normal left submucosal ureter. Vesical mucosa removed except for collar around ureteral meatus. Fascia (black arrows) incised longitudinally from collar to hiatus, exposing white wall of ureter. (Cut edges of mucosa indicated by white arrows and white lines.) (Reprinted, by permission, from Stephens, F.D. (1979), The vesicoureteral hiatus and paraureteral diverticula. J. Urol. 121, 786, Fig. 1.)*

muscle layers, the ureter then runs a short course in the submucosal plane to issue on the cornu of the trigone. Cussen (1967a, 1979) has provided normal values for the length of the submucosal segment of the ureter (Appendix 1, Number 5) and the position of the orifice relative to the internal urinary meatus according to age, length and weight (see trigonal measurements, Appendix 1, Number 10). The more detailed anatomy of the normal and abnormal ureterovesical hiatus is described in Chapter 12.

Embryology of the bladder and trigone

When the flat, discoid embryo turns itself into cylindrical form, it does so by folding in both longitudinal and transverse planes. The head and tail ends grow rapidly, forming the head and tail folds. With rapid growth of the tail fold, the allantois, body stalk and cloacal membrane rotate 180° to a ventral position, and part of the yolk sac is incorporated in the tail forming the future hind gut and cloaca. The urorectal septum then partitions the cloaca in the coronal plane into the vesicourinary canal anteriorly and the rectum posteriorly. Partition begins and ends between the fourth and sixth week (4-16-mm crown-rump length) (see Fig. 1.2).

Incorporation of wolffian ducts and ureters into the urinary tract

Early in the fourth week, the solid growing end of the wolffian (mesonephric) duct turns medially from the back wall of the embryo across the nephrogenic cord. It courses obliquely around the side wall of the cloaca to enter it anterolaterally near the cloacal membrane. Soon after penetration of the cloacal wall, the duct canalizes. The original entry point of the wolffian ducts into the cloaca is close to the anterior border of the cloacal membrane, and at the completion of partition of the cloaca, the orifices lie together high on the posterior wall of the anterior chamber at Müller's tubercle (the future verumontanum in the male) (Figs 1.3 and 1.10). Rathke's folds, which complete the subdivision of the cloaca, carry the duct orifices from lateral to posterior orientations, and atrophy of the roof of the orifice and duct transposes the orifice cranially.

The ureteric bud on each side arises from the wolffian duct posterior, but close to, the tubercle. The terminal end of the duct to a point cranial to the bud widens in trumpet shape and exstrophies into the vesicourethral canal, forming the provisional trigone and providing separate entry of wolffian duct into the urethra and of the ureter into the bladder (Fig. 1.10).

The vertex and allantoic contribution

The vesicourethral canal above the entry points of the wolffian ducts expands in globular fashion to create the vertex or reservoir of the bladder, and the terminal parts of both expanded wolffian ducts let in trigonal gussets in the fundus.

The vertex of the bladder is in continuity with the allantois and the site of junction between allantoic and cloacal parts of the bladder and urethra is a debated issue among embryologists (page 403). The allantois undergoes atrophy in the body stalk and adjoining vertex, and all that remains is a fibrous, cord-like connection between bladder dome and the umbilicus, called the 'urachal ligament'.

The muscle layers

After the visceral epithelial structures have attained their near final configuration at about 10–12 weeks (40–56-mm crown–rump length; Arey, 1974), the loose mesenchyme around these organs differentiates into smooth muscle. In the bladder, the muscle is laid down in three distinct layers (Felix, 1912a). The outer longitudinal layer of muscle appears first from the apex to the ureteric orifices on the dorsal wall, and is more thinly disposed elsewhere. A little later, in the loose mesenchyme between this muscle layer and the epithelium, the circular muscle layer develops in the apical region and gradually extends throughout the bladder. Later still, the inner incomplete longitudinal layer appears. Both the inner and outer longitudinal layers give off interlacing fascicles into the circular layer forming a feltwork over the dome of the bladder. Below the level of the ureteric orifices, circular muscle is oriented around the bladder base and forms the sphincter at the internal meatus. Later, the two longitudinal muscle coats are added to the bladder base though both are incomplete, especially laterally. The mesenchyme around the ureter and superficial trigone is transformed into the intrinsic musculature at a later stage.

The shape of the bladder and urethra is conditioned by a number of factors. First, the inherent embryological capacity of modelling a sphere from a tube; if the expansion and modelling lack the normal restraining influences, the bladder may exhibit overgrowth, irregular shapes or hourglass constrictions. Second, the taking up of the terminal ends of the wolffian ducts into the bladder base and trigone adds a gusset into the fundus, and if exaggerated, the prostatic urethra and trigone become enlarged. The normal dimensions of the trigone according to the age of the child have been determined by Paquin *et al.* (1960) and Cussen (1979). Third, the degree of regression of the allantois modifies the shape of the vertex and its proximity to the umbilicus.

If the kidneys are absent, and urine is not formed, the bladder conforms to the shape of the vertex and fundus of the bladder, but because of the lack of urine content, the bladder remains somewhat tubular, fails to expand and lags in growth during fetal life.

Bladder capacity was calculated from nuclear cystogram studies by Berger *et al.* (1982). The simple formula for bladder capacity in ounces according to age in years of the child is age plus 2 ounces (60 ml), up to 11 years. (Appendix 1.8)

Obstructive and non-obstructive diverticula

Gaps of weakness in the muscle meshwork lead to narrow or wide neck diverticula, depending on the size of the muscle defect. Bladder mucosa is forced by normal or abnormally raised voiding bladder pressures through the gap in the muscle of the bladder wall. Though in the past all diverticula were considered to be secondary to bladder neck or urethral obstruction, many are now known to occur in the absence of obstruction (Johnston, 1960; MacKellar and Stephens, 1960). In both instances, a primary pocket of weakness is essential to the development of a diverticulum.

Non-obstructive diverticula

Non-obstructive diverticula rarely cause symptoms directly resulting from the diverticulum itself. Most often, the diverticulum is small, paraureteral, and associated with vesicoureteral reflux which promotes stasis and infection. Large isolated diverticula without reflux may also promote infection. Rarely, the diverticulum may induce dysuria, which is the only symptom, and which is attributable to distension or overdistension of the herniated bladder mucosa.

Radiographic features of non-obstructive diverticula

Cystography and voiding cystourethrography are the usual means by which diverticula are first diagnosed. The cystogram as shown by excretory urography may demonstrate the presence of a diverticulum, though voiding cystourethrography will demonstrate the full size and declare others that do not show on passive filling of the bladder.

Voiding cystourethrography also provides a clear outline of the bladder neck and urethra and either discloses or excludes evidence of obstruction or vesicoureteral reflux.

It should be noted that, in children, spontaneous cures of small diverticula and bladder weaknesses occur over several years as the coats of the bladder gain muscle and strength.

Bladder and urethral pressures during voiding were recorded in patients with non-obstructive diverticula by MacKellar and Stephens (1960). The pressures were well within normal limits and the gradients between bladder and urethra in two patients were also normal.

Cystoscopic features

Cystoscopically, the narrow-neck diverticula, globular in shape, constituted the common variety and occurred mainly in relation to the lateral cornu of the trigone and the hiatus. They impinged on, or engulfed, the ureteric orifice or were entirely separate. Others were located in the lateral wall or dome of the bladder. Wide-neck diverticula were dish-shaped bulges in the lateral wall contiguous with the ureterovesical hiatus and were difficult to recognize cystoscopically, even when very obvious radiographically (see Fig. 12.5e).

Correlation of the cystoscopic and radiographic studies showed a relationship between the location of the diverticular orifice and competence of the uretero-vesical valve (Fig. 12.1). If the ureteric and diverticular orifices were completely separate, there was no reflux; if the orifices were contiguous, limited reflux into the lower part of the ureter occurred; if the ureteric orifice was engulfed in the diverticulum, there was free reflux (MacKellar and Stephens, 1960). It appears that lack of muscle may be responsible for both the diverticulum and the reflux (Fig. 12.1b). The intrinsic qualities of muscle and length of the submucosal ureter determine the state of continence of the ureterovesical junction when the orifice of the diverticulum was well clear of the ureteric orifice (Fig. 12.1).

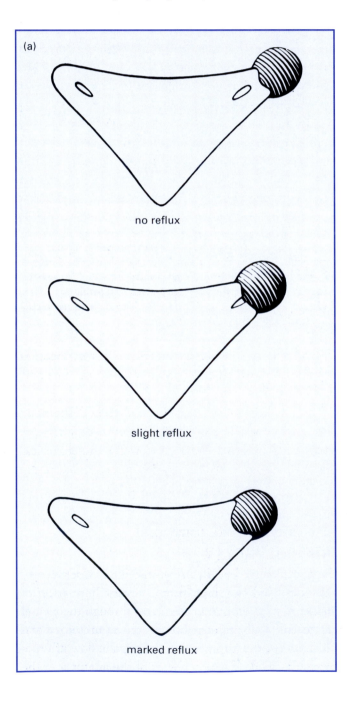

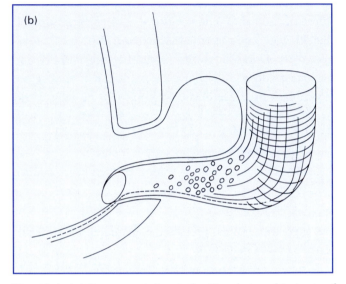

Fig. 12.1 (**a**) *Paraureteral diverticula. Correlation of intimacy of orifice of diverticulum and ureter to the vesicoureteric reflux.* (**b**) *Structure of intravesical ureter of Baby H., with paraureteral diverticulum and urethral valves. Muscle is absent in roof, then patchy, then thin and finally thick laterally. ((**a**) (**b**) reprinted, by permission, from MacKellar, A. and Stephens, F.D. (1960), Vesical diverticula in children. Aust. N.Z. J. Surg. 30: 20, Fig. 5. (b)*

Structure of non-obstructive diverticula

Most diverticula contain muscle around the neck and some muscle in the side walls, but in the dome of the expanded diverticulum, the muscle may be absent, or present only as sparse strands. The walls of several wide-neck diverticula exhibited either a thin but complete covering of muscle or, as in one specimen, a tissue-paper thickness of fibrous tissue in the centre with a surround of thin and incomplete smooth muscle.

Microscopic studies indicate that both narrow-neck and wide-neck diverticula have similar pathology, which MacKellar and Stephens (1960) describe as 'congenital failure of normal muscle development in a given area of bladder wall'. The narrow-neck diverticulum occurred most in the vicinity of the ureteric orifice (Fig. 12.3), but the wide-neck type characteristically occurs as deficiencies in the lateral wall, which is normally composed of interlacing bundles of circularly disposed muscle, and lacks the support of the internal and external longitudinal coats (Fig. 12.2).

Diverticula associated with urethral obstruction

The high intravesical pressures engendered by urethral obstruction cause generalized hypertrophy, sacculation and trabeculation of the bladder musculature. If the muscle of the bladder and Waldeyer's fascia are intact and undergo hypertrophy, diverticula do not occur. Areas of relative weakness or congenital absence of muscle develop into pulsion diverticula, which, unlike sacculations, protrude beyond the outside margin of the bladder wall. In children, after removal of the obstruction and the subsequent reduction of vesical pressures, many of the small and large diverticula disappear spontaneously.

Urachal diverticula

The urachus may fail to regress, or share the expansion stimulus of the bladder anlage, creating a diverticulum that may be so large it resembles the dome of an oversized bladder, or may be demarcated by a circumferential constriction. The muscle in the urachal segment may be irregularly disposed or absent, the coat being composed of mucosal lining reinforced by collagen and fibroblasts and sparse muscle cells. The dilated urachus may retain

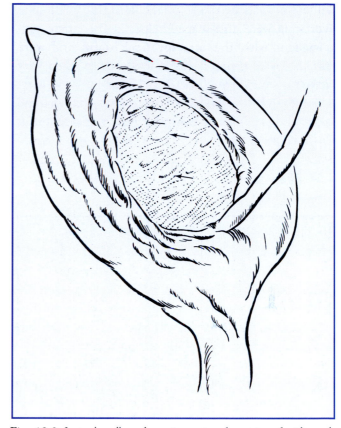

Fig. 12.2 *Lateral wall weakness promoting formation of wide neck diverticulum. Note the circular muscle coat with deficiencies (arrows) and ureter entering bladder at lowest point. Absence of longitudinal muscle in the lateral window. (Reprinted, by permission, from MacKellar, A. and Stephens, F.D. (1960), Vesical diverticula in children. Aust. N.Z. J. Surg. 30: 20, Fig. 6A.)*

free communication with the umbilicus or a connection by a fine cord, which may exhibit a lumen in some part of its course.

Abnormalities of size and shape, muscle deficiencies with or without collagen substitution in place of muscle, urachal anomalies and defects of the ureterovesical junction, all occur in infants with the so-called prune belly or triad malformation (Chapter 37).

The normal and abnormal vesicoureteral hiatus

The portal of entry of the ureter into the bladder is especially designed anatomically to prevent herniation of bladder mucosa alongside the ureter through the tunnel and to enhance the competence of the ureterovesical sphincter yet not to impair the antegrade flow of urine through it. The present concepts of the anatomy of the ureterovesical junction are made from contributions by many research workers, beginning in 1892 with Waldeyer who observed a muscular sheath derived from the vesical musculature around the extravesical ureter. Observations of others on the general and particular structure of the normal hiatus and ureter, together with defects and paraureteral diverticula, are added to elaborate the morphology of the junctional area.

The hiatus

The ureter enters the bladder through a cleft in the posterior longitudinal muscle at the posterolateral corner of the bladder where the labile wall meets the stable platform of the bladder base. The posterior external longitudinal muscle bundles radiate from the centre of the bladder base cranially and laterally and, at the cleft, diverge around the ureter and converge again cranial to it. In some bladders, the bundles fail to converge, leaving a thin area cranial to the tunnel covered only by the inner circular muscle layer (Gil-Vernet, 1948; Uhlenhuth *et al.*, 1953a). Once through the outer layer, the ureter dips between the rungs of the circular muscle coat and then lies on the circular muscle of the bladder base for a distance of up to 2 cm, depending on the age of the subject (see Fig. 11.1).

Muscle fascicles from the tenuous inner longitudinal muscle coat descend over the anterolateral wall to mesh into the arching rungs of circular muscle of the roof and sides of the hiatus, and some dip under the submucosal segment to mesh into the circular rungs in the bed of the ureter. Another set of delicate fibres separate from the circular muscle of the *bas fond* into a submucosal plane and converge on, and mesh into, the circular and inner longitudinal muscular components of the roof and sides of the mouth of the hiatus. Some fibres in this same plane emerge from the network at the hiatus, cross over the roof of the ureter, and turn anteromedially on the bladder base, completing the inverted 'U' arrangement. These intermeshing multidirectional muscle bundles form a scaffold that maintains a non-constricted tunnel in the bladder wall (see Fig. 11.2).

Uhlenhuth *et al.* (1953a,b) described the bundles of longitudinal muscle that arch over the submucosal ureter, contiguous with the hiatus as a sphincter of the ureter. Elbadawi *et al.* (1973) found a meshwork of muscle reticulum over the roof of the submucosal ureter

and also claimed for them some ureterosphincteric action. This muscle reticulum may supplement the main intrinsic sphincteric mechanism of the normal ureter to some extent but its main function is to seal the potential space between the ureter and bladder wall.

Waldeyer's fascia or superficial sheath of the ureter

The ureter enters the bladder through the tunnel clothed in a fibromuscular sleeve that attaches firmly to the tunnel walls and embraces the juxtavesical ureter laterally and the submucosal ureter medially. The lateral sleeve gains attachment to the ureteral wall and the medial sleeve clings to the submucosal ureter as far distally as the orifice and flows beyond into the trigone (Fig. 12.3). This sleeve or fascia of Waldeyer tethers the ureter to the walls of the tunnel, permits movement and expansion of the ureter, and prevents the occurrence of pulsion saccules alongside the ureter in the tunnel.

This sheath contains smooth muscle that can be traced from the muscle of the bladder wall in the tunnel to the juxtavesical ureter laterally. The medial sleeve of the sheath can be identified easily on dissection, but it is difficult to recognize this structure histologically in specimens taken from young children (Elbadawi, 1972). Diverging sparse muscle bundles can be traced medially from the hiatus to the trigone to either side of the ureteral orifice but no separate fibromuscular sheath can be identified histologically over the roof of the submucosal ureter.

Tanagho and Pugh (1963) found that Waldeyer's fascia was a close-fitting sheath belonging to the ureter, with only minimal delicate adherence to the muscle of the tunnel (Fig. 12.3a). Woodburne (1964) found a lateral but no medial component of Waldeyer's fascia and considered that the muscle fascicles arose directly from the detrusor muscles bordering the hiatal tunnel and gained only lateral attachments to the juxtavesical ureter. Elbadawi (1972) found the lateral and medial components of the sheath each integrating with the bladder muscle of the tunnel and termed this 'Waldeyer's fascia,' or the superficial sheath of the ureter (Fig. 12.3b).

Felix (1912a) observed that the ureter entered the bladder end-on until the 70-mm (head–foot length)

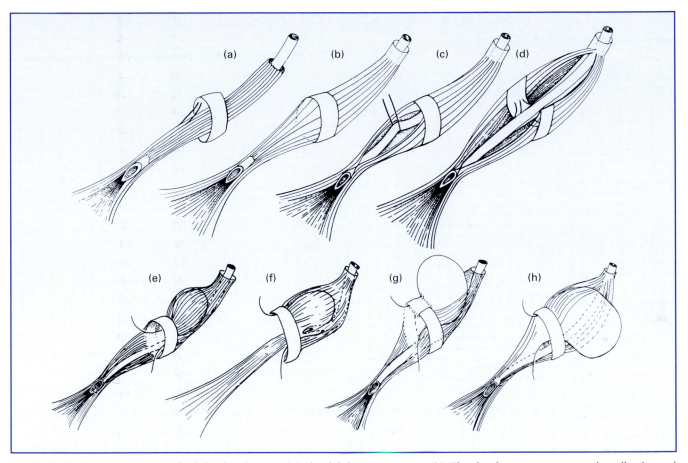

Fig. 12.3 *Waldeyer's fascia (superficial sheath) of ureter. (a) Sheath belonging to ureter. (b) This sheath integrates into muscle walls of tunnel and grips deep sheath of ureter laterally, and meatus and trigone medially, and gains delicate attachments to ureter in tunnel. (c), (d) Separation of fibres of sheath exposing nude body of ureter in its bed of fascia medially and laterally after incision of roof of hiatus. (e), (f) Defects of medial sleeve with ureteral orifice in normal position and in wall of hiatal diverticulum, respectively. (g), (h) Medial and lateral sleeve and hiatal muscle defects with large herniations directed cranially and caudally, respectively. (Reprinted, by permission, from Stephens, F.D. (1979), The vesicoureteral hiatus and paraureteral diverticula. J. Urol. 121: 786, Fig. 2.)*

embryo and that it had obtained an oblique course at full term. He also noted that when the circular muscle coat of the bladder was laid down in the vicinity of the hiatal tunnel, it gave a sleeve-like extension of longitudinally oriented muscle on the juxtavesical part of the ureter. This muscle presumably is that which was recognized as Waldeyer's 'fascia'.

The deep sheath of the ureter

The ureter in the juxtavesical segment is ensheathed by an additional close-fitting, thin, see-through fascia that can be separated cleanly from the muscle coat of the ureter. This loose sheath extends cranially around the ureter, but at the hiatus, it blends firmly with the adventitia of the ureteral wall, where it can only be displayed as such by sharp dissection. It continues distally to the ureteral meatus. Elbadawi traced it beyond the meatus into the trigone of the bladder. This sheath in the extravesical course of the ureter can be identified more readily in fresh specimens and at operation than in the formalin fixed state. Elbadawi (1972) termed this the 'deep sheath of the ureter', which, together with the superficial sheath or Waldeyer's fascia, led him to propose the dual-sheath concept of the ureterovesical fascia (Fig. 12.4).

The arrangement of longitudinal, circular, and oblique muscle of the extravesical ureter ceases abruptly at the hiatus. The muscle of the intravesical ureter is composed of longitudinal fibres only. This longitudinal muscle coat extends to the rim of the orifice and, in the floor, it passes beyond into the superficial trigone.

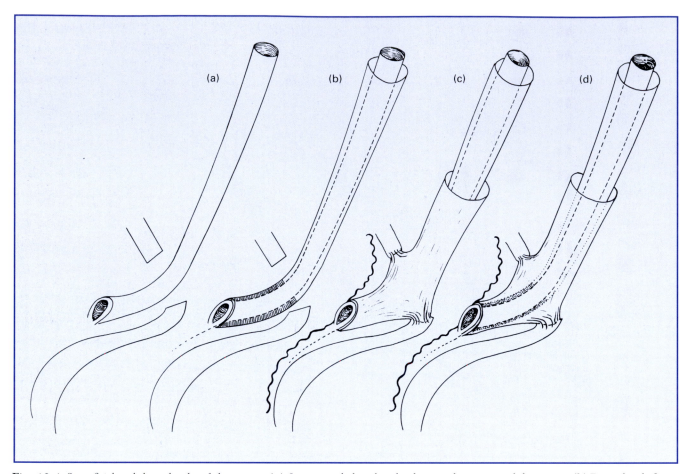

Fig. 12.4 *Superficial and deep sheaths of the ureter. (**a**) Juxtavesical, hiatal and submucosal segments of the ureter. (**b**) Deep sheath fitting loosely around juxtavesical ureter, but firmly attached to hiatal and submucosal segments. (**c**) Sock-like superficial sheath (Waldeyer's fascia) with medial and lateral components having continuity of muscle with the bladder muscle walls of the hiatal tunnel. (**d**) Composite section showing both sheaths. (Reprinted, by permission, from Stephens, F.D. (1978), The normal and abnormal ureterovesical hiatus: methods of correction of vesicoureteral reflux and paraureteral diverticula. J. Cont. Ed. Urol. Fig. 6.)*

The ureteral musculature and competence

The competence of the ureterovesical valve is chiefly dependent on intact ureteral musculature and its intrinsic tone that actively closes the lumen of the submucosal ureter (Stephens and Lenaghan, 1962; King and Stephens, 1977). Competence may be impaired if the submucosal ureter is deficient in muscle, shorter than normal, or absent, in which event, the orifice lies in a lateral position, the so-called 'lateral ectopy' of Ambrose and Nicholson (1962). To denote degrees of ectopy, the location of the normal orifice position is called the 'A' position, 'B' is midway to the hiatus and 'C' is at the hiatus, while 'D' denotes an orifice in the wall of a hiatal diverticulum. These positions are determined with the bladder full at 50 cmH₂O at the time of cystoscopy, or in specimens after fixation in the distended state (Lyon *et al.*, 1969; Mackie and Stephens, 1975).

The combination of the vesical musculature around the tunnel and the superficial and deep sheaths of the ureterovesical junction seals the hiatus against pulsion herniations of the bladder mucosa, while the intrinsic musculature of the submucosal segment of the ureter seals the lumen of the ureter from vesicoureteral reflux.

Hiatal and perihiatal hernias

Saccules or diverticula of the bladder mucosa that protrude through defects of Waldeyer's fascia along the ureterovesical tunnel are hiatal hernias (Figs 12.3 and 12.5). The orifice of the ureter may be located on the trigone or bladder base, on the neck of the diverticulum,

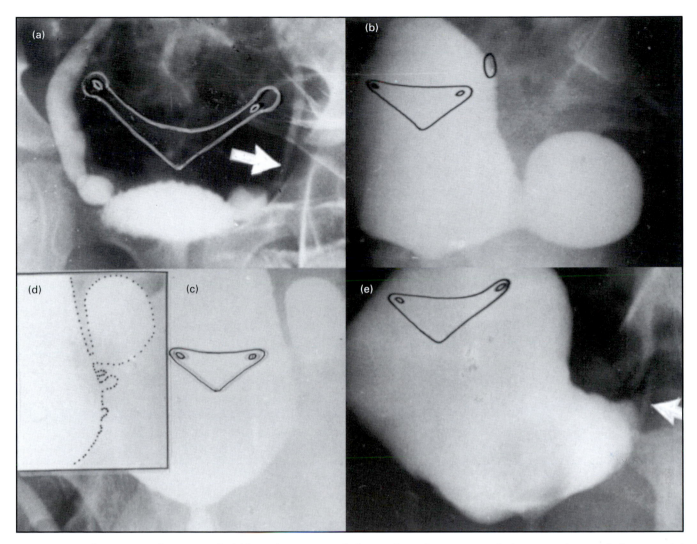

Fig. 12.5 *Voiding cystourethrograms of children showing vesical diverticula with superimposed diagrams of trigonal features. (**a**) 5½-year-old boy (J.P.) with hiatal hernias filled to capacity near end of micturition; right ureteral orifice in diverticulum and free reflux; left ureteral orifice in bladder contiguous with ureter and limited reflux (arrow). (**b**) Six-year-old boy (A.T.) with left combined hiatal and perihiatal diverticulum; large hiatal tunnel and no reflux. (**c**) Seven-year-old boy (G.D.) with honeycomb defects of left lateral wall and nest of perihiatal diverticula; ureteral orifices in normal position. (**d**) Tracing of diverticula vaguely outlined in (c). (**e**) Five-year-old girl (J.G.) with wideneck perihiatal diverticulum owing to weakness of lateral vesical wall; left ureteral orifice midway to hiatus and limited reflux. Arrow points to limited reflux. (Reprinted, by permission, from Stephens, F.D. (1979), The vesicoureteral hiatus and paraureteral diverticula. J. Urol. 121: 786, Fig. 3.)*

or outside the bladder on the floor or dome of the diverticulum.

Diverticula arising in defects of the muscle meshwork contiguous with or adjacent to the hiatus on the lateral wall of the bladder are termed here, 'perihiatal herniations' (Figs 12.5 and 12.6).

Sometimes the muscle defects occur in Waldeyer's fascia and the muscle of the bladder wall, resulting in a compound hiatal and perihiatal hernia (Fig. 12.5b). The term 'paraureteral diverticula' comprises hernia-

tions through and close to the hiatus and is appropriate for herniations in the vicinity of the ureterovesical junction when the precise anatomy is not clearly identified.

Hiatal hernias

Congenital weakness or absence of Waldeyer's fascia over the roof or sides of the submucosal ureter causes a pouting of vesical mucosa in the potential space alongside the ureter in the hiatus. The resulting hiatal hernia-

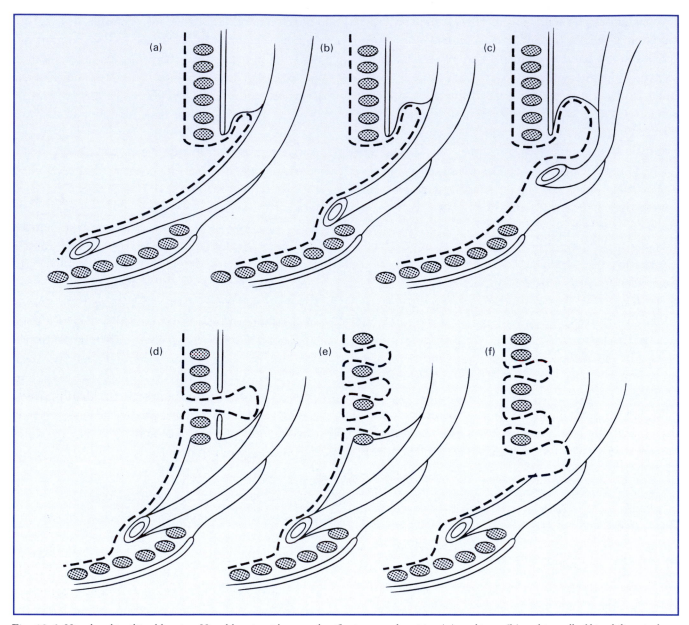

Fig. 12.6 *Hiatal and perihiatal hernias. Hiatal hernia with ureteral orifice in normal position (**a**), at hiatus (**b**) and in wall of hiatal diverticulum. (**c**, **d**) Perihiatal hernia hiatus, and ureteral orifice normal. (**e**) Honeycomb deficiencies with hernias of lateral bladder wall. (**f**) Hiatal and perihiatal hernias. (Bladder mucosa represented by dotted line Waldeyer's fascia by fine black line, and circular vesical muscle bundles by shaded egg shapes.) (Reprinted, by permission, from Stephens F.D. (1979), The vesicoureteral hiatus and paraureteral diverticula. J. Urol. 121: 786, Fig. 4.)*

tion of bladder mucosa that is more pronounced during voiding is characteristically small and about the size of a pea. The diverticulum has a narrow neck and usually is restrained from further enlargement by the intact lateral extension of Waldeyer's fascia around the juxtavesical ureter (Fig. 12.3a).

With a hiatal hernia that accompanies a submucosal ureter of normal length and 'A'-position orifice, the medial extension of Waldeyer's sheath is lacking. With 'D'-position orifices, this medial component of Waldeyer's sheath is also lacking.

With hiatal hernias, reflux usually is absent when the ureteral orifice is normally situated in the 'A' position. If a similar defect of Waldeyer's fascia is associated with 'B'-, 'C'- or 'D'-position orifices, the size and position of the diverticulum or Hutch saccule (Hutch, 1961a), are similar, but the submucosal ureter may lack muscle in its roof or be short or absent and vesicoureteral reflux ensues.

Wickramasinghe and Stephens (1977) found by dissection that, if the diverticulum and ureter had independent orifices in the bladder, each had an independent fascial sheath. When the ureter entered the wall of the diverticulum, however, the fascial sheath of the ureter was continued over the diverticulum to gain attachment to the muscle coats of the bladder around the hiatus. They did not make a distinction as to whether the fasciae were derived from the superficial or deep sheaths.

The hiatal diverticulum conforms in shape and position to the extent of the deficiency of Waldeyer's fascia. If the fascia is lacking over the roof and sides of the submucosal ureter, the neck of the diverticulum forms a crescentic crease straddling the submucosal ureter when the bladder is partly filled, and a globular shape with the ureter tenting the floor when the bladder is distended.

When the ureteral meatus is located lateral to but separate from the orifice of the diverticulum, the ridge formed by the underlying submucosal ureter can be seen on probing to emerge from the bladder under the floor of the diverticulum through the hiatus. If the meatus is balanced on the floor of the hiatus, the orifices of the ureter and the diverticulum are separate, and both emerge separately from the bladder through the hiatus. However, when the orifice of the ureter opens into the diverticulum, the ureter lies entirely outside the wall of the bladder beyond the margins of the hiatus (Fig. 12.6c).

The sac of the hiatal hernia usually withdraws into the bladder and appears as redundant mucosa in the region of the hiatus when the bladder is opened surgically. If the mucosa is incised and undercut to expose the hiatus and ureter, the oval gap in the fascia of Waldeyer overlying the ureter leading into the hiatal tunnel is thrown into relief by the sharp, selvaged edges of the fascia bordering the defect. The arching stretched muscle bundles of the roof of the tunnel face wear smooth and shiny with the in–out movement of the sac, and the nude body of the submucosal ureter lies clean and glistening in its deep sheath on the floor of the tunnel.

Perihiatal hernia

On the lateral wall of the bladder, cranial to the hiatus, the outer longitudinal muscle coat may be deficient, the area then being covered only by the circular muscle layer (Uhlenhuth *et al.*, 1953a). Then local defects in the circular muscle meshwork lead to single or multiple discrete pulsion diverticula (Figs 12.3 and 12.5), while a more extensive defect leads to a wide-neck bulge in the bladder wall (Fig. 12.5c,d,e). The local defects may be single or multiple, small or large, and near or far from the hiatus. The defect may impinge on the wall of the hiatus, in which event, the hiatal and perihiatal defects merge, forming the compound diverticulum (Fig. 12.5b). If the ureteral orifice is placed laterally, vesicoureteral reflux may be an additional feature.

The neck of the perihiatal diverticulum may be narrow or wide, depending on the extent of the muscle defect. The neck is surrounded by muscle, which turns abruptly outward as a short collar, through which vesical mucosa protrudes. Perihiatal and composite diverticula are not contained by a restraining fascia and hence are usually larger than the hiatal diverticula (Fig. 12.5b,c).

The wide-neck bulge of the weak lateral wall (Uhlenhuth *et al.*, 1953a,b; MacKellar and Stephens, 1960) becomes more apparent with bladder distension or during voiding cystourethrography and emptying may be incomplete. Some muscle trabeculae may crisscross its dome causing indentations or loculi (Fig. 12.5e).

Combined perihiatal and hiatal hernia

When the defects involve the hiatal muscle and Waldeyer's fascia, the neck of the hernia is large as well as hiatal and perihiatal and may exhibit a discrete or shelving neck and a deep pocket or a shallow, wide bulge. Reflux may be expected if the submucosal ureter is abnormally short and the orifice is contiguous with or in the compound diverticulum.

Compound diverticula enlarge presumably because the roof of the hiatus and roof attachments of the lateral extension of Waldeyer's fascia are defective. The diverticulum may enlarge during voiding cranially and caudally or only caudally, in which event it may protrude into the pelvis and obstruct the urethra (Fig. 12.3g,h and Fig. 12.7).

Embryogenesis of diverticula

Most hiatal and perihiatal herniations of the bladder in children result from the aforementioned congenital muscle or fibromuscular defects. However, one type

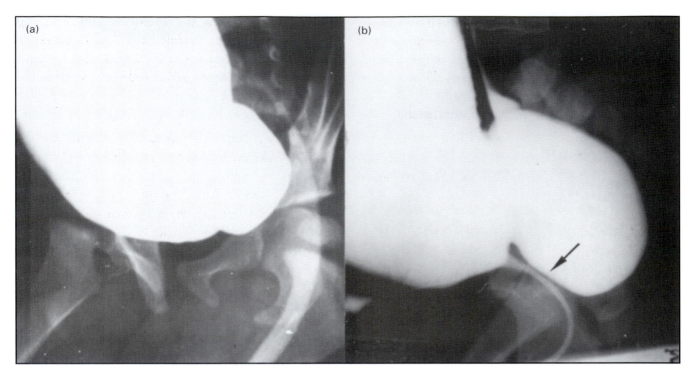

Fig. 12.7 *Combined hiatal and perihiatal diverticulum shown on cystourethrography. (**a**) Diverticulum partially filled during filling of the bladder. (**b**) Diverticulum fully distended and extending caudally behind and obstructing the urethra, causing arrest of micturition. Note catheter in urethra demonstrating the location and the flattening of the diverticular wall against the wall of the urethra, arrow. ((**a**) Reprinted, by permission, from Stephens, F.D. (1983), Congenital Malformations of the Urinary Tract, New York, Praeger, Fig. 9.7A, p. 181. (**b**) reprinted, by permission, from Smith, E.D. (1980), Malformations of the bladder and urethra, and hypospadias, in Pediatric Surgery, T.M. Holder and K.W. Ashcraft (eds). Philadelphia, Saunders, Fig. 58.3B, p. 753.)*

appears to be of a different origin and may be described more correctly as a diverticulum than a herniation (Fig. 12.6c). This is the hiatal hernia or diverticulum that shares with the ureter a common opening into the bladder. Hutch and Amar (1972) believed that some hiatal diverticula occurred as the result of normal urodynamic pressures forcing a mucosal saccule through the Waldeyer's fascia (primary saccule), and that others were induced by high intravesical pressures of vesical-outlet obstruction which stretched the hiatus and forced a saccule (secondary saccule) through the relatively weak hiatus of the bladder. They considered that the distending saccule dragged mechanically the ureteral meatus from its feeble trigonal anchorage through the neck of the diverticulum into the saccule.

The extreme lateral positions of the ureteral orifices in the diverticula, however, may be explained embryologically (Mackie *et al.*, 1975; Wickramasinghe and Stephens, 1977). The ureteral orifice gains its lateral intradiverticular position because the origin of the ureteral bud from the wolffian duct is far caudal compared with the situation of a normal bud. In the process by which the wolffian duct is absorbed into the bladder, the abnormally sited bud is projected laterally beyond the normal location of the ureteral orifice to the far lateral location even beyond the bladder wall. Its orifice comes to lie within a collar of opened-out wolffian duct, which forms the floor of the diverticulum, the sides and roof of which are made up of bladder mucosa. The fascia over the diverticulum was found by Wickramasinghe and Stephens (1977) to be continuous with the fascial sheath of the ureter. The abnormal embryology accounts for the laterality of the ureteral orifice, whether on the bladder base or in a hiatal diverticulum. The apparent movement of a ureteric orifice from the bladder base into the diverticulum during filling of the bladder merely returns it to its original abnormal position from that which it takes up when the diverticulum is collapsed and prolapsed in the hiatus.

Whereas small herniations associated with defects of the superficial sheath of the ureter may in time undergo spontaneous repair by natural strengthening of the sheath and the muscle of the bladder wall around the tunnel, it is unlikely that the diverticulum that engulfs the ureteral orifice would do so because of the developmental origin of this far laterally placed orifice.

Surgical management of diverticula

Hiatal diverticula and those perihiatal diverticula located so close to the hiatus that their repair involves the muscle of the hiatal tunnel are usually repaired in combination with reimplantation of the ureter (Fig. 12.8).

Diverticula readily apparent when the intravesical pressure is raised on voiding cystourethrography may be invisible when the pressure is low or atmospheric at the time of cystoscopy or cystotomy. The exact location should be identified and documented carefully at prior cystoscopy. The site of the diverticulum may be recognized at cystotomy by a saddle-like groove in the vesical mucosa over the ureter near the hiatus, by redundancy of mucosa that prolapses in the bladder or by the pout of mucosa through the deficiency.

Transhiatal repair of paraureteral diverticular and vesicoureteral incompetence

A racquet incision of the vesical mucosa is made around the ureteral orifice and extended cranially through the loose redundant mucosa overlying the hiatus and site of the diverticulum. The mucosa is undercut widely and cleanly to demonstrate the undisturbed muscle coat of the bladder wall and the deficiencies. The ureter is freed from strands of the defective fascia of Waldeyer and its attachments to the trigone and walls of the tunnel, and

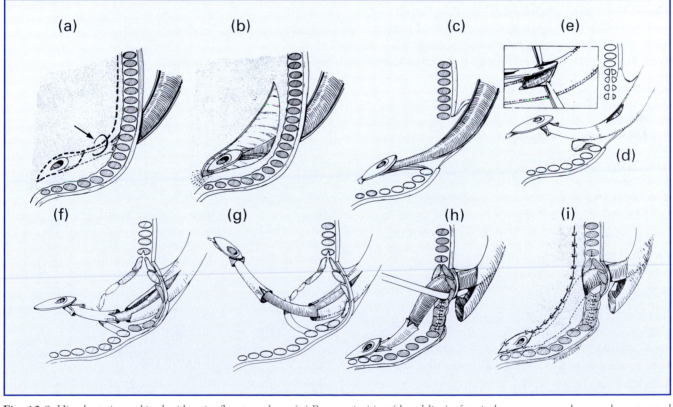

Fig. 12.8 *Hiatal repair combined with anitreflux procedure.* (**a**) *Racquet incision (dotted line) of vesical mucosa around ureteral meatus and across hiatal diverticulum (arrow) and along posterior bladder wall.* (**b**) *Mucosa widely undercut exposing bladder muscle and defective fascia of Waldeyer.* (**c**) *Roof of hiatal tunnel cleared exposing see-through sheath of juxtavesical ureter.* (**d**) *Division of roof of tunnel and posterior bladder wall, and incision of see-through deep sheath by precise scissor cut of tented sheath and gentle development of plane of separation between sheath and ureter.* (**e**), (**f**), (**g**) *Mobilization and release of ureter from deep sheath.* (**h**) *Repair of caudal part of enlarged hiatus and cinching of muscle around 8F calibrator to ensure adequate dimension of new hiatus.* (**i**) *Advancement of meatus with its collar of vesical mucosa onto trigone and reapposition of vesical mucosa.* (Reprinted, by permission, from Stephens, F.D. (1979), The vesicoureteral hiatus and paraureteral diverticula. J. Urol. 121: 786, Fig. 5.)

is lifted out of its bed in the bladder and hiatus. The cranial rim of the tunnel is then defined and together with the adjoining muscle and attachments of Waldeyer's fascia incised cranially for 1–2 cm (Fig. 12.3d). By this means, the juxtavesical ureter is exposed and freed readily from the then bivalved lateral extension of Waldeyer's fascia. If more mobilization is necessary to permit ureteral advancement on the trigone, the filmy, see-through, deep ureteral sheath that tethers the ureter cranially is picked up over the juxtavesical ureter and incised first longitudinally then delicately separated from the ureter and divided circumferentially. The ureter, thus, is disengaged from its deep sheath, from which it slips readily and without recoil. The ureter is brought through the new hiatus, located at the cranial end of the incision in the bladder wall, the bladder muscle being repaired caudal to the ureter to provide a firm muscular wall at the site of the original hiatus and diverticulum (Fig. 12.8) (Stephens, 1979a).

The new hiatus is made to accommodate the ureter together with an 8F gauge metal sound. The metal sound when removed ensures adequate dimension of the new hiatus. The ureteral meatus and the cuff of the bladder mucosa are then relocated on the trigone. To ensure a 2.5-cm length of the submucosal ureter, an advancement on, or across, the trigone may be required for those ureters with laterally placed orifices lying close to the neck or actually in the diverticulum. For large perihiatal diverticula the dome may need an extravesical dissection preliminary to inversion of the mucosa and excision, followed by repair of the bladder wall deficiency.

Honeycomb diverticula

Honeycombing of the lateral wall of the bladder requires clear exposure of the multiple gaps in the muscle mesh by wide elevation of the mucosa. Isolated defects can be repaired individually, but those closely clustered should be run together by cutting the interlacing muscle bridges, trimming the cut strands and suturing healthy muscle edge to edge. The wide bulge of the lateral wall may need repair. If the bulge is several centimetres in diameter, the edges of the defect may not be well defined even after wide clearance of the vesical mucosa. It may be expedient

to incise the muscle wall radially from the hiatus through the weak area, free the thin muscle coat from contiguous perivesical tissues, excise redundant thin tissue of the dome and repair the defect by overlapping the more robust and muscular walls near the base.

Bladder exstrophy*

Classic exstrophy of bladder and urethra

In classic vesical exstrophy, the bladder lumen opens widely onto the surface of the abdomen. The mucosa of the pelvic urethra is exposed between the divaricated pubes, the two sides of the pelvic girdle are rotated outwards and in the male the penile urethra is represented by a dry mucosal covered plate on the dorsum of the penis and glans. Other genital anomalies coexist.

A new and successful technique of surgery that has been designed by Kelly (1995) to achieve physiological continence in classical vesical exstrophy is based on new concepts of anatomy of the potential urethral sphincter muscles.

This technique involves extensive dissection of the pelvic urethral muscles, the position, importance and location of which have not been fully appreciated hitherto in regard to their role in the reconstruction of the voluntary sphincter mechanism. A brief account of the pathological anatomy of these muscles as identified by Kelly (1995) follows.

Urethra

In both sexes, the urethra is laid open and represented by an exposed wet epithelial covered strip as far distally in the male as the verumontanum and in the female as the narrow bridge between urethra and vagina. In the male, the rudimentary urethra continues on the dorsum of the penis and glans in the form of a dry strip of cornified mucosa called the urethral plate.

There is a gradual transition between the exposed bladder and urethral plate and on dissection it has not been possible to identify a specific thick internal urethral sphincter muscle other than the continuum of the wall of the bladder and urethra. Passing from one pubis to the other behind the bladder neck region is a taut band of tissue which may represent the puboprostatic fibromuscular ligaments.

Author: Mr J.H. Kelly—Personal communication.

Male genitalia and urethral plate

For convenience of description, the urethra can be divided into three sections: (i) from bladder neck to verumontanum; (ii) from the verumontanum to the coronal sulcus; and (iii) in the glans. The verumontanum is a convenient reference point in vesical exstrophy as it lies on the mucosal surface and is obvious as a short midline ridge and marks the point of divergence of the urethral plate on the dorsum of the penis from the potential external sphincter muscles lying toward the back of the pelvis.

1. The narrow urethra proximal to the verumontanum gradually merges with the mucosa of the bladder trigone without a change in the mucosal appearance. The urethral wall is ridged in a longitudinal direction to a varying degree and at its margins blends with smooth red hairless skin that extends alongside the junction of the bladder mucosa and urethra toward the level of the verumontanum.
2. The urethral plate between the verumontanum and the glans is smooth and convex from side to side, covering about two-thirds of the dorsal surface of the penis. In the newborn it is seldom more than 2 cm in length, and the shortness of this segment of urethral plate contributes to the formation of the dorsal curvature of the penis. This section replaces the membranous urethra and the bulbar and part of the penile urethra which are absent in classic vesical exstrophy.
3. The urethral plate on the glans is continuous with the penile segment but instead of being smooth and convex is concave in transverse section and exhibits longitudinal ridges and grooves; the erectile tissue of the glans is grooved longitudinally into two roughly equal halves, each of which surmounts its corpus cavernosum. Deep to the groove is the skin on the ventral surface of the penis and the ventral prepuce.

Penis

The individual variation in overall dimension and the length of the shaft of the penis is often proportional to the severity of the abnormality. For example, with the most severe types of cloacal exstrophy the penis is represented by two very small half penises, separated by several centimetres. In most babies with vesicourethral exstrophy the penile shaft may appear much shorter than normal but the overall dimension of the crura and corpora cavernosa is normal.

In classic vesical exstrophy, the crura of the penis are attached to the ischiopubic rami as in the normal child. As each pubis and ischium are widely separated from the midline, each crus traverses a greater distance to meet its fellow of the opposite side to form a foreshortened penile shaft. The glans has an abnormal shape, being flatter than normal and divided by the urethral groove and plate into halves. The coronal sulcus is present on the dorsal and lateral aspects and on the ventral aspect overlying the distal penile shaft there is a cuff of loose preputial skin. The penis exhibits a severe dorsal curvature or 'chordee' which is contributed to by the shortness of the urethral plate and abnormal shape of the corpora cavernosa.

Scrotum

The scrotum is flat and wide and very variable in its state of development and it usually contains the testes, although maldescent is not uncommon. However, even when descended, the testes tend to be widely separated within the scrotum. A flat band of smooth skin lies between the scrotum and the base of the penis in place of the usual penoscrotal junction.

Female genitalia and urethral plate

In classic exstrophy the vulva is cleft and the mons is absent. The clitoris is in halves, separated by up to several centimetres, and each half clitoris is located at the anterosuperior end of each labium minor. Between the anterior ends of the divaricated labia minora is the introitus of the vagina. The vaginal orifice is sometimes obscured by a prominent hymen. The vagina passes posteriorly from the introitus rather than posterosuperiorly, and is short. At laparotomy no unusual features of the internal genitalia have been observed.

The urethral plate in the female is short and not well defined. The junction between trigone and urethra is gradual and indistinct and there is no abrupt transition between wider bladder and narrower urethra. Smooth mucosa covers the slightly concave surface from trigone to the vaginal orifice, a total distance of about 1 cm in the newborn. Laterally, the everted urethral strip joins the smooth abnormal skin strip alongside the margins of bladder and clitoris.

Anus and perineum in males and females

The perineum is wide and the medial surface of each thigh is far from the midline. The anus has the appearance of being anteriorly located, but this may be more apparent than real, as the distance between the anus and the coccyx is normal. Although rectal prolapse is common, the contractions of the external anal sphincter muscle as detected by electrical stimulation at operation are strong.

Pelvic sphincter muscles

Levatores ani muscles

The anterior border of the levatores ani muscles in the normal child is formed by the puborectalis muscle attached to the posterior surface of the pubis on either side. It forms narrow muscle slings around the pelvic viscera. In classic vesical exstrophy, with the separation of the pubic bones, the anterior attachments of the slings are widely divaricated and they lose much of the mechanical advantage as a sphincter. More posteriorly, as in the normal pelvis, the pubococcygeus and ischiococcygeus muscles (the levator diaphragm) arise from the pubis and the condensation of obturator internus fascia known as the 'white line' and the ischial spine. The muscles pass medially to support the pelvic viscera and posteriorly to form the pelvic diaphragm. The direction of their fibres is altered by the open nature of the pelvis.

Urogenital diaphragm

Normally the diaphragm is orientated in the transverse plane of the pelvis but because of the pubic separation in exstrophy the diaphragm is tilted towards the vertical. Hence it has superior (rostral), inferior and lateral borders.

The urogenital diaphragm in the normal male is a narrow triangular structure between the pubic bones and the ischiopubic rami and perforated by the membranous urethra. It is a layer of skeletal muscles sandwiched between two layers of delicate fascia. The fascia and ischiocavernosa and sphincter urethrae muscles surround the crura of the corpora cavernosa laterally and the urethra medially, respectively. The external sphincter muscle blends with the capsule of the prostate rostrally and with the bulbocavernosus muscle inferiorly. The posterior limit of the urogenital membrane is the transversus perinei muscle passing from one ischiopubic ramus to the other and in the midline blending posteriorly with the perineal body and the anterior fibres of the external anal sphincter and superficially with the bulbocavernosus muscle.

The urogenital diaphragm in vesical exstrophy in males is rectangular rather than triangular as the ischiopubic rami run anteroposteriorly rather than towards the midline in front. The attachments of the crura of the corpora of the penis are widely separated and the urogenital diaphragm is much wider than normal. The urethral plate is on the dorsum of the penis, and deviates anteriorly away from the urogenital diaphragm. The bulb of the urethra is lacking in part. The ischiocavernosa muscles surround the crura and base of the corpora cavernosa, but otherwise the muscles of the urogenital diaphragm are a transversely oriented blend of opened out and stretched skeletal muscle of the external urethral sphincter, bulbocavernosus and transversus perinei backed by pubourethralis musculature. Because this skeletal muscle mass has the potential to be utilized as a voluntary sphincter of a reconstructed urethra, it will be termed 'voluntary urinary sphincter'.

Voluntary urinary sphincter musculature

Male vesical exstrophy anomaly. In the newborn male with bladder exstrophy, the voluntary urinary sphincter is a quadrangular sheet of skeletal muscle oriented in the coronal plane between the pubic rami approximately 3 cm in width, 1.5 cm in height and 1–2 mm in thickness with a transverse clearly defined superior margin and an inferior transverse margin which is continuous in the midline posteriorly with the perineal body.

Superficial and anterior to the voluntary urinary sphincter is the scrotum and its contents. Posterior to it is the rectum in the midline and lateral to the rectum the fat of the ischiorectal fossa. Laterally it is attached to the ischiopubic ramus, to the crura of the penis and to the ischiocavernosus muscles.

The pudendal neurovascular bundle in Alcock's canal passes along the medial aspect of the ischiopubic ramus at the attachment of the crura in a compartment of the periosteum. Pudendal nerve branches pass out from the canal into the sphincter musculature.

On the superior margin of the voluntary urinary sphincter a fascial band stretches between the corpora cavernosa, and deep to this band are the prostatic vascular plexus, the capsule of the prostate gland and the back of the urethral plate. As the plate passes along the dorsum of the dorsally curved penis from the verumontanum, it becomes increasingly remote from the voluntary urinary sphincter.

The pudendal nerve and vessels to the voluntary urinary sphincter. Using a nerve stimulator it is possible to demonstrate at operation that the pudendal nerve is the motor supply of the voluntary urinary sphincter, and it is assumed that the proprioceptive sensory supply is also via the pudendal nerve. The pudendal nerve, having entered the pelvis from behind the ischial spine on the medial aspect of the ischial tuberosity in the periosteal compartment known as 'Alcock's canal', passes along the medial aspect of the ischiopubic ramus and ends as the dorsal nerve of the penis. This nerve is also readily identified at operation on the dorsal surface of the corpus cavernosum, from the pubic end of attachment of the crus and its branches can be followed on the superolateral surface of the corpus. Because of the nature of the operative dissection, the branches of the pudendal nerve to the voluntary urinary sphincter have not been identified but it is likely that they enter it posterolaterally.

The pudendal artery and veins accompany the nerve and contribute to the blood supply of the voluntary urinary sphincter, but there is a rich midline vascular network around the prostate gland which provides an important venous drainage and may also contribute to the arterial supply.

Female vesical extrophy anomaly. The urogenital diaphragm in the normal female is a triangular structure between the pubic bones and the ischiopubic rami and perforated by the urethra and the vagina. It is a layer of skeletal muscles sandwiched between two layers of delicate fascia. The fascia and muscle laterally surround the crura of the clitoris as the ischiocavernosus muscles, and medially surrounds the urethra as the sphincter urethrae and the vagina as the sphincter vaginae. The posterior limit of the urogenital membrane is formed by the transversus perineii muscles passing from one ischiopubic ramus to the other and blending posteriorly in the midline with the perineal body and with the anterior fibres of the external anal sphincter.

The ischiopubic rami are parallel with one another and the urogenital diaphragm is a wide rectangle. The vagina is more anterior than normal and the urethra is laid open so that the individual muscles of the urogenital diaphragm form a single sheet of transversely oriented bundles extending from the vaginal orifice in the urogenital diaphragm back to the perineal body. This sheet of muscle is similar to the muscle complex described for the male. It is composed of outstretched external voluntary muscle of the urethra rostrally and the muscle bundles of transverse perinei and pubovaginalis posteriorly.

Superficial to the voluntary urinary sphincter is a flat plane of skin between the vagina and the anus with a layer of vascular connective tissue between. More laterally are the labia minora and the labia majora.

Posterior to the voluntary urinary sphincter is the rectum and more laterally the fat of the ischiorectal fossa. Laterally on either side is the crus of the clitoris surrounded by the blended bulboischiocavernosus muscle and attached to the ischiopubic ramus with the pudendal neurovascular bundle on the posteromedial aspect.

Posteroinferiorly the voluntary urinary sphincter muscle meets the perineal body in the midline and with the anterior fibres of the external sphincter of the anal canal.

Principle of the Kelly repair of classic vesical exstrophy anomaly

In classic vesical exstrophy the pelvic structures and the individual urethral sphincter muscles have different relationships from normal but they are all present in modified form and it is their presence that makes anatomical reconstructive repair successful in achieving physiological urinary continence and a favourable genital and cosmetic result.

Kelly (1995) has described his successful operation based on a new appreciation of the pathological anatomy described here. Its success lies in the technique of stripping the periosteum with all attached structures attached from the insides of the pelvic bones including the neurovascular bundles in Alcock's canals and the crura of the corpora cavernosa. By so doing, the lateral attachments of the opened-out voluntary urinary sphincter muscles are mobilized and wrapped around the tubularized and redirected urethral plate. No attempt is made to approximate the pubic bones by any of the forms of osteotomy. This urethral plate is detached from the dorsum of the penis, tubularized and rotated posteriorly to be enveloped by the sphincter muscles. The new 'posterior urethra' then issues anterior to the scrotum as a perineal urethrostomy, later to be advanced along the under surface of the reconstructed penis and glans. In the female, the wrap of muscle embraces the tubularized urethra with vaginal introitus attached.

The ureter

IV

The wolffian duct derives its name from the famous German embryologist, Caspar Friedrich Wolff (1733–1794) who at the age of 26 years, in 1759, challenged the prevailing ideas and 'preformation' theory of embryonic development (Aulie, 1966). At the Halle University, Wolff studied the developing chick embryo with the aid of the rather crude microscope of the day and observed the growth and migration of the mesonephric duct and the coming and going of the mesonephros and the formation of the metanephros. He was responsible for debunking the popular theory that organisms existed completely formed in the egg or sperm and for substituting in its stead, and reviving, the concept that embryos develop as differentiating and growing organs.

Wolff noted that the kidney starts as a pronephros in the thorax, continues as the mesonephros in the lumbar region, and ends as the metanephros in the pelvis, all of which at one stage share a common duct. It is fitting that this duct be named after Wolff (Fig. 13.1).

Wolff's observations and theory ran contrary to contemporary views of the preformation theorists, especially the very influential Swiss scientist, and embryologist, Albrecht von Haller, who was completely blind to Wolff's concept of embryonic development. So fierce were the arguments raised against those of the lone Wolff that he was ostracized from German academic medicine. He turned to the army and served for four years in the Seven Years' War only to return to Berlin and the same condemnation by his superiors. Catherine the Great of Russia invited him, in 1766, to become a member of the Russian Academy of Sciences in St Petersburg, where he spent the remainder of his life studying and writing embryology.

The wolffian duct and wolffian body from which the three kidneys and the entire upper urinary tract are derived, are monuments to the man who redirected human thought to the new and modern concept of embryology. It is sad that he died at 61 years, 18 years before his theory, which he knew to be correct, was finally accepted and propounded by Johan Friedrich Meckel.

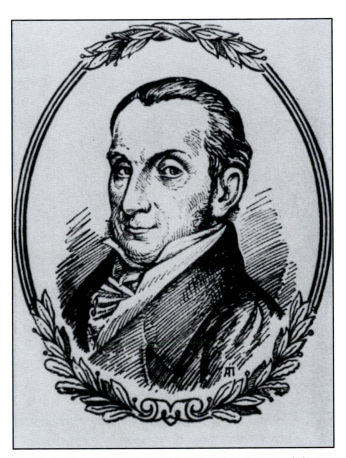

Fig. 13.1 *Casper Friedrich Wolff (1733–1794). (Reprinted, by permission, from Speert, H. (1958), 'Essays in eponymy', in* Obstetric and Gynecologic Milestones. *New York, Macmillan, Fig. 3.1.)*

Embryology

From 21 to 28 days, the mesoderm, from which the urogenital systems are derived, is recognizable in the wings of the flat embryonic disk. It is fed out during the third week between the ectoderm and endoderm from the epiblast of the primitive streak, which generates all the mesoderm of the body of the embryo. The mesoderm, which is arranged longitudinally, between the somites medially and the lateral mesoderm, is called the intermediate mesoderm. It forms a ridge on the dorsal wall of the coelomic cavity, known as the 'wolffian' body, most of which is nephrogenic, but part of which is gonadal (see Fig. 1.9). As the embryo elongates, the ridge grows caudally by additions of segments or nephrotomes, which coalesce to form the nephrogenic cord. At first, in the thoracic region in the dorsolateral wall of this intermediate mesoderm, a longitudinal condensation of cells canalizes *in situ* to form the wolffian duct. Caudal to the 14th somite, the blind end then activates and grows distally to reach and penetrate the cloaca. Canalization follows closely behind the solid growing end.

Several pairs of nephric tubules form in the future cervicothoracic region of the cord, but do not communicate with the wolffian duct. They are vestigial and represent all that there is of the pronephros in man (see Fig. 1.9).

In the future thoracolumbar region, the mesonephric tubules are much more numerous and voluminous. Each tubule gains independent connection with the wolffian (mesonephric) duct, elongates, and forms a glomerulus within the nephrogenic cord. The mesonephros is a transient excretory organ in the human until about the 10th week. It involutes progressively from the cranial to the caudal end, and function in the caudal portion overlaps that of the oncoming metanephros.

The caudal end of the wolffian body lies in the future sacral zone and gives rise to the metanephros or permanent kidney. It begins development in the fifth week when the ureteric bud grows out from the wolffian duct at the level of the 28th somite. At this point, the duct bends ventrally, lifting off the posterior wall crossing the metanephros from lateral to medial sides to reach the cloaca. At this bend, the ureteric bud penetrates the adjacent metanephros. The metanephric mesenchyme differentiates into the secretory and excretory parts of the kidney, and the bud forms the urine-transport systems, which include ureter, pelvis, calyces and collecting ducts. That part of the wolffian body between the mesonephros and the metanephros is called the nephrogenic cord.

The distal end of the wolffian duct from the ureteric bud to the vesicourethral tract is called the common excretory duct. The common excretory duct plus a short length of the wolffian duct above the bud expand in trumpet fashion and evert into the bladder and urethra to form one-half of the trigone. The trigone is formed chiefly by the integration and differential growth of the upper lip of the common excretory duct into the bladder base (Brockis, 1952) (Fig. 13.2). The attachment of the ureter to the wolffian duct switches from posterior to anterolateral locations and, by the expansion and absorption of the common excretory duct into the urinary tract, the orifices of the ureter and wolffian ducts become independent and move away from each other and settle in the bladder and urethra respectively (Fig. 13.2).

At the time that the ureters are separating from the wolffian ducts, the tubular vesicourethral canal undergoes an accelerated expansion to form the bladder and prostatic urethra. This takes place in embryos of 6–66-mm crown–rump length.

The metanephros, or permanent kidney, develops in a specific section of the nephrogenic ridge alongside the angulated section of the wolffian duct from which the ureteral bud arises and enters the metanephric blastema. The metanephric blastema differentiates around the bud and then the developing kidney moves cranially to the loin, while the ureteral bud orifice migrates caudally as described.

The wolffian ducts act as the guides to the müllerian ducts, which arise near the gonads on the wolffian ridge and come to issue into the urethra, between the orifices of the wolffian ducts near the bladder neck, at or about the 30-mm stage (Fig. 13.3). In the male, the wolffian duct develops into the vas deferens and the müllerian ducts atrophy, except for the utriculus prostaticus. In the female, the wolffian ducts wither and become incorporated, as Gartner's ducts, in the lateral walls of the müllerian ducts. They may eventually disappear altogether.

The müllerian ducts meet in the midline of the pelvis at the 28-mm stage, descend side by side to Müller's tubercle in the urogenital sinus at the 35-mm stage, and migrate distally, shifting the orifice from the original level of Müller's tubercle to the vestibule (see Fig. 4.1). The contacting walls of the two tubes break down with the formation of one uterovaginal canal. This takes place almost immediately after the tubes reach the sinus.

Ureter of infants and children

In order to study congenital malformations of the ureter, especially such lesions as stenoses, valves and megaureters, it was first necessary to measure the dimensions

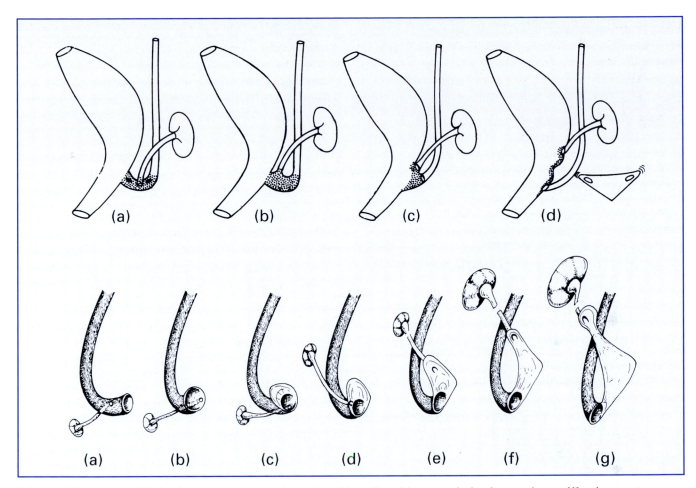

Fig. 13.2 Upper row. (**a**) *Embryologic rearrangement and migration of the orifices of the ureteric bud and ureters from wolffian duct to urinary tract and formation of the trigone. Lateral projection:* (**a**) *single ureter arising from normal site on wolffian duct (middle black dot) and migrating to the lateral cornu of the trigone* (**d**). (**b**) *and* (**c**) *Show the expansion or trumpeting of the common excretory duct and the adjoining short segment of the wolffian duct to be turned into the urethra and bladder as the trigone (stippled area). Lower row.* (**b**) *Anteroposterior projection showing rotation of the orifice of the ureteric bud from posteromedial to anterolateral orientations and the taking up and integration of the upper lip of the common excretory duct into the trigone* (**a**)–(**e**). *Shown also are hyperelongated trigones with lateral ectopy of the ureteric orifice* (**f**) *and hiatal diverticulum with ureteric orifice on the extended cornu in the diverticulum.* (Upper row, reprinted, by permission, from Stephens, F.D. (1979), Bifid and double ureters, ureteroceles and fused kidneys, in Pediatric Surgery, 3rd edn, M.M. Ravitch et al. (eds). Chicago, Year Book, Fig. 108.1, p. 1189. Lower row, Reprinted, by permission, from Stephens, F.D. (1983), Congenital Malformations of the Urinary Tract, New York, Praeger, Fig. 10.3B, p. 191.)

and quantitate the muscle and elastic constituents of normal ureters throughout the growth period from birth to adolescence. The calibre and muscle cell populations are different at different levels in the ureter and Cussen (1967a,b) made comprehensive scales for comparison with abnormal states.

Dimensions

Cussen (1967a) measured the length and diameters of 276 normal ureters in the fresh postmortem state obtained from fetuses of 20 weeks upwards, through infants and children to the age of 12 years. Those parts of the ureter within the wall of the bladder, namely the

intravesical, the intramural and submucosal segments, were determined microscopically from serial sections. The length of the extravesical ureter and the diameters of the ureteropelvic junction, middle spindle, distal end of the ureter and ureteric orifice were measured macroscopically. Blunt-nosed cylindrical probes measuring 0.03–1.00 cm in diameter were used to calibrate the ureters. The measurements were plotted against age, height, weight, crown–rump length, and surface area and a 'ready reckoner' of approximate ureteric dimensions was constructed for convenience of endoscopists and urosurgeons. The lengths and diameters of normal ureters were determined according to ages at 30-weeks'

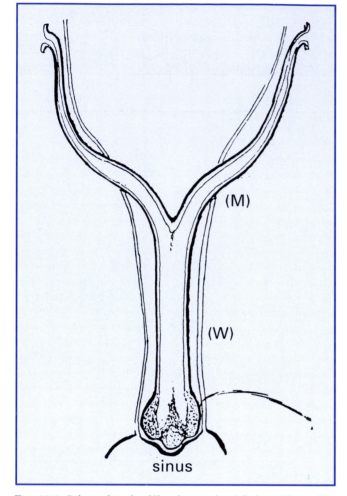

Fig. 13.3 *Relationship of wolffian ducts and pathfinders of the müllerian ducts, which penetrate the vaginal bulbs at the urogenital sinus (W = wolffian ducts; M = müllerian ducts). (Reprinted, by permission, from Frazer, J.E. (1931), A Manual of Human Embryology. London, Baillière, Tindall and Cox, Fig. 264, p. 436.)*

gestation, three months, three years, six years and 12 years of age, and the corresponding heights and weights (Appendix 1, No. 5). These data were essential to other studies on the aetiology of megaureters, strictures and vesicoureteral reflux ureters.

Structure

Cussen (1967b) also made a study of the population numbers and average size of the smooth-muscle cells and elastic fibres of 380 normal ureters from 200 subjects, whose ages ranged from 12 weeks' gestation to 12 years. Having determined the muscle cell numbers and size and the elastic component of the ureters at the uretero pelvic junction, middle spindle, distal end and submucosal segment, he plotted these measurements against age, height and weight and found good correlations. Conclusions based on these data were that the population of muscle cells varied at different levels in the ureter, being maximal in the middle spindle and minimal in the submucosal ureter. No smooth muscle was observed in the fetal ureter at 12 weeks' gestation, but at 16 weeks' gestation, smooth muscle extended throughout the length of the extravesical ureter but not into the intravesical ureter. At 20 weeks' gestation, muscle was seen partly surrounding the submucosal ureter and, by 36 weeks, smooth muscle formed a complete layer down to the orifice. The muscle cell population increased in each part with increasing age up to 12 years and probably beyond this age. The most rapid increase in numbers occurred in the first year. In the middle spindle, it was calculated that the population increased by 50 per cent in the first four years from birth and doubled in the first 12 years.

The average size of the smooth-muscle cell increased from birth to 12 years by only 10 per cent.

Elastic fibres were not demonstrable in the fetal ureter, but appeared first at the time of birth in the middle spindle and in the submucosal segment and showed a general increase with age up to 12 years. Elastic fibres were fewer in the region of the ureteropelvic junction than elsewhere in the ureter.

A 'ready reckoner' was constructed showing the muscle cell population, sizes, and areas in the different parts of the ureter according to ages up to 12 years (Appendix 1, No. 7). The data provided material essential to the studies of the aetiology and nature of the various types of megaureter.

Cussen (1972) measured the response of smooth muscle to incomplete obstruction in the ureter of the adult dog and showed considerable increase in size of the muscle cells (hypertrophy) and numbers (hyperplasia). Cussen and Lenaghan (quoted by Stephens, 1974), measured the muscle cell size of ureters of adult dogs in which vesicoureteral reflux was induced by incision of the roof of the submucosal ureter. It was found that increase in muscle cell size was a more accurate indicator of obstruction of the urinary tract than hyperplasia of muscle cells, and that hyperplasia without increase in cell size beyond the range of normal occurred with increased work load but without obstruction (Stephens, 1974).

The ureteric bud, with its inherent powers of moulding to shapes and sizes of the ureter, pelvis, calices and ducts of Bellini, may develop abnormally. The bud may be single but divide to form a bifid ureter, or may fail to develop, or may arise from the wolffian duct but fail to grow, or, having grown, may become atretic. Its site of origin may be ectopic with subsequent ectopic locations of the ureteric orifice in the urinary or genital tracts. On rare occasions, the orifices of the wolffian duct and ureter may be ectopic, giving rise to persisting mesonephric duct and vas ectopia anomalies. Buds may be multiple, forming duplicated or triplicated ureters. Intrinsic anomalies of calibre may be focal or general creating stenoses or other forms of obstruction or ectasia of the ureter without obstruction. Some malformations such as bifid systems are prone to other anomalies. Lenaghan (1962) found urinary tract anomalies (including vesicoureteral reflux) in 16 of 29 patients with bifid ureters, an incidence of 55 per cent. Other unusual abnormalities in the bifid systems include ectasia of the branches, ureterocele, ureteral atresia and multicystic kidney, ureteral stenosis, ureteropelvic obstruction and vesical exstrophy (Fig. 14.1). Complete double systems are prone to irregular sites of entry of the upper pole ureter into the urethral and genital systems, in addition to the array of anomalies listed for bifid systems. These developmental errors of budding will be discussed here.

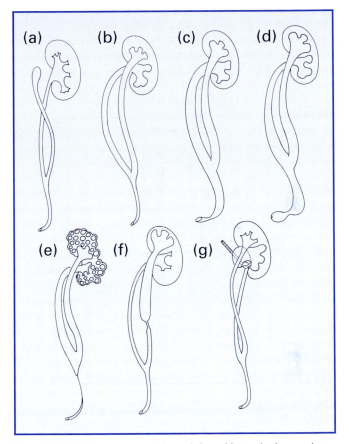

Fig. 14.1 *Bifid ureters complicated by additional abnormalities. (a) Blind ending ectopic ureter. (b) Megaureters and normal calibre stem. (c) Megaureter with vesicoureteral reflux. (d) Ureterocele. (e) Atresia. (f) Ureteral stenosis. (g) Lower hilar vessel obstructing the lower pole ureter. (Reprinted, by permission, from Stephens, F.D. (1983), Congenital Malformations of the Urinary Tract, New York, Praeger, Fig. 11.1, p. 202.)*

Agenesis and blind ureter

The ureteric bud may fail to develop either because of absence of the wolffian duct or because the bud does not arise from it. The malformation of bilateral bud agenesis leads to oligohydramnios, the Potter facies and deformities caused by compression.

In six examples of congenital bilateral absence of the ureter, the vas deferentia were present in all but one. Absence of the ureter therefore may result from agenesis of the ureteric bud or from failure of the wolffian anlage to develop.

Absence of a ureter occurs not infrequently in association with cloacal anomalies, especially when combined with lumbosacral scoliosis or sacral agenesis. The ureteric bud may develop but fail to reach and induce the neighbouring metanephric mesenchyme. The ureter may be short or long and usually exhibits a bulbous cranial end (Fig. 14.1a).

Atresia of the ureter

Ureteric atresia is generally accompanied by an ipsilateral multicystic or dysplastic kidney and sometimes by atresia, stenosis or stenoses, megaureter or vesicoureteral reflux in the contralateral ureter. Filmer and Taxy (1976) found a 16 per cent incidence of contralateral upper-tract anomalies in patients who had nephrectomy for multicystic kidney and an incidence of 50 per cent in an autopsy series.

The atretic segment may be focal or short or long; it may be found in upper, middle, lower or all parts of the ureter, and the atresia may affect a ureter that is initially of normal or larger-than-normal calibre (Fig. 14.2e,f).

Focal atresia may be accompanied by marked dilatation with hypertrophy of the muscle of the ureter and dilatation of pelvis and calyces in communication with collecting ducts and small regular macrocysts (Fig. 14.2d). The wall of the ureter with extensive atresia may be reduced to a fine cord, or thread- or hair-like strand that may be so fine as to be unrecognizable macroscopically (Fig. 14.2a). A segment of the ureter

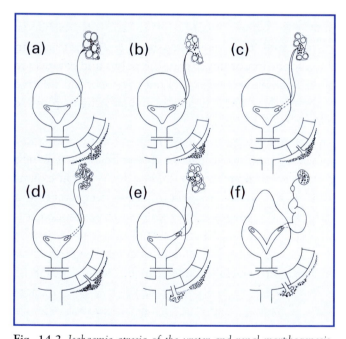

Fig. 14.2 *Ischaemic atresia of the ureter and renal morphogenesis. The wolffian duct, ureteric bud and metanephros are represented in the lower half of each diagram, and the trigone, ureter and kidney as seen in the newborn baby are represented in the upper half.* (**a**) *to* (**d**) *Normal bud and metanephros with ureteric ischaemia resulting in renal dysplasia and total, graduated, focal and segmental atresia, respectively.* (**e**) *Abnormal bud and metanephros with segmental atresia and lateral ectopy of the ureteric orifice, megaureter caudal to the atresia and renal dysplasia.* (**f**) *Abnormal bud and metanephros in prune belly syndrome with multiple ischaemic atresias, megaureters, lateral ectopy and reflux and renal dysplasia. (Reprinted, by permission, from Stephens, F.D. (1983), Congenital Malformations of the Urinary Tract, New York, Praeger, Fig. 11.2, p. 203.)*

may even be absent. The atretic process may extend into the pelvis and some of the calyces and collecting ducts, obliterating part or whole of the lumens of these structures (Fig. 14.2b,c).

These atresias affecting the lower end of the ureter are more likely to be accompanied by lesions in the contralateral ureter (DeKlerk *et al.*, 1977). The lesions include single or multiple stenoses, or atresia and megaureter with reflux.

In most examples of ureteral atresia, the ureteric orifice and adjoining ureter are normal in calibre and structure but taper toward the site of obliteration of the lumen (Fig. 14.2b). In some, the distal ureter and meatus may also be involved in the atretic process, in which event the ureteric orifice may be a dimple only or unrecognizable (Fig. 14.2a). The ureter, which obliterates its lumen by the acquired atretic process, usually tapers from below upward (Fig. 14.2a). This tapered end contrasts with the bulbous upper end, which is characteristic of the developmentally blind ureter (Fig. 14.1a). Megaureters with reflux are not absolved from atresia; the lumen of the distal ureter may be very large yet obliterate suddenly at some point where the ureter becomes atretic up to the kidney, which exhibits dysplasia (Fig. 14.2e). The ureters in the prune belly triad may be gigantic distally, but also exhibit one or more short or long atretic segments and dysplastic kidneys (Fig. 14.2f).

Structure of atretic ureter

The morphology of the atretic segment of ureter may be:

1. A fibrous membrane.
2. A fibrous 'string' meeting a tapered ureter at the vesical end in which the epithelial and muscular walls diminish progressively in amount and are extinguished giving place to fibrous tissue only in the string.
3. Absence of a segment between the vesical and renal ends of the ureter and the kidney.
4. Multiple atretic segments.
5. Segment of ureter of microdimensions but with a microlumen and total functional obstruction.

Embryogenesis of atresia

The bud and metanephric components may be normal structures initially, but during the migration of the developing kidney from the sacral to lumbar locations, the shifting network of mesonephric vessels and capillaries that establish the blood supply of ureter and metanephric kidney obliterates or fails to maintain adequate blood supply to the rapidly elongating and migrating structures. The changeover of segmental vessels and anastomosing capillaries supplying the elongating ureter and migrating kidney is defective creating an avascular loophole in the 'mesentery' of the ureter. A zone of ureter, short or long, then becomes totally or relatively ischaemic, incurring the characteristic morphologies of the atretic ureter as described by Cussen (1971a). This may be the ureteral counterpart of intestinal atresia which was shown experimentally to be ischaemic in origin by Louw and Barnard (1955). This explanation accounts not only for atresia and stenosis, long or short, but also for the postnatal disappearances of the multicystic dysplastic kidney. Furthermore, the same process may operate to create the defects in the contralateral ureter.

The nature of the defect of the vascular supply may be a simple accident of formation or a teratogenic impairment of the shifting capillary links that accompany the migrating ureter and kidney.

The aetiology of the multicystic and dysplastic kidneys and the ureteral atresias and the long stenotic segments of near-atresias is attributed by Potter (1972) to one and the same pathological disturbance. Suffice to say that complete ureteric occlusion of the ureter or a long shelving impermeable stenosis and dysplastic kidneys, usually multicystic, are mutual lesions.

Unduplicated ectopic ureter

Unduplicated ureters that issue by an orifice located elsewhere, but in the corner of the normal trigone, may be considered to be ectopic. Those orifices that lie within the confines of the bladder but lateral or caudal to the normal sites are examples of lateral or caudal intravesical ectopy respectively (page 286). Other orifices are termed urethral, vestibular or genital (vasal or vaginal) ectopy depending on their location and the sex of the individual. The urogenital tract may be otherwise normal except for the ectopic ureter and its junction with the genital tract, or it may exhibit local malformations in the urethra or the ipsilateral genital organs, or it may be combined into a urorectogenital malformation of the cloaca.

Ectopy associated with duplex systems is approximately four times as common as unduplicated ectopic ureters.

Lateral ectopy

The ureteral orifice gains a lateral or even intradiverticular position because the origin of the ureteral bud from the wolffian duct is far caudal compared with the normal bud. To denote degrees of ectopy, the location of the normal orifice is called the 'A' position, 'B' is a position midway to the hiatus through which the ureter enters the bladder, 'C' is at the hiatus and 'D' denotes an orifice in the wall of a hiatal diverticulum (Lyon et al., 1969). With lateral ectopy, the ureter may be of larger than normal calibre and often demonstrates vesicoureteral reflux (Ambrose and Nicholson, 1962).

When the reflux ureter is larger than normal in calibre, the orifice is often in the 'B', 'C' or 'D' position, is wider than normal, is 'stadium', 'horseshoe' or 'golfhole' in shape, respectively, and is patulous. Furthermore, the ureter may show focal expansions in the midportion or upper end, the pelvis and calyces are often large and rounded and out of proportion relative to the ureter, and the kidney is thin and oligonephronic and may be dysplastic.

In lateral ectopy, the ureteric bud arises from the most caudal and expanded part of the wolffian duct, which becomes incorporated into the bladder, and that expansion process is continued into the ureter, creating a 'megabud'—megaureter, megacalyces and expanded collecting ducts. The bud arising so distally penetrates the nephron-deficient tail end of the metanephric mesenchyme and lacks inducer capability. The enlarged lateral orifice, ureter and calyces, and the renal dysmorphia indicated that the reflux associated with a wide ureter is incidental to the underlying pan-bud malformation.

Caudal ectopy

When the ureteric orifice lies caudal to the normal location on the trigone, the ureteric bud is presumed to have arisen from a point more cranial on the wolffian duct than normal. When the terminal section of the duct is absorbed into the vesicourethral canal, the ureteric orifice falls short of the normal position at the corner of the trigone. In the male, it may lie toward the bladder neck or in the prostatic urethra, or it may be attached to some part of the ejaculatory duct, seminal vesicle or vas deferens; in the female, the orifice may lie near the bladder neck, in the urethra, on the urethrovaginal bridge in the vestibule, or in the vagina (Fig. 14.3).

Kesavan *et al.* (1977) described 19 unduplicated urethral or vulval ectopic ureters in 15 children. Four ureters were bilateral and 11 unilateral, of which eight were right- and three left-sided: of the 15 patients, seven were females and eight males. These patients exhibited chiefly urethral and vestibular ectopy, and six of the 15 children had additional malformations of the penile urethra or vagina.

Intravesical caudal ectopy

When the ureteric orifice lies caudal to the normal site but within the bladder, the ureter and kidney are generally normally formed but may exhibit a stenotic ureterocele. The hiatus in the bladder wall, however, is also ectopic, being more caudally placed than normal.

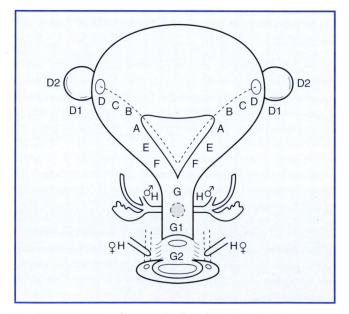

Fig. 14.3 *Composite diagram of male and female genitourinary tracts denoting normal and abnormal UO positions; trigone (A, E, and F); lateral ectopy (B, C); diverticulum (D, D1, D2); urethra above the verumontanum in male (G); vas or vesicle (H); upper half of female urethra (G); lower half (G1); urethrovaginal bridge (G2); and hymen of Gartner's duct (H). (Reprinted, by permission, from Schwarz, R.D., Stephens, F.D. and Cussen, L.J. (1981), The pathogenesis of renal dysplasia. II. The significance of lateral and medial ectopy of the ureteric orifice. J. Invest. Urol. 19: 97, Fig. 1.)*

Urethral ectopic ureter

Urethral ectopic ureters share most of the clinical features of duplex ectopic ureters that issue in corresponding locations. These features are described on page 222. Most urethral non-duplicated ectopic ureters run a short submucosal course in the bladder base to reach the urethra and exhibit ureteropelvic ectasia and some measure of renal hypoplasia. The orifice may be normal in size, stenotic or large. The intravesical part of the ureter is short and the hiatus in the bladder lies close to the vesical outlet. The ureter may be evenly dilated or exhibit a ureterocele that may be large and incompletely muscularized. When the anomaly of urethral ectopy of non-duplicated ureter is bilateral, the vesicourethral hiatuses at bladder neck may disrupt the vesical sphincter causing urinary incontinence. Infection and wetting are the chief clinical features. The ipsilateral kidney may have good, impaired or no evidence of function.

Vestibular ectopic ureter

In vestibular ectopic ureter, the orifice may lie to one side of the external urinary meatus or posterolateral lip, on the urethrovaginal bridge or the hymen. The ureter from its hiatus at the bladder neck runs a submucosal course along the urethra, but rarely, it grooves the muscle wall of the urethra possibly impairing muscle control. Its orifice may be stenotic or normal and visible especially if urine jets at the time of examination.

Vaginal ectopic ureter

In vaginal ectopic ureter, a very rare type, the symptoms are those of infection, flank or pelvic pain, or wetting. The orifice from which urine leaks may not be discovered but may lie at the base of the hymen or in the lateral wall of the vagina or cervix. In either instance, the ureter bypasses the bladder and enters the side wall of the vagina. If it joins Gartner's duct, the urine is led in the duct to the base of the hymen; if the duct atrophies proximal and distal to the junction, a soft cystic swelling composed in part of ureter and Gartner's duct may project into the lumen of the vagina. If a direct opening is found in the side wall of the vagina, it may result from rupture of the cyst or possibly by amputation of the high ectopic bud from the wolffian duct by the migrating müllerian duct, which incorporates the ureter and its lumen into its wall and lumen, respectively.

Associated cloacal abnormalities

Upper urinary-tract anomalies are common in cloacal malformations in both males and females. In a study of the so-called 'persisting mesonephric duct', in which the unduplicated ureter remains attached to the vas, Schwarz and Stephens (1978) found cloacal anomalies to be associated in five of the eight cases described. Gibbons *et al.* (1978), in their review of previously reported cases, found that four of eight patients with the single ectopic ureter joining the vas (persisting mesonephric duct) had supralevator imperforate anus malformations. Johnston and Davenport (1969) reported a case of rectovestibular fistula complicated by unduplicated urethral ectopic ureters. One female patient with a rectocloacal fistula under the author's (F.D.S.) care had a leaking urethral ectopic ureter.

The diagnosis of the urological component may be readily made during the investigations initially undertaken to elucidate the cloacal deformities. However, leakage of urine in such patients requires special assessment to determine whether it results from an excessively short urethra, neuropathic impairment, or ureteral ectopy, or a combination of these factors.

Voiding cystourethrography displays the bladder and urethra and often the ureters and vas by reflux; antegrade and retrograde pyeloureterography or vasography may give additional information, and a flush vaginogram may display and localize the ectopic ureter by reflux (Katzen and Trachtman, 1954). Treatment is very much a matter of making on-the-spot decisions for each patient because of the many variants and combinations of urorectal and genital malformations.

Wetting

Three different circumstances in the case of single ectopic ureter may give rise to wetting.

1. The ectopic orifice may lie distal to the midpoint of the urethra (this occurs in females only) (group A).
2. The ectopic orifice may lie in the vagina or cervix (group B).
3. The ectopic ureter may issue in the urethra in male or female, but the hiatus through which the ureter enters the urinary tract is located in the bladder neck

region disrupting the involuntary sphincter mechanism (group C).

The disruption is more severe if the contralateral ectopic ureter also issues in the urethra; urine then leaks directly to the exterior and the bladder remains empty and small. Wetting can be effectively stopped by reimplantation of the ureter or if the ectopy is unilateral by nephrectomy in groups (A) and (B). Wetting, however, may persist in group (C) because of an accompanying defect in the sphincters of the bladder (see Fig. 22.9).

One specimen of a single ectopic megaureter issuing into the bladder neck with the orifice in the upper urethra was available for histological study of serial sections. In this newborn baby, the contralateral ureter issued in the normal situation on the hemitrigone, and the bladder was normal in size. The muscle of the bladder base and upper urethra was well formed, but on the side of the ectopic ureter, the muscle fibres deviated around the tunnel formed by the hiatus in the sphincteric wall of the bladder neck. The hiatus occupied a wedge sector of the posterolateral quadrant and interrupted the muscle ring in the greater part of this quadrant. After entering the hiatus, the ureter took a short, oblique course in the submucosa to its orifice in the upper urethra.

Wetting may result from the fortuitous location of the hiatus in the vicinity of the internal sphincter, or from the distal ectopic positions of the orifice of the ureter, or both.

If the hiatus lies in the bladder base, the sphincteric action is unlikely to be impaired. If, however, the hiatus verges on the bladder neck and the ureter is bulky, the internal sphincter is deranged, as in the specimen described here, and enuresis may be troublesome. If the ectopy is bilateral and symmetrical, the derangement would be more extensive, the bladder neck wide and relaxed, and wetting continuous and the bladder capacity small.

The location of the ectopic ureteric orifice may be in the upper or lower urethra in females. Wetting is unusual if the orifice is high in the urethra and cranial to the high point in the urethral pressure profile unless the hiatus disrupts the bladder neck. Wetting is usual if the orifice is 'beyond' this point, but the sphincter in such patients may also be impaired if the hiatus disrupts the bladder neck.

In boys, the orifice may be located in the upper urethra or contiguous with the ejaculatory duct, but wetting occurs only if, in addition, the ectopic hiatus deranges and impairs sphincter function.

Surgical significance of urethral ectopic ureters and wetting (group C)

Wetting that persists after reimplantation of unduplicated urethral ectopic ureters or after heminephrectomy in unilateral conditions, is likely to result from derangements of the posterior quadrants of the bladder neck. The results of surgical repair of the sphincters are, in the main, unsatisfactory and especially for bilateral ectopic ureters with a very small capacity bladder. Occasional successes have been reported by epispadiac types of repairs (Williams and Lightwood, 1972) and by bladder neck sling derived from the levatores ani (Chun and Braga, 1965). Successful repair of the bladder neck of one child with bilateral single urethral ectopic ureters was achieved using a technique devised for stress incontinence (Stephens, 1970). On the basis of this experience and the microscopic studies of the specimen described, the following recommendations can be made:

1. The ureteric stump including the submucosal segment should be removed, and the hiatal tunnel occluded at the time of reimplantation of the ureters.
2. The repair should be directed to the posterior quadrants of the bladder neck.
3. When ectopy is bilateral, the posterior wall of the bladder neck requires extensive plication.

The rationale and technique of the operation devised for repair of the bladder neck for a form of stress incontinence resulting from anatomical defects follow below. The procedure was successful in four patients (Stephens, 1970b).

Anatomical arrangement of the muscle of the bladder and urethra

Normal bladder neck

The bladder has three incomplete muscle coats, consisting of a circular arrangement sandwiched between outer and inner longitudinally disposed layers. The circular muscle lies, tier upon tier, over the dome and all sides of the bladder, and tier within tier on the flat trigonal base. The internal urethral meatus being situated at the anterior extremity of the trigone, the tiers spread out posteriorly from it, whereas anteriorly the tiers wrap around the vesicourethral junction in collar fashion, one caudal to the other, but interwoven with longitudinal muscle around the neck. It is presumed that the outer tiers of the bladder base support and aid the action of the inner tiers, and that the combined effect is to create a sphincteric muscle mass at and below the internal meatus. During the reservoir and detrusor periods of bladder activity, the tiers contract and relax; the bladder base is a platform during filling and tilts when the sphincteric rings reorientate during voiding, transforming the base of the bladder into a funnel called by Hutch (1972) the 'trigonal canal'. This tilt of the trigone tubularizes the bladder base into the trigonal canal which incorporates in it the fundus ring of Uhlenhuth *et al.* (1953).

Distal to the internal sphincter mass, the circular muscle is continued in the wall of the urethra as a thin layer to the perineal membrane. On its inner aspect is the inner, longitudinal smooth-muscle layer, extending over the same length of urethra, which is then adequately equipped for peristalsis. Presumably, its function is to express the last drops of urine in antegrade direction from the urethra (see Figs 6.11 and 10.4).

The inner longitudinal muscle of the urethra corresponds to the inner longitudinal muscle of the bladder, though the continuity around the bladder base and neck is incomplete.

The outer longitudinal muscle coat of the bladder is most complete and strongest over the dome and anterior and posterior walls. It gains strong attachment to the pubis in front through the pubovesical ligaments, and its tendinous coat-tails penetrate the circular muscle of the internal sphincter. Posteriorly, this muscle divides, joining a fibromuscular knot of tissue caudal to the internal sphincter, and other tendrils penetrate the circular muscle of the bladder neck from behind.

The voluntary external muscle surrounds the distal half to three-quarters of the pelvic urethra outside the smooth-muscle layers. It has a powerful voluntary sphincteric action on the distal three-quarters of the pelvic urethra, arresting or preventing micturition on demand.

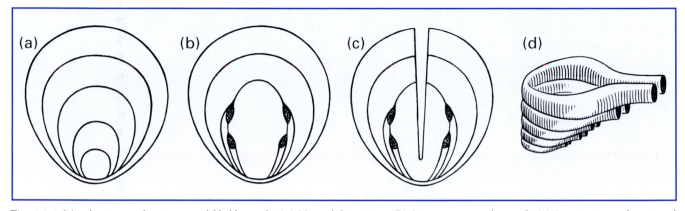

Fig. 14.4 *Muscle rings in the trigone and bladder neck. (**a**) Normal disposition. (**b**) Innermost rings damaged. (**c**) Incision in urethrotrigonal muscle. (**d**) Bipennation and keeling to show the V-type narrowing of the trigone and internal meatus, and the direction of the pull of the reorientated fibres towards the pubes. (Reprinted, by permission, from Stephens, F.D. (1970), A form of stress incontinence in children: another method of bladder neck repair. Aust. N.Z. J. Surg. 40: 125, Fig. 4.)*

Total continence depends on intact inner rings of the vesicourethral internal sphincter together with the external sphincter. Wedge defects of the internal sphincter cause impairment of the innermost rings. The long rings of the trigonal muscle are effective for control of small volumes with low pressure within the bladder, but are inadequate to resist the higher pressures induced by larger volumes or by stress.

Abnormal bladder neck

The posterior gap in the bladder neck caused by the ectopic hiatus for the single ectopic ureter on one or on both sides interferes with the shortest circular rings of the bladder base (Figs 14.4a and 22.9). The gaps may not be identifiable macroscopically, but radiographically, leakage of contrast material exposes either a conical shape of the bladder neck or a streak through it into the distal urethra (Fig. 14.5).

Surgical correction of 'stress' incontinence

Restoration of the circular vesicourethral muscle rings is the aim of surgery.

The plan of surgical reconstruction of the bladder neck in children with posterior defects is to convert the arrangement of the muscle rings of the trigone and bladder neck into a bipenniform keel, at the same time repairing and diminishing the diameter of the rings. The combination of bipennation and keeling of the urethrotrigonal muscle reduces the size of the loops and

effects a pincer action by posteroanterior compression of the bladder neck.

The bladder is opened in the midline, and the stump of the ectopic ureter is excised. The mucosa of the bladder and urethra is then widely undercut on both sides of the wedge-shaped bed of the ureter. If the stump has previously been removed or the weakness of the

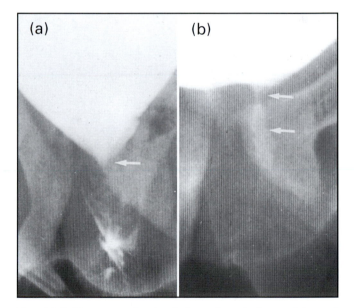

Fig. 14.5 *Cystogram showing leakage through damaged internal sphincter. (**a**) Case A.N., female aged seven years, with wide evagination of bladder neck after division of the roof of the urethral ectopic ureter. (**b**) Case S.W., contrast leaking into urethra and slight evagination of bladder neck. (Reprinted, by permission, from Stephens, F.D. (1970), A form of stress incontinence in children: another method of bladder neck repair. Aust. N.Z. J. Surg. 40: 125, Figs 2 and 6.)*

bladder neck was caused by previous trauma, the healed mucosa of the bladder base is incised in the midline into the depth of the cup-shaped patulous urethral meatus (Fig. 14.6a, b). The mucosa is then widely undercut on both sides of the incision throughout its whole length, but especially around the two posterior urethral quadrants. The freed mucosal flaps are retracted laterally by guy stitches.

The whole thickness of the trigonal muscle and scar is then incised in the same line as the mucosal incision (Fig. 14.6c). The front of the wall of the vagina or cervix is then exposed to view. The cut edges of the trigonal muscle are then everted posteriorly, and the muscle rings bipennated with 4/0 chromicized catgut Cushing

sutures (Fig. 14.6d). The suturing is started at the cranial end of the incision, and gentle tension on the thread rucks up the muscle ahead of each succeeding stitch, thus facilitating the insertion of the stitches along the trigone and into the urethra.

A second and a third layer of continuous Lembert sutures are then inserted to keel and narrow the trigone, still further shorten the effective rings of muscle, and constrict the internal urethral meatus almost to the point of occlusion (Fig. 14.6f,g).

At this stage, the excess mucosal lining is trimmed and approximated with fine absorbable sutures (Fig. 14.6h). The bladder is drained suprapubically for two weeks to permit sound healing in the undistended state.

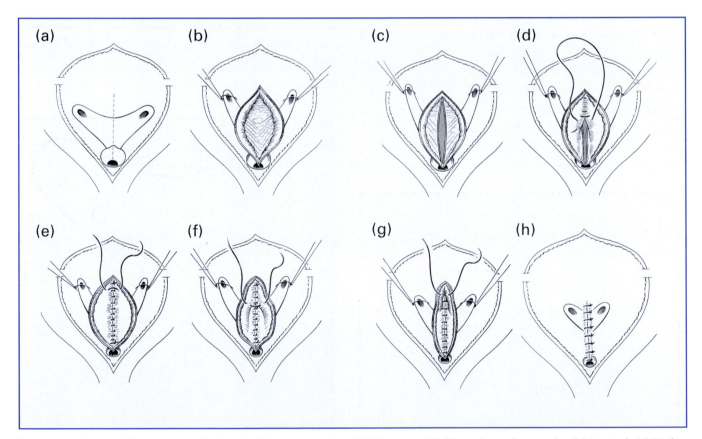

Fig. 14.6 *Technique of bipennation and keeling. (**a**) Incision in mucosa. (**b**) Trigone and bladder neck muscle exposed and (**c**) incised. (**d**) Keeling by Cushing suture. (**e**), (**f**) Insertion of row of Lembert sutures to elongate the keel and to draw in the V of the bladder neck to make a smaller aperture. (**g**) A third row of Lambert sutures. (**h**) Mucosal sutures. Note narrowing of trigone and urethral meatus. (Reprinted, by permission, from Stephens, F.D. (1970), A form of stress incontinence in children: another method of bladder neck repair. Aust. N.Z. J. Surg. 40: 125, Fig. 5.)*

The wolffian duct between the ureteric bud and the urinary component of the cloaca (the common excretory duct) is absorbed into the urinary tract in normal embryos. Rarely, however, this absorption does not occur or is incomplete and the common excretory duct carrying the ureter and vas persists, its orifice translocating to, or towards, the lateral cornu of the trigone and its structure simulating that of a ureter. An extraordinary example of a duplication of a vas that mimicked in many respects an ectopic ureter will also be described in this chapter. An explanation for the embryogenesis of both these anomalies is proposed.

Schwarz and Stephens (1978) described case reports of eight patients (or specimens) exhibiting nine persisting mesonephric duct (PMD) units. Five of the patients had coexisting rectal anomalies (Fig. 15.1).

Level of junction of ureter and wolffian duct

In one instance, the vas joined the ureter at a point less than 0.5 cm from the ureteropelvic junction in the right loin (Fig. 15.1, Case 1). In three others, the junction occurred above the common iliac artery (Fig. 15.1, Cases 3, 5 and 7). Two of these kidneys were ectopic, located at the level of the iliac crest. In one, the junction was at the renal pelvis (Fig. 15.1, Case 5). In the remaining five units, the junction was in the more usually described position, that is, behind the bladder base.

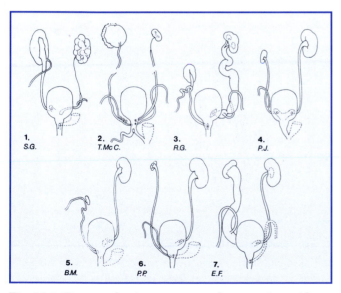

Fig. 15.1 *Diagrams showing uroanatomy of seven patients with persisting mesonephric duct anomalies and one with contiguous orifices of vas deferens and ureter; orifice of right PMD in Case 7 not known; Cases 1, 2, 4, 5 and 6 have associated rectal deformities. (Reprinted, by permission, from Schwarz, R. and Stephens, F.D. (1978), The persisting mesonephric duct: high junction of vas deferens and ureter. J. Urol. 120: 592, Fig. 2.)*

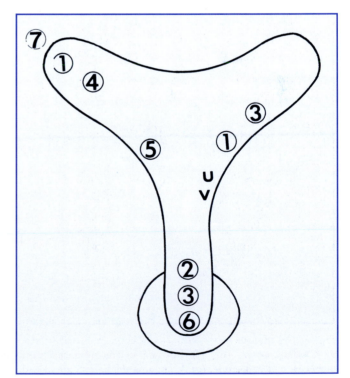

Fig. 15.2 *Trigonal and urethral positions of persisting mesonephric duct orifices. Numbers refer to case number in Fig. 15.1; U and V refer to orifices of left ureter and vas in Case 2. (Reprinted, by permission, from Schwarz, R. and Stephens, F.D. (1978), The persisting mesonephric duct: high junction of vas deferens and ureter. J. Urol. 120: 592, Fig. 4.)*

Termination of the persisting mesonephric duct

The position of the orifice of the persisting mesonephric duct ranged from the verumontanum to the lateral cornu of the trigone (Fig. 15.2).

Structure

The gross and microscopic examination of the persisting mesonephric duct showed it to be similar to that of the ureter above its junction with the vas (Fig. 15.3). In those units in which the persisting mesonephric duct was dilated abnormally, the ureter also was dilated above the junction. The epithelial lining and musculature were indistinguishable above and below the junction with the vas in the five instances that were examined. The vas seemed to join the ureter rather than the ureter joining the vas. In none of the nine instances of persisting mesonephric duct could a seminal vesicle be identified positively. In one of the two units exhibiting separate contiguous orifices, the seminal vesicle was present (Fig. 15.1, Case 2).

Obstruction

Of the persisting mesonephric ducts, two ended blindly (Fig. 15.1, Cases 1 and 5), one had a valve-like obstruction above the junction with the vas (Fig. 15.1, Case 3) and there was one ureteropelvic junction obstruction (Fig. 15.1, Case 2). An atretic ureteropelvic junction was found in one of the examples of contiguous orifices (Fig. 15.1, Case 2).

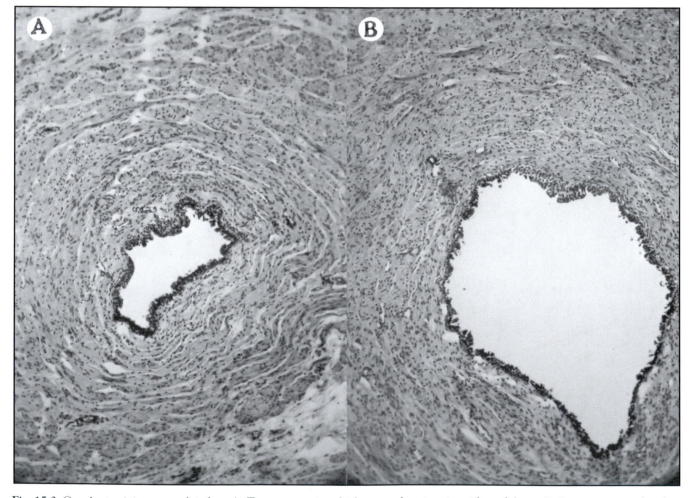

Fig. 15.3 *Case 1—persisting mesonephric duct.* **A.** *Transverse section of right ureter above junction with vas deferens.* **B.** *Persisting mesonephric duct below junction with vas deferens. Note similar musculature but wider lumen of PMD. Reduced ×35. (Reprinted, by permission, from Schwarz, R. and Stephens, F.D. (1978), The persisting mesonephric duct: high junction of vas deferens and ureter. J. Urol. 120: 592, Fig. 5.)*

Reflux

Of the five persisting mesonephric duct units tested, four exhibited reflux that filled the persisting mesonephric duct, ureter and vas (Fig. 15.4).

Kidney function

The kidneys in five PMD units were non-functioning on IVP. One showed faint function, one moderate delayed function and one good function.

The histological features reflected the functional differences. Four kidneys showed major degrees of hypodysplasia and three showed milder histological changes, only one of which demonstrated urographic function. The two other functioning kidneys showed near normal structure.

Complete obstruction of the persisting mesonephric duct or ureter was accompanied by non-functioning hypodysplastic kidneys (one multicystic and two small,

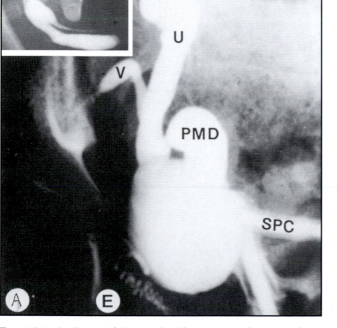

Fig. 15.4 **A.** *Post-void X-ray of voiding cystourethrogram, shows reflux into right persisting mesonephric duct, tortuous megaureter, vas deferens and epididymis.* **B.** *Bifid urethra. (SPC = suprapubic catheter; PMD = persisting mesonephric duct; U = ureter; V = vas deferens; E = epididymis.) (Illustration courtesy of J.H. Johnston; reprinted, by permission, from Schwarz, R. and Stephens, F.D. (1978), The persisting mesonephric duct: high junction of vas deferens and ureter.* J. Urol. 120: 592, Fig. 3.)

solid nubbins). Neither the site of junction of the vas with the ureter, the position of the persisting mesonephric duct orifice, nor the demonstration of reflux bore relationship to renal histological or functional quality.

Associated anorectal anomalies

Of the eight children with a persisting mesonephric duct, one had a rectobulbar fistula (Fig. 15.1, Case 5), two had rectourethral fistulas (Fig. 15.1, Cases 1 and 6), one had an H-type urethroanal fistula (Fig. 15.1, Case 2), and in one, the urethra issued on the perineum in conjunction with the anus (Fig. 15.1, Case 4).

There were two patients who demonstrated separate contiguous ectopic orifices of the ureter and vas (Fig. 15.1, Cases 2 and 7). In one, the left ureter opened at the bladder neck and showed reflux on the voiding study. The vas opened high in the posterior urethra just distal to the internal urethral orifice (Fig. 15.1, Case 2).

There were multiple anomalies, including an imperforate anus with a rectovesical fistula in one specimen (Fig. 15.1, Case 8). On the right side, the ureter and ejaculatory duct issued into the bladder together beside the orifice of the fistula. On the left side, the ejaculatory duct orifice lay beside the fistula, but the left ureter opened onto the lateral cornu of the trigone.

Embryogenesis of the persisting mesonephric duct (PMD)

If the ureteral bud originates at a far more cranial ectopic position than normal, the ureter and genital ducts may not achieve separate orifices when the distal part of the wolffian duct becomes absorbed into the urinary tract, leaving a persisting common duct (Williams and Royle, 1969). Presumably, the more cranial the ectopic bud, the longer the PMD would be. If the ureteral bud arises from a less distant cranial ectopic position, the absorption of the caudal wolffian duct may just reach the point of origin of the ureteral bud, in which event the orifices would be contiguous in the urinary tract. The two units in this series in which the vas and ureter had separate, contiguous, ectopic orifices represent less cranial ectopy of the bud than those with PMD deformity.

Another possible explanation of the PMD anomaly is that the ureteral bud originates from its normal position opposite the metanephric blastema adjacent to the urogenital sinus (Alfert and Gillenwater, 1972). The common excretory duct, rather than the ureter, then elongates. The caudal end of the wolffian duct would remain unexpanded and would not be absorbed into the urinary tract, causing the persisting mesonephric duct to issue at the verumontanum. There are several objections to this theory. In seven of nine instances of persisting mesonephric duct, the ureter did elongate. Also, that the caudal portion of the wolffian duct was absorbed into the urinary tract is shown by the trigonal position of the persisting mesonephric duct orifice. Finally, the persisting mesonephric ducts with double kidneys (Riba, et al., 1946) and the two instances of separate contiguous orifices of the vas and ureter are not easily explained by this theory.

If the ureteral bud arose from the wolffian duct at a cranial ectopic location, the resulting kidney should be extremely dysplastic (Mackie and Stephens, 1975). Kidneys of good quality, however, were found in our series of PMD deformities and have been reported previously (Riba et al., 1946; Alfert and Gillenwater, 1972). There are two possible explanations for the rare good kidneys found with this anomaly. First, the ureteral bud and the metanephric blastema may lie together in a cranial ectopic position. The persisting mesonephric duct may be part of a pancloacal anomaly as in the five children with anorectal anomalies. In these circumstances, the bud, blastema and rectum may all be dislocated equally in a cranial direction. Second, the ectopic ureteral bud may induce a good metanephric kidney in the nearby undifferentiated and non-involuted mesonephric blastema. This mechanism is supported by the experiments of Wolff and associates who showed that explants of a chicken ureteral bud induced metanephric tubules in the uninduced mesonephric blastema of another chicken embryo (Wolff et al., 1969).

In none of the cases of persisting mesonephric duct was a seminal vesicle positively identified grossly or microscopically, and in the two instances of separate contiguous orifices, one had a seminal vesicle. The absence of seminal vesicles together with the gross and histological appearance of the PMD suggests that the duct differentiates along ureteral lines. In our series, the orifices of the PMD and contiguous ureter and vas were located along the embryologic ureteral pathway from the verumontanum to the cornu of the trigone (Fig. 15.2). The duct differentiated structurally as a ureter rather than a vas, and, presumably, the persisting mesonephric duct was incorporated into the urethra and bladder as a ureter.

Vas ectopia

Gibbons et al. (1978), reported two case histories illustrating 'vas ectopia' in association with unduplicated ureters. They also proposed an embryological explanation for the PMD and vas ectopia abnormalities.

They found that in their two patients, the vas issued onto the trigone inferomedial to the ureteric orifices and exhibited free vesicovasal reflux. In one patient with anorectal malformations, the left vas was very dilated and exhibited active peristalsis visible externally between the scrotum and the inguinal canal, and the right was normal in calibre. Both ureters issued in 'B' position, were non-reflux in type and subtended normal upper tracts. In the other patient who had in addition a laryngeal cleft, the left ectopic vas was normal in calibre; the left ureter was in 'A' position, exhibited free reflux and served a radiographically normal kidney.

Proximal vas precursor

Gibbons et al. (1978) proposed that the normal terminal end of the wolffian duct can theoretically be divided into sections including the common excretory duct, next to it the proximal vas precursor (PVP) and more cranial to it the upper wolffian duct. The common excretory duct becomes incorporated into the urinary system as the vesicourethral trigone and ureter and the PVP incorporates itself into the vicinity of the verumontanum and forms the ejaculatory duct, vesicle and juxtaurethral vas. The situation of the PVP between the upper wolffian duct which forms the vas and the lower wolffian or common excretory duct which buds a ureter, gives a bipotential capability to this zone. This segment may either follow the normal embryogenesis and form ejaculatory duct, vesicle and vas (vasation), or it may encroach onto the ureteric budding zone of the common excretory duct, ureterize and migrate into the urinary tract to a site located along the embryologic pathway in the bladder neck or trigone of a normal ureter

(Fig. 15.5). If the ureterization encroaches onto the bud site or beyond, then the common excretory duct ureterizes and follows the migratory path of the ureter to the bladder. The vas becomes structurally an appendage of the ureter. If the PVP ureterizes and encroaches on the common excretory duct, theoretically it is unlikely that the seminal vesicle will develop and this fits the facts provided in the review of other case reports.

Ureterization of the PVP causes vas ectopia and may not influence the quality of the kidney, which is predetermined by the initial location of the ureteric bud on the common excretory duct (Mackie and Stephens, 1975).

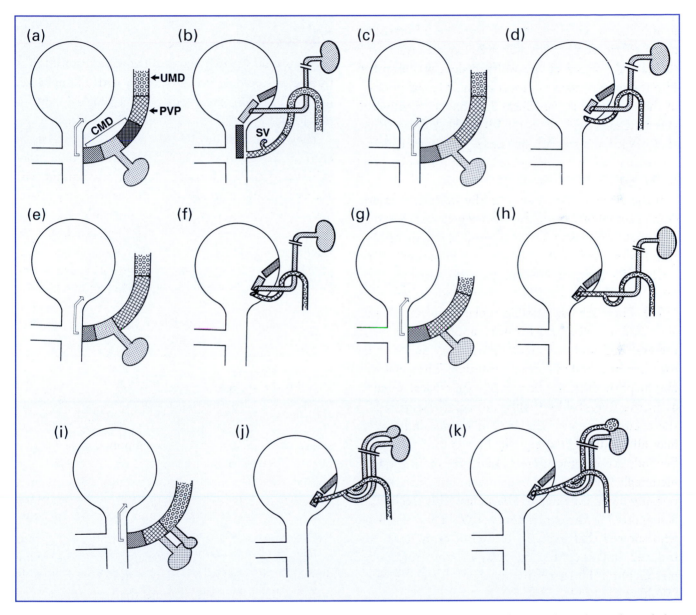

Fig. 15.5 *Ureterization of the wolffian duct and vas ectopia. (**a**) Three segments of the common mesonephric duct (CMD), together with their incorporation and repositioning in the bladder base and urethra. (**b**) Segment of the proximal vas precursor (PVP) moves to the juxtaurethral location; and forms the ejaculatory duct, seminal vesicle (SV) and the ampulla of the vas; UMD, upper mesonephric duct. (**c**), (**d**) 'Ureterization' by the PVP of the cranial segment of the CMD resulting in vas ectopia and suppression of the SV. (**e**), (**f**) Encroachment and ureterization to the ureteric bud and migration of both orifices to the midtrigone. (**g**), (**h**) PVP overrides the middle zone completely and migrates to the cornu of the trigone with ureter conjoined. (**i**), (**j**) PVP ureterizes the middle section and migrates to the trigone carrying both ureters of a duplex system with it. (**k**) Similar to (**j**) except that the upper pole ureter is 'vasated'—that is, part or all of it resembles vas or epididymal structure. (Reprinted, with permission from, Stephens, F.D. (1995), Embryology of the upper genitourinary tract, in Paediatric Urology, 3rd edn. S. Koff and B. O'Donnell (eds). London, Butterworth Heinemann.)*

The theory may explain the occasion of the good-quality kidney accompanying high vas–ureter junction in either an unduplicated or duplex ectopic system (Fig. 15.5 I–K). The ureterized PVP and common excretory duct lengthen with ascent of the kidney in the manner of an elongating ureter instead of giving rise locally to ejaculatory duct and vesicle. The authors emphasize the difference in the anatomical arrangement between the 'H'-position ectopic ureter draining into the vas and the vasoureteral malformation, in which the vas and ureter join.

The 'H'-position ureter arises from a vas issuing into the normal site of the verumontanum whereas in 'C' vasoureteral ectopia, the orifice of the vas is ectopic.

Unique variant of vas ectopia

Brown *et al.* (1988) describe a rare anomaly in a male aged 30 years with urinary infection in whom the regular vas and another structure resembling a ureter and issuing from the lowermost minor renal calyx inosculated in the epididymis or rete of the scrotal testis. Apart from the lowermost minor calyx, the kidney and pyelon were otherwise normal (Fig. 15.6). The question arose as to whether this extra structure was an ectopic duplex ureter or a limb of a duplicate or bifid vas deferens. Four theories were advanced, three being unlikely because explanations did not conform to present concepts of embryology. In the fourth theory, the extra structure, the orchiorenal connecting tube was considered to be one limb of a bifid mesonephric duct, the main limb and the common stem being the regular mesonephric duct.

The ureteric bud presumably arose at the junction of the two limbs of the bifid duct close to the point of entry of the common stem into the urinary tract (Fig. 15.7). The bud elongated carrying with it the limb of the mesonephric duct attached to the lower polar division of the future renal pelvis. At its other end this orchiorenal duct with its several vasa efferentia gained

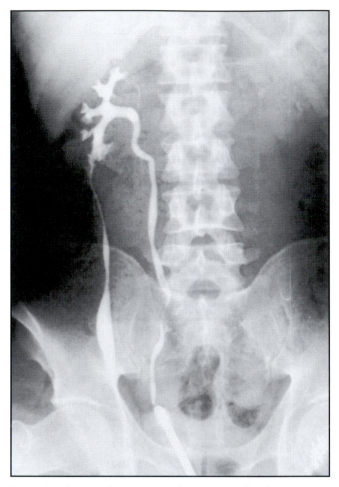

Fig. 15.6 *Retrograde pyelogram showing normal right ureter and calyceal system except for the caudal most minor calyx from which escaped the radiopaque medium into an orchiorenal tube resembling a ureter. (Reprinted, with permission, from The Williams and Wilkins Co., from Brown, D.M., Peterson, N.R. and Schultz, R.E. (1988), Ureteral duplication with lower pole ectopia to the epididymis. J. Urol. 140: 139–141, Fig. 1B.)*

attachment to the upper polar region of the rete testis. The kidney migrated rostrally and the testis descended through the inguinal canal to the scrotum.

The very short common stem of the bifid duct became incorporated into the urinary tract to form the hemitrigone, at the same time reorientating the ureteric bud orifice to the lateral cornu and the orifice of the regular

Fig. 15.7 *Bifid mesonephric duct. (a) Split or separate mesonephric (inset) ducts and vasa efferentia to testis at rostral end and short common stem at distal end. (b) Ureteric bud arises from the regular mesonephric duct at its junction with duplicate mesonephric duct. (c) The bud induces the metanephric blastema. (d) Ureter elongates with kidney and orchiorenal duct attached to lower pole of renal pelvis; kidney migrates rostrally and the common stem of the bifid mesonephric duct is incorporated into the urinary tract. (e) Kidney reaches loin and testis migrating towards the scrotum on elongated orchiorenal and orchiourethral ducts. Note seminal vesicle diverticulum on orchiourethral duct. (f) Scrotal testis and junction of both ducts in the epididymis or in the rete testis via the vasa efferentia (inset). (Reprinted, with permission, from Brown, D.M., Peterson, N.R. and Schultz, R.E. (1988), Ureteral duplication with lower pole ectopia to the epididymis. J. Urol. 140: 139–141, Fig. 4.)*

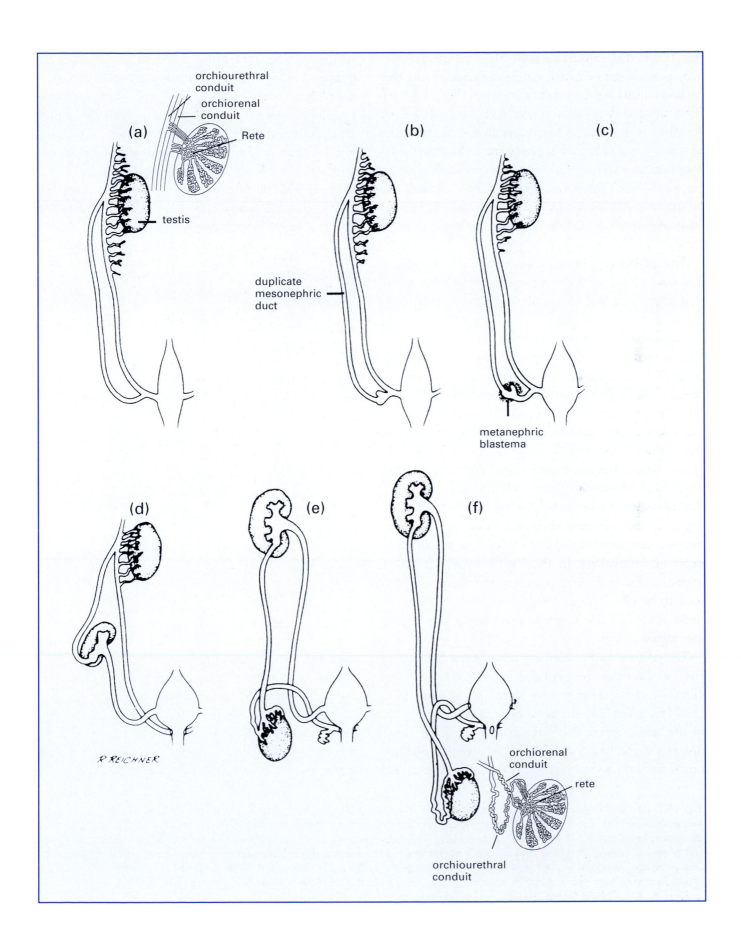

vas into the urethra. The seminal vesicle was shown radiographically to be formed in association with the regular vas deferens.

This regular vas deferens or orchiourethral duct at its cranial end gained the major connection but with the rete testis through its dominant vasa efferentia. It was shown radiographically by injection that radiopaque fluid passed from one duct to the other through either the rete testis or by a junction between the two limbs before the vasa efferentia joined the rete testis (Fig. 15.6).

The orchiorenal duct was found to resemble a ureter radiographically and histologically. Gibbons *et al.* (1978) and Schwarz and Stephens (1978) have shown that persisting mesonephric ducts acquired ureteric dimensions and structure thus masquerading as a ureter. This same phenomenon provides the explanation of the 'ureterized' orchiorenal limb of the bifid mesonephric duct.

Embryologically, the orchiorenal duct is mesonephric in origin and does not conform to anatomical features one would expect of an ectopic duplex ureter.

The ureterocele with a stenotic orifice is the most common type of ureterocele in association with single ureters. It may also occur on the ectopic ureter of a duplex system. The orifice is located on the trigone, the ureter dilates in proportion to the degree of stenosis, and the kidney is usually of good functional quality in children. It occurs unilaterally and bilaterally in the proportion of 1:1. The size of the ureterocele varies from side to side when bilateral and from patient to patient (Fig. 16.1). The ureterocele may be less than 5 mm in diameter and so small that it can be recognized radiographically or cystoscopically only when distended at the ending of ureteric propulsive peristaltic wave and only about 3–5 mm in diameter. Others range up to about 2.0 cm in diameter and remain distended. The very small orifice may be readily identified resting on the trigone or subterminal on the upside or downside of the distended ureterocele (Fig. 16.1).

Other types of ureterocele such as cecoureterocele and sphincteric types occur rarely with single ureters. They will be described in Chapter 35.

Infection, haematuria, dysuria resulting from prolapse of the ureterocele into the urethra, and suprapubic and flank pains cause the patient to seek medical advice, but two ureteroceles were symptomless and undiagnosed during life and were incidental findings at necropsy.

Radiologic features

The classical radiological appearance on excretory urography of a dense, round structure in the bladder base surrounded by a contrast-free halo was present in three patients (Fig. 16.2). The common finding of a plain filling defect without a halo was noted in most of the others (Fig. 16.2). The halo effect is apparent only when there is sufficient contrast medium inside both the ureterocele and the bladder to demonstrate a filling defect caused by the wall of the ureterocele.

The affected renal segment appeared hydronephrotic in one-third of the patients. Absence of renal function on intravenous pyelography was noted in two patients, and in the remainder, function appeared to be satisfactory.

Sixteen patients had micturition cystourethrograms and were specifically tested for vesicoureteric reflux. No patient had reflux into the ureterocele.

In two male patients, the ureteroceles prolapsed from the bladder into the posterior urethra during voiding (Fig. 16.3). The ureterocele remained in evidence in the base of the bladder after voiding because of its inability to empty through the stenotic orifice.

It was possible to distinguish the ureterocele as stenotic in type on the radiographic appearances when the ureterocele could be seen, by virtue of its radiopaque content, to be lying well within the bladder and in continuity with the adjoining ureter. When a ureterocele appeared as a filling defect, it could generally be diagnosed as stenotic or sphincterostenotic if it remained visible after micturition.

Cystoscopic findings

The stenotic orifice was visible only in those few ureteroceles in which the location was flush or nearly flush

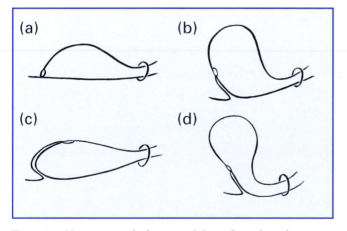

Fig. 16.1 *Variations in the location of the orifices of simple ureteroceles: terminal (**a**) and subterminal (**b**), (**c**), (**d**). Note also sessile and polypoid expansions of the ureteroceles. (Reprinted, by permission, from Subbiah, N. and Stephens, F.D. (1972), Stenotic ureterocele. Aust. N.Z. J. Surg. 4: 267, Fig. 1.)*

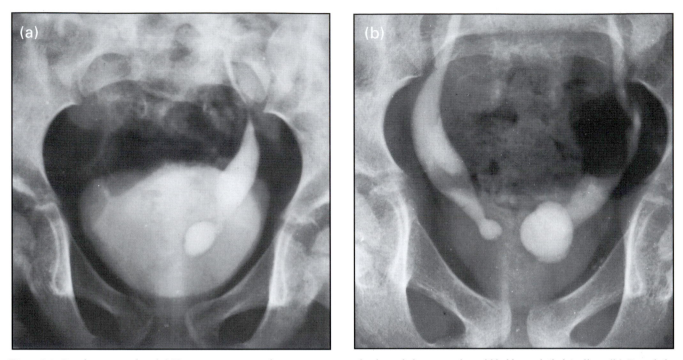

Fig. 16.2 *Simple ureteroceles.* (**a**) *Excretory urograms showing contrast in the distended ureterocele and bladder with 'halo' effect.* (**b**) *Faint halo on right side in bilateral ureteroceles. Note absence of halo if contrast is too dilute in bladder (or in ureterocele).* ((**a**) *reprinted, by permission, from Stephens, F.D. (1963), Congenital Malformations of the Rectum, Anus and Genito-Urinary Tracts. Edinburgh, Livingstone, Fig. 91B, p. 179.* (**b**) *reprinted, by permission, from Subbiah, N. and Stephens, F.D. (1972), Stenotic ureterocele. Aust. N.Z. J. Surg. 4: 257, Fig. 2.)*

with the trigone. In those patients in whom the orifice was perched on the dome, it was usually not identified.

In the course of the cystoscopy, a study was made of the peristalsis of the ureterocele. In those with extreme stenosis, the ureterocele remained globular and full; in others with less obstruction, the ureterocele appeared to distend and collapse; and in still others, the dome-like ureterocele suddenly vanished from view in a peristaltic flurry.

If peristalsis was clearly seen and differentiated by the characteristic movement of the wall from mere distension and collapse of the ureterocele, it was presumed that the wall was well muscularized.

Histology

Histological examination of eight stenotic ureteroceles was undertaken by Dr L.J. Cussen. Stenotic ureteroceles were found to exhibit three different arrangements of the muscle in their walls. The direction of muscular fibres in the ureteroceles was longitudinal in five, longitudinal and circular in one, circular in one and not determined in one.

Where the muscle coat was complete throughout the ureterocele, it was thickened and strong, but in others, the muscle was extremely thin. Of those in which the muscle was incomplete, the deficiency occurred in the distal half including the wall around the meatus of the ureterocele (Fig. 16.4). In one, the muscle bundles throughout were evenly distributed, but were regularly interrupted by gaps containing connective tissue.

If the orifice was at the end of the ureterocele and the muscle was complete, both hypertrophy and hyperplasia were present, but if the muscle was deficient in the distal part, the remaining myocytes showed no hypertrophy or hyperplasia. If the orifice was subterminal, the fibres were longitudinal and might show deficiencies (bundle isolated, but not continuous), or be complete but not hypertrophic, or be complete with hypertrophy and hyperplasia. There was no evidence that an eccentric bulge in the wall of the ureterocele was caused by a relative weakness of that portion of the wall of the ureterocele. Furthermore, the size of the ureterocele could not be correlated with the amount of muscle in the wall. It appears that neither the muscle content nor

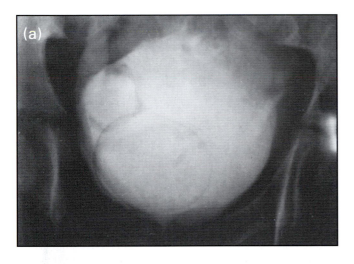

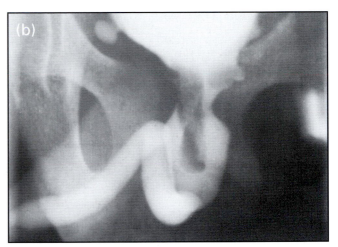

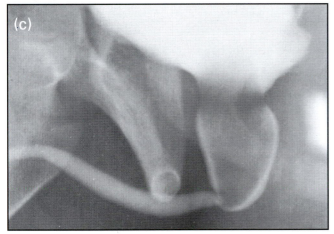

Fig. 16.3 *Prolapse of simple ureterocele into the urethra. Case O'T. Excretory urography showing simple polypoid ureterocele with 'halo' in bladder (**a**), prolapsing into urethra during voiding (**b**), and prolapsed and plugging posterior urethra (**c**). (Reprinted, by permission, from Subbiah, N. and Stephens, F.D. (1972), Stenotic ureterocele. Aust. N.Z. J. Surg. 4: 257, Figs 2B and 3.)*

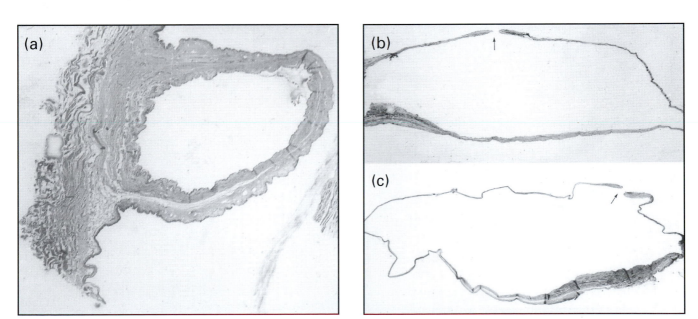

Fig. 16.4 *Histologic structure of three simple ureteroceles. (a) Muscle walls hypertrophic. (b) Attenuated and incomplete muscular wall (arrow denotes the orifice). (c) Muscle only in the floor (arrow denotes the orifice). (Reprinted, by permission, from Subbiah, N. and Stephens, F.D. (1972), Stenotic ureterocele. Aust. N.Z. J. Surg. 4: 257, Figs 4, 5 and 6B.)*

the size nor location of the orifice could be explained on the basis of obstruction alone, and that the eccentric bulge on many of the ureteroceles did not occur at sites that histologically seemed thinner or weaker than elsewhere in the ureterocele.

Subterminal location of the orifice of the ureterocele

The stenotic orifice was found to be perched either on the convexity of the ureterocele or on the caudal underhung aspect of a polypoid type of expansion. It was found histologically that it was not a focal 'blowout' of the muscle coat that determined the site and size of the bulge of the ureterocele, because the muscle was no more deficient there than anywhere else. The shape of the ureterocele and the location of its orifice appear to be better explained on an embryological basis. The ureter within the bladder shares the same expansion process and expands from a tubular to a globular shape as occurs with the formation of the bladder. Depending on the form of expansion, the orifice will be flush on the trigone or tilted onto some part of the convex surface of the ureterocele.

Prolapse

In the two male children in whom the ureterocele prolapsed into the posterior urethra, the ureterocele was pedunculated, its orifice was subterminal and underhung on the caudal aspect of the pedicle, and the muscle in one was complete but extremely thin, and in the other showed a tessellation of muscle separated by fine septa of collagenous tissue. This weak muscle, together with the pedunculated shape, probably accounted for the reten-tion of urine in the ureterocele, the presence of a bolus and prolapse into the urethra during voiding.

Choice of surgical technique

Treatment is initially directed to the kidneys and ureters if the function is minimal, and to the ureterocele when the renal function is salvageable.

From this small series of ureteroceles treated in different ways, it is apparent that several types of operations can be used to overcome the obstruction without inducing reflux. Treatment included enlargement and partial excision or incision of the orifice in nine patients, seven of whom showed no persisting reflux.

The ureterovesical mechanism was efficient after enlargement of the meatus in seven, presumably because the muscle in the remaining walls of the ureteroceles was adequate to activate the flap-valve mechanism, even though in some the orifice was much larger than normal. Hence, observations of the active contractility of the ureterocele may be important in the decision whether or not enlargement of the orifice is a suitable form of treatment.

Though the ureterovesical valves were competent in seven out of nine patients treated by enlargement of the orifice, the result in individual patients is unpredictable. A ureteral reimplantation procedure is probably more certain to create a competent valve and may be carried out as a primary procedure. There is, however, a place for primary transurethral enlargement of the orifice in the first instance, especially when the orifice is clearly visible, the urine is not infected, and active peristaltic contractility is visible in the ureterocele.

'Megaureter' is a term now used to include all ureters of abnormally wide dimensions. Since some measure of agreement on nomenclature and classification of megaureters was reached by a working party (Smith, 1977), which reported an International Pediatric Urological Seminar in Philadelphia in April 1976, the schema (Table 17.1) has been adopted provisionally. It provides simple descriptive terms for the three major groups:

A. Reflux megaureter.
B. Obstructed megaureter.
C. Non-reflux, non-obstructed megaureter.

All have primary and secondary subgroups. Other terms, such as 'megaloureter', 'hydroureter', 'ureterectasis', 'wide ureter' and 'macroureters' were not used or given specific connotations. In this 'ABC' classification, 'secondary'

Table 17.1 *Classification of megaureters**

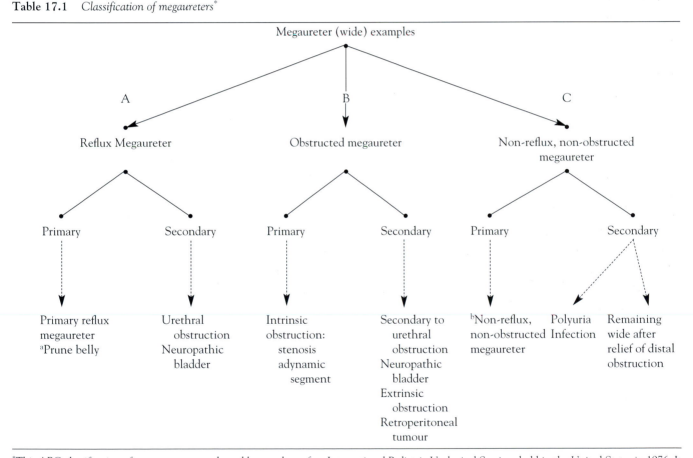

*This ABC classification of megaureters was adopted by members of an International Pediatric Urological Seminar held in the United States in 1976. It was a combined meeting of the Urological Section of the American Academy of Pediatrics, the Society of Pediatric Urological Surgeons and the Society of Pediatric Urology, and held at the Philadelphia Children's Hospital. (Reprinted, by permission, from Smith, E.D. (1977), Report of Working Party to establish an international nomenclature for the large ureter, in *Urinary System Malformations in Children*, D. Bergsma and J.W. Duckett, eds. New York, Alan R. Liss for National Foundation—March of Dimes. BD:OAS, XIII:3, No. 5.)
[a]Some conditions (e.g. prune belly, ureteroceles, ectopic ureters, etc.) may appear under several other columns.
[b]As proved not to be obstructed.
Note: An occasional megaureter may show reflux and apparent obstruction.

denotes a reaction of the ureter to lesions elsewhere inside or outside the urinary tract, such as urethral obstruction, neuropathic bladder, obstruction of the ureter by external compressions or enlargement due to the polyuria.

The classification in its present form is simple, but improvements to it may eventuate to incorporate some of the following examples, which may cause confusion. First, a ureter may be Type A on one side and Type C on the contralateral side or, rarely, Types A and B in the same ureter—for example, primary reflux megaureter and primary distal intrinsic ureteral obstruction as well. Second, a patient may exhibit Type A primary megaureter on one side, Type C megaureter on the opposite side and urethral valves that severely obstruct the urinary tract. Third, the grotesque megaureters of the prune belly triad occur concomitantly with such a bizarre array of other urinary-tract anomalies that the ureter falls into A, B or C types, or combinations of AB or AC with or without a secondary component in addition. For example, the megaureter may exhibit reflux due to congenital absence of the submucosal ureter, an intrinsic partial or complete obstruction in mid-ureter, and congenital obstruction (partial or complete) of the posterior or anterior urethra, which adds a secondary component to the Type A primary reflux megaureter.

The classification as it stands, however, is workable and defines the entities about which much confusion has arisen because of the semantics involved.

Morphometric study

A megaureter may be large because of obvious or presumptive evidence of obstruction in the ureter or urethra, but enlargement may occur without obstruction and with no known cause. To provide some objective criteria on the causes of enlargement of the ureter, the size and numbers of smooth-muscle cell components of the walls were measured. Meaningful patterns have emerged on the basis of cell size, clarifying the role and sites of obstruction and providing logical explanations for the obscure, non-obstructive examples.

The muscle components of the walls of 380 normal ureters and 300 megaureters from infants and children were studied by Dr L.J. Cussen (1971a) (Table 17.2). He found the muscle coats of the megaureters to be thick, normal, thin or absent, and a close correlation was apparent between the state of the muscle and the diagnoses based on clinical, biopsy and autopsy investigations. These investigations included accurate calibrations of the suspect sites for comparison with normal values and perfusion of the isolated ureters to test for impairment of flow.

Of the 300 megaureters, 201 were obstructive (129 Class B exhibiting primary and 72 secondary megaureters), 72 were Class A reflux megaureters, three were bifid ureters with normal common stems and with ureter-to-ureter reflux around the Y junction, 18 were Class C primary non-reflux, non-obstructed megaureters and six were from babies who died of the triad or prune belly syndrome. The type of megaureter commonly associated with gross spinal deformities, such as myelomeningoceles, was not included in the study.

The area of muscle and the number of nuclei in a transverse section of 10-μm thickness were estimated, using a graduated grating on the ocular of a microscope,

Table 17.2 *The structure of the normal human ureter in infancy and childhood: ready reckoner of approximate microscopic measurements of ureters*

Age	Height (cm)	Weight (kg)	Muscle cell population				Muscle cell size (μm^3)	Area of muscle in section of ureter (mm^2)			
			P-U*	M-S	D-E	U-V		P-U*	M-S	D-E	U-V
30 weeks' gestation	40	2	1200	1600	1400	900	1500	0.2	0.3	0.2	0.1
3 months	60	5	1700	2200	1500	1000	1500	0.2	0.5	0.2	0.2
3 years	90	13	2000	2600	1900	900	1500	0.4	0.5	0.3	0.2
6 years	120	20	2700	3200	2500	1400	1700	0.5	0.8	0.5	0.3
12 years	150	35	3300	4000	3100	2000	1700	0.6	1.0	0.8	0.3

*P-U, Pelviureteric junction; M-S, middle spindle; D-E, distal end of extravesical ureter; U-V, ureterovesical junction.

†Reprinted, by permission, from Cussen, L.J. (1967), The structure of the normal human ureter in infancy and childhood: a quantitative study of the muscular and elastic tissue. *Invest. Urol.* 5: 179, Table 6.

and the cell size and numbers were estimated from these data. Muscle thickness can be seen macroscopically, but the ratio of hypertrophy to hyperplasia is calculated by microscopic methods (Fig. 17.1).

'Hypertrophy' is the term used here for cell enlargement and 'hyperplasia' for cell proliferation.

Correlation of cell size and numbers in six types of megaureters

The muscle cells of 380 normal ureters were quantified. The muscle cell size ranged from 800 to 3300 μm³ with a mean of 1600 μm³. The cell population per transverse section of 10-μm thickness was 900 to 4700 with a mean of 2800 (values cover the age range from birth to 12 years) (Table 17.2).

Hypertrophy of muscle cells

One hundred and twenty-nine dilated ureters with identifiable intrinsic obstruction had moderate cell hypertrophy (mean 3300, μm³, range 2400 to 5900 μm³) up to two to three times the normal average, and 72 megaureters secondary to clear-cut urethral obstruction showed muscle cells even larger, being three to five times normal (mean 4000 μm³, range 2900 to 7700 μm³).

Reflux, whether it occurred as vesicoureteral reflux (mean 2200 μm³, range 1500 to 4300 μm³) or ureter-to-ureter reflux (mean 2600 μm³, range 1500 to 4300 μm³), evoked minimal cell hypertrophy, if any, and then, with only one exception, within the normal range. The 18 idiopathic or primary non-reflux, non-obstructed megaureters (mean 2300 μm³, range 2100 to 3300 μm³) and the six triad (prune belly) ureters (mean 2000 μm³, range 1800 to 2100 μm³) showed muscle cells within the normal range for size (see Fig. 19.4).

Hyperplasia of muscle cells

Intrinsic ureteral obstructions caused moderate hyperplasia of up to three to five times the normal numbers of muscle cells, and urethral obstruction induced a gross degree of up to 5–50 times normal (mean 12 500 cells per transverse section, range 4800 to 26 000; mean 34 800, range 6800 to 101 000, respectively).

Ureters subjected to vesicoureteric reflux showed only minimal hyperplasia of one to three times the normal numbers of muscle cells (mean 6100 cells per transverse section, range 1800 to 11 000).

The Type C primary non-reflux, non-obstructed megaureters exhibited no hyperplasia, the cells being thinly spread and forming a tenuous coat around the enlarged ureter (mean 3100, range 2500 to 4000).

The triad or prune belly ureters were thick-walled structures comprised predominantly of collagenous matrix and sparse fibrocytes. The ureters lacked muscle, or exhibited isolated fibres or unorganized clumps of muscle cells.

Muscle cell size in experimental obstruction and reflux

Cussen tested the reaction of adult canine muscle cells to chronic ureteral obstruction, urethral obstruction and reflux by the same cell measuring techniques (Cussen, 1972; Stephens, 1974). Degrees of hypertrophy and hyperplasia in chronic ureteral obstruction and reflux were similar to those in human ureters. With prolonged urethral obstruction, however, the size of ureteral muscle cells did not achieve the degree of enlargement found in babies with congenital urethral valves.

Primary megaureters

Primary obstructed megaureter

Three types of intrinsic obstruction were recognized, and their presence was confirmed by the occurrence of proximal muscle cell hypertrophy and hyperplasia of the dilated ureter: atresia, stenosis and a third variety more common than usually realized, the ureteral valve. All

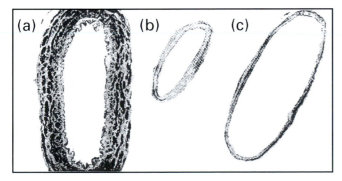

Fig. 17.1 (a) *Transverse section of dilated, obstructed ureter with muscular hypertrophy and hyperplasia (darker areas) (Masson trichrome, ×10).* (b) *Transverse section of normal ureter.* (c) *Transverse section of dilated, non-obstructed, non-reflux ureter, with a continuous but attenuated muscular coat (dark lines) (Masson trichrome, ×10). (Reprinted, by permission, from Cussen, L.J. (1971), The morphology of congenital dilatation of the ureter: intrinsic ureteral lesions. Aust. N.Z. J. Surg. 4: 185, Fig. 1.)*

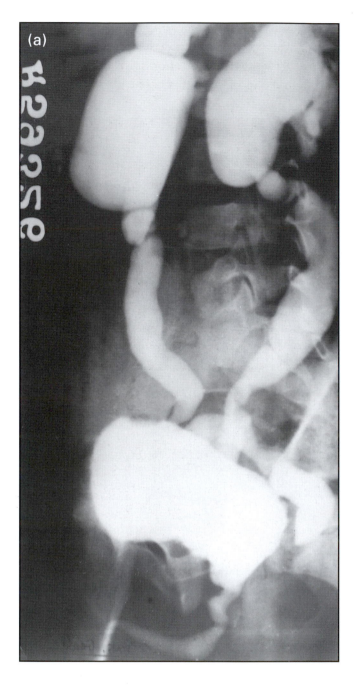

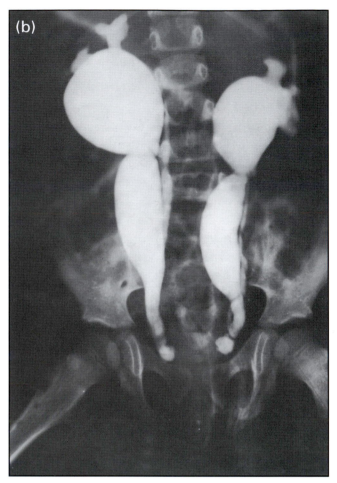

Fig. 17.2 *Focal overgrowth of upper urinary tracts.* (**a**) *Voiding cystoureterography and urethrography demonstrating focal hyperexpansions (during voiding) of the upper and lower spindles of the left ureter and both pelves.* (**b**) *Cystoureterogram of duplex ureters (at end of voiding) show focal enlargements of the upper spindles and pelves of both lower pole ureters. Note the relatively undilated caudal spindles.* ((b) *reprinted, by permission, from Stephens, F.D. (1963),* Congenital Malformations of the Rectum, Anus and Genito-Urinary Tracts. *Edinburgh, Livingstone, Fig. 62, p. 126.)*

three types were readily distinguished in the upper end and middle parts of the ureter, but special preparation and examination were required to identify these types at the lower end in the vicinity of the ureterovesical junction. Here the macroscopic anatomy of the ureter and its lumen were hidden within a thick ureteral sheath of fascia, and even after dissection, the cause may not be apparent. However, necropsy specimens provided undisturbed material which was appropriately fixed and

studied qualitatively and quantitatively by microscopy of serial sections.

Valves of the ureter similar to the high take-off valve at the pelviureteral junction were found to occur in 42 (33 per cent) of the total number of megaureters: 18 with and 24 without an associated stenosis. Ostling (1942) considered that the valve action of the ureter and pelvis was common in the genesis of hydronephrosis, and it appears to be a contributing factor in the genesis of megaureters (see discussion on valves of the ureter, page 212).

Primary reflux megaureter

The minimal hypertrophy and hyperplasia in human ureters were comparable with the measurements obtained after surgical induction of reflux in canine experiments (Stephens, 1974). By inference, these cell changes were attributable to the increased workload imposed by reflux rather than suspect obstructions of the bladder neck or urethral outlet.

Primary non-reflux, non-obstructed megaureter

The primary non-reflux, non-obstructed megaureter exhibited abnormal dilatation, but no hypertrophy or hyperplasia. Hence, the muscle coat was thin and tenuous, but complete, and no organic cause could be found for the dilatation.

Hitherto, the primary obstructed megaureter, caused by ureteral valve formations and the non-obstructed, non-reflux megaureters of the prune belly syndrome may have been regarded as neuromuscular incoordinations, a diagnosis in children now effete.

Morphometric criteria of primary megaureters

Obstruction as a group induced cell enlargement of approximately 100 per cent of the mean normal values in intrinsic obstructions and 200 per cent in ureters associated with chronic urethral obstruction. Cell numbers in ureters were increased in ureteral and urethral obstructions by approximately four and 12 times normal, respectively. The combination of large cells and high numbers served to distinguish ureters as obstructive (Stephens, 1974).

For practical purposes, the upper limit of normal range for size, namely 3300 μm^3, divides the cell sizes for obstructed ureters not only from cells of normal ureters but also from those of other types of non-obstructive megaureters.

By this morphometric study of muscle cells it was possible to identify the megaureters that were caused by obstruction not only in the excised specimen but also by a frozen-section biopsy technique during surgery. It was also possible to show the minimal cell reaction that takes place in the reflux ureter and to exclude obstruction as a cause of the dilated megaureters of the bifid

type, the Type C megaureter and the prune belly megaureter. Since these non-obstructive types of megaureters are congenital, the explanation for the dilatation was sought from theories and studies of embryology.

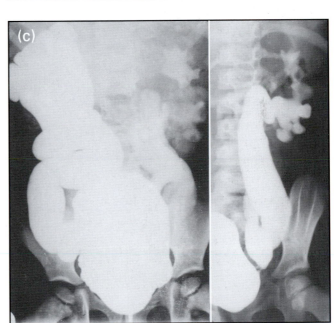

Fig. 17.3 *Bilateral reflux and tubular megasystems with unequal shapes and sizes of calyces, pelves and ureters in patients with no obstructive components.* (**a**) *Male aged four months, right ureter moderately large, left near normal.* (**b**) *Female aged four years, right ureter and calyces very large, left ureter and calyces moderately large.* (**c**) *Female aged* $3\frac{1}{2}$ *years with four megaureters (right ectopic not shown by reflux) and right lower pole ureter pelvis and calyces extremely large; left upper pole ureter and calyces only mild dilation; left lower pole ureter and calyces intermediate between left upper pole and right lower pole systems. (Reprinted, by permission, from Stephens, F.D. (1983), Congenital Malformations of the Urinary Tract, New York, Praeger, Fig. 14.5, p. 232.)*

Embryogenesis of non-obstructive megaureters

Differential expansion is a normal quality and function of the developing bladder, the pelvis, and calices and spindles of the ureter. It is also a process by which the terminal ends of the wolffian ducts and ureters become incorporated into the vesicourethral canal. Aberrations of the programming of the developing bud and ureter may prevent expansion resulting in stenosis or give rise to overexpansion producing megaureters or hydro-nephrosis. The expansion may be sudden or gradual, focal (Fig. 17.2) or tubular (Fig. 17.3) and concentric or eccentric accounting for the many variations of shape and size of the reflux megaureter. It may also explain the eccentric expansions leading to intrinsic valves of the ureter and the high or eccentric insertions of the ureter into the pelvis (Fig. 20.1). The degree of expansion of each reflux megaureter is independent of that of another in the same child (Fig. 17.3).

Vesicoureteral reflux is a phenomenon resulting from defects of the intravesical ureter and is associated with ureters of normal or greater than normal calibre. Free reflux occurring during early filling of the bladder (low-pressure reflux) or during late filling and micturition (high-pressure reflux) into normal or large-calibre ureters is common, and rarely, if ever, does persisting reflux cause those ureters to increase in size. Reflux, however, may distend a megaureter during vesical filling or emptying, and such ureters may exhibit wide diameters of ≥ 2–3 cm, as measured on standard radiographs. These ureters, when observed over many years and with persisting reflux, show decrease rather than increase in calibre. The dilatation of the primary reflux megaureter is *associated* with vesicoureteral reflux rather than *caused* by it.

The boundary line between a normal-calibre ureter and a megaureter is somewhat indefinite. Cussen (1967a) calibrated the mid-ureters of infants and children (Table 18.1; the upper limits of the ranges from birth to 12 years were as follows: 0.4 cm, 3 months; 0.6 cm, 3–12 months; 0.5 cm, 1–3 years; 0.4 cm, 3–6 years; 0.5 cm, 6–9 years; 0.64 cm, 9–12 years. If allowance of 10 per cent were made for X-ray magnification with standard 105-cm (42-inch) distance and supine position, the outside limit of diameters of mid-ureters for ages over one year and up to 12 years as measured radiographically would be no greater than 0.66 cm. The upper limit of normal was thus set at 0.7 cm and for the purposes of this discussion, a ureter with a diameter above 0.7 cm demonstrated radiographically on standard films taken at 105 cm (42 inches) by IVP or voiding cystourethrography is defined as a megaureter. Reflux ureters may not fully expand during the phase of bladder filling until voiding ensues. Then maximum dilatation becomes apparent. Hence ureters opacified by contrast during routine IVP or plain cystograms may appear normal, though when put to the stretch test of micturition, may be surprisingly large in diameter (Fig. 18.1).

Since reflux occurs in association with normal-calibre ureters or megaureters, the aetiology of the underlying defect in the ureterovesical junction will be described first, and the aetiology of the accompanying megaureters and renal morphology will be discussed on pages 208 and 307.

Table 18.1 *Dimensions of the normal ureter in infancy and childhood: ready reckoner of approximate ureteric dimensions*[*]

Age	30 weeks' gestation	3 months	3 years	6 years	12 years
Height	40 cm	60 cm	90 cm	120 cm	150 cm
Weight	2 kg	5 kg	13 kg	20 kg	35 kg
Total length of ureter	5 cm	10 cm	15 cm	20 cm	25 cm
Length of intravesical ureter histologic	0.4	0.6	0.8	1.0	1.2
Length of submucosal ureter histological	0.2	0.3	0.4	0.5	0.6
Diameter and Charrière gauge[†‡]					
P-U[†] diameter	0.05 [2]	0.15 [4]	0.20 [6]	0.25 [8]	0.30 [10]
M-S diameter	0.15 [4]	0.35 [10]	0.40 [12]	0.45 [14]	0.50 [16]
D-E and U-V diameter	0.05 [2]	0.10 [3]	0.15 [4]	0.18 [5]	0.20 [6]

[*]All measurements are in centimetres.
[†]P-U, pelviureteric junction; M-S, middle spindle; D-E, distal end of extravesical ureter; U-V, ureterovesical junction.
[‡]French (Charrière) catheter gauge indicated in brackets.

Reprinted, by permission, from Cussen, L.J. (1967a), Dimensions of the normal ureter in infancy and childhood. *J. Invest. Urol.* 5: 164, Table 6.

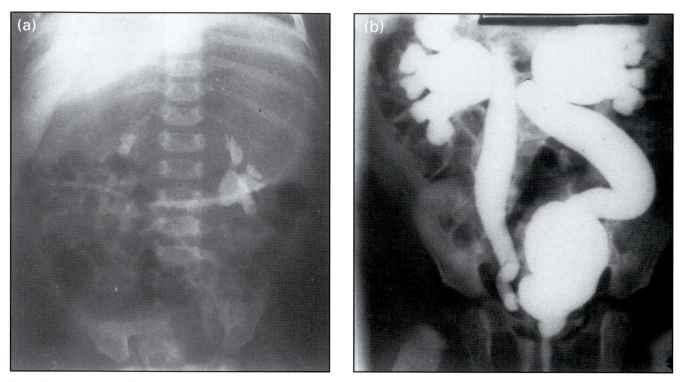

Fig. 18.1 *Contrasting calibres of reflux ureters under low and high pressures in the same female infant, as shown by excretory urography (***a***) and voiding cystourethrography (***b***). (Reprinted, by permission, from Stephens, F.D. (1983),* Congenital Malformations of the Urinary Tract, *New York, Praeger, Fig. 15.2, p. 243.)*

The ureterovesical lock mechanism

Anatomically, the ureter consists of two parts, the long extravesical ureter and the short intravesical segment which lies within the wall of the bladder. The intravesical portion is subdivided into an intramural segment which lies in the muscular tunnel of the bladder wall and a submucosal segment which runs beneath the vesical mucosa, supported between the tunnel and the orifice by muscle of the base of the bladder.

The theory of action of the ureterovesical lock mechanism as described by Sampson (1903) has been widely accepted. He considered that a flap valve is extrinsically operated by compression of the roof of the ureter against the floor by the intravesical tension, and that this effect is enhanced by the obliqueness of the ureter as it traverses the muscular and submucosal layers of the bladder wall. This view gained support from the work of Gruber (1929).

Gruber, working on postmortem specimens of animals, found that vesicoureteral reflux occurred in animals such as the rabbit, which he showed have very short submucosal segments and, therefore, defective flap valves. Moreover, the theory gained further support by the fact that tests for reflux in the human postmortem specimens revealed a mechanism, which, of necessity, depended upon this extrinsic mechanical flap valve action for its efficiency.

Two observations of double ureters cast some doubts on this theory and suggest that other factors intrinsic in the ureters themselves must play an important role in prevention of reflux (Stephens and Lenaghan, 1962). In three patients who exhibited double ureters, two ureters lay side by side, entered the bladder through the same intramural tunnel, coursed without crossing for the same distance in the submucosal plane of the bladder, and issued into the bladder through independent orifices sited side by side on the trigone: one ureter exhibited reflux and the other did not. Furthermore, in two other patients with double ureters, the submucosal portion of the ectopic component of the double ureter in each patient traversed a course much longer than normal, and both exhibited free reflux, but the shorter orthotopic ureters were competent (Fig. 18.2).

These two phenomena of reflux are not compatible with an extrinsic mechanism acting alone, because it

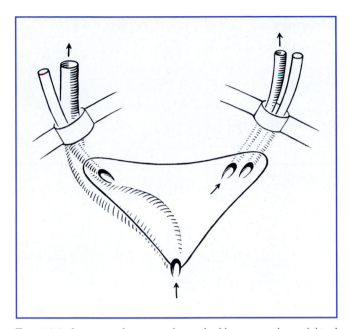

Fig. 18.2 *Intravesical course of two double ureters that exhibited reflux, and which invalidate the simple mechanical flap valve theory of action of the ureteral valve. Reflux occurred into the right extra long megaureter and into the left ectopic ureter, which is of similar length to its accompanying competent orthotopic ureter. (Reprinted, by permission, from Stephens, F.D. and Lenaghan, D. (1962), The anatomical basis and dynamics of vesicoureteral reflux. J. Urol. 5: 669, Fig. 1.)*

would exert similar effects on both of the duplicated ureters with resulting inhibition of reflux on each.

The normal ureterovesical sphincter

Thirty ureters of newborn infants were studied histologically by serial section (Stephens and Lenaghan, 1962). These babies had not been tested for reflux, but the organs of the lower urinary tract appeared normal. Four hypertrophied ureters that did not permit reflux in patients exhibiting severe urethral obstruction were also examined to show in greater relief the detail of the muscle, and the transition between the extravesical and intravesical parts of the ureters. In two other specimens, the direction of the muscle bundles of the intravesical ureter was traced by microdissection.

The calibre and structure of the vesical segment differ from those of the remainder of the ureter. The lumen is slightly smaller. At the outer margin of the bladder wall, the extravesical ureter shed its circular coat and the longitudinal muscle continues in parallel bundles along the whole length of the intravesical ureter to insert into the edges of the ureteric orifice. A few delicate strands inter-

mingle with the muscle of the bladder at the outer end of the tunnel. The muscle on the floor of the ureter is thickest and is continued distally beyond the orifice into the submucosa of the trigone, tethering the ureter and its orifice.

We suggest that the sphincter action is effected by contraction of the longitudinal muscle laying back the margins of the orifice and roof upon the floor of the submucosal ureter, thus apposing roof and walls to floor. Muscle contraction causes rotation of any cross-section of the intravesical ureter about the floor, which is anchored to the trigone. This neuromuscular action is the primary and essential agency by which sudden closure is effected. Its efficiency is enhanced by hydrostatic pressures which create a flap-valve effect upon the roof of the submucosal segment (Fig. 18.3).

Cystoscopic examination of the orifices of normal ureters reveal that, during the resting phase of the ureter, the lumen is occluded. Intermittently, urine jets from the orifice which either remains immobile or

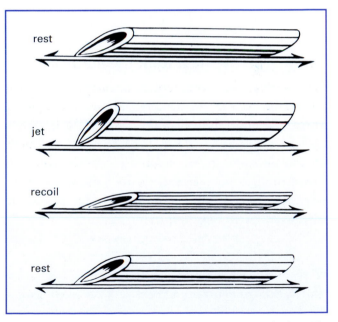

Fig. 18.3 *Intrinsic muscular 'activation' of ureterovesical valve. The drawings represent the intravesical ureter: the muscle arranged longitudinally contracts causing rotation of any cross-section about the floor that is tethered. The lumen is lightly occluded in resting phase, distended during the jet phase, and tightly occluded in the resetting, or recoil, phase of contraction. (Reprinted, by permission, from Stephens, F.D. and Lenaghan, D. (1963), The anatomical basis and dynamics of vesicoureteral reflux, in Congenital Malformations of the Rectum, Anus and Genito-Urinary Tracts, F.D. Stephens (ed.). Edinburgh, Livingstone, Fig. 67, p. 134.)*

widens with the force of the stream. When the jet stops, the ureter may remain immobile, or it may be snapped back momentarily in the line of the ureter and resume its previous resting state. It seems that the jet is propelled by the peristalsis of the invisible extravesical ureter along the immobile intravesical ureter, the lumen of which is regulated by the tone of the muscle on its wall. Some jets may evoke no visible enlargement of the lumen or movement of the ureter; others may prize open the lumen, which then becomes visible, and excite the recoil action. The jerk of the submucosal ureter ensures instantaneous closure of the lumen by the action already described. After this jerking movement, the tone is adjusted and restored to the needs of the resting phase of the ureter and its orifice, which resume the quiescent appearance. It is presumed that the muscle is the 'activator' of the sphincter mechanism, which requires a side-on or oblique course for efficiency, which is still further enhanced by hydrostatic pressures. The combined effect is a highly efficient 'activated' flap valve (Fig. 18.3).

Whereas Stephens and Lenaghan (1962) considered the ureterovesical valve to be activated by the intrinsic muscle of the ureter, Tanagho et al. (1965) attribute this function to contraction of the muscle of the superficial trigone, which is in direct continuity with the longitudinal muscle coat of the ureter and thereby increases the contractile tone of the muscle of the submucosal ureter. Hutch and Amar (1972) consider that Waldeyer's sheath enhances the activation of the ureterovesical junction even more than does the superficial trigone. Stephens (1979a) attributed a different function to Waldeyer's fascia (page 148).

The intravesical segment of the reflux-permitting ureter

Postmortem studies on the intravesical segments of those ureters that were known to have exhibited primary and secondary reflux in life were conducted in order to test the validity of the view that the sphincter resided in the intrinsic muscles of the ureter (Stephens and Lenaghan, 1962). Some megaureters that showed free reflux when tested at necropsy examination were also examined.

Primary vesicoureteral reflux

There were four ureters in which reflux was proved to have occurred in life and seven ureters in which vesicoureteral regurgitation was demonstrated after death only. The survey of these specimens revealed three types of congenital abnormalities, viz. defects in length or deficit of muscle of submucosal ureter, or combinations of both (Figs 18.4 and 18.5).

Congenital absence or shortening of the submucosal segment

One boy (G.O'S.), aged eight years, was observed for $4\frac{1}{2}$ years, after having presented with urinary tract infection.

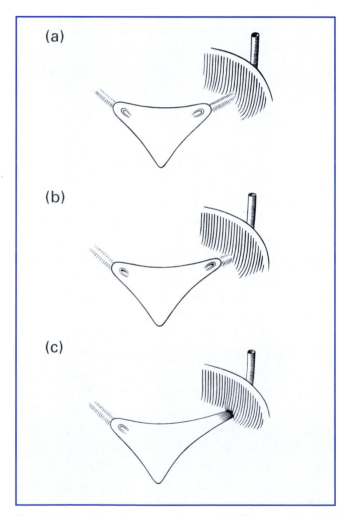

Fig. 18.4 *Drawings of trigone and ureter. (**a**) The normal length of the submucosal segment of the ureter. (**b**) Congenital shortening. (**c**) Absence of this segment. (Reprinted, by permission, from Stephens, F.D. and Lenaghan, D. (1962), The anatomical basis and dynamics of vesicoureteral reflux. J. Urol. 5: 669, Fig. 3.)*

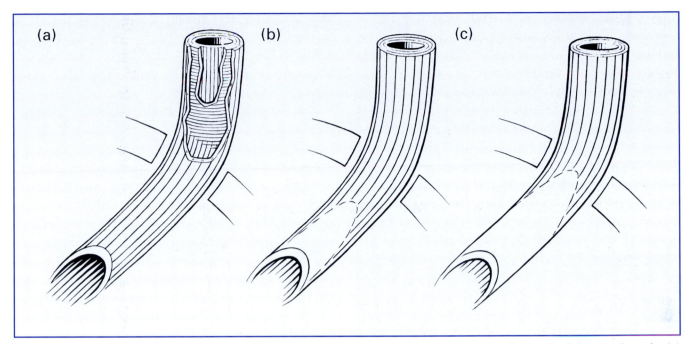

Fig. 18.5 *Intravesical segments of the ureter. (**a**) The extent of normal longitudinal muscular coat. (**b**) Short wedge deficiency of muscle. (**c**) Long defect of muscle. (Reprinted, by permission, from Stephens, F.D. and Lenaghan, D. (1962), The anatomical basis and dynamics of vesicoureteral reflux. J. Urol. 5: 669, Fig. 4.)*

During life, reflux occurred into the right and left megaureters and into the enlarged pelves, but the urethra was not obstructed. Both ureteric orifices were very large and patulous. Postmortem examination revealed free reflux and deficient submucosal segments of the ureters. The large extravesical ureter entered the intramural tunnel of the bladder wall and ended flush with the inner end of the tunnel. The large and gaping orifice in the collapsed state measured 0.3 and 0.7 cm when gently distended. There was no submucosal segment on either side and its absence caused two changes in appearance of the trigone. The cornua were elongated, and the ureteric orifices were widely separated, raised, upright and lay partly in the bladder base and partly in the posterolateral wall.

Three other postmortem specimens (stillborn males P.M. and McK. and female K.S., aged 14 years) exhibited free reflux into five of their ureters and absence of submucosal segments and trigonal appearances similar to that of G.O'S. (Fig. 18.4c).

Microscopic examination of one ureter from each of the four revealed longitudinal and circular muscle in the very dilated extravesical segments, and a short length of longitudinal muscle only in the intramural hiatal seg-

ments. The muscle of the ureteric floor continued distally as very fine, longitudinally arranged fibres into the submucosa of the trigone but the muscle disappeared from the sides and roof at the orifice, which lay flush with the inner end of the intramural tunnel (Fig. 18.4c).

The macroscopic appearances of the trigone and ureteric orifices of this type of congenital anomaly were so characteristic on examination at postmortem that it can safely be presumed that reflux would have occurred during life.

Congenital absence of muscle in the submucosal segment

In this group, only two patients in whom reflux was demonstrated during life subsequently died. Reflux was unilateral, and the calibre of the involved ureter of each child was normal, as shown by reflux of iodide in the course of micturition cystourethrography.

Baby B. (female, aged three months) displayed in life reflux into the right normal-calibre ureter, and a stenotic ureterocele and bifid megaureters on the left side.

The submucosal segment of the right ureter was apparent as a mucosal ridge in the fixed specimen and the orifice lay ajar. Microscopy showed: that the distal end of the submucosal segment lacked muscle in its roof and both side walls; that the longitudinal muscle bundles formed a complete coat at the proximal end of the submucosal segment, though thinnest in the roof; and that along the 3.7-mm length of the submucosal segment, as measured by compilation of section thicknesses, the muscle deficiency assumed a zone that was narrowest cranially and widest distally (Fig. 18.5). Furthermore, the muscle in the roof of the ureter in the intramural segment remained comparatively thin until the ureter became extravesical (Fig. 18.6); longitudinal

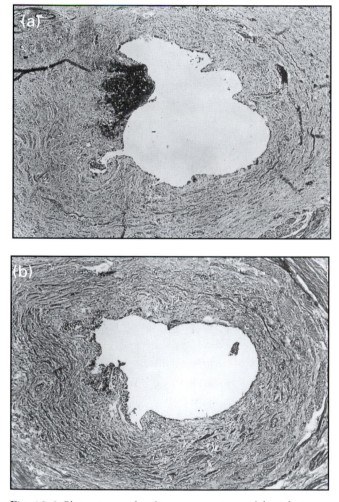

Fig. 18.6 *Photomicrographs of transverse sections of the right intravesical ureter (reflux type) of Baby B. The roof of the ureter is at the top.* (**a**) *The submucosal ureter 3 mm from the orifice. Note absence of muscle in the roof and scanty muscle in the sides. (The dark area is a small haematoma.)* (**b**) *The ureter in the intramural tunnel 6 mm from the ureteric orifice. Note complete muscle coat thinnest in the roof. (Reprinted, by permission, from Stephens, F.D. and Lenaghan, D. (1962), The anatomical basis and dynamics of vesicoureteral reflux.* J. Urol. 5: 669, Fig. 5.)

muscle bundles were present in the floor of the ureter and beyond it in the ureteral groove of the trigone.

The roof and walls of the submucosal segment, which lacked muscle, were composed of fibrocytes, intercellular connective tissue and collagen.

This is a clear-cut example of a congenital deficiency of muscle in the distal end of the ureter, and this anomaly may well account for reflux.

The second example is not so clearly defined, but may represent a combined lesion responsible for reflux. Baby D.H., female aged nine months, exhibited Turner's syndrome. The right ureter, which was continuously infected, permitted free reflux of urine (Fig. 18.7).

The right and left submucosal ureters were of normal and equal length macroscopically, but microscopically, the right submucosal ureter contained in its walls a less complete layer of longitudinal muscle as compared with that of the left side. Large, discrete clumps of small, round cells disrupted the muscle coat, though the muscle fibres showed no degenerative or inflammatory reaction. These aggregations of cells were in evidence also in the trigonal mucosa. Here muscle discontinuity and cell masses combined to impair function, but the relative importance of each in the weakening of the lock mechanism is debatable.

Combined deficiency in length and absence of muscle in the submucosal segment

One postmortem specimen of bilateral megaureters was obtained from Baby L., a newborn female, and the bladder and ureters exhibited reflux under low pressure. The urethral outflow was unobstructed. The submucosal segments on both sides were very much shorter than normal, the orifices were widely separated, and the cornua of the trigone were correspondingly elongated.

The short submucosal, the intramural, and the adjacent extravesical ureters revealed a wedge-shaped deficiency in the muscle of the roof of the caudal part of the ureter. The deficiency was maximal caudally and became extinguished cranially in the extravesical part of the ureter (Fig. 18.8).

This is an example of a combined anomaly in which deficiency in length of the submucosal segment and of deficit of muscle in the wall of the remaining part enhance the likelihood of vesico-ureteral reflux.

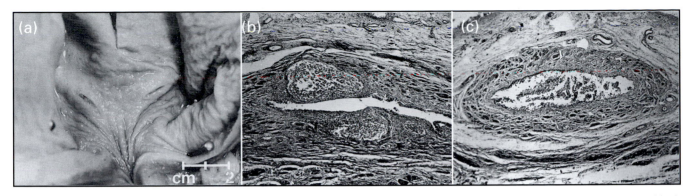

Fig. 18.7 *Reflux and infection. Trigone of Baby D.H., aged nine months (**a**) and histological sections through submucosal segments of both ureters—right swollen and permitting reflux (**b**) and left not permitting reflux (**c**). (**a**) Symmetrical trigone and raised submucosal segment of right side. (**b**) Lymphoid collection partially disrupting the mucosal and muscular coats of the right ureter. (**c**) Normal muscle coats of the left ureter. (Reprinted, by permission, from Stephens, F.D. and Lenaghan, D. (1963), The anatomical basis and dynamics of vesicoureteral reflux, in Congenital Malformations of the Rectum, Anus and Genito-Urinary Tracts, F.D. Stephens (ed.). Edinburgh, Livingstone, Fig. 71, p. 139.)*

Absence of the submucosal ureter and of its muscle may be anticipated in less severe combinations—the length may be reduced, the muscle deficiency may be only partial; infinite degrees are likely, and the existence of such variants would readily account for the many individual reflux peculiarities.

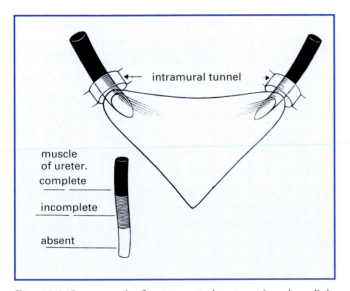

Fig. 18.8 *Structure of reflux intravesical ureters of newborn Baby L. Lateral wedge defects of muscle in the submucosal segment. On medial side muscle sweeps medially into the intertrigonal ridge. (Reprinted, by permission, from Stephens F.D. and Lenaghan, D. (1963), The anatomical basis and dynamics of vesicoureteral reflux, in Congenital Malformations of the Rectum, Anus and Genito-Urinary Tracts, F.D. Stephens (ed.). Edinburgh, Livingstone, Fig. 72, p. 139.)*

Experiments denoting the mode of activation of the ureterovesical valve

Lenaghan *et al.* (1972a) showed that division of one-third of the roof of the canine submucosal ureter, which exhibited the same structures as in the human, induced reflux in 50 per cent of the ureters; division of one-half and three-quarters of the roof induced reflux in 70 per cent and 100 per cent of the ureters respectively. A critical length of approximately two-thirds the normal length (normal in 25-lb dog = 1.5 cm) was required for efficient function.

Hannan and Stephens (1973) studied the function of the canine trigone in the mechanism of the normal ureterovesical valve. They transposed submucosal ureters and their orifices, preserving the normal ureterovesical hiatuses to sites cranial to the trigone on the posterior wall of the bladder. The trigone was then excised, except for the mucosal layer, which was used to close the gap in the muscle of the bladder base (Fig. 18.9). In a total of 11 trigonectomies, one only of the 22 ureters exhibited reflux in the postoperative periods of 4–11 weeks. The investigators concluded that the ureterovesical valve mechanism was not dependent on the interaction of the intrinsic muscle of the submucosal ureter and trigone even though normally there is a coordinated muscular ureterotrigonal interplay (Tanagho and Pugh, 1963). The intrinsic activated flap valve of the submucosal ureter provided an efficient and effective one-way antireflux mechanism.

King and Stephens (1977) conducted experiments to study the intrinsic action of the muscles of the canine

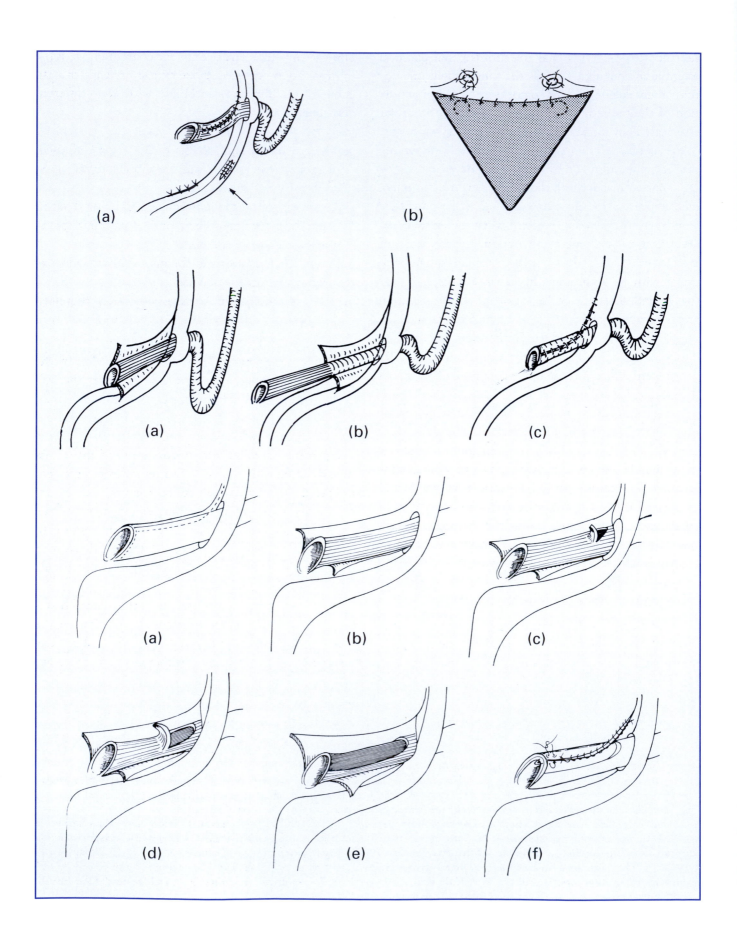

submucosal ureter: (1) Was the firm trigonal platform essential as backing?; (2) was the longitudinal orientation of muscle essential for competence?; (3) was activation of the valve by muscle in the wall of the ureter essential? They found, first, that by simple transposition of the submucosal ureter to the bladder wall, preserving the original hiatus or by creating a new hiatus, the unsupported bladder wall did not impair the antireflux mechanism of the ureterovesical valve. Second, they found that the valve was efficient when the extravesical ureter, with its circular and oblique arrangement of muscle, was substituted for the normal submucosal ureter with its longitudinally disposed muscle. Third, they found that the valve action of the submucosal ureter became inefficient when the roof was denuded *in situ* of its muscle (Fig. 18.9). Furthermore, the bladder muscle surrounding the ureter in the hiatal tunnel did not prevent reflux in those ureters denuded of muscle in the submucosal segment.

It was concluded that the canine sphincter mechanism operated intrinsically in the wall of the submucosal ureter, that either circular or longitudinal orientations of the muscle coat could activate the valve, that an end-on entry of ureter into the bladder and defective muscle in the wall of the submucosal ureter were conducive to reflux, and that the tonic action of the smooth muscle was the activator that ensured the continuous closure of the flap valve between peristaltic waves.

Secondary vesicoureteral reflux

The aetiology of ureterovesical incompetence has been a contentious issue, chiefly because of the mixing of primary and secondary reflux conditions under the one clinical umbrella. The reasons for contention were the interpretations brought about by the presence of vesicoureteral reflux in association with four different clinical entities.

1. Obvious congenital defects of the submucosal segments of the ureter and of accompanying para-ureteral diverticula.
2. Obstruction of the posterior urethra by Young's valves or erroneous radiologic interpretations of narrow-calibre vesical outlet.
3. Spinal cord injuries and the neuropathic bladder of myelomeningocele patients.
4. The association of ureterectasis with presumed bladder-outlet dysfunction.

Stephens now considers that primary reflux in the paediatric age group is due to a local defect in the wall of the submucosal ureter—partial or total absence, a muscle deficit, a combination of both, with or without an accompanying hiatal diverticulum or, in infants, a delay in the neuromuscular maturation; and that reflux in association with Young's valves results from a congenital defect additional to the urethral valves, viz. a partial or total absence of the submucosal segment of the ureter. After relief of the obstruction, many ureters with partial deficits regain competence, though those with total deficit and those engulfed by hiatal diverticula usually remain incompetent.

Saccules acquired in the vicinity of the ureteral hiatus following spinal-cord injury focused attention on the bladder-wall weakness as a cause of the reflux. The common association of reflux with congenital myelodys-

Fig. 18.9 *Designs of three surgical procedures used in studies of the mechanism of the canine ureterovesical valve.*
*Upper row. (**I**) Transportation of submucosal ureter from trigone to bladder wall. (**a**) Original submucosal ureter brought through new bladder hiatus and reimplanted in submucosal tunnel onto posterior bladder wall, original tunnel and orifice oversewn (arrow). (**b**) Ureters transposed from trigone to bladder wall using original hiatus.*
*Second row. (**II**) Replacement of submucosal ureter with circular muscle coat for that with original longitudinal coat. (**a**) Bladder mucosa incised and reflected from submucosal ureter. (**b**) Ureter dissected free and advanced through original bladder hiatus. (**c**) Terminal ureter with longitudinal muscle cut off and subterminal ureter with circular muscle coat reimplanted in original trigonal site.*
*Third and fourth rows. (**III**) Resection of longitudinal muscle coat of roof of the submucosal ureter. (**a**) Bladder mucosa over submucosal ureter incised as shown by dotted line. (**b**) Bladder mucosal flaps reflected away from submucosal ureter. (**c**) Longitudinal muscle coat incised and plane between muscle and ureteric mucosa developed. (**d**) Ureteric muscular roof dissected off ureteric mucosa (**e**). (**f**) Bladder mucosa re-apposed. (I (**a**) reprinted, by permission, from Hannan, Q.H.A. and Stephens, F.D. (1973), The influence of trigonectomy on vesicoureteral reflux in dogs. J. Urol. 10: 469. I(**a**), II(**b**), III(**c**) reprinted, by permission, from King, P.A. and Stephens, F.D. (1977), Ureteral muscle tone in the prevention of reflux. j. Invest. Urol. 14: 488.)*

plasia supported a neuropathic cause for the ureterovesical incompetence. Though the bladder saccules and the neuropathy are associated pathological lesions, which may be conducive to reflux in patients with congenital spina bifida with myelodysplasia, an accompanying congenital deficiency of the length and muscularity of the submucosal segment of the ureter is also a cause of the reflux in some instances (Smith, 1965; Stephens, 1983c).

Paquin (1959) calculated the length of the submucosal ureter versus the diameter of its orifice and considered that a 5 : 1 ratio was required in the prevention of reflux. It is not uncommon to see abnormally wide, gaping ureteric orifices with short, submucosal segments associated with high grades of reflux. In such otherwise normal children, the wider the orifice, the shorter is the length of the submucosal ureter and the more marked is the degree of ureteral and calyceal ectasia. These combined morphologies point to an abnormal embryogenesis of the ureteric bud rather than to bladder-outlet dysfunction.

Study of ureterovesical junction associated with severe urethral obstruction

Reflux occurs so commonly in association with urethral obstruction in male children that it is widely believed that it is caused by 'back-pressure' effects of obstruction. But the reflux may be only unilateral and, in many patients with severe chronic urinary retention, the ureters remain competent even to overflow vesical pressures of up to 75 mmHg. Factors local to the ureterovesical junction and additional to the distal urethral obstruction must be postulated to account for the variants that occur. Some infants in this group, who were investigated for reflux in life by micturition cystourethrography, subsequently died. Postmortem specimens obtained from them, and especially the regions of the ureterovesical junction of both the reflux and non-reflux ureters were studied anatomically and histologically.

Morphology of competent ureterovesical junctions with urethral valves

In four patients, seven ureters, all of which resisted reflux during life, showed evidence of hypertrophy. The intravesical and extravesical ureters were examined macroscopically in five instances and microscopically in serial section in four.

The intravesical ureter was clearly apparent in the bladder as a submucosal ridge. Four orifices were oblique or crescentic slits, and one was upright and end-on to the thickened submucosal ureter. Microscopic examination of serial sections demonstrated that, in three, the longitudinal muscle in the intravesical ureter was thicker than normal and extended throughout the whole length of the intravesical ureter. In the extravesical ureter, the thickened circular coat ended abruptly at the outer wall of the bladder, beyond which point, the thickened longitudinal coats continued alone as the muscle of the intravesical ureter.

The fourth ureter showed, in the intramural tunnel, the same arrangement of muscle as the other three, but in the submucosal segment, the longitudinal fibres in the roof dwindled and stopped well short of the rolled, collar-like thickening of the orifice. The roof of the distal half of the submucosal ureter was incomplete, but the proximal half was complete and was sufficient to maintain competence in the ureter.

Morphology of incompetent ureterovesical junctions with urethral valves

In a group of megaureters, abnormalities of the submucosal segments were found to account for the reflux.

Congenital absence of the submucosal segment. Two children died as a result of the destructive effects on the kidney of prolonged, severe urethral obstruction. Both children exhibited posterior urethral valves. One ureter of each child was found to be deficient in its submucosal segment, and the cornu of the trigone was correspondingly enlarged. In one child, Baby C., micturition cystourethrography in life demonstrated reflux into this defective ureter, while in the other, Baby I., no test for reflux was made, but upon the pathological appearances of the intravesical ureter, reflux would be expected to have occurred.

Serial transverse sections of both ureters were examined microscopically to study the muscle of the intramural parts. In one ureter (Baby I.), in which the submucosal segment was absent, the hiatal part exhibited a wedge deficiency of muscle in the roof and side walls extending to the extravesical ureter. Only on the floor was muscle present for the short length of this intramural segment. In the other ureter (Baby C.), the submucosal segment was deficient, and muscle was absent from the entire circumference in the region of the ureteric orifice and from the roof of the adjoining intramural segment.

Baby X., a premature baby, died at birth, and necropsy revealed gross dilatation of bladder, upper urinary tract and prostatic urethra. Congenital valves of the urethra caused severe urethral obstruction. The trigone was enlarged at the expense of a considerable length of the submucosal segments of the ureters, the roof of each being represented by a lip-like projection of the rim of each orifice into the bladder; postmortem radiographic studies revealed free reflux up each ureter.

Serial transverse sections of the left ureteric orifice and the adjoining ureter showed that in the very short submucosal lip, and in the entire intramural part of the vesical ureter, the longitudinal muscle was deficient. The wall of the ureter was composed of fibrocytes, and intercellular matrix, and ureteral epithelium. At the junction with the enlarged extravesical ureter, muscle fibres, sparse at first, and thicker more proximally, were recognized.

The ureter associated with paraureteral diverticula of the bladder. Reflux in the absence of outflow obstruction was shown by MacKellar and Stephens (1960) to be closely related to the location of the ureteric orifice with reference to that of the diverticulum. When the two orifices were separate, there was no reflux; when contiguous, the reflux was limited, but when the ureteric orifice was engulfed by the diverticulum, reflux was free. This same relationship applies in patients with congenital urethral obstruction.

Histological studies revealed that the longitudinal muscle clothed the intramural ureter and was present in part of the submucosal segment, when the orifices were well separated. When the ureteric orifice was engulfed, the submucosal ureter lying in the diverticulum was short and its muscle was deficient. In one patient (Baby H.) with urethral valves, who exhibited, in life, reflux into the lower reaches of both ureters, the orifices lay contiguous with those of the diverticula. Both ureters showed similar features. In their submucosal courses, they were not entirely deficient in muscle, the floor containing longitudinal muscle fibres, which continued beyond the orifices into the trigone; there was a wedge-shaped deficiency of muscle in the roof of each ureter, extending from its orifice to the floor of the diverticulum. For a very short zone in the submucosal segment inside the diverticulum, discrete, tiny flecks of muscle formed an incomplete muscle layer in the roof, which became complete, though thin, before the ureter became extramural. It seems that arrest of myogenesis occurred, leaving small clumps which failed to coalesce and lay between the zone of absent muscle near the orifice and the muscularized zone laterally.

Reflux rarely occurred when the orifices of the ureter and diverticulum were separate, because in such case, the intravesical segment was long and contained an adequate coat of longitudinal muscle in the greater part of its length; reflux was limited when the orifices were contiguous, in which event the submucosal ureter was intermediate in length and contained muscle, albeit patchy and thin, in the proximal reaches of the submucosal and intramural parts. When the orifice of the ureter was engulfed by the diverticulum, reflux was free, because the submucosal ureter was short, nearly end-on to the lumen of the diverticulum, and almost completely deficient in muscle. This rule holds true for reflux associated with paraureteral diverticula, whether or not urethral obstruction coexists.

This interpretation of the relation of reflux to paraureteral diverticula is somewhat different from that of Hutch (1958) who considered that the diverticulum undermined the flap-valve action of the intravesical ureter. It now appears that reflux results from defects in the length and musculature of the submucosal segment and that the diverticulum is an incidental anomaly. If the submucosal ureter is intrinsically normal, the ureterovesical valve remains continent even in the presence of the paraureteral diverticulum.

19

The reflux ureter

Normal calibre ureters and megaureters both exhibit vesicoureteral reflux. It occurs more commonly into ureters at or below the borderline mid-spindle ureteral diameter of 0.7 cm when measured at the site of greatest width as determined by ureterography.

It is proposed here to describe normal calibre and wide-calibre reflux ureters separately. The associated renal morphology will be described in Chapter 30.

Reflux ureter of normal calibre

The abnormality in a reflux ureter of normal calibre is in the ureterovesical junction; the extravesical ureter is normal in all other respects.

The ureteric orifice is usually in the near-normal position; the submucosal segment may be normal in length or slightly shortened. The orifice, instead of being closed in the resting phase, lies open in a pit, a slit or under the crescentic lateral lip of the meatus. Peristalsis in the ureter is active, producing regular jets from the orifice which remains relatively immobile. The patulous orifice permits a two-way flow of urine in and out of the ureter.

The aetiology of the incompetence of the ureterovesical valve of normal ureters is presumed to be a deficit in the intrinsic musculature, which has already been described, or possibly a delay in the maturation of the neuromuscular synapses. This neuromuscular defect is usually temporary and matures in the first year or two. Within the first five years of life, the muscle population increases or the submucosal ureter lengthens with growth sufficiently to permit spontaneous arrest of reflux. Smellie and Normand (1979) found that over 80 per cent of undilated ureters that initially exhibited reflux developed a competent ureterovesical junction and the reflux ceased spontaneously.

It is likely that reflux ureters of normal calibre would pass unnoticed were it not for the interception of infection resulting from stasis and the ready access of infection from the urethra and bladder to the kidney.

Reflux megaureters

When the ureter is larger than normal, not only is the ureterovesical valve abnormal, but also the ureter and very often the pelvis, calyces and renal parenchyma are abnormal.

The ureteric orifice and the length of the submucosal segment are abnormal. The orifice may be larger than normal, laterally situated on an elongated cornu of the trigone, patulous and open. It may be immobile or exhibit lazy retraction of iris-like contractions. It exhibits four standard shapes, which are likened on cystoscopic examination, when the bladder filling pressure approximates 60 cmH$_2$O, to a cone, stadium, horseshoe or golf hole (Fig. 19.1A); some orifices lie on a shallow, saucer-like saccule on the trigone or out of sight in a hiatal diverticulum. Other minor variations of shape of the orifice are recognizable (Fig. 19.1B). These may have some significance embryologically, though most can be placed into one of the broad types described by Lyon *et al.* (1969). They described the cone, the stadium, the horseshoe and the golf hole orifices. One additional variant is the congenital absence of the lateral pillar of the ureteral meatus (Fig. 19.1B). The muscle of the ureter is located in the medial pillar and in the Mercier's bar of the trigone. The orifice is usually laterally located and permanently incompetent.

The submucosal segment is sometimes absent. Then the ureter may issue by an end-on vertical orifice at the hiatal tunnel or issue at an orifice balanced on the edge of, or in, a diverticulum. All the orifices may lie between the normal situation and the extreme locations and are labeled 'A' when judged to be located normally, 'C' when at or near the hiatus and 'B' when halfway between (Lyon *et al.*, 1969; Stephens, 1979c) (Fig. 18.4). 'D' denotes an orifice in a diverticulum. Lyon *et al.*, (1969) found a clear correlation between ureteric-orifice configurations and the degrees of lateral ectopy of the ureteric orifices and the higher grades of vesicoureteric reflux and renal scarring. Heale

A

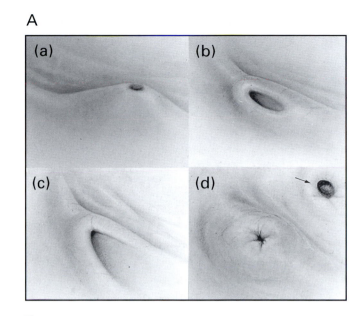

B

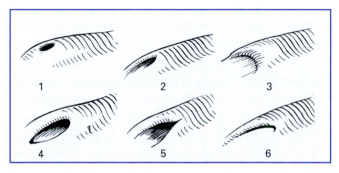

Fig. 19.1 A. *Shapes of the ureterovesical meatus and orifice.* (**a**) *Cone.* (**b**) *Stadium.* (**c**) *Horseshoe.* (**d**) *Golf-hole when bladder nearly empty—so-called 'anal' appearance and when bladder full (arrow). (Reprinted, by permission, from Lyon, R.P., Marshall, S. and Tanagho, E.A. (1969), The ureteral orifice: Its configuration and competency. J. Urol. 102: 504, Fig. 1.)* **B.** *Other variations of shape of the normal and abnormal ureteric orifice. 1, The pit; 2, the slit; 3, and the crescent. All are variants of normal. 4, Stadium; 5, fissured horseshoe; and 6, lateral pillar defect. (Reprinted, by permission, from Stephens, F.D. (1983), Congenital Malformations of the Urinary Tract, New York, Praeger, Fig. 16.1B, p. 260.)*

(quoted by Stephens, 1979d) correlated the ureteric orifice configurations (Table 19.1) and positions (Table 19.2) (assessed by two cystoscopists, Drs F.D. Stephens and J.H. Kelly) and the occurrence of reflux and renal scars (Tables 19.3 and 19.4) in 208 children with 308 reflux ureters, including some duplex systems and 115 non-reflux ureters. These correlations support the findings of Lyon *et al.* (1969) that vesicoureteric reflux and renal scarring were more common and severe with the more abnormal orifice configurations

Table 19.1 *Correlation of vesicoureteral reflux with ureteric orifice configuration*[*]

Parameter	Normal (0)	Stadium (1)	Horseshoe (2)	Golf-hole (3)	Total
Numbers of reflux ureters	11/43	61/101	156/199	80/80	308/423
Percentage reflux ureters	26%	60%	78%	100%	73%

[*]208 children with 308 reflux and 115 non-reflux ureters.

Source: Stephens, F.D. (1979d), Cystoscopic appearances of the ureteric orifices associated with reflux nephropathy, in *Reflux Nephropathy*. C.J. Hodson and P. Kincaid-Smith (eds), p. 122, Table II. New York, Masson. Correlations provided by courtesy of Dr W.F. Heale.

Table 19.2 *Correlation of vesicoureteral reflux with ureteric orifice position*[*]

Parameter	A	B	C	Total
Numbers of reflux ureters	17/69	188/247	103/107	308/423
Percentage reflux ureters	25%	76%	96%	73%

[*]208 children with 308 reflux and 115 non-reflux ureters.

Source: Stephens, F.D. (1979d), Cystoscopic appearance of the ureteric orifices associated with reflux nephropathy, in *Reflux Nephropathy*. C.J. Hodson and P. Kincaid-Smith (eds), p. 121, Table I. New York, Masson. Correlations provided by courtesy of Dr W.F. Heale.

Table 19.3 *Correlation of renal scars with ureteric orifice configuration*[*]

Parameter	Normal (0)	Stadium (1)	Horseshoe (2)	Golf-hole (3)	Total
Numbers of kidneys with scars	2/43	5/101	65/199	65/80	237/423
Percentage of kidneys with scars	5%	5%	33%	81%	32%

[*]208 children with 308 reflux and 115 non-reflux ureters.

Source: Stephens, F.D. (1979d), Cystoscopic appearances of the ureteric orifices associated with reflux nephropathy, in *Reflux Nephropathy*. C.J. Hodson and P. Kincaid-Smith (eds), p. 123, Table IV. New York, Masson. Correlations provided by courtesy of Dr W.F. Heale.

and lateral positions of the orifices (Figs 19.2A and 19.2B).

Table 19.4   *Correlation of renal scars and ureteric orifice position**

Parameter	A	B	C	Total
Numbers of kidneys with scars	4/69	56/247	77/107	137/423
Percentage of kidneys with scars	6%	23%	72%	32%

*208 children with 308 reflux and 115 non-reflux ureters.

Source: Stephens, F.D. (1979d), Cystoscopic appearances of the ureteric orifices associated with reflux nephropathy, in *Reflux Nephropathy*. C.J. Hodson and P. Kincaid-Smith (eds), p. 123, Table III. New York, Masson. Correlations provided by courtesy of Dr W.F. Heale.

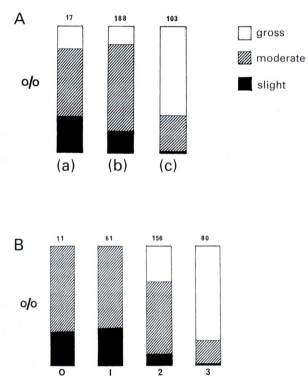

Fig. 19.2 A. *Correlation of orifice position (graded (**a**) (**b**) and (**c**) as in Table 19.2) with grade of vesicoureteral reflux in 308 reflux ureters.* **B.** *Correlation of orifice configuration (graded 0–3 as in Table 19.1) with grade of vesicoureteral reflux. (Courtesy of Dr W.F. Heale. Reprinted, by permission, from Stephens, F.D. (1979d), Cystoscopic appearances of the ureteric orifices associated with reflux nephropathy, in* Reflux Nephropathy. *J. Hodson and P. Kincaid-Smith (eds), pp. 123–124, Fig. 1. New York, Masson.)*

Investigations

Radiographic appearances

The dilatations of the ureters may be mild, moderate or gross. The degree is assessed radiographically during vesicoureteral reflux of opaque medium. The ureters

undergo maximum dilatation when the vesical pressures are highest and reflux of urine greatest during voiding. A series of ten radiographs (Fig. 19.3[1–10]) were taken in the course of micturition cystourethrography as described in Chapter 6. The patient was a girl, D.A., aged seven years. This series of radiographs embodies most of the information to be gained from cysto-urethrography in the presence of megaureter with reflux. From this patient, together with others, the following observations can be made:

1. Reflux occurred early in the course of filling of the bladder in some cases; in others, not until the full stage approached; and in others again, during emptying. The reflux was often carried further up on one side than the other (Fig. 19.3[1]).

2. With continued filling of the bladder, the ureter might partly empty its content back into the bladder and spontaneously refill (Fig. 19.3[2]), an occurrence suggestive of free efflux and reflux.

3. The bladder outlines were smooth. In one patient, two very small juxtaureteral diverticula, each the size of a split pea, were apparent. The urethra and bladder neck were normal in outline (Fig. 19.3[3, 4]).

4. During micturition, further reflux occurred, usually up both ureters (Fig. 19.3[5]). The amount of reflux varied from patient to patient, and in some individuals from one side to the other.

5. The ureters were dilated and elongated, and somewhat tortuous, but the enlargement was mainly in the lateral, as opposed to the longitudinal, dimension. The pelves and calyces frequently escaped dilatation, and in three children, on one side only, the calyces were bunched together in a manner that suggested some degree of hypoplasia of the kidneys. During the cystourethrography studies, clubbing frequently occurred during stages of maximum reflux, and reverted to a cupped appearance in the more empty phases (Fig. 19.3[5, 9]).

6. The bladder emptied completely in cooperative children (Fig. 19.3[9]).

7. The bladder expelled its contents through the urethra, but also into the ureters, to an amount depending on the dimensions of an individual ureter and the degree of incompetence of its ureterovesical orifice. This reflux content of the

"Fig. 19.3 Micturition cystourethrogam—D.A., female, aged seven years. Micturition cystourethrogram series showing ureteral reflux. This series of pictures is representative of the findings in megaureter with vesicoureteral reflux. 1. Bladder containing 90 ml of 16 per cent Uriodone showing free reflux up left ureter. 2. Bladder containing 180 ml and no effort made to micturate. Left ureter is emptier than in film (1). 3. Bladder contains 180 ml and micturition begun. Left ureter as before, and urethrogram normal. 4. Bilateral ureteric reflux and normal urethrogram. The lower end of the left ureter is narrow at its intramural portion. With the sustained effort of micturition, the reflux distends both ureters. 5. Bladder decreasing in size and ureters and pelves and calyces distended to capacity. Normal urethrogram. Normal opening of bladder neck. 6. Air bubble in empty bladder immediately after cessation of micturition. The ureters and pelves are distended to capacity and the lower ends of the iodide columns are abruptly terminated at the sites of entry into the bladder wall. 7. Distribution of iodide 30 seconds after micturition terminated as seen in film (6). The ureters and pelves are partially emptied and the bladder is filling. 8. Distribution of iodide immediately after further few millilitres voided. The bladder is again empty but iodide is still in moderate quantity in the upper urinary tract. 9. Three minutes after film (6), the ureters have discharged most of their content into the bladder. 10. After film (9), a further 10 ml of urine were passed and this film demonstrates that practically the whole urinary tract has been emptied. (Reprinted, by permission, from Stephens, F.D. (1954), Megaureter. Aust. N.Z. J. Surg. 23: 197, Figs 1–10.)"

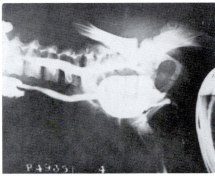
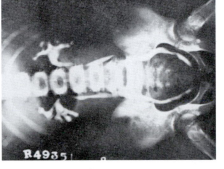
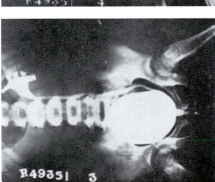
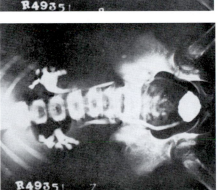
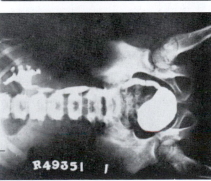
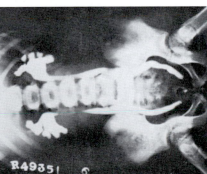
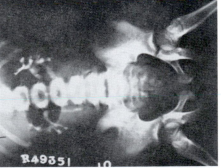
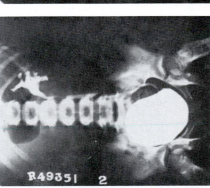
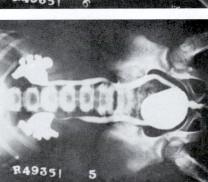
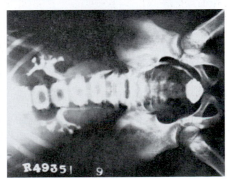

Fig. 19.3 Micturition cystourethrogam—D.A., female, aged seven years. Micturition cystourethrogram series showing ureteral reflux. This series of pictures is representative of the findings in megaureter with vesicoureteral reflux. **1.** Bladder containing 90 ml of 16 per cent Uriodone showing free reflux up left ureter. **2.** Bladder containing 180 ml and no effort made to micturate. Left ureter is emptier than in film (1). **3.** Bladder contains 180 ml and micturition begun. Left ureter as before, and urethrogram normal. **4.** Bilateral ureteric reflux and normal urethrogram. The lower end of the left ureter is narrow at its intramural portion. With the sustained effort of micturition, the reflux distends both ureters. **5.** Bladder decreasing in size and ureters and pelves and calyces distended to capacity. Normal urethrogram. Normal opening of bladder neck. **6.** Air bubble in empty bladder immediately after cessation of micturition. The ureters and pelves are distended to capacity and the lower ends of the iodide columns are abruptly terminated at the sites of entry into the bladder wall. **7.** Distribution of iodide 30 seconds after micturition terminated as seen in film (6). The ureters and pelves are partially emptied and the bladder is filling. **8.** Distribution of iodide immediately after further few millilitres voided. The bladder is again empty but iodide is still in moderate quantity in the upper urinary tract. **9.** Three minutes after film (6), the ureters have discharged most of their content into the bladder. **10.** After film (9), a further 10 ml of urine were passed and this film demonstrates that practically the whole urinary tract has been emptied. (Reprinted, by permission, from Stephens, F.D. (1954), Megaureter. Aust. N.Z. J. Surg. 23: 197, Figs 1–10.)

ureters was expelled in part back into the bladder within 30 seconds to 2 minutes of micturition (Fig. 19.3[7, 9]). The volumes passed were measured, and the second and third amounts found constant in repeated estimations. In some cases, the ureters were emptied in two successive efforts. Without the assistance of gravity, the ureters had the power of completely expelling their contents within a period of approximately 4 minutes, provided the bladder was voluntarily emptied in successive attempts spaced at 2-minute intervals (Fig. 19.3[10]).

8. The columns of iodide in the lower ends of the ureters were obliterated in their intramural courses (Fig. 19.3[4]). In one child, a spiral narrowing approximately 0.5-cm long preceded the final obliteration of the column at the intramural site.

9. Over periods ranging from six months to two years, repetition of cystourethrographic studies indicated no noticeable increase in the ureteric dilatation. In some, the ureters had diminished in calibre and the volume of refluxed urine was much reduced or reflux had ceased spontaneously.

Intravenous pyelouretrography

The opacification in the pelves and calyces was, in most cases, good in the early films, and the medium appeared in the bladder within 10 minutes. It is to be noted that when ureters permit reflux, interpretation of function from the later pyelograms of the series must be guarded because of reflux of contrast material, which is an admixture of that secreted by the kidneys from both sides. A free-draining, in-dwelling catheter during intravenous pyelouretrography procedure prevents reflux and avoids possible misinterpretation.

Cystoscopic appearances

In this group of patients, the bladder showed none of the trabeculation so conspicuous in the hypertrophied bladder of urethral obstruction. The ureteric orifices were clearly and easily seen on the pale, smooth background of trigone and bladder.

The cystoscopic appearances of the ureteric orifices in this series varied from patient to patient, and from side to side in some of the individual children: some orifices appeared normal in all phases; others, though at first sight normal, at the moment of discharge of fluid displayed a small central, dark spot which denoted a wider calibre than usual; a winking, incompetent, thin, iris-like diaphragm, which never completely occluded the lumen, was occasionally observed; or the orifice was frankly enlarged, patulous and exhibited a dark lumen. Occasionally, a saddle-like wrinkle of the bladder mucosa overlies the submucosal section near the meatus indicating the presence of a small hiatal diverticulum, which becomes evident radiographically only during micturition when the bladder pressure is high.

In the correlation of the cystoscopic appearances with the radiographic evidence of reflux, it appeared that the less the deviation from normal presented by the ureteric orifice, the less the reflux, and that such reflux occurred mainly during micturition, while with the patulous type of orifice, reflux occurred early or late in the process of filling of the bladder, and to an even greater extent during micturition.

Aetiology of reflux ureterectasis

With lesser grades of reflux and a range of dilated ureters that may be classed subjectively as normal ureters or borderline megaureters, the dilatation is usually uniform when the ureter is filled and shares vesical pressures during voiding. These include (Appendix, page 444):

Heikel and Parkkulainan (1966), grades 1 to 3.
Smellie (1967), grades 1, 2 and 3.
Rolleston et al. (1970), grades mild and moderate.
Dwoskin and Perlmutter (1973), grades 1 to 3.
The International Study Classification, Levitt (1981), grades 1 to 3.

The megaureters of the highest grades of reflux exhibit many variations of calibre, length and tortuosity. Some are uniformly wide and straight, others are widest in the middle zone, others in the distal one-third, and yet others in the upper half with near-normal calibre in the lower reaches (see Figs 17.2 and 17.3). All show relative narrowings at the ureteropelvic junction and ureterovesical junction with often a redundance near the junction. The modelling of the ureteric shape and length of the gross megaureters are disorganized and haphazard.

Nunn (1964) has shown that the vesicourethral pressures of patients with primary reflux were not elevated above normal and that the gradient between bladder and urethral voiding pressures was normal. Whitaker *et al.* (1969) demonstrated that the urethral resistance in primary reflux patients, as determined from the equation

$$\text{Resistance} = \frac{\text{Bladder pressure} - \text{Exit pressure}}{(\text{Flow rate})^2}$$

was not abnormally elevated. Furthermore, it must be assumed that reflux in most children began prenatally and continued to the age at which it was recognized. It is unlikely therefore that normal vesical pressures, either *in utero* or afterwards, would create the wide variety of megaureters in some and not in the majority of others. The highest grades of ureterectasis are found in patients with the prune belly syndrome, many of whom exhibit vesicoureteral reflux as one of many non-obstructive malformations of size and calibre occurring elsewhere in the urinary tract (see page 391).

Congenital meatomegaly

It was observed that the ureteric orifice of most very dilated reflux ureters was also ectatic, sometimes meas-uring ≥ 1.0 cm in diameter and sometimes accompanied by megacystis. The likely explanation for meatomegaly associated with vesico- and ureteromegaly in the absence of obstruction is an organizer disorder resulting in devel-opmental overgrowth of these structures. The orifice of the ureteric bud may share the same expansion stimulus resulting in the trumpeting and integration of the termi-nal end of the wolffian duct and the large bud orifice into the urinary tract.

Muscle cell dimensions in reflux megaureters

Cussen (1967b, 1971a) measured the size of the muscle cells and found that in 18 primary reflux megaureters and six reflux megaureters of prune belly babies, cell hypertrophy was lacking in all except one (Stephens, 1974). In contrast, the muscle cells of megaureters asso-ciated with ureteral or urethral obstruction exhibited hypertrophy of two to five times normal size. It was con-cluded that the size of the muscle cells of primary reflux ureters did not increase beyond the normal range and that the lack of hypertrophy indicated that obstruction was not the primary cause of the reflux (Fig. 19.4).

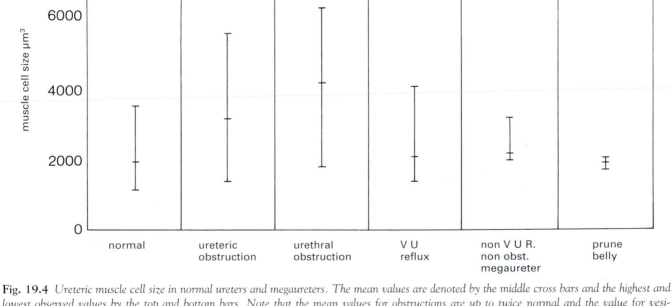

Fig. 19.4 *Ureteric muscle cell size in normal ureters and megaureters. The mean values are denoted by the middle cross bars and the highest and lowest observed values by the top and bottom bars. Note that the mean values for obstructions are up to twice normal and the value for vesi-coureteral reflux only slightly above normal. (Reprinted, by permission, from Stephens, F.D. (1983), Congenital Malformation of the Urinary Tract, New York, Praeger, Fig. 16.4, p. 265.)*

Asymmetrical dilatations

Although long-term free reflux may be bilateral, on one side the ureteric dimensions may be near normal, and on the contralateral side, several centimetres in diameter. With free reflux occurring on each side, it must be assumed that the pressures equalize in the ureters.

The explanation of the ureterectasis lies therefore not in the abnormal urodynamics so much as in the defective programming and prototyping of the ureteric bud. The phenomenon of reflux in normal calibre ureters is a consequence of a localized defect in the submucosal ureter, whereas with the reflux megaureters, the abnormal ureteral dimensions result from an organizer disturbance in the bud.

Spontaneous repair of ureterovesical valve

Stephens (1970a) observed 101 children with 165 reflux ureters uncomplicated by duplication, urethral obstruction, paraureteral diverticula or neuropathic disturbance over periods ranging from 5 to 15 years. He found: (1) that the ureterovesical valves of 68 per cent of 79 ureters of maximum width of $\leqslant 1$ cm, measured on standard radiographs demonstrated by micturition cystoureterograms, became competent spontaneously; and (2) that the ureterovesical valves of 33 per cent of 86 megaureters of diameters > 1.0 cm underwent spontaneous repair, 27 per cent were showing improvement in efficiency of the valve and 40 per cent remained unchanged. Normand and Smellie (1979) observed the rate of natural repair of the ureterovesical valve in 112 reflux ureters in children over periods ranging from 8 to 15 years. The valve became competent in 85 per cent of undilated and 41 per cent of dilated ureters.

The nature of the repair is conjectural. Three possible reasons for the improvement are:

1. Elongation of the submucosal ureter with growth (Hutch, 1961). Hutch found that the normal submucosal ureter elongated from 5 to 13 mm from birth to 12 years, and postulated that natural elongation or maturation may convert a marginal incompetence into competence.

2. Muscle deficiency in the intravesical segment of the ureter may be due to delayed conversion of mesenchyme into muscle. Progressive muscularization occurs normally during the early years of childhood and may operate to enhance the efficiency of the valve. Cussen (1976b) found muscle normally appears first in the body of the ureter and last between the eighth and ninth month of fetal life in the intravesical ureter. Muscle cell numbers increased up to 12 years, though this increase was maximal just before and after birth (Fig. 19.5a). Delayed muscularization is a rational explanation for the occurrence of reflux in infancy, and late muscularization for improvement in competence of the ureterovesical mechanism.

3. Late appearance of muscle may be accompanied by late maturation of the neuromuscular connection. Torbey and Leadbetter (1963) demonstrated that division of the nervi erigentes was accompanied by ipsilateral vesicoureteral reflux and proved that the valve was influenced by parasympathetic nerves. This neuromuscular maturation and link between nerves and muscle in the intravesical ureter may be immature in the first months or years of postnatal life, and on maturation, the valve gains competence.

Infection and reflux

Submucosal ureters of marginal competency may be tipped into incompetence by urinary infection in the bladder permeating the submucosal segment of the ureter and its muscle coat (see Fig. 18.7). With cure of infection and resolution of the inflammation in the ureter, the valve may regain competence.

Those ureters in which the submucosal ureter is too short or absent, too wide in diameter proportional to length, and too lightly clad with muscle may never gain competency with growth of the individual.

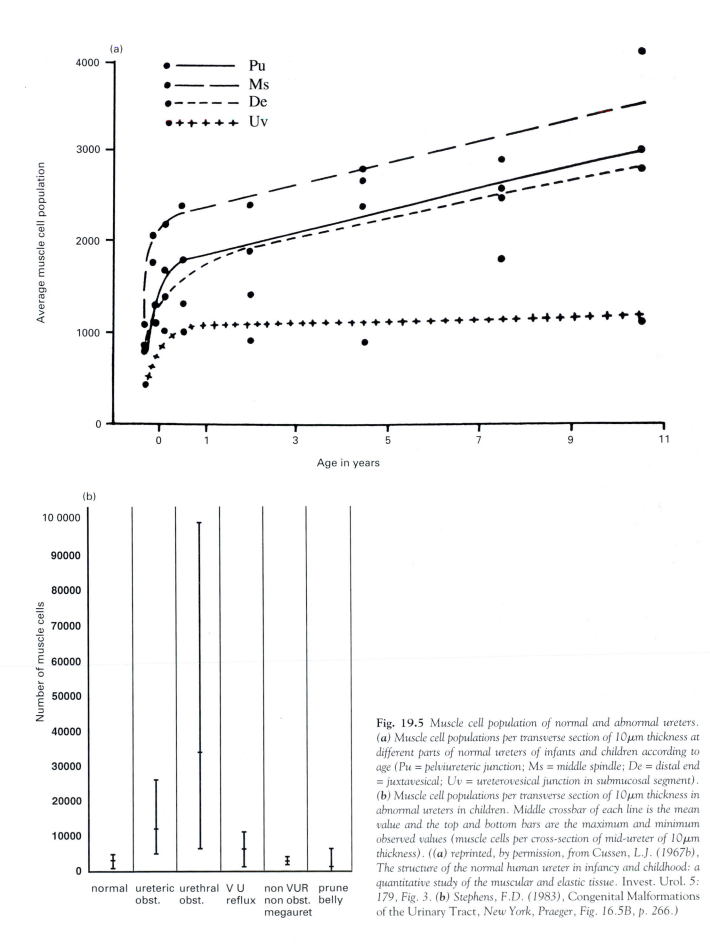

Fig. 19.5 *Muscle cell population of normal and abnormal ureters.* (**a**) *Muscle cell populations per transverse section of 10 μm thickness at different parts of normal ureters of infants and children according to age (Pu = pelviureteric junction; Ms = middle spindle; De = distal end = juxtavesical; Uv = ureterovesical junction in submucosal segment).* (**b**) *Muscle cell populations per transverse section of 10 μm thickness in abnormal ureters in children. Middle crossbar of each line is the mean value and the top and bottom bars are the maximum and minimum observed values (muscle cells per cross-section of mid-ureter of 10 μm thickness). ((***a***) reprinted, by permission, from Cussen, L.J. (1967b), The structure of the normal human ureter in infancy and childhood: a quantitative study of the muscular and elastic tissue. Invest. Urol. 5: 179, Fig. 3. (***b***) Stephens, F.D. (1983), Congenital Malformations of the Urinary Tract, New York, Praeger, Fig. 16.5B, p. 266.)*

20

Primary obstructed megaureter

Megaureter develops as a secondary reaction of the muscular tube to distal obstruction, much in the same way the pelvis of the kidney enlarges above an obstruction at the ureteropelvic junction. It is probable that the causes of obstruction at the ureteropelvic junctions and the distal ureterovesical junctions are similar, but more readily detected, investigated and understood at the upper end of the ureter (Fig. 20.1).

The symptomatology of obstructive megaureter is similar to that of obstruction at the ureteropelvic junction—the lesion may be present for years without symptoms. Grumbling pains, haematuria, or the symptoms of urinary infection or calculus may bring the condition to notice. The obstruction may be uni- or bilateral and radiological investigations disclose the dilated urinary tract above the point of obstruction. The ureter below the dilated segment is usually normal in calibre, but rarely seen radiographically when the obstruction is close to the bladder wall. The ureterovesical junction is competent and the ureteric orifice is located in the cornu of the trigone.

Cussen (1971a) studied 124 dilated ureters that were not associated with vesicoureteral reflux, lower urinary-tract obstruction, or lesions of the spinal cord, such as myelodysplasia. In the segment caudal to the dilated part of the urinary tract, an obstruction was found in the majority of specimens in the upper, middle or lower parts of the ureter. Stenosis was the cause of the obstruction in 81 specimens and valves of the ureter in 42. In addition to these 124 obstructive lesions, there were 18 non-reflux, non-obstructed megaureters and five examples of atresia.

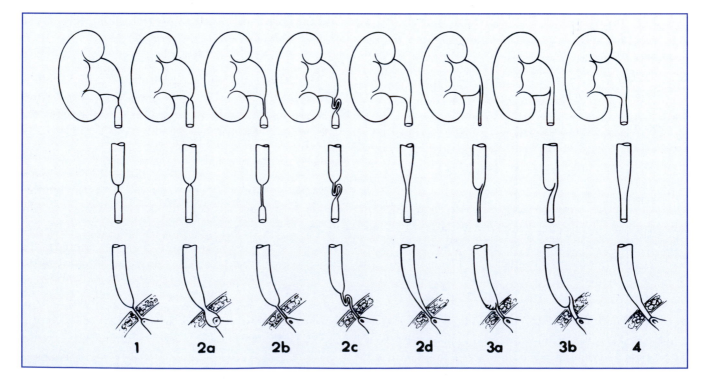

Fig. 20.1 *Intrinsic obstructions of the ureter. 1, atresia; 2a, stricture including meatal stenosis with ureterocele; 2b, segmental stricture; 2c, serpiginous stricture; 2d, shelving stricture; 3a, stricture with ureteral valve formation; 3b, ureteral valve; 4, non-reflux, non-obstructive megaureter. All lesions occur in any part of the ureter. (Reprinted, by permission, from Cussen, L.J. (1971a), The morphology of congenital dilatation of the ureter: intrinsic ureteral lesions. Aust. N.Z. J. Surg. 41: 185, Fig. 2.)*

Stenosis

Stenoses were of four types: stricture, segmental, serpiginous or shelving. All four types were found in the proximal, middle or distal parts of the ureter (Fig. 20.1). In all of these specimens, the diameter of the lumen at the site of stenosis was diminished to less than 60 per cent of the lower limit of normal for age, while the diameter of the proximal dilated portion was increased up to 13 times the normal value for age. There was muscular hypertrophy (up to three times normal) and hyperplasia (up to 4.3 times normal) in the wall of the proximal dilated part of the ureter (Cussen, 1971a). At the site of the stenosis, the lumen was lined by the usual transitional epithelium and was surrounded by smooth muscle with a smaller population of leiomyocytes than normal. However, the individual leiomyocytes were of normal size. There was no increase in the amount of fibrous tissue in the wall of the stenotic zone of any of the 81 ureters.

Parts of the ureter adjoining an atretic segment may exhibit a diminishing muscle coat with substitution of fibrous tissue culminating in a fine fibrous strand at the atretic segment. Occasionally, the strand is thicker and a microlumen persists in a fibrous sheath. These changes may represent the effects of ischaemia on the developing ureter. Stenosis in the contralateral ureter, or isolated stenosis, especially the shelving type in other patients, may sometimes have a similar aetiology and morphology.

An isolated shelving stenosis may be so gradual and slight that it may simulate ureterographically a zone of peristalsis and evoke only dubious pelvic or calyceal fullness.

A 4F ureteric catheter may pass in retrograde direction through the suspect zone. A 3F Fogarty balloon catheter distended minimally with contrast medium can be used to determine and isolate the suspected stricture zone. The balloon is expanded in the normal-calibre part of the ureter to a preset dimension using a tuberculin syringe locked to the catheter. The balloon is then advanced cranially to the suspect site. If the advance is arrested, a radiograph is obtained and the balloon is emptied and refilled in the pelvic or wider-calibre ureter above the site and then withdrawn in antegrade direction. If the balloon arrests, a further radiograph is obtained and the length of the strictured zone can be gauged from the radiographs. The stricture may be quite long, requiring surgery, and the same catheter procedure should be adopted at the time of repair in order to determine the exact site and length, which may not be apparent from external examination of the ureter.

Furthermore, because the narrowing may measure several centimetres, the narrow segment should not be excised in the first instance. The ureter is better divided in the middle of the stricture and spatulated longitudinally in both directions into the non-strictured zones. The shelving ends may then be used in the anastomosis to overcome a possible length discrepancy (Fig. 20.2). The narrow and shelving ends are dovetailed up and down into the spatulated contiguous healthy ureter. They act as toeholds and add welcome gussets that augment the calibre at each end of the anastomosis and incorporate all of the usable ureter to avoid tension.

Valves of the ureter

Forty-two of the 147 ureters (29 per cent) were of this type. There were two subtypes of ureteral valves, one associated with ureteral stenosis at the site of the valve and the other in a ureter of normal calibre (Fig. 20.1). In both subtypes, the orifice and long axis of the distal part of the ureter were eccentrically situated with respect to the lumen and long axis of the proximal dilated part of the ureter. The diameter of the proximal part of the ureter was increased up to eight times the normal value for age. In the subtype with distal stenosis, the luminal diameter of the distal segment of the ureter was less than 60 per cent of the normal value for age while, in the subtype without stenosis, the luminal diameter of the distal part of the ureter was within the normal range for age. In both subtypes, there was muscle cell hypertrophy (up to twice normal) and hyperplasia (up to 5.8 times normal) in the wall of the proximal dilated part of the ureter. The degree of muscular hypertrophy and hyperplasia was similar in both subtypes. At the site of change of calibre, microscopic sections of the ureter revealed two lumina side-by-side, one in the axis of the proximal and one in the axis of the distal part of the ureter (Fig. 20.3). The lumina were separated by a strip of tissue containing all the layers of the ureter and lined on either side by transitional epithelium.

A

(a) (b)

(a') (b')

Fig. 20.2 A. *Shelving stricture of upper ureter mimicking peristaltic wave; also secondary obstructive caliectasis mimicking megacalycosis. Two pyeloureterograms of suspect narrow site. (*a*) Ureteral lumen at end of peristaltic wave. (*b*) Ureteral lumen at beginning of peristaltic wave. (*a'*), (*b'*) A technique of identifying the stricture and its limits (arrows) by a Fogarty catheter (3F) and an opacified balloon arrested in its advance from below and above after evacuating, advancing, refilling and retracting the balloon (see text). B. Technique for repair of shelving stenosis: conservation of length of ureter by using the tapering ends to augment the lumen of the anastomosis (*a*)–(*d*)* (Reprinted, by permission, from, Stephens, F.D. (1983), Congenital Malformations of the Urinary Tract, New York, Praeger, Fig. 17 2A, p. 275 and Fig. 17.2B, p. 276)

B

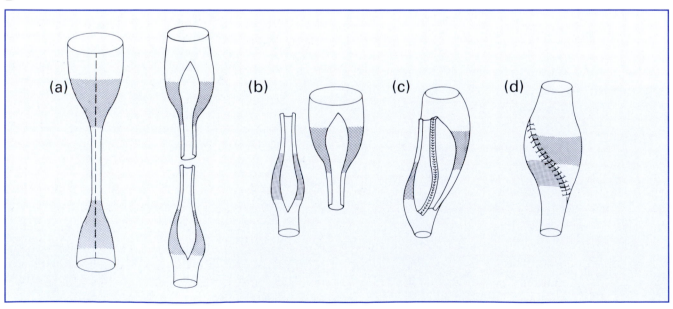

(a)   (b)   (c)   (d)

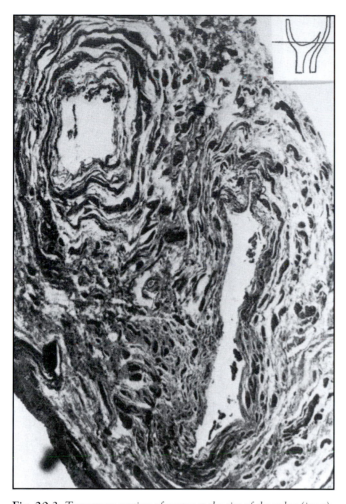

Fig. 20.3 *Transverse section of ureter at the site of the valve (inset). The upper lumen is the distal bulge of the proximal part of the ureter and the lower is the lumen of the distal ureter. The intervening strip of tissue is the flap of the valve (Masson trichrome, ×42). (Reprinted, by permission, from Cussen, L.J. (1971a), The morphology of congenital dilatation of the ureter: intrinsic ureteral lesions. Aust. N.Z. J. Surg. 41: 185, Fig. 12.)*

Orthograde perfusion of the proximal dilated ureter of postmortem or biopsy specimens in both subtypes demonstrated an obstruction to flow at the site of the valve, which could be overcome if very high perfusion pressure was used. Presumably the walls of the dilated ureter became overstretched permitting leakage through the valve. Flow from the distal to the proximal part of the ureter, however, was unimpeded in those valves without distal stenosis. The obstruction caused by the valve may be intermittent, particularly in the subtype with a distal ureter of normal calibre.

Anatomy of ureteral valves

Maizels and Stephens (1980) studied 15 specimens of megaureter with ureteral valves. These specimens included the kidneys, bladder and urethra of babies dying from other causes and also segments of ureter excised at operation.

The sites of the valvular obstructions included the ureteropelvic junction in five, the upper ureter in one and the lower ureter adjacent to the bladder in nine. The valves were present in infants and older children, of whom 11 were boys and four were girls. The valves were unilateral and occurred on the left side in 12 instances and on the right side in three. Two of these children had the prune belly syndrome.

Externally, the dilated ureter or pelvis tapered abruptly at the site of obstruction (Fig. 20.4A,B). At this site, the ureter was enveloped by an adherent loose or dense connective tissue, which was later found by radiographic and histological preparations to conceal and belie the actual course of the underlying ureter. In 11 of the 15 specimens, the longitudinal axis of the distal undilated segment lay oblique to that of the dilated proximal segment. In the remaining four specimens, both segments were aligned externally in the same longitudinal axis. Inspection of the lumen, however, demonstrated that the lumen of the narrow distal segment emerged tangentially or eccentrically from the lumen of the proximal dilated ureter (Fig. 20.4A,B). The lining of the dilated segment at the junction with the narrow segment was raised as a 'lip' or cusp. The margin of the lip was crescentic (Fig. 20.4A) or circular.

Ureteral reflux was documented in only four of these specimens, including two in which the ureteral orifices were determined cystoscopically to be laterally situated in the bladder. The orifice location was not available in the other two specimens.

Radiography

Of the 15 specimens, 12 were examined by ureterography to demonstrate the undilated and dilated segments of each ureter. The valves occurred at the junction of the dilated pelvis or ureter with the undilated ureter. These junctions had characteristic radiographic appearances.

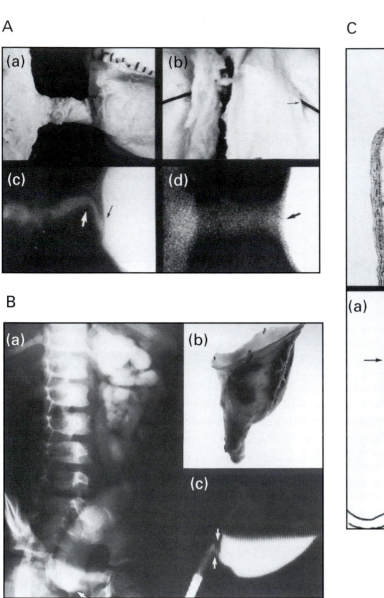

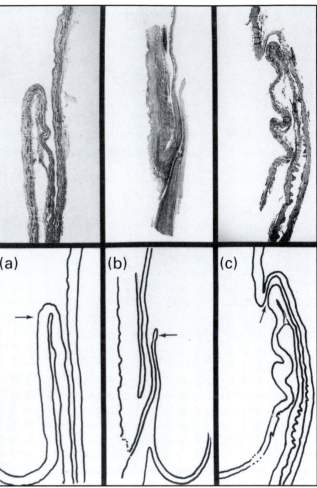

Fig. 20.4 A. *Valve of lower ureter causing partially obstructed megaureter in patient D.P. (male stillbirth, autopsy specimen). (**a**) External appearance of lower ureter (right) at the site of obstruction adjacent to bladder (left). Ureter angulates acutely at site of obstruction. Overlying fascia disguises true course of lumen of ureter demonstrated radiographically. (**b**) Appearance of valve (arrow) as seen through lumen of ureter, reduced from ×10. Bristle spans from intravesical ureter (left) to cusp of valve (right). (**c**) Retrograde ureterogram of specimen demonstrates single acute angulation of course of lumen (white arrow). Valve appears as single filling defect (black arrow). (**d**) Drainage film reveals complete obstruction of ureter at site of valve (arrow).*
B. *Valve of lower ureter causing obstruction of reflux megaureter in patient, J.C., five-year-old boy. (**a**) Pyelogram demonstrates left hydroureteronephrosis with site of obstruction at lower ureter (white arrow). (**b**) External appearance of excised segment of ureter at site of obstruction. Overlying fascia disguises true course of lumen. (**c**) Retrograde ureterogram of specimen demonstrates true course of lumen and two acute angulations (arrows). Valves appear as pair of filling defects angulating ureter wall within adventitious sheath of the ureter.*
C. *Longitudinal histological sections (top) of three ureters obstructed by valves (low power) and schematic drawings (bottom) demarcating valves (arrows) reconstruct anatomy of valves. (**a**) High insertion valve (arrow) at ureteropelvic junction. (**b**) Single-pleat valve (arrow) of lower ureter; pleat overlies lumen of ureter to produce valve mechanism. (**c**) Double-pleat valve at ureteropelvic junction (overlapping pleats indicated by arrow).*
*(**A**, **B**, **C**, respectively, reprinted, by permission, from Maizels, M. and Stephens, F.D. (1980), Valves of the ureter as a cause of primary obstruction of the ureter: anatomic, embryologic and clinical aspects. J. Urol. 123: 742, Figs 1, 3 and 4.)*

1. The lumen of the ureter apposed the wall of the pelvis or dilated ureter to create the typical 'high-insertion' type of obstruction (one specimen).

2. A single-filling defect originated from one wall of the ureter to indent the lumen of the narrow segment as a spur (Fig. 20.4A). This spur or pleat corresponded

to the lip demonstrated anatomically and separated the dilated segment above from the undilated segment below (nine specimens). As a result, the course of the undilated ureter adjacent to the spur lay oblique to the longitudinal axis of the ureter. Beyond the pleat, the lumen of the ureter resumed its axial alignment. The spur allowed free retrograde passage of fluid, but the pressure developed during orthograde injection of the dilated segment apposed the spur against the opposite wall of the undilated segment, occluding the lumen and preventing antegrade flow.

3. A double-pleat valve, created by an elbow bend of the undilated ureter emerging from the ectatic segment, permitted free retrograde but obstructed orthograde flow (Fig. 20.4B).

Histology

Nine specimens were suitable for morphometric determination of the muscle cell size. The average muscle cell size of the ectatic ureter was larger than the upper limit of the range of normal for age in eight of the specimens, as determined by the method described by Cussen (1967b). These measurements substantiated the presence of obstruction at the suspect site (Stephens, 1974).

The obstructing segments exhibited three different morphologies: the high-insertion valve at the ureteropelvic junction in one specimen, the single-pleat valve in nine and the double pleat valve in five (Fig. 20.4A,B). In the high-insertion valve, the upper ureter was bound to, and angulated against, the pelvis by fascia to induce a valve mechanism at the ureteropelvic junction. In the single-pleat valve, which simulates the high insertion at the ureteropelvic junction, part of the wall of the ureter was folded upon itself into the lumen of the ureter as a pleat. This pleat corresponded to the single spur that was observed radiographically to be responsible for obstruction. The pleat was covered by mucosa and was composed of the infolded muscle of the ureter. The muscle fibres became attenuated toward the free edge of the pleat. At the base of the pleat, the infolded muscle coats were bound to each other by the adventitia of the ureter. The walls of the ureter opposite the spur were not indented and showed continuity of its muscle layers from the dilated through the undilated segments. In the double-pleat valve, co-apting walls of the undilated ureter were folded into the lumen

as a pair of interlocking pleats that corresponded with the spurs observed radiographically. The pleats were covered by mucosa and were composed of the infolded muscle coats of apposing walls of the dilated and undilated segments. The pleats formed a hairpin bend of the ureter that was held in place by the adventitial coat (Fig. 20.4C). The pleats occurring at the upper end of the ureter were similar to those at the lower end.

Of the 15 examples of ureteral valves, seven were in patients who were investigated urologically. The valve was suspected before surgery because obstruction to antegrade, but not retrograde, flow was present and was demonstrated radiographically as a filling defect (four patients) or because the excised specimen allowed retrograde but not antegrade flow (three patients) (Figs 20.4B and 20.5).

Historical review

Fenger (1894) described a flap valve as the cause of obstruction at the ureteropelvic junction. Since then, 99 examples of valves of the ureter have been reported, and this entity presently is regarded as a rarity (Maizels and Stephens, 1980). In 69 ureters, the valves occurred in infants, children and adults and were located at the ureteropelvic junction and upper ureter (60 per cent), mid-ureter (20 per cent) and lower ureter (20 per cent). Upper ureteral valves were described as a 'flap', while lower ureteral valves were described as 'annular'. In 21 ureters, the valves were complicated by the presence of stenosis at or below the valve, and in nine, the valves lacked muscle in the flap and may be regarded as a variant of the valve as defined herein. Ureteral valves that caused obstruction have been treated by excision of the valve leaflet, reduction of the ureteral fold and resection of the segment of ureter containing the valve.

Embryogenesis of ureteral valves

By five weeks of gestation, the ureteral bud develops as a posterior diverticulum arising from the caudal end of the mesonephric duct. The bud grows out into the renal blastema and subdivides to form calyces and parts of the renal collecting systems. By eight weeks, the ureter has elongated *pari passu* with ascent of the kidney. At 12 weeks, the ureter demonstrates relative intrinsic narrowings at the ureteropelvic junction, pelvic brim and ureterovesical junction, and intrinsic dilatations of the upper, middle and lower spindles (Fig. 20.6). However,

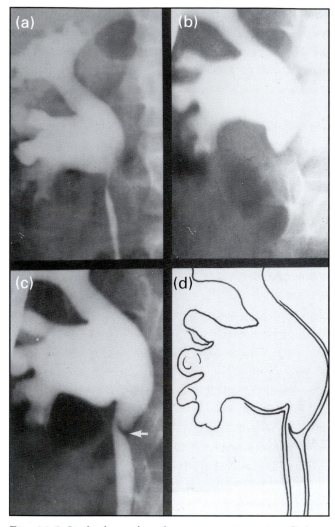

Fig. 20.5 *Single-pleat valve of upper ureter in patient G.A., a 10-year-old boy whose intravenous pyeloureterogram demonstrated right hydronephrosis. (a) Retrograde pyelogram with patient in supine position reveals apparent stricture of upper ureter. (b) Drainage film confirms obstruction. (c), (d) Retrograde pyelogram and drawing with patient in right anterior oblique position show single filling defect of valve in lumen of ureter (arrow). Presence of valve was confirmed surgically. (Reprinted, by permission, from Maizels, M. and Stephens, F.D. (1980), Valves of the ureter as a cause of primary obstruction of the ureter: anatomic, embryologic and clinical aspects. J. Urol. 123: 742, Fig. 5.)*

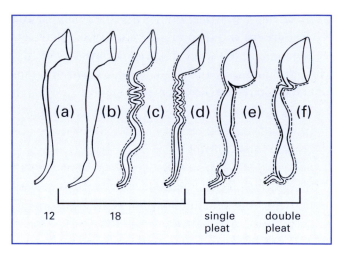

Fig. 20.6 *Possible embryogenesis of valves of ureter. (a) By 12 weeks of gestation, uniform calibre of ureter. (b) At 18 weeks, pelvic and abdominal spindles of ureter appear. If elongate growth of ureter occurs faster than that of trunk ureter may become tortuous (c) or acquire pleats (d). (e), (f) Pleats are normally not obstructive but may persist as valves. (Reprinted, by permission, from Maizels, M. and Stephens, F.D. (1980), Valves of the ureter as a cause of primary obstruction of the ureter: anatomic, embryologic and clinical aspects. J. Urol. 123: 742, Fig. 6.)*

the ureter may elongate faster than the ascent of the kidney. To absorb this excess length, the ureter may assume either a tortuous course or 'concertina' its wall as pleats—the 'fetal folds' of Ostling (1942). The pleats, together with the ureter, become muscularized and enveloped by an outer adventitial coat. Postnatally, the infant's growth rate exceeds that of the ureter and the ureter may lose its tortuosity and unfold its pleat or retain the pleat or pleats permanently. Although these folds occur more commonly near the junction of the ureter and pelvis, Cussen has described similar pleats giving rise to obstruction in the lower end of the ureter.

Many other aetiologies have been proposed to explain the obstructed primary megaureter but a valve is only rarely mentioned. A valve mechanism may arise at the ureteropelvic junction 'from distortion of the pelvic dilatation' (Campbell, 1970a). A mucosal pleat may lie concealed at other levels of the ureter beneath a thick adventitia that masks the angulation within (Fowler and Kesavan, 1977).

Ostling (1942) reported three examples of ureteropelvic junction obstruction, caused by mucosal lips in ledges containing muscle, which he believed were caused by retention of fetal folds of the ureter. Mering *et al.* (1972) agreed with the point of view. This pleat theory provides an explanation for the presence of a valve at any level and for multiple valves. The extreme focal ureterectasis characteristic of the prune belly syndrome may have predisposed the ureters of two of the patients to develop extreme and multiple valve-like obstructions.

Chwalle's membrane has been held responsible for the development of ureteral valves. Chwalle (1927) claimed that the membrane occludes temporarily the ureteral meatus and is a normal feature of development of the ureter. Subsequently, it ruptures under the hydraulic pressure of urine secretion. A partially ruptured membrane may be retained as a ureteral valve or a ureterocele.

Surgical management

Fowler and Kesavan (1977), having studied the work of Cussen (1971a), considered that a valve of the ureter near the ureterovesical junction was one cause of primary obstructive megaureter. Fowler and Kesavan (1977) preferred ureteroureteral anastomosis to reimplantation, when possible, and performed an intraoperative Whitaker test to prove obstruction. They then transected the dilated segment of the ureter and inspected the junction site from within the lumen of the dilated ureter to confirm the presence of an eccentric placement of the distal orifice before undertaking the anastomosis. Seven of nine ureters so treated showed marked improvement, and two of the ureters were considered to be unimproved. The results indicate that the obstruction is localized and not operating throughout the length of the segment. However, many urologists prefer to reimplant the ureter into the bladder after excision of the undilated segment, although if the abnormality occurs higher in the ureter, a well-executed ureteroureteral anastomosis suffices with relief of obstruction.

A valve as the cause of the obstruction would be strongly suspected by the surgeon if the dilated ureter remained large and obstructed after transection of the distal non-dilated ureter about 2–3 mm below the terminal end of the dilated segment. Further transections of the undilated segment much closer to the dilated ureter demonstrate persistence of the obstruction and further evidence of a strictly focal valve action.

Tortuosities and kinks of the ureter

Tortuosities of the ureter are distinguished from valves of the ureter. Ureters that dilate and hypertrophy in response to distal obstruction elongate, fold and become tortuous within their fascial envelopes. The lumen of the ureter at the site of folding is flattened but not constricted and all coats of the ureter follow the folds. Hypertrophy of the muscle coats is present above, below, and at the site of a fold, and the ureter remains unobstructed.

Ureters that are kinked by external structures may angulate (for example, over the lower polar vessels). One side of the ureter is pressed against the other to form an obstructing kink (see Fig. 26.2). Valves of the ureter, however, involve a structural anomaly of the muscle coat. A lamina of the muscular wall infolds to create a one-sided tuck from the dilated to the undilated segment. This lamina is permanently tucked in by the remaining coats of the ureter, which bridge the base of the tuck. Hydrostatic pressure that is developed during peristalsis presses the tuck against the wall of the non-dilated segment obstructing the lumen of the ureter. This arrangement of muscle indicates the congenital developmental anomaly of the valve and explains the obstructive mechanism.

21

Non-reflux, non-obstructed megaureter

The non-reflux, non-obstructed megaureter occurs less commonly than the primary reflux type and has been often wrongly bracketed with the primary obstructed megaureter. This megaureter may be found incidentally or because of stasis and urinary-tract infection or as a component of the prune belly syndrome (see Chapter 37).

Morphology

In 18 of the 147 megaureters (12 per cent) studied in the postmortem state by Cussen (1971a) the ectatic ureter was dilated to an internal diameter of up to four times the normal value for age, but the most distal part of the ureter was of normal dimensions (80–150 per cent of the normal diameter for age), and no obstructive lesion was demonstrated at the site of change of calibre (Figs 20.1 and 21.1). No evidence of muscular hypertrophy or hyperplasia was found in the wall of the proximal ureter; the average size of the leiomyocytes varied from 85 to 120 per cent of the normal value for age, and the average population of leiomyocytes in a cross-section of ureter from 90 to 140 per cent of normal. The wall of the dilated part of the ureter was found to contain the same muscular coats as the wall of the non-dilated part, but the muscle was more sparsely distributed around the wider lumen. Hence, the muscle was relatively thinner than normal, but the absolute amount of muscle present was within the normal range.

Aetiology

The non-reflux, non-obstructed, congenitally dilated ureter presumably represents a localized lateral overgrowth of the developing ureteral bud. The growth stimulus may be similar, though misplaced, to that which normally induces the formation of the renal pelvis. Simple overexpansion has already been proposed by Ostling (1942) as an explanation for some examples of congenital hydronephrosis. Alternatively, the ectasis is the lingering ureteral dilatation associated with vesicoureteral reflux, which has since abated spontaneously. It is important to recognize this group of non-obstructed dilated ureters in the clinical setting, as surgical inter-

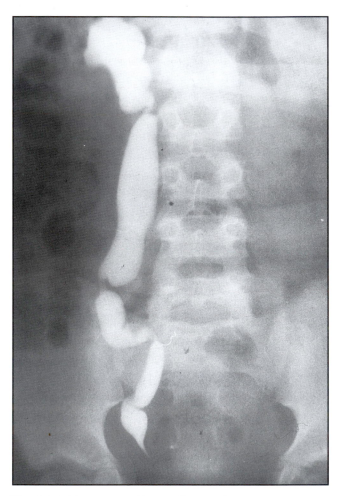

Fig. 21.1 *Megaureter without reflux or obstruction—excretory urogram showing the large calibre of the ureter and the similarity to primary obstructive megaureter. (Reprinted, by permission, from Stephens, F.D. (1983), Congenital Malformations of the Urinary Tract, New York, Praeger, Fig. 18.1, p. 285.)*

vention is rarely, if ever, necessary for these patients. This non-reflux, non-obstructed, congenitally dilated ureter, with growth of the child and time, gradually assumes normal functional diameter.

Non-reflux megaureter: terms and trends and achalasia

The terms 'neuromuscular incoordination', 'achalasia' and 'functional obstruction' have been used in the past to explain the dilated, non-reflux ureter with the distal short normal or narrow calibre juxtavesical segment. One school of thought (Creevy, 1970) considered that the dilated ureter exhibited faulty peristalsis resulting in dilatation above a normal narrow segment. Another school (Pfister *et al.*, 1971; Hanna and Wyatt, 1975) considered that the juxtavesical narrow segment was adynamic, causing secondary obstructive dilatation of the ureter above. Until recently, the non-reflux, non-obstructed megaureter has been included in the obstruction category, mainly on the basis that abnormal dilatation in itself was conclusive evidence of obstruction.

Demonstration of the course, calibre, and length of the distal 'narrow' segment either by prograde or retrograde ureterography has been unsuccessful in the clinical setting. Fluoroscopic studies of the dynamics of the megaureter and emptying times have been helpful subjective means of indicating obstructive or non-obstructive qualities of the enigmatic distal segment.

The Whitaker perfusion pressure–flow test (1973) and diuretic radionuclide radiography (Koff *et al.*, 1979, 1980) determine more objectively the presence or absence of obstruction in the distal short segment. It is now possible to recognize clinically in most instances the two types of non-reflux megaureters—the primary megaureters with and without obstruction.

With calibration of the narrow segment, perfusion fixation techniques, and special radiographic methods of demonstrating the course of the lumen of postmortem or biopsy specimens, it is now possible to distinguish strictures and occult ureterovalves (Cussen, 1971a; Maizels and Stephens, 1980), in some, but not all, of the primary obstructed megaureters.

The term 'adynamic narrow segment' is now very commonly used to describe the so-called adynamic narrow segment in most primary obstructive megaureters and little credence is given to the entity of 'occult ureterovalves'. Objective urodynamic recordings of intraluminal pressures or peristaltic activity in the walls of the narrow segments, however, are lacking. Excised specimens of proven obstructing distal segments have been studied by light and electron microscopy. In some, the muscle and adventitia were normal, or the circular, instead of helical, muscle formed an obstructing band around the lumen (Murnaghan, 1957; Tanagho *et al.*, 1970). In others, a paucity of muscle or excess fibrous tissue or collagen with separation of the nexus bands (Notley, 1972; Hanna *et al.*, 1976) were demonstrated. Few such microscopic studies have been correlated with perfusion fixation methods or precise ureterography of the excised undissected narrow segment. More examples of non-reflux, non-obstructed megaureters and ureterovalves will be recognized in the future and the so-called 'functional' or 'adynamic' obstruction will become a rarity. Furthermore, the importance of correctly diagnosing valves of the ureter is threefold. First, the ureter distal to the valve is non-obstructive. Second, ureteroureteral anastomosis is a sound method of management and is the technique of choice if the segment distal to the valve is long. Third, the valve lip may be amenable to minimally invasive intraureteral endoscopic resection or dilatation.

22

Duplex ureters

When two ureters issue from a double kidney, they may join at a Y-junction with long or short common stems, or at a V-junction with negligible stem, in both cases being referred to as 'bifid ureters', or they may open separately into the urinary or genital tracts as 'double ureters'. These are common developmental and often inherited abnormalities and, as such, may be entirely symptom-free (Whitaker and Danks, 1966; Atwell *et al.*, 1974). Some have defective insertions into the bladder or the urethra, resulting in vesicoureteral reflux; others exhibit obstructive lesions that promote stasis and infection; in females, the ectopic component may cause wetting.

Duplex ureter systems are prone to many additional anomalies of the upper tracts and may occur in association with cloacal or lower urinary tract deformities. The introduction of ultrasonography and micturition cysto-urethrography in the routine clinical investigation of urinary tract disease in children has led to much clearer understanding of the defects of the double or bifid ureters.

Excretion urography is usually the first radiographical procedure that brings to notice the presence of double ureters. Micturition cystourethrography is now a routine radiological test of competence of the ureterovesical-valve mechanisms, which, in normal children, resists vesicoureteral reflux of urine, but which in subjects with double ureter, is frequently incompetent. Hence, the test may demonstrate one or both components of a double system by reflux of contrast medium from the bladder. The nuclear cystogram procedure is a more sensitive test of competence because the test is carried out with continuous monitoring of the upper tracts during the whole of the filling phase and after voiding.

The ureter draining the upper portion of the double kidney is termed the 'upper pole ureter' (UPU); that draining the lower portion is the 'lower pole ureter' (LPU). When these ureters form cranial to the bladder to form a common stem, it is described as a bifid ureter. The part of the orthotopic or ectopic ureter or common stem that lies within the walls of the bladder is called the 'intravesical ureter', which includes the hiatal or intramural segment in the muscular tunnel and the submucosal segment.

The orifice of the LPU is located on the cornu of the trigone. The cornu may be elongated so that the orifice, which lies in a more lateral position, is described as lateral ectopia. The orifice of the UPU is usually located medial and caudal to the LPU. It is termed simply 'ectopic' but may be qualified by such terms as 'vesical', 'urethral', 'vestibular', 'vasal' or 'vaginal' to denote the general location (Fig. 22.1). More specific locations within these anatomical regions are indicated by letters of the alphabet, A to H (see Fig. 14.3).

Anatomical vagaries

The position of emergence in the genitourinary tract of each component of a double ureter has long held anatomical and embryological interest. Generally, an ectopic orifice will lie caudal to the LPU orifice (Weigert, 1877). Meyer (1946), however, claimed that the position of the UPU orifice may be medial or caudal, and that the relative positions of the orifices were so constant that he formulated a law—the Weigert–Meyer law. This law, that the UPU orifice lies caudal and medial to the LPU orifice, incorporates the observations of both Weigert and Meyer.

However, it has been found that the positions of some UPU orifices violated the Weigert–Meyer 'law' and lay on an embryological 'ectopic pathway' (Fig. 22.2). By plotting the locations of the orifices, which were examined in postmortem specimens or identified by cystourethroscopy, and which were accurately described in published case reports, this ectopic pathway was established.

The situation of the orifices

Postmortem series

Thirteen specimens were available for this study. The double ureter anomaly was bilateral in three and conjoined in four. The positions of the 12 ectopic orifices are shown in Fig. 22.2.

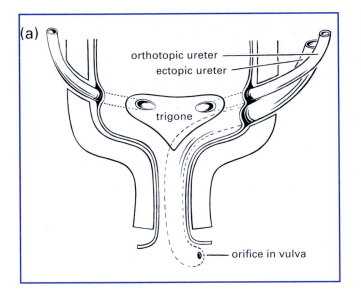

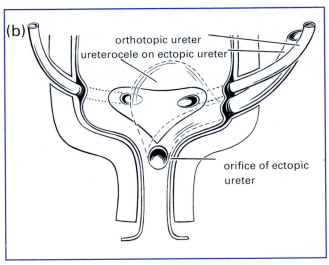

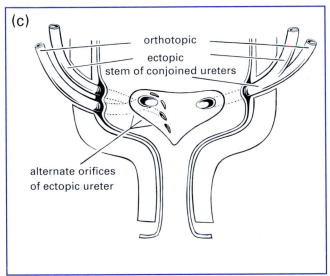

Fig. 22.1 *Connotations of orifices of ectopic ureters according to regional location. (**a**) Vulval or vestibular ectopic. (**b**) Urethral ectopic. (**c**) Vesical ectopic. (Reprinted, by permission, from Stephens, F.D. (1963), Congenital Malformations of the Rectum, Anus and Genito-Urinary Tracts. Edinburgh, Livingstone, Fig. 77, p. 155.)*

Orifice of the LPU

In 12 specimens, the LPU orifice was normally situated in the lateral extreme of the cornu of the trigone. In one, the orifice lay in a diverticulum, which corresponded in position to the LPU orifice of the opposite side. In all the double-ureter anomalies in this post-mortem series, the LPU orifice was found to lie on the trigonal platform and it was the UPU that lay in abnormal positions relative to the LPU orifice.

Combined LPU and UPU orifice

In one specimen, the LPU orifice was shared by the UPU orifice. Here the cranial portion of the lumen of the common orifice was that of the UPU. From within the bladder, the dividing septum was not visible but when traced from above, the ureters were found to join within 0.2 cm of the orifice.

Caudal orifice of the UPU

The UPU orifices, usually appearing as dimples or fine, elongated grooves, were smaller than their corresponding LPU orifices.

Seven lay medial to the LPU orifice. They were close to the medial half of the circumference of the LPU orifice—a distance of 0.2 cm from it in the newborn, and 0.6 cm in the adult specimen. Three orifices were seen in the cranial and medial quadrant. In one instance, the UPU orifice was found in the caudal and medial quadrant; three were situated directly medial to the LPU orifice. In four other double-ureter specimens,

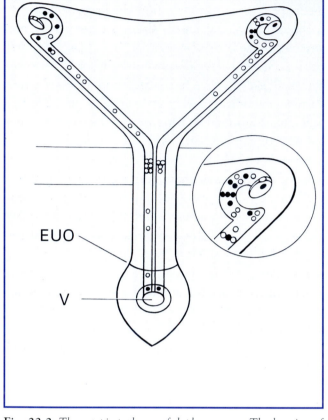

Fig. 22.2 *The ectopic pathway of duplex ureters. The location of orifices of ectopic ureters is plotted on the diagram depicting the trigone, urethra and vestibule. Black dots represent those orifices studied in postmortem specimens and open circles those in clinical examinations. The two horizontal lines demarcate the internal sphincter zone. (EUO = external urethral orifice and V = vagina). Inset shows a composite view of the positions of all the orifices both right and left lying in close proximity to the orthotopic orifice. The 'arcway' pivoting on the orthotopic orifice is valid even when the orthotopic orifice is itself laterally or medially ectopic. (Reprinted, by permission, from Stephens, F.D. (1958), Anatomical vagaries of double ureters. Aust. N.Z. J. Surg. 28: 27, Fig. 2.)*

the UPU orifices lay beyond the LPU orifice—one lay exactly caudal to its lower lip, another lay on the inferior margin of the trigone, and the other two, after a long submucosal course, opened in the vagina on the cranial surface of the hymen (Fig. 22.2).

Cystourethroscopy series

The pathway along which 35 UPU orifices were found to lie was plotted from the study of 27 children (Fig. 22.2).

In eight instances, the UPU orifice lay in very close proximity to the medial margin of the LPU orifice. One,

slit-like in appearance, lay in the rolled-out upper lip of the LPU orifice and the other three were situated craniomedially. Two were situated in the caudomedial arc and two were directly caudal.

Thirteen orifices were distributed along the lower border of the trigone as far distally as the internal meatus. In the urethra, the orifice of the UPU opened most frequently into the internal sphincter zone; at this site in the female children, the orifice was characteristically larger than normal. There were 10 ectopic orifices in this zone. Only two lay in the external sphincter zone of the female urethra. One child exhibited an ectopic orifice posterolateral to the external urethral orifice in the vestibule. In one male child, the orifice, small in size, could be recognized on the cranial side of the verumontanum but close to it.

In some male patients, who are additional to this series, the UPU joined the ejaculatory duct system. The orifice was not visible endoscopically.

The course of the 'ectopic pathway'

The line connecting all these UPU orifices, which were visualized not only at operation but also in the series of postmortem specimens, had a devious course, which could appropriately be called the 'ectopic pathway'. It arose tangentially from the upper margin of the circumference of the orthotopic orifice. It was directed craniomedially and then followed closely the medial hemicircumference of this orifice until it reached the most caudal point. The pathway then deviated from the arc of the circle to follow the inferolateral border of the trigone into the urethra.

In the female, it coursed along the posterior wall of the urethra to the ipsilateral side of the midline, as far as the external urethral orifice. The pathway in the vulva lay on the posterolateral aspect of the urethral orifice or continued posteriorly to the side of the midline on the urethrovaginal bridge to the base of the hymen. The ureters with orifices located on the pathway take a submucosal course within the bladder, urethra and vulva as depicted in Figs 22.3 and 22.4.

In the male, the ectopic pathway was traced on the posterior wall of the urethra to the side of the midline, cranial to the verumontanum. No proven caudal extension beyond the verumontanum occurred in this series.

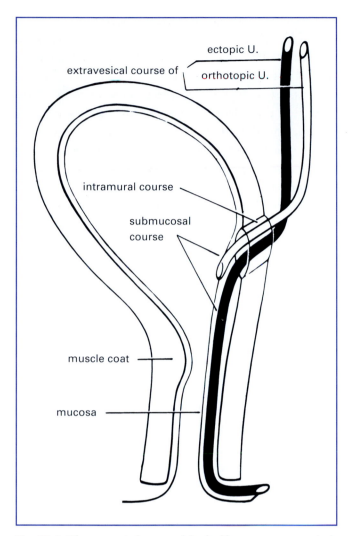

Fig. 22.3 *The anatomical course of the double ureters—extravesical, intramural in the vesical hiatus, and submucosal in bladder, urethra and urethrovaginal bridge. (Reprinted, by permission, from Stephens, F.D. (1958), Anatomical vagaries of double ureters. Aust. N.Z. J. Surg. 28: 27, Fig. 1.)*

The UPU, however, may join the ejaculatory-duct system or wolffian derivatives (Eisendrath, 1938; Way and Popper, 1946; Campbell, 1951c) (Fig. 22.5).

Case report series

Weigert (1877) described seven specimens with complete duplication of the ureter. He made the pronouncement that, in all cases, the lower-lying orifice in the bladder corresponded to the ureter coming from the upper renal pelvis. Weigert (1878) reported six more cases of completely duplicated ureters that conformed to this pattern. He observed also an exceptional case of double monster in which the ureter from the upper

pelvis of a double kidney opened into the bladder in a higher place than the ureter from the lower pelvis.

Meyer (1946) elaborated Weigert's observations, and formulated the Weigert–Meyer 'law', viz. that the ureter from the upper kidney characteristically ends more caudally and medially than the ureter from the lower kidney. At the same time, Meyer was prepared to allow that this generalization would be better regarded as a rule than a law because a few exceptions had been recorded.

Since Weigert's first passing reference to a case that violated this rule, there have been reports of at least two postmortems (Kerr, 1911; Mills, 1939) and two cystoscopic (Lund, 1949; Dougherty, 1954) studies of double ureters exhibiting ectopic orifices lying higher in the bladder than the corresponding orthotopic orifice.

Seven cases in Stephens' investigation, including three in a postmortem series and four in patients being examined cystoscopically, also revealed a more common incidence of this so-called anomalous positioning of the UPU orifice (Fig. 22.6). There was an incidence of seven in 36 patients with complete duplication of the double ureters. When both complete double ureters in bilateral cases were included in the total, the incidence was seven nonconforming in 47 complete double ureters.

It would seem fair on the evidence to extend the pathway beyond the limits described by Weigert and Meyer in order to include all the deviations from the recognized ectopic pathway described in this communication, and in those of Kerr (1911), Mills (1939), Lund (1949) and Dougherty (1954) (Fig. 22.6a,b).

Lateral 'ectopy' of the orthotopic orifice and the ectopic pathway

In this study of postmortem specimens of duplex systems, the orifices of the LPUs were located on the otherwise normal cornu of the trigone. The LPU, however, is commonly located at a more lateral site, or even in a hiatal diverticulum. If the UPU is also laterally located, it takes up a position at some point on the pathway that is orientated around the laterally placed LPU orifice (Fig. 22.6b).

Duplex ureter anatomy
The extravesical course

The extravesical courses of the duplex ureters both in the bifid and double forms exhibit regular relationships,

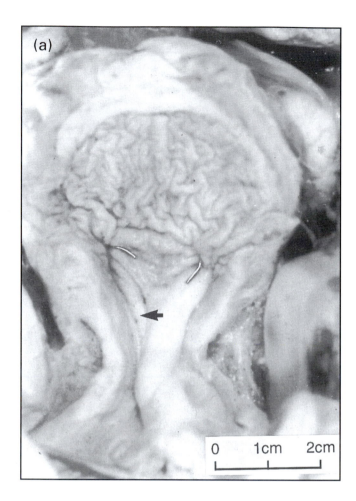

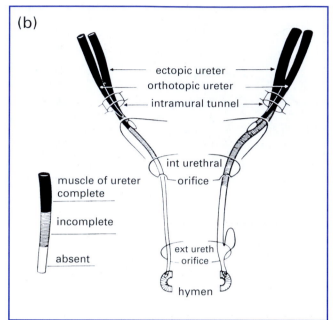

Fig. 22.4 *Specimen and diagram of bilateral duplex systems of Baby W., depicting course and muscularity of the intravesical and urethral segments of ectopic ureters. (**a**) Bristles demarcate LPU orifices. Left ectopic megaureter is the long white structure in the trigone and urethra. Right ectopic ureter is much smaller (arrow). (**b**) Note the long amuscular urethral and partially muscularized vesical segments of the ectopic ureters. Muscle coats fully constituted in the extravesical ureters. Also diverticulum near external meatus on left ureter. (Reprinted, by permission, from Stephens, F.D. (1963), Congenital Malformations of the Rectum, Anus and Genito-Urinary Tracts. Edinburgh, Livingstone, Fig. 89, p. 175 (**a**); Fig. 74, p. 144 (**b**).)*

which are complicated, but not basically altered, by elongation or tortuosity of one or both or the site of the Y-junction in bifid systems. Both ureters reside in the same fascial compartment.

In six postmortem specimens of bifid ureters, the upper pole component was found to lie in a plane anterior to its accompanying LPU. Frontal crossings of this UPU varied; but all the upper pole components of the Y-ureters, including those bifid ureters that became conjoined at the common orifice in the bladder, joined the anterior aspect of the LPU in forming the common stem (Fig. 22.7).

With double ureters, the UPU lies anterior to the LPU in the major part of its course, but a definite pattern of rotation of the lower end of the UPU around the LPU in the vicinity of the vesical hiatus was noted.

Intravesical course

The distribution of the UPU orifices has already been plotted along the ectopic pathway. For ease of description of the relationship of the two ureters as they enter the hiatus, three points on this pathway are selected, namely, the cranial, the medial and the caudal points in close proximity to the medial border of LPU orifice.

When the ectopic orifice was cranial, the UPU was anterior to the LPU and the two ureters did not cross; when the orifice was medial, the UPU lay medial in the intravesical course; a caudal orifice was associated with a UPU that crossed behind the LPU in the hiatus to get to its destination (Fig. 22.7). Intermediate positions of the orifice were indicative of graduated degrees of rotation of the UPU about the LPU (Fig. 22.8).

Even when the UPU orifice lay still more caudal at any point along the LPU pathway, the UPU crossed the

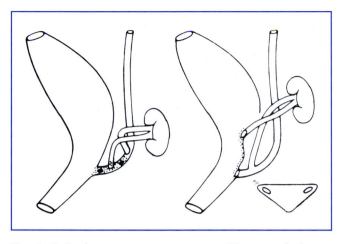

Fig. 22.5 *Duplex ectopic ureter joining vas. The ectopic bud arises outside the zone of the wolffian duct that is incorporated into the bladder or urethra (shaded zone) and remains attached to the seminal duct. Ipsilateral trigone present with orifice of orthotopic ureter only on it. Heavy black dots on wolffian duct denote points of origin of the buds that would come to lie in the bladder or urethra. (Reprinted, by permission, from Stephens, F.D. (1974), Idiopathic dilatations of the urinary tract. J. Urol. 112: 819, Fig. 1.)*

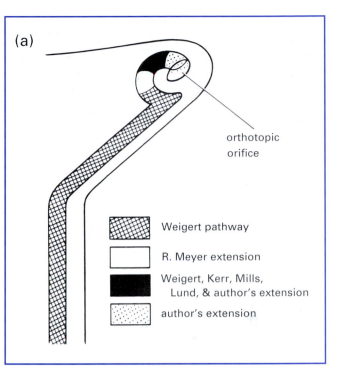

orthotopic orifice

Weigert pathway

R. Meyer extension

Weigert, Kerr, Mills, Lund, & author's extension

author's extension

LPU orifice posteriorly and appeared caudal to the orifice in the submucosal plane (Fig. 22.7). When the UPU orifice lies level with or cranial to the LPU orifice, the two ureters may be totally uncrossed. Lund (1949) reported a case of uncrossed double ureters. After careful analysis of the literature on this unusual arrangement, he considered that uncrossed double ureters could occur in approximately 8 per cent of complete duplications.

When the orifice of the UPU lies on the medial arc of the ectopic pathway, the intravesical segments of both the ureters are closely bound together and cannot be separated without causing ischaemia of one or both ureters. If the UPU lies on the distal trigone near the internal urinary meatus or beyond, the two ureters are separate in their intravesical course and can be separated without impairment of blood supply to the LPU.

Unusual intramural and extravesical caudal paths taken by upper pole ureters

In both males and females, the UPU may enter the bladder together with the LPU, but instead of lying in the submucosal plane, the ectopic ureter grooves and weakens the muscle wall (Williams *et al.*, 1964). The groove may be in continuity with the hiatus and extend partially or all the way to the verumontanum in the

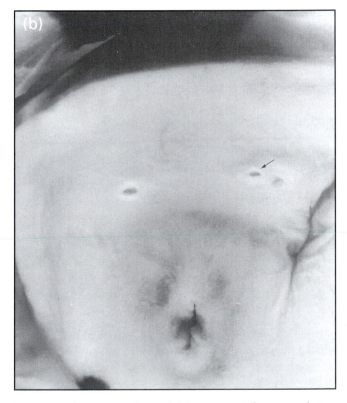

Fig. 22.6 *The ectopic pathway. (a) Diagram to indicate contributors and their contributions to the ectopic pathway. (b) Specimen of the trigone showing the left ectopic orifice (arrow) of a duplex system lying in the black zone cranial and medial to the orthotopic orifice. (Reprinted, by permission, from Stephens, F.D. (1958), Anatomical vagaries of double ureters. Aust. N.Z. J. Surg. 28: 27, Fig. 3.)*

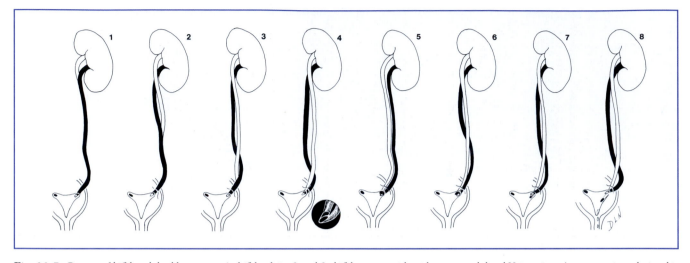

Fig. 22.7 *Course of bifid and double ureters: 1, bifid pelvis; 2 and 3, bifid ureters with mid-ureter and distal Y-junctions (note anterior relationship of UPU; 4, intravesical V-junction; 5, uncrossed double ureters with UPU orifice cranial to orifice of LPU; 6 and 7, junctional bud ureters on medial arc of ectopic pathway (note that in 7 the UPU crossed behind the LPU in the intramural tunnel to achieve an opening caudal to the orifice of the LPU); 8, locations of UPU orifices on lateral border of trigone and in urethra. (Reprinted, by permission, from Stephens, F.D. (1979c), Bifid and Double Ureters, Ureteroceles and Fused Kidneys, 3rd edn, M.M. Ravitch et al. (eds), Fig. 108.4, p. 1190. Chicago, Year Book.)*

male or to the external urinary meatus in the female. The groove may completely interrupt the muscle coat of the trigone or urethra creating urinary incontinence. When the UPU is complicated by ureterocele formation, the ureterocele may expand both inside and outside the bladder or urethral wall. The extramural expansion is most noticeable on voiding cystourethrography and was especially noticeable with cecoureteroceles (Figs. 24.7 and 24.18).

In males, if the ureter joins the vas or vesicle, it may not enter the hiatus, but takes a direct course bypassing the bladder and urethra (Fig. 22.5).

Rarely in females, the ectopic ureter may part company with the orthotopic ureter at the juxtavesical region to enter the side wall of the ipsilateral vagina bypassing the bladder and urethra. The ureter then joins Gartner's duct (persisting remains of the wolffian duct) in the side wall of the vagina (Fig. 24.18). If Gartner's duct remains patent, urine is conducted to the base of the hymen, but if this duct undergoes atrophy a cystic swelling may develop and project or ulcerate into the lumen of the vagina.

It is possible that the ureter may gain a direct entry into the vagina, in which case the müllerian duct, when it advances alongside the wolffian duct, may cut through and incorporate the ectopic ureter, giving it a direct entry into the lumen of the genital passage. This may be a valid and alternative explanation for the ectopic ureter that gains entry into the fornix of the vagina or cervix of the uterus.

Embryology

The translocation of double ureteric buds from wolffian duct to bladder base follows closely the procedure described for the single bud (Fig. 1.10). The common excretory duct with buds attached trumpets and exstrophies to form the trigone (Fig. 22.8). The most caudal bud on the common excretory duct is integrated first followed by the second bud which is disposed at some point along the ectopic pathway.

Junctional ectopic buds may lie on the medial arcway disposed close to the LPU orifice revealing the initial relationship between the two twin buds at their points of origin from the common excretory duct.

The LPU orifice in all instances was placed in the lateral cornu of the trigone and it was the UPU orifice that was disposed about it. This relationship is maintained when the LPU orifice lies in an abnormally lateral position.

The terminal end of the UPU, lying anterior to the LPU when conjoined, and posterior when its orifice is caudal, may be said to have undergone a developmental somersault about the orthotopic orifice. The following is proposed:

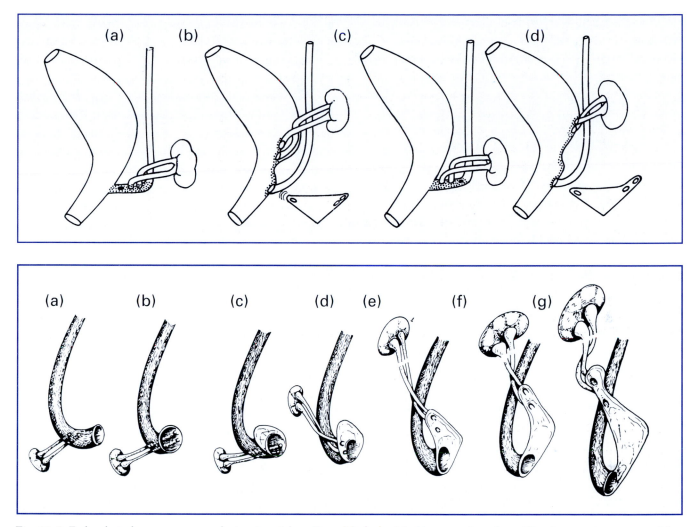

Fig. 22.8 *Embryological rearrangement and migration of the orifices of the buds of double ureters from the wolffian duct to urinary tract and formation of the future trigone.*

Upper row. *Lateral projection.* (**a**) *Two ureteric buds arise from common excretory duct (stippled area) and migrate to trigone with LPU orifice normally sited and ectopic orifice caudal to it* (**b**). (**c**) *LPU bud arises from a point caudal to UPU bud, which arises from the normal site, and both buds migrate to trigone. LPU orifice abnormally sited laterally and the UPU ureter located in the normal position* (**d**). *(Upper row: Reprinted, by permission, from Stephens, F.D. (1974), Idiopathic dilatations of the urinary tract. J. Urol. 112: 819, Fig. 1.)*

Lower row. *Embryological rearrangement of the ureteric bud around the wolffian duct and onto the trigone. Anteroposterior projection showing rotation of the orifices of two buds from posteromedial to anterolateral orientations around the wolffian ducts and the taking up and integration of the upper lip of the common excretory duct into the trigone* (**a**)-(**e**); *shown also are hyperelongated trigones with lateral ectopy of both orifices* (**f**), *and hiatal diverticulum with LPU orifice on the extended cornu in the diverticulum and ectopic orifice on the trigone in the bladder* (**g**). *Note also the crossings of the ureters resulting from the migration. (Lower row: reprinted, by permission, from Stephens, F.D. (1983), Congenital Malformations of the Urinary Tract, New York, Praeger, Fig. 19.8, p. 304.)*

1. Bifid ureters arise from the wolffian duct as a single bud.
2. UPUs, whose orifices lie along the pathway caudal to the LPU orifice, arise as two independent ureteric buds from the wolffian duct.
3. UPUs issuing on to the medial arcway in close proximity to the orthotopic orifice originate as junctional buds.
4. The UPU, which shares a septate orifice with the LPU, represents the true bifurcated ureteric bud arising from the wolffian duct.

When both the LPU and UPU orifices are situated in abnormal lateral positions, the UPU orifice lies on a similar ectopic pathway orientated to the LPU orifice.

The upper pole ureteric orifices on the pathway trace all levels of origin of the second ureteric bud to the point where it is no longer an independent but a single bud.

Surgical import of duplex ureters

There is a surgical import in all this intricate anatomical relationship of double ureters.

In the first place, the lowermost crossing of complete double ureters in their submucosal course, unlike the more proximal crossings in the extravesical parts of the ureters, may be obstructive to the LPU. Obstruction ensues only if the UPU itself is obstructed, when the distended, turgid UPU compresses the LPU orifice at the point of crossing within the confines of the hiatus (Fig. 24.11). Release of the obstruction of the UPU creates a spontaneous decompression of the LPU.

Second, ureteric crossings are non-obstructive when both ureters are normal in calibre. This is important in the assessment of the common complaint of periodic, short-lived peri-umbilical colic in children in whom normal calibre double ureters coexist. In one child in this study, the colic was indeed severe, but the ureters did not cross from their origins to their terminations in the bladder.

Third, pain of double ureters is most often attributable to infective crises. It is the pain of acute pyelonephritis; it is situated in the loin; it may persist for hours or days, sometimes with exacerbations. It subsides when the infection subsides.

The principal factor promoting infection is urinary stasis; for example, ureter-to-ureter reflux in conjoined ureters, vesicoureteral or urethroureteral reflux in complete duplications, or ureteral obstruction (Stephens, 1956a, 1957). These children were remarkably free from pain in the absence of infection.

Clinical implications

In the great majority of duplex ureter systems, both components are functionally normal in all respects and the child is symptom-free, but when either component is abnormal, pain, symptoms of infection, wetting and failure to thrive may ensue. The LPU may have defects of the submucosal segment associated with reflux, reflux megaureter and renal malformations. The UPU, when

abnormal, may exhibit similar anomalies but also ureterocele formation, prolapse of the ureterocele, ureteral obstruction and malformation of the male and female genitalia.

The same congenital defects of the submucosal ureter, especially that of lateral ectopy of the orifice as described for single ureters, may afflict the LPU of the duplex system (page 169). The occurrence of dilatation of the ureter, pelvis and calyces, together with a degree of renal hypodysplasia, is a common accompaniment of the defects of the submucosal segment and the double-ureter malformation. It is uncommon to find ureterocele formation or intrinsic obstructions of the duplex LPU.

The UPU is often the more conspicuous pathological component of the double-ureter malformation, and may therefore be assumed to be the only site of infection. Though an infected UPU is, in many cases, the main cause of symptoms, the LPU and to some extent the opposite ureter may also contribute to the clinical status of the patient.

Effect of urethral sphincters on the urethral ectopic upper pole ureter

Perineal and urethral upper pole ureters, which track in the submucosal plane of the bladder and urethra to their orifices, become partially obstructed by the circumferential grip of the internal urethral sphincters during the reservoir phase of bladder filling; it is only during micturition phases that this sphincteric obstruction is released. Obstruction of the UPU orifice by an intrinsic stenosis may occur giving rise to a ureterocele within the bladder or in the urethra, where the sphincter squeeze aggravates the obstruction. The UPU is usually dilated and tortuous, and the upper pole of the kidney may be hypodysplastic.

Position of ectopic orifice and wetting

The level of the orifice of the UPU in relation to the highest resting pressure zone of the urethral pressure profile determines the presence or absence of wetting (Fig. 22.9). Leakage may be profuse, minimal, absent or intermittent, depending on the renal excretory function, the status of infection and the reservoir capacity of the UPU. Wetting, when a symptom of UPUs, has special features: (1) leakage occurs apart

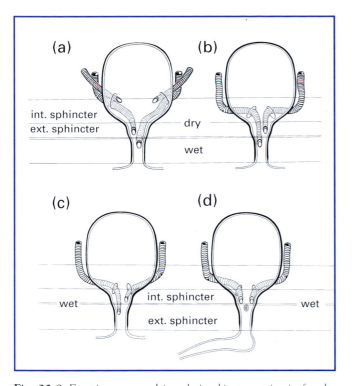

Fig. 22.9 *Ectopic ureter and its relationship to wetting in females and, rarely, in males. Double transverse lines represent the normal highest resting pressure zone of the urethral pressure profile. Urine from orifices cranial to it spills back into the bladder; urine from orifices caudal to it drain uncontrollably to the exterior. (a) Orifice positions of ectopic ureters of duplex systems; wetting unique to females; urethral sphincters normal. (b) Orifice positions of single ectopic ureters; when ureterovesical hiatus normally located in bladder, wetting occurs as in (a). (c) and (d) When hiatus is at bladder neck, the internal sphincter and continence are disturbed in females and males irrespective of location of ureteric orifices. (Reprinted, by permission, from Stephens, F.D. (1983), Congenital Malformations of the Urinary Tract, New York, Praeger, Fig. 19.9, p. 305)*

from acts of normal micturition; (2) it occurs in females; (3) it is induced by the position of the orifice of the upper pole ureter being distal to the middle of the urethra; and (4) reports indicate that it may be nocturnal or diurnal or become apparent for the first time later in childhood or after a pregnancy when it is then likely to be caused by free passage of pus from the functionless ectopic ureter.

1. Wetting and acts of micturition. Normal micturition can be expected, because the bladder fills normally from the other ureters and its detrusor and sphincter mechanisms are normal, but urine from the ectopic orifice escapes by ureteric propulsion, past the sphincters during the resting phases of bladder function.

2. Wetting confined to females. The sex characteristic is explained on the basis of the embryology of the female urogenital sinus. The müllerian ducts, the caudal ends of which are known as the müllerian bulbs, first join the urethra between the openings of the wolffian (ejaculatory) ducts, at the site of the verumontanum or Müller's hillock. The bulbs then migrate caudally from this site to the normal position of the outlet of the vagina (Fig. 24.18). If the orifice of a UPU lies in close proximity to the original site of the müllerian bulbs, it may become incorporated and carried part or all of the distance to the new site of the vaginal outlet. The ureteric orifice then lies on the posterolateral wall of the urethra, on the vulval bridge between urethra and introitus, on or near the hymen, or in the vagina. By virtue of the embryological process of migration, the orifice of the ureter in conjunction with that of the müllerian ducts may be shifted from the dry side to the wet side of the urethral watershed or into the vagina or even to the contralateral side on very rare occasions (Figs 24.11 and 25.4).

3. Urethral ectopic UPU and wetting. The ectopic orifice, which lies in the urethra cranial to the verumontanum in the male or mid-urethra in the female is above the urethral watershed. Urine is held back in the ureter by the compression of the ureter by the urethral sphincters. When the urine fills the ureter and overflows into the urethra, it takes the path of least resistance and spills back into the bladder. If, however, the ectopic orifice of the UPU lies distal to the urethral watershed, urine from the ureter overflows or jets to the exterior.

4. Diurnal or nocturnal characteristics of wetting. If a muscular defect, either partial or total, occurs in the wall of the UPU, the power of the internal sphincter may prevail over the weakened or non-peristaltic ureter. The child may then be dry during the day when the ureter is intermittently decompressed during the acts of micturition, but wet at night when the ureter fills to overflow during the long, uninterrupted sleep.

Intermittent periods of wetting may occur from non-functional renal segments, which from time to time become infected, seeping purulent discharges from the ureter.

Impairment of the urethral sphincters

Duplex systems may occur in patients with myelodysplasia or other neuropathic causes of urinary incontinence. The UPU may then be only incidental or contributory to the neuropathic wetting.

The ectopic ureter of the duplex system may split the musculature of the urethral sphincters leading to wetting from sphincter derangement. This may be suspected as a cause of wetting in males or in females with ectopic orifices sited cranial to the mid-urethral watershed and especially with non-duplicated urethral ectopic orifices (Fig. 22.9). In one patient, the large ectopic ureter appeared to split the urethral musculature throughout its length (Fig. 22.10). After excision of the urethral segment, it was necessary to suture together the free edges of the whole length of the posterior urethra. This child gained complete continence postoperatively.

Contralateral ureter

The opposite ureter is prone to exhibit abnormalities. In 20 per cent of patients, the duplex system is bilateral. If the contralateral ureter is single, the ureterovesical valve may be incompetent, or the ureter may be larger than normal, with or without reflux, or may exhibit additional anomalies.

Duplex ureters and vesicoureteral reflux

Reflux is a common and most important cause of morbidity in patients with a double-ureter malformation. It occurs in normal calibre ureters or megaureters, and its importance lies in the fact that refluxed urine is residual urine, notorious in promoting infection.

Ureteral reflux bears no causal relation to megaureter. Investigations show that ureters of normal calibre with free reflux for many years show no progression to megaureters. Furthermore, repeated radiographical examina-

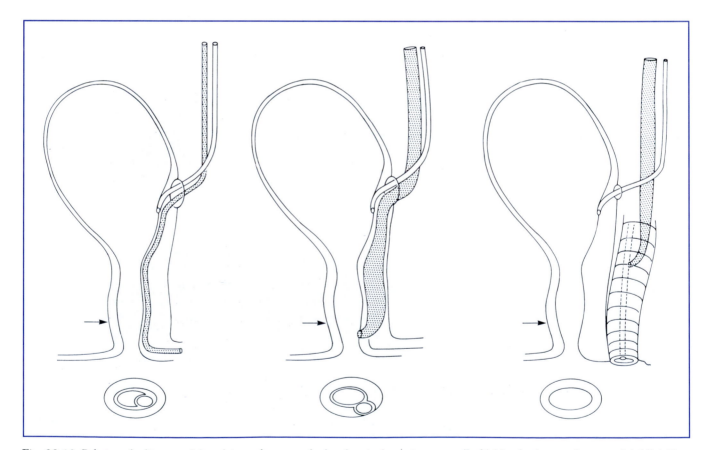

Fig. 22.10 *Relation of sphincters of the pelvic urethra to urethral and vaginal ectopic ureters. (Left) Usual submucosal course. (Middle) Very rare sphincter splitting course and inset shows the ectopic ureter disrupting the ring of muscle. (Right) Vaginal ectopic ureter is unrelated to the urethra sphincters. (Insets show cross-sections of urethras at the level of the arrows.) Reprinted, by permission, from Stephens, F.D. (1983),* Congenital Malformations of the Urinary Tract, New York, Praeger, *Fig. 19.10, p. 306)*

tions of megaureters that show marked reflux, have shown no increase in the calibre of such ureters. It is doubtful, therefore, that vesicoureteral reflux is the cause of megaureter. The term 'reflux megaureter' implies a cause-and-effect relationship, but it is more likely that megaureter anomaly in association with reflux is a specific intrinsic entity in itself.

Reflux of urine from bladder or urethra to the ureter is determined by the competence of the valve mechanism in the submucosal segment of the ureter. This, in turn, is dependent on orifice position, length of the submucosal segment, and muscle component of the wall of the ureter. Hence reflux is more frequent in the LPU ureter because its orifice is more frequently laterally ectopic. The length of the submucosal section of the UPU may be normal in length, occasionally shorter and usually longer than normal; reflux is uncommon and results from lack of the intrinsic muscle and defective activation of the mechanical flap valve.

Ureteroureteral reflux

Whether the components of a bifid ureter are normal or larger than normal in calibre, yo-yo reflux from one to the other occurs around the Y-junction leading to stasis. The larger the Y and calibre of the ureters above the normal calibre stem, the more prolonged is the emptying time and the greater the chances of episodes of infection or calculus formation (see page 235). It should be remembered that cystitis is very common in female children, and that a non-reflux bifid ureter may be a completely innocent non-infected bystander. If the ureterovesical mechanism of the common stem is defective, vesicoureteral and ureteroureteral reflux ensue.

Urethroureteral reflux

Urethroureteral reflux is limited to the urethral UPU and occurs only during micturition, since in the intervals the bladder is excluded from the urethra by the contracted urethral sphincter muscles. In one patient, the ureter, which contained the refluxed urine, remained distended for at least an hour after micturition (Fig. 22.11). This urine was retained in the ureter because its orifice became obstructed by the urethral sphincter in the quiescent phases between voidings. This possibly should be remembered in searching for

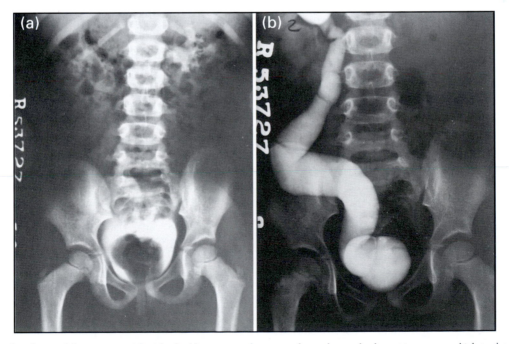

Fig. 22.11 *E.B., female, aged four years, with right double ureter and ureterocele on the urethral ectopic ureter, which prolapsed externally on three occasions.* (**a**) *Filling defect of ureterocele in bladder in the 50-minute intravenous pyeloureterography series.* (**b**) *Micturition cystourethrogram series showing iodide locked in the ectopic ureter and ureterocele by the grasp of the internal sphincter. This radiograph was taken one hour after micturition had emptied the bladder but filled the ureterocele and ureter by reflux. Note that the obstruction to the ureter caused by the internal sphincter was complete during the filling phase of bladder function. (Reprinted, by permission, from Stephens, F.D. (1958), Ureterocele in infants and children. Aust. N.Z. J. Surg. 27: 288, Fig. 3.)*

features predisposing to chronic infection in a given instance of ureteral duplication.

Morphology of urethral ectopic ureters of duplex ureters without ureteroceles

Eleven ectopic ureters that traversed the urethra were available for special studies. Two of their orifices lay in the internal sphincter zone and seven in the external sphincter zone and two upon the hymen. Infection supervening on stasis was the reason for investigation in most of these children, but in seven, wetting was an additional symptom or sign.

These ureters all ran the same submucosal course in the bladder and urethra as has already been described, but did not exhibit ureterocele formation.

Seven of the 11 ureters in the submucosal segments have been removed and have been subjected to further scrutiny. One baby (Baby W.) was stillborn, and provided a valuable specimen of bilateral double ureters with long upper pole ureters (UPUs). It is from this collection of material that some of the conclusions concerning the behaviour of intravesical ureters and of ureteroceles have been reached.

Pathological features of necropsy specimen

The specimen of Baby W. displayed bilateral double kidneys and ureters. The caudal parts of the kidneys had normal calibre ureters, which issued into the bladder at the lateral cornua of the trigone. The cranial parts were drained by ureters that ran a course in relation to the lower pole ureters as shown in Fig. 22.4. These ureters, on entering the ureterovesical hiatus, lay in the submucosal plane of the bladder and urethra and in the bridge in the vestibule between the urethra and vagina; the right ureter opened onto the outer, and the left onto the inner surface of the hymen. The extravesical course of the right UPU was straight and appeared normal in calibre, and the left was enlarged and tortuous. In its intravesical course, the right UPU was not enlarged, but the left formed a conspicuous ridge along the trigone and urethra.

The most pertinent histological features of the specimen relate to the muscular components of the ureters. In the segments distal to the bladder neck, the muscle was absent from the walls, which were composed of fibrous tissue and transitional epithelium. At the internal urethral meatus, muscle fibres first appeared on the floor of the ureter and, as the ureter coursed proximally, more muscle fibres and bundles were added to the floor, then to the side walls, and finally near the cornua of the trigone to the roof (Fig. 22.4b). On the right side, the whole of the extravesical ureter was mainly fibrous with muscle bundles difficult to identify and scattered irregularly. On the left side, the muscle walls were more complete, though the fibrous component was exaggerated.

These long ectopic ureters exhibited dysplastic walls, as indicated by absence or deficiencies of muscle in parts of the walls, and excessive amounts of fibrous tissue. Their renal segments also exhibited parenchymal dysplasia.

Excised intravesical stumps

Seven ureters were excised by the suprapubic route. It was noted at operation that all the submucosal ureters within the bladder were sturdy structures which could be readily handled and dissected. This was in sharp contrast with the majority of ureteroceles, which were flimsy and readily fragmented.

Histological sections revealed that the walls of the ureters in the submucosal coats of the bladder and urethra had the following characteristics:

They were fully muscularized, exhibiting three layers—a middle circular between two longitudinal layers, or they were thick-walled, with some muscle, especially in the floor, and thick fibrous tissue components, or they were composed of fibrous tissue and collagen.

It is apparent from the histology of this newborn specimen and of biopsy specimens that the submucosal ureter, which normally is endowed only with longitudinal muscle fibres, may in the long ectopic ureters be supplied with two or three muscle coats similar to those of the extravesical ureter, or may be partly or completely deficient in muscle, or may have an excessive admixture of fibrous and collagenous tissue or fibrous tissue only (Fig. 24.15).

Bifid ureters: an anatomical, physiological and clinical study*

Some bifid ureters may never cause symptoms and are noted only as incidental findings in life or at routine autopsy examination. Others, however, are clinically important because of associated pyelonephritis. The anatomical and physiological investigations described herein establish reasons that explain why some cause infection while others do not.

Bifid ureters may be of normal calibre, although not uncommonly they show enlargement compared with the normal calibre of the common stem. Both normal and dilated types have been studied; anatomical, histological and radiological examinations were made of the junctional zone and pressure tracings recorded of the ureteral activity, with a view to identifying defects of structure and function. By these means, the existence of inefficient and delayed emptying of the contents of the ureters, predisposing to infection, has been established. A rationale of management based on the findings is outlined in this chapter.

The descriptions that follow apply first to those bifid ureters that join to form a common stem outside the bladder wall, and second to those uncommon forms that join at a Y-junction within the bladder (Fig. 23.1).

The term 'bifid ureter' refers to the congenital anomaly of partial duplication of the ureter. The two ureters from the duplex kidney unite caudally to form a single stem that issues into the bladder by one ureteral orifice.

The junction of the bifid ureters is termed 'extravesical' when it occurs outside and 'intravesical' when it takes place inside the bladder wall (Fig. 23.1). The zone demarcating the junction of the bifid ureters and the common stem is a three-way chamber that models the two ureters into one, and that is called the 'fork', the 'Y-junction' or for brevity, the 'Y'.

The investigation was made on 29 children, 21 girls and eight boys, who provided in all 33 bifid ureters. Eight bifid ureters occurred on the right side, 17 on the

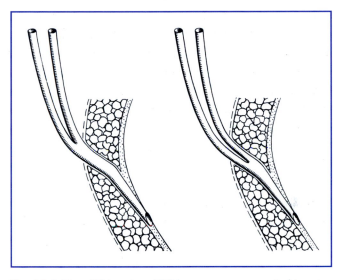

Fig. 23.1 *Site of Y-junction of bifid ureters: an extravesical junction occurring in lower one-third of ureter (left), and the less common intramural junction (right). (Reprinted, by permission, from Lenaghan, D. (1962), Bifid ureters in children: an anatomical, physiological and clinical study. J. Urol. 87: 808, Fig. 1.)*

left, and four were bilateral. Clinical investigations were conducted in 20 patients; in three children, morbid anatomical studies of the bifid ureter specimens supplemented the clinical, and in a further six in whom the anomaly was found incidentally at autopsy, the investigation was of necessity limited to the study of the morbid anatomy.

Bifid ureters with extravesical Y-junctions

The two limbs of a bifid ureter united outside the bladder wall. Their anatomical relations were found to be constant, their calibre varied, the Y-junction varied in size and shape from patient to patient, and other developmental anomalies coexisted. All of these aspects deserve special mention, as they are of significance in the production of stasis in the bifid ureter.

*Reprinted by permission of the Williams and Wilkins Co., from Lenaghan, D. (1962), Bifid ureters in children: an anatomical, physiological, and clinical study. J. Urol. 87: 808.

Levels of junction

The two limbs of the bifid ureter united to form a 'Y' in the extravesical course in 28 instances and in the intravesical course in five. The site of the 'Y' in this series showed a preponderance of junctions in the lower third of the ureteral course, a figure that concurs with the findings of Campbell (1951d). However, in another large series examined by Nation (1944), the site of the junction was uniformly distributed.

The site of the 'Y' is significant in two ways: (1) with respect to the volume of urine contained in the two limbs, and (2) in relation to the technique of surgery used in the management. Both these features are discussed later in this chapter.

Anatomical relations

Usually, the ectopic ureter crossed the orthotopic ureter from medial to lateral sides in its upper portion and recrossed from lateral to medial sides at the lower end; the ectopic ureter lay anterior to the orthotopic ureter at both points of crossing in all specimens (Fig. 22.7; Stephens, 1958). In eight patients, the ureters were uncrossed, the ectopic ureter being medial to the orthotopic ureter throughout its course.

The lower the fork, the more intimately the two ureters became bound together near their caudal ends; it was difficult to separate them by sharp dissection without damaging the walls. When the ureters joined within the wall of the bladder, as was seen in two dissected postmortem specimens, the ectopic ureter lay medial and joined the anteromedial aspect of the orthotopic ureter to form an ultrashort stem.

Surgeons may be faced with dissection of one ureter from another in a bifid system and should be aware of the intimacy of contact in those ureters that join in their lower halves.

Dilatation

Not infrequently, dilatation of some part of the bifid ureters occurred. This additional anomaly is significant because of the proneness to infection it entails.

In 17 instances, the ureters were of normal diameter, but in 12 of the 29, abnormal dilatation was observed. In only two was an organic cause of dilation present. One patient exhibited a stenotic ureterocele, and the other a neuropathic bladder and urethra. In the others,

the dilation was idiopathic and occurred in both limbs of the bifid system cranial to the fork. The three-way junctional chamber served to mould the calibre of the two dilated branches to that of the normal calibre single stem.

The Y-junction

Anatomical studies have revealed considerable variation in size of the Y-junction. The dimensions of the junction were determined by the calibre of the bifid limbs and the position of the crescentic septum formed by their union. Three possible variations of the junction region have been noted.

1. In 11 examples with normal calibre ureters, the Y-junction was a scarcely noticeable dilation (Figs 23.2 and 23.3).
2. The junction was an elongated, enlarged structure in seven instances. The ureters, which were of normal calibre, united to form a common chamber whose lumen was the sum of those of the ureters forming it. Cranially, it was limited by the position of the septum; caudally, the chamber narrowed to the calibre of a single ureter (Fig. 23.2).
3. The Y-junction was grossly enlarged in seven instances. Dilated upper ureters contributed to its formation, and the common chamber was larger than the ureters forming it. At its lower end, it narrowed disproportionately into a common stem (Fig. 23.2).

The existence of a considerable enlargement of the lumen at the junction as described in the two latter types results in the upper ureters communicating widely with each other before draining into the common stem.

In the event of obstruction at the lower end of the ureter, a dilated common stem would be expected. Such an obstruction was not seen in the extravesical junctions studied, but it did occur in one intravesical junction, owing to the presence of a stenotic ureterocele. Ectasia of the common stem, the 'Y' and the bifid ureters may be associated with lateral ectopy of the ureteric orifice and vesicoureteral reflux.

The structure of the chamber, the septum and of the adjoining ureters was examined by microscopy of serial sections of one dilated and two normal calibre specimens. In all, the muscle of the upper ureters was con-

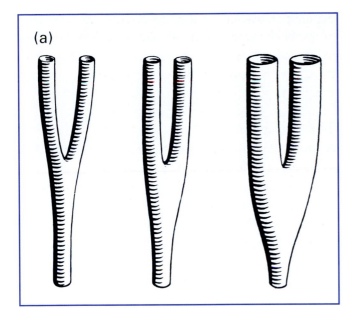

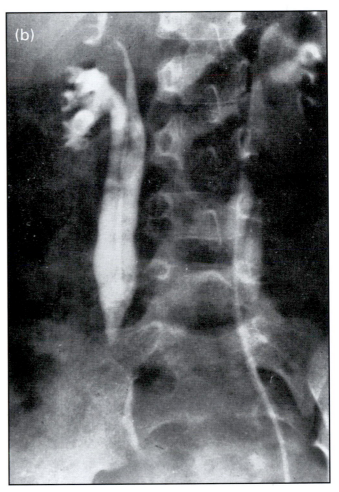

Fig. 23.2 (*a*) *The Y-junction and normal calibre common stem: three variations. (Left) The ureters are of normal calibre and do not form an enlarged union. (Centre) Normal calibre ureters with a dilated junction. (Right) The upper ureters are wide and there is an even larger common chamber. The larger the dimensions of the Y-junction, the greater the shunt of urine from one branch to the other.* (*b*) *Ureterogram of bifid ureter with wide branches; wide-calibre bifid ureters and normal-calibre stem.* ((*a*), (*b*) reprinted, respectively, by permission, from Lenaghan, D. (1962), Bifid ureters in children: an anatomical, physiological and clinical study. J. Urol. 87: 808, Figs 4 and 3.)

tinuous through the junction with that of the stem below. The septum in all three was composed of the separate muscular coats of both ureters down to the distal edge, around which the muscle coats fused with one another.

The Y-junctions exhibited the important anatomical variations noted above and these, together with physiological dysfunction, predisposed to stasis. The stasis was mainly caused by shunting of urine from ureter-to-ureter across the chamber. The larger the calibre of the ureters and the size of the junction, the greater the volume of the shunt.

Associated anomalies and vesicoureteral reflux

The occurrence of other urinary tract anomalies together with duplication has been emphasized by Campbell (1951d) and Gross (1953), both of whom found that the incidence of such anomalies was 15–20 per cent.

In the examples studied, 12 of 29 were associated with other urinary tract anomalies. These mainly involved the ureters and included two instances of the rare blindly ending bifid ureter, which has been described already by Kretschmerm (1933), Harris (1937), Hanley (1945), Culp (1947) and several others (Table 23.1 and Fig. 14.1).

The high incidence of associated anomalies makes it incumbent on the surgeon to demonstrate and examine all parts of the urinary tract in patients with bifid ureters, which in themselves may be only a contributory factor in the whole disease.

Vesicoureteral reflux, either into the stem of the bifid ureter or the opposite single or reduplicated ureter, occurred in more than one-third of the patients investigated for such reflux. Four of the eight patients found to have vesicoureteral reflux also fell into the group of 12 patients with associated structural anomalies. Vesicoureteral reflux is, in its own right, a precursor of

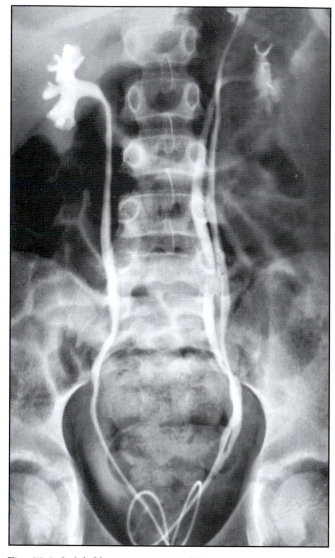

Fig. 23.3 *Left bifid ureter; extravesical Y-junction. Retrograde injection of opaque medium into the ectopic branch outlines both branches and calyceal systems due to ureter-to-ureter reflux. (Reprinted, by permission, from Lenaghan, D. (1962), Bifid ureters in children: an anatomical, physiological and clinical study.* J. Urol. 87: 808, Fig. 7.)

Table 23.1 *Anomalies associated with bifid ureters*

Anomaly	Patients (n)	Percentage of sample
No other anomalies detected	17	58%
Other anomalies detected	12	42%
Renal hypoplasia	1	
Complete double ureters (contralateral side)	4	
Blindly ending bifid ureters	2	
Ureterocele	1	
Hydronephrosis (pelviureteric obstruction)	2	
Myelomeningocele	1	
Ectopia vesicae	1	

Source: Lenaghan, D. (1962), Bifid ureters in children: an anatomical physiological and clinical study. *J. Urol.* 87: 808, Table 2.

was delayed thereby from the normal time of a few to 10 minutes to more than 1 hour. The larger the calibre of the limbs, the longer is the delay in emptying. Campbell (1951d) observed that the two limbs of a bifid ureter can usually be outlined at retrograde ureteropyelography by dye flowing from one branch around the junction to the other. This ureter-to-ureter reflux was noted in six cases with an extravesical junction (Fig. 23.3). Electromanometric pressure recordings of peristaltic activities in the ureter offer explanations for the reflux.

Ureteral peristalsis

Important features in relation to ureter-to-ureter reflux were noticed, namely differential resting pressures in upper and lower ends of the ureters, the timing and direction of propagation of the peristalsis and the possibility of functional obstruction in the common stem.

1. Resting pressures. By placing ureteral catheters in the lower and upper ends of a ureter, respectively, it was found that the resting pressure caudally was usually 2–3 mmHg higher than cranially (Fig. 23.4a). The same finding obtained in bifid ureters, in which the pressure in the stem was higher than that in the limbs. This pressure difference offers resistance to flow along the common stem and facilitates lateral shunting in the fork.

infection because of the stasis it involves. The inclusion of this phenomenon among the list of associated anomalies raises the incidence from 42 to 55 per cent.

Physiology

The physiological action and dysfunction of bifid ureters were studied radiographically, at operation, and by electromanometric recordings of intraluminal pressures.

Observations showed that, around the junction, contrast medium or coloured fluid regurgitated from one limb to the other and that the emptying of the ureter

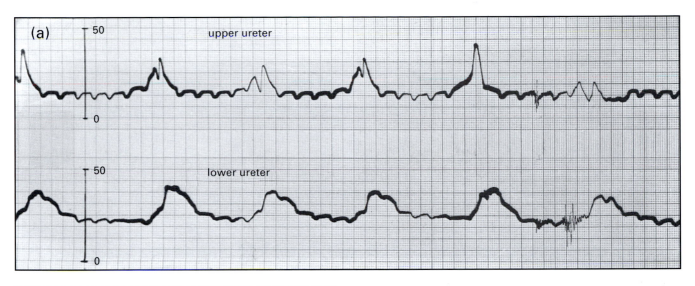

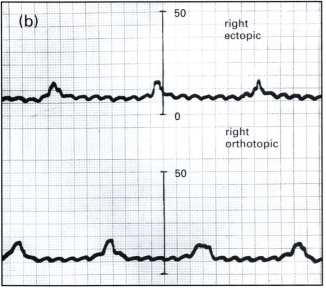

Fig. 23.4 (*a*) *Electromanometric recording in normal ureter. Simultaneous recording from two catheters, one placed 15 cm and the other 5 cm from the ureteral orifice. Pressure range 0–50 mmHg. Horizontal scale of one square equivalent to 2 seconds. Note ureteral resting pressure is 12 mmHg mercury in upper end and 21 mmHg in lower, and ureteral peristaltic waves are clearly shown in both tracings. Bladder was full of fluid during these recordings. (**b**) Electromanometric recording in completely duplicated ureters of normal calibre. Catheters at identical levels in each ureter. Pressure range 0–50 mmHg. Horizontal scale of one square equivalent to 2 seconds. Peristaltic waves occur asynchronously and at slightly different frequencies. (Reprinted, by permission, from Lenaghan, D. (1962), Bifid ureters in children: an anatomical, physiological and clinical study. J. Urol. 87: 808, Figs 8 and 9.)*

2. Timing of peristaltic waves. During surgery and radiography, peristaltic waves were observed to be asynchronous in the two limbs of a bifid ureter. This observation has been made also by electromanometric pressure recordings in completely duplicated ureters. Catheters were introduced into the separate orifices lying side-by-side on the trigone, and simultaneous recordings were obtained from similar levels in both ureters. In three patients, the recordings showed asynchronous peristaltic contractions, except for rare occasions when they were momentarily in phase (Fig. 23.4b).

3. Propagation of peristaltic waves in bifid ureters. Irregularity in the propagation of waves from the bifid ureters to the common stem was noted.

In two patients, catheters were introduced through a cystoscope, one into a limb of a bifid ureter and a second into its common stem to record peristalsis in each simultaneously. The following observations were made.

The nature of the peristaltic wave in the components of the bifid ureter appeared normal. In one patient, some of the peristaltic waves that were recorded in the upper pole branch of the bifid ureter were transmitted to the common stem. Others recorded in the upper pole ureter did not appear in the lower single ureter. Radiographical evidence suggests that these peristaltic waves were propagated in a reverse direction in the second limb of the bifid ureter. Occasionally, a peristaltic contraction was seen in the common stem independently of a contraction in the upper pole ureter. Presumably, such a peristaltic wave originated in the lower pole limb, which did not contain a recording catheter.

In the second patient, all the waves recorded in one upper limb were present also in the common stem. However, the time relationship between the waves was variable (5–9 seconds apart). This variability suggested that the waves were subjected irregularly to delay in their propagation through the junction.

Cineradiography confirmed that reversal of flow from one limb to the other took place. This was actuated by a peristaltic wave, which emptied fluid from one limb into the flaccid adjacent limb. Peristalsis then travelled in a retrograde fashion in the second limb.

Physiological reasons for ureter-to-ureter reflux

There are several physiological reasons for ureter-to-ureter reflux: (1) the resting pressure in the stem is higher than the resting pressures in the upper limbs; (2) the peristaltic waves from one limb are propagated into the other limb rather than down the stem; (3) the asynchronicity of the peristalsis in the upper limb presents a low pressure in one limb at a moment of high pressure in the other; furthermore, the ease and magnitude of the shunt are, to some extent, determined by the anatomical dimensions of the three-way chamber and the calibre of the ureters that join it; (4) the stem may be obstructed.

The free ebb and flow of fluid from limb to limb through the 'Y' in preference to the onward movement down the ureter implies an obstruction. To evaluate this hypothesis, certain observations were made on ureteral calibre and peristalsis.

In several bifid ureters of normal calibre, despite the presence of reflux from limb to limb and delayed emptying, no dilation has developed. If obstruction were the cause of such reflux, one would expect some ureterectasis. Its absence renders unlikely obstruction in the stem.

In the bifid ureters with dilated upper components and junction regions, obstruction seems more apparent. However, electromanometric recordings showed normal peristaltic waves in the stem of the ureter from its origin to the vesical orifice. This suggests that there is no functional disturbance in such ureters. Furthermore, observations have been made on the activity and calibre of the ureter after surgical excision of the upper pole limb in three patients. Peristalsis was found to be conducted uniformly along the whole length of the ureter, and no enlargement has taken place in the remaining ureter.

The bifid ureter of a girl aged seven years was studied at operation. Electromanometric pressure recordings were made simultaneously from both limbs of the bifid ureter and the common stem. In this way, the origin and course of every peristaltic wave could be seen and recorded. It was noted that contractions in one limb were often conducted around the limb of the Y-junction to the other limb, and not down the common stem. There was a greater number of peristaltic contractions in the upper ureters than in the common stem. When one limb was occluded by means of a bulldog clip placed close to the bifurcation, it was observed that all peristaltic contraction waves from the other limb of the ureter proceeded without interruption down the ureter and along the common stem. This showed that if the shunt was occluded, peristalsis in the remaining components was normal. This phenomenon is further evidence that excision of one limb of the bifid system, when indicated, is a suitable form of treatment.

From these facts, it seems that ureter-to-ureter reflux is induced for reasons other than obstruction of the common stem, but when the dimensions of the fork and limbs are enlarged in comparison with that of the stem, a peristaltic aberration exists that favours branch-to-branch reflux and stasis.

Bifid ureters with intravesical Y-junctions

Radiological investigations revealed one highly significant feature distinctive of the bifid ureter that unites within the walls of the bladder: in two thoroughly investigated patients, whose bifid ureters so united, there was no demonstrable ureter-to-ureter reflux. This feature is significant both in diagnosis and treatment.

Retrograde ureterography displays the exact site of junction satisfactorily in the extravesical junction by taking advantage of ureter-to-ureter reflux (Fig. 23.3). In intravesical junctions, such reflux does not occur and, therefore, this method of ureterography will not display both limbs. It is rarely possible to pass ureteral catheters into both parts of the bifid ureter, as the catheter glides freely into one limb only and may not be manoeuvred into the other. It may be possible to outline the 'Y' of bifid ureters with an intramural junction by injecting contrast medium through a bulb-tipped or cut-off catheter placed in the ureteral orifice. If however, the common stem and orifice are incompetent, the 'Y' can be seen radiographically by reflux of contrast medium (Fig. 23.5). It would be anticipated that in the absence of demonstrable vesicoureteral reflux, infection would be unlikely to occur. One of the two children, the limbs of whose bifid ureters united intramurally, had recurrent cystitis presumably unrelated to the bifid system.

In addition to these two patients, there was one who exhibited a simple stenotic ureterocele on the single stem of a bifid system and one postmortem specimen that was available for dissection and microscopy.

Serial microscopic sections of the intravesical junction were examined. Both longitudinal and circular muscle fibres were seen in the fused edge of the septum. In the single ureter below this point, the muscle coat was longitudinally arranged, as is normal for the intravesical ureter. The length of the common stem determined by compilation of the serial sections of known thickness was 4.5 mm.

The following reasons for the absence of ureter-to-ureter reflux in this type of junction are: (1) the short length of the common stem; (2) the effect on the walls of the ureter of the surrounding bladder muscle; and (3) the presence of longitudinal muscle fibres only in this part of the ureter.

The special longitudinal arrangement of the muscle coat in the intravesical ureter is associated with a distinctive mode of action (Stephens and Lenaghan, 1961). The peristaltic waves recorded in this portion of the ureter are of low amplitude and altered from the same waves recorded higher in the ureter. The submucosal ureter is immobile during the efflux of urine from its orifice and only retracts after the urine has been expelled. It is proposed that the low pressure in the common stem and the passive role played by the intramural ureter explain why urine escapes along the short common stem in preference to the other limb of the bifid system.

If the submucosal segment of the stem is abnormally short or wide or lacks muscle, vesicoureteral reflux will occur into both ureters, and the intramural 'Y' can then be demonstrated by cystoureterography (Fig. 23.5).

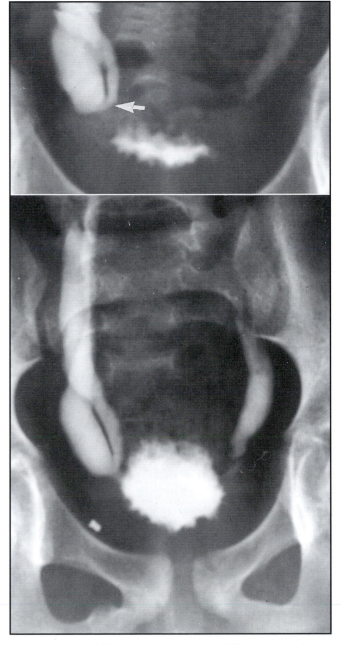

Fig. 23.5 *Right bifid ureter with intramural Y-junction and vesicoureteral reflux; intramural junction demonstrated by reflux of contrast medium. Note nipping of both ureters at the vesical hiatus when bladder is temporarily contracting at the end of micturition (arrow, top). (Reprinted, by permission, from Lenaghan, D. (1962), Bifid ureters in children: an anatomical, physiological and clinical study. J. Urol. 87: 808, Fig. 6.)*

Principles of management of bifid ureters

Treatment is aimed at the elimination of factors causing stasis. The amount of stasis depends on the amount of ureteroureteral reflux. Slight reflux such as is found in normal calibre ureters with the junction in the upper one-third is unlikely to lead to serious infections. Dilated ureters and junctions situated in the lower portions of the ureter are prone to induce greater stasis and episodes of infection.

Occasional or mild infection requires only chemotherapy to control isolated attacks, but more frequent episodes necessitate surgical treatment designed to eliminate stasis caused by the ureteroureteral reflux. When both parts of the duplex kidney are healthy, anastomosis of the ectopic ureter to the orthotopic pelvis or ureter together with excision of the remainder of the ectopic ureter is the treatment of choice (Gibson, 1957; Sandegard, 1958; Ratner et al., 1961). Excision of one of the limbs of the bifid ureter and its corresponding renal segment is indicated if one part of the kidney or ureter is impaired beyond repair.

Abdominal pain

In this series, three patients presented with abdominal pain, and, in the course of searching investigations, bifid ureters were noted. The pains were cyclical and occurred with no definite evidence of infection, stone formation, ureterectasis, or kidney disease, apart from this one malformation. The cause of the pain was a mystery, but there was some evidence in these children to suggest that the pain originated as crises of abdominal migraine or recurrent intestinal colic of children for whom appropriate medical treatment resulted in alleviation of symptoms.

Recurrent abdominal pain associated with bifid or double ureters has been attributed to ureteric colic. In the absence of infection, calculus, or other anomalies, the pain is more likely to be extraurinary in origin. It is unlikely that ureteral crossings of normal calibre ureters cause symptoms, as there is no evidence of obstruction or constriction at these sites.

Colosimo (1938), Dees (1941) and Gutierrez (1944) believe that malcoordinated peristalsis causes pain. In our patients, all of whom have been shown to exhibit ureter-to-ureter reflux around the 'Y', pains have occurred irregularly and do not constantly accompany the reversal of flow. It is possible that hyperdiuresis producing increased peristalsis and an overfull bifid system may result in attacks of pain, but it seems that pain is unlikely to arise in bifid ureters unless some additional malformation or complication can be demonstrated.

Ureteroceles on duplex ureters

Ureterocele is a well-defined entity associated with the upper pole ureter of duplex ureters or, more rarely, a single ureter in children. It may be discovered in the course of a search of the urinary tract for the cause of urinary tract infection, or, in the female, it may effect a dramatic entrance to the clinical stage by presenting as a red, fleshy mass at the urethral orifice.

'Ureterocele' is the term applied to the ballooning of the ureter in its course in the submucosal layer of the base of the bladder. The ureterocele is located on the upper pole ureter (UPU) of the duplex system, rarely on the common stem of a bifid ureter, and very rarely on the lower pole ureter (LPU).

Classification

In preference to the more complete and complex classifications of Gross and Clatworthy (1950), Campbell (1951e), the anatomical classification of Ericsson (1954a) and the groupings according to the clinical evidence of ureteral and urethral obstruction as advocated by Uson (1961), ureteroceles are classified here by the following morphological types: stenotic, sphincteric, sphincterostenotic, blind, cecoureterocele and non-obstructive (Fig. 24.1). An analysis of 60 such ureteroceles showed 25 stenotic (including six bilateral) ureteroceles, 21 sphincteric, four sphincterostenotic, three blind, three non-obstructive, three cecoureteroceles and one not classified (Stephens, 1971; Friedland and Cunningham, 1972).

Stenotic ureterocele

The stenotic ureterocele has its narrow orifice within the bladder and has similar qualities to those on single ureters (Chapter 16).

Sphincteric ureterocele

In sphincteric ureteroceles, the ureter has a wide, long and sometimes sinuous course in the submucous layer of the bladder. In the urethra, the ureter usually becomes

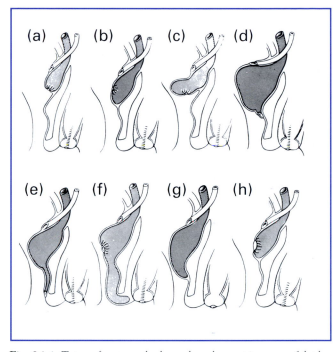

Fig. 24.1 Types of ureteroceles located on the ectopic ureter of duplex systems, showing also the anatomical relation of the expansion to the orifice. (**a**), (**b**), (**c**) Stenotic ureteroceles: terminal expansions with orifice raised off the trigone (**a**), perched on the dome (**b**) and underhung (**c**). (**d**), (**e**) Sphincteric ureteroceles: subterminal expansion, with the orifice, large or small, resting on the posterior wall of the urethra. (**f**) Cecoureterocele: terminal expansion with long drawn-out caudal extension forming a 'cecum' in the submucosal plane of the urethra. (**g**) Blind ureterocele: subterminal expansion with atrophy of the ureter distal to the ureterocele. (**h**) Non-obstructed ureterocele: terminal expansion with large orifice lying within the confines of the bladder. (Reprinted, by permission, from Stephens, F.D. (1971), Cecoureterocele and concepts on the embryology and aetiology of ureteroceles. Aust. N.Z. J. Surg. 40: 239, Fig. 1.)

near normal in calibre, but may continue to its orifice at some point in the urethra as a dilated prolongation of the ureterocele (Fig. 24.1e; see also Fig. 24.7).

In the analysis of 60 specimens, ureterocele formation was much more common when the ureter terminated within, rather than beyond, the internal sphincter zone of the urethra. Of the 19 ureters that terminated in this zone, 17 exhibited ureterocele formation, whereas of the nine ureters that terminated in the external sphincter zone and perineum, only two displayed ureterocele formation. This form of ureterocele is usually large and sometimes nearly fills the bladder. Its shape may be globular or lobulated, or the dilation may be elongated with tortuosities folded one upon the other in the intravesical segment. Contrasting with the lateral position of the stenotic type, the sphincteric ureterocele is more often located both laterally and centrally in the base of the bladder.

The orifice is situated posteriorly in the urethra, and is not usually obstructive; on the contrary, the orifice in 13 patients was larger than normal. When the orifice lay in the internal sphincter zone, it was compressed by the internal sphincter muscle of the urethra in the resting periods of bladder inactivity. With the relaxation of the sphincter during micturition, the orifice became

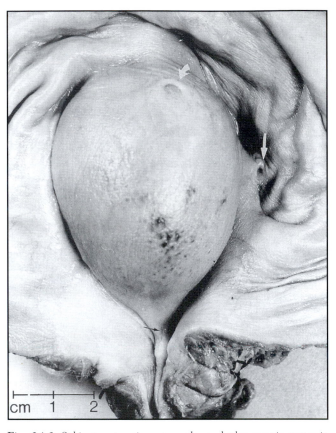

Fig. 24.3 *Sphincterostenotic ureterocele on duplex ectopic ureter in male, aged 12 years. Dome expands and undermines right hemitrigone and minute orifice lies in urethra 3 mm cranial to verumontanum (small black arrow). Right orthotopic orifice (curved arrow) raised upon ectopic ureterocele. Left single orifice is tucked back on left hemitrigone (white arrow). Black arrow denotes a longitudinal crease in which ectopic orifice is located. (Reprinted, by permission, from Stephens, F.D. (1983), Congenital Malformations of the Urinary Tract, New York, Prager, Fig. 21.3, p. 337.)*

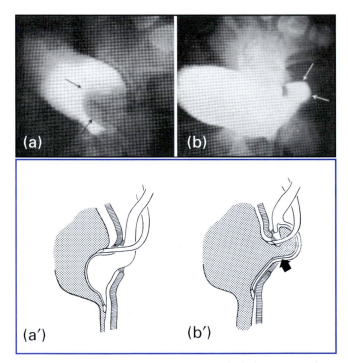

Fig. 24.2 *Intra-extravesical ectopic ureterocele (sphincteric type), in female, aged 1½ years. (a) Cystogram with filling defect in the bladder base (black arrows) and reflux into the orthotopic ureter. (b) During voiding, the convex intravesical wall herniates backwards through a large hiatus and muscle gap in the bladder base (white arrows). (a'), (b') Presumed anatomic arrangement of ureterocele and ureters in relation to the hiatus and urethra in response to reservoir and voiding bladder pressures (black arrow depicts lumen of compressed empty ureterocele). (Reprinted, by permission, from Stephens, F.D. (1963), Congenital Malformations of the Rectum, Anus and Genito-Urinary Tracts. Edinburgh, Livingstone, Fig. 92, p. 182.)*

unblocked and the urine passed without let or hindrance. This observation was also made by Ericsson (1954b) who considered, however, that the chances of emptying the ureterocele were limited.

The sphincteric ureteroceles expand to retain the urine excreted by the corresponding kidney. When voiding starts, some ureteroceles contract, expel their content, and assume the shape and size of a ureter and form a ridge beneath the trigonal mucous membrane of the base of the bladder. Others are less contractile and, on emptying, merely flatten and become invisible, or may be pressed posteriorly through an abnormally wide hiatus that extends toward the bladder neck or urethra (Fig. 24.2).

Sphincterostenotic ureterocele

The orifice of the ureter is concealed in a sphinc-terostenotic ureterocele because of its small calibre. The narrow orifice is still further obstructed by the internal sphincter. The ureterocele remains distended and effect-ively obstructs the vesical outlet (Fig. 24.3).

Blind ureterocele

In blind ureteroceles, the expanded intravesical ureter swells over the trigone and beyond into the bladder neck and lacks an orifice into the bladder or urethra. These 246 ureteroceles in the series plugged and severely obstructed the urethra (Fig. 24.4).

Cecoureterocele

The cecoureterocele expands beneath the mucosal layer of the trigone and urethra, creating a dome-like protru-sion into the lumen of bladder and urethra. The lumen of the ureterocele extends beyond its orifice as a long tongue or cecum in the urethral submucosal layer (Figs 24.5, 24.6 and 24.7). The tongue may reach the level of the external urinary meatus. The orifice may be located on the dome in the bladder or urethra and be large, permitting free to-and-fro movement of urine in and out of the ureterocele. During voiding, the tongue of the ureterocele between the mucosal and muscle layers of the urethra fills by reflux and compresses the urethral lumen. If the orifice of the ureterocele is small, the ureterocele with its caudal tongue fills by urine from its own kidney segment and, when full, partially obstructs the urethra.

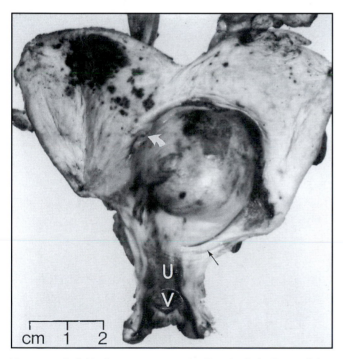

Fig. 24.4 *Left blind ectopic ureterocele. Female, Baby P., aged four weeks. Ureterocele undermines trigone and encroaches into bladder neck causing retention. Left orthotopic orifice not visible; right orifice set back on cornu of trigone (white arrow); V = vaginal orifice; U = urethra; black arrow denotes expanded bladder neck). (Reprinted, by permission, from Stephens, F.D. (1963), Congenital Malformations of the Rectum, Anus and Genito-Urinary Tracts. Edinburgh, Livingstone, Fig. 93, p. 183.)*

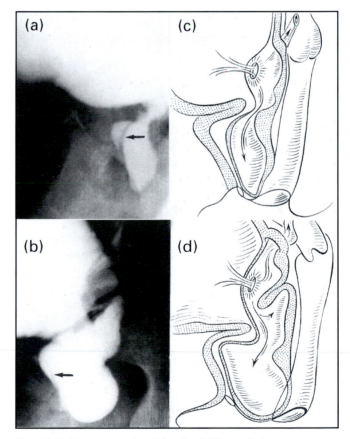

Fig. 24.5 *Cecoureterocele of female, S.W., aged three years: mic-turition cystourethrogram, showing opaque medium filling the tongue of the cecoureterocele and compressing the urethra (arrows), early (a) and late (b) during efforts to void. Diagrammatic drawings on the right show the manner in which the opaque medium regurgitated through the large orifice of the ureterocele from the bladder and thence into the tongue and the ureter at early (c) and late (d) stages. (Reprinted, by permission, from Stephens, F.D. (1971), Cecoureterocele and concepts on the embryology and aetiology of ureteroceles. Aust. N.Z. J. Surg. 40: 239, Fig. 2.)*

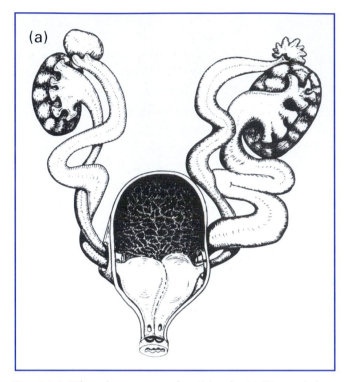

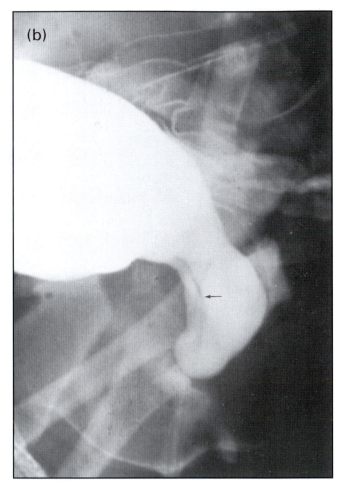

Fig. 24.6 *Bilateral cecoureteroceles of female, N.W., aged three months. (**a**) The large ureteral orifices are located in mid-urethra (composite diagram drawn from cystoscopic radiographic and operative findings). (**b**) Voiding cystourethrogram of same patient showing cecoceles filled with contrast medium and obliterating urethral lumen. The linear filling defect (arrow) was caused by overlapping walls of the cecoceles. (Reprinted, by permission, from Stephens, F.D. (1983), Congenital Malformations of the Urinary Tract, New York, Praeger, Fig. 21.6, p. 339.)*

Non-obstructed ureterocele

The non-obstructed type of ureterocele lies entirely within the bladder, its orifice is large, permitting to-and-fro movement of urine, and its walls are crenated from lack of distention (Fig. 24.7). Cecoureteroceles and non-obstructed ureteroceles each comprise 5 per cent of the total.

Variant of sphincteric ureterocele

Some ectopic megaureters enter the bladder at the hiatus in company with the orthotopic ureter and run caudally in the submucosal plane to issue into the urethra or beyond without forming a ureterocele (Fig. 22.4). Others exhibit tortuosities in the bladder base, which, when superimposed, give the appearance radiographically of a ureterocele (Fig. 24.8). This tortuosity which was included in the sphincteric category of ureteroceles was termed the 'seventh radiologic type' by Friedland and Cunningham (1972) and was challenged by Cumes *et al.* (1981) as mas-

querading as a ureterocele. Other ureters expand as a ureterocele in the bladder but abruptly change to ureter dimensions in the urethra (Fig. 24.1e), and yet others maintain the expansion of the ureterocele throughout their course in the urethra (Fig. 24.7).

Effects on urethra, ureter, hiatus and bladder base of urethral obstruction by the ureterocele

The simple sessile ureterocele is usually small, laterally situated and non-obstructive to the urethra. Rarely, the ureterocele is polypoid whence prolapse and plugging of the urethra may occur. When large, tense and located close to the internal meatus, as with the ectopic ureter of a duplex system, it may lean into and partially obstruct the bladder outlet.

The sphincteric ureterocele is large and often may nearly fill the bladder. It lies over the internal urethral

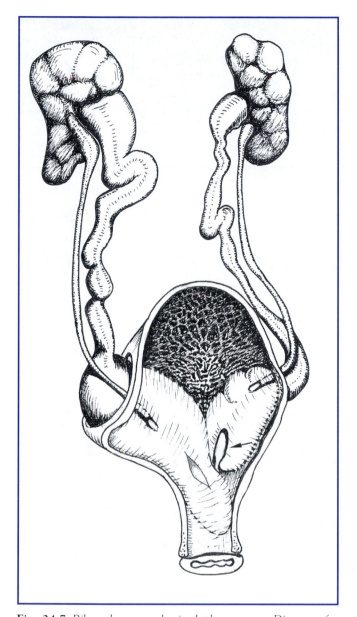

Fig. 24.7 *Bilateral ureteroceles in duplex systems. Diagram of a specimen of the urinary tract from a newborn, Baby M., showing the left non-obstructive ureterocele with elongate orifice in the bladder (arrow) and the right cecoureterocele with large orifice in bladder neck and submucosal cecal extension along the urethra. Note the wide hiatus and extravesical extension of the ureterocele on the right side. (Reprinted, by permission, from Stephens, F.D. (1983), Congenital Malformations of the Urinary Tract,* New York, Praeger, *1983, Fig. 21.7, p. 340.)*

orifice only when the ureterocele is distended, and synchronously with relaxation of the internal sphincter at the beginning of micturition, the wide orifice of the ureterocele is unblocked. Both bladder and ureterocele then empty together, unimpeded by any obstruction to either.

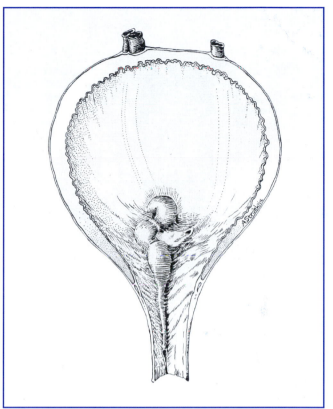

Fig. 24.8 *Right ectopic ureter of a duplex system of female C.W., aged four months, with tortuosities that, when superimposed, give an appearance radiographically of a ureterocele. (Reprinted, by permission, from Stephens, F.D. (1963), Congenital Malformations of the Rectum, Anus and Genito-Urinary Tracts. Edinburgh, Livingstone, Fig. 100, p. 191.)*

The most dangerous ureteroceles are the sphincterostenotic type, in which the stenosis is extreme, and the blind ureterocele, which encroaches on the urethra. The continuously distended ureterocele plugs the bladder outlet and so causes retention of urine and general impairment of kidney function, in addition to extreme damage to the corresponding kidney segment. The less severely stenosed orifices permit a degree of emptying on voiding and a correspondingly reduced urethral blockage.

Prolapse of the ureterocele may occur from the bladder into the urethra and cause obstruction for the duration of prolapse. It seems that factors conducive to maintaining distention of the ureterocele during voiding, together with the intrinsic encroachment of the ectopic ureter into the urethra, promote prolapse. These factors are: (1), refilling from below during voiding–urethroureteral reflux (Fig. 22.11); (2), retention because of stenosis of the orifice; (3), rapid refilling of the ureterocele from above

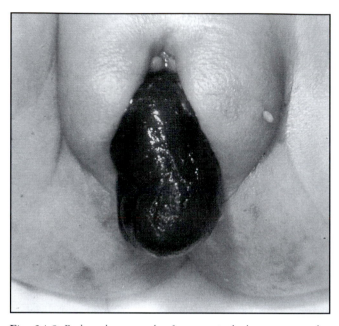

Fig. 24.9 *Prolapsed ureterocele of an ectopic duplex ureter together with a caudal slide of the trigone and other ureters into the bladder neck and urethra. (Reprinted, by permission, from Klauber, G. and Crawford, B. (1980), Prolapse of ectopic ureterocele and bladder trigone. Urology 15: 164, Fig. 1.)*

by peristalsis of the enlarged full ureter; (4), polypoid nature of the ureterocele (Fig. 16.3). It seems that some ureteroceles have a loose attachment to the trigone, making it possible for the ureterocele and the overlying urethrotrigonal mucosa to slide through the urethra occasionally, dragging the LPU orifice caudally with them (Fig. 24.9).

In the female, the prolapsed ureterocele appears suddenly as a red or black fleshy mass protruding from the external urethral orifice and receives early treatment. It may retract back into the bladder spontaneously or remain prolapsed (Fig. 24.9). Klauber and Crawford (1980) identified the nature of the fleshy mass, first by aspiration of urine and then injection of contrast medium displaying a free connection with the UPU more cranially. Other structures that may share some of the features of a prolapsed ureterocele are urethral cysts, bulging imperforate hymen with hydrocolpos, prolapse of Gartner's duct cyst or sarcoma botryoides.

In the male, prolapse or partial prolapse is occult and symptomless *per se* and may be identified late either

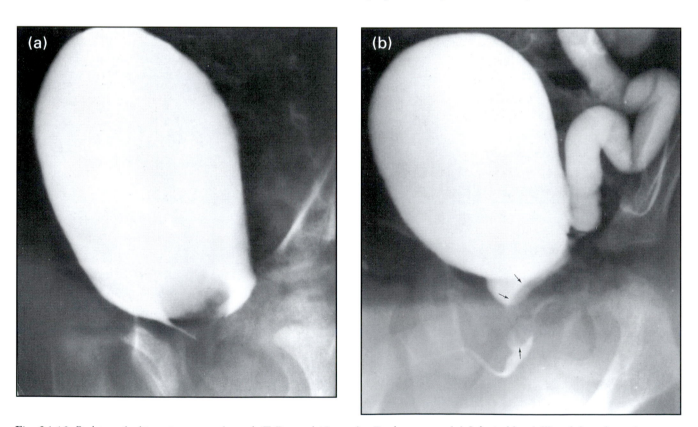

Fig. 24.10 *Prolapse of sphincteric ureterocele, male T.R., aged 19 months. Duplex ureters. (a) Spherical basal filling defect of ectopic ureterocele. (b) During voiding, dome of the ureterocele (arrows) prolapses into and plugs the urethra: reflux into lower pole ureter. (Reprinted, by permission, from Stephens, F.D. (1963), Congenital Malformations of the Rectum, Anus and Genito-Urinary Tracts. Edinburgh, Livingstone, Fig. 94, p. 184.)*

endoscopically or radiographically as a filling defect in the posterior urethra on micturition cystourethrography (Fig. 24.10). Reduction of the prolapse relieves the obstruction, though recurrence is likely. Insidious renal impairment ensues in the undiagnosed and untreated occult type.

The cecoureterocele obstructs the urethra in the manner previously described (Fig. 24.5). The cecal tongue is submucosal and, when distended, encroaches on and may obliterate the lumen of the urethra. It is a developmental anomaly, which is very different from intraluminal prolapse of the other types of ureterocele.

Ureter obstruction

Obstruction of ipsilateral lower pole ureter (LPU) in the duplex system

The actual course of the ectopic ureter within the walls of the bladder may be conducive to obstruction of the LPU. The UPU traverses the muscular wall of the bladder through a tunnel in common with, but posterior to, the LPU and orifice, lying in the submucous plane between this orifice and the muscle wall of the bladder (Fig. 24.11). The UPU and ureterocele, when turgid, compress the LPU orifice and the adjoining ureter in the tunnel. The orifice may become tilted and raised on the wall of the distended ureterocele. The ultimate effects are ureterocaliectasis and renal impairment from obstruction of the LPU, both of which may improve after decompression of the ureterocele.

Vesicoureteral reflux in the ipsilateral LPU occurs when the orifice is lateral, or when the submucosal ureter is short or lacks muscle or is distorted by the ureterocele. The flattened orifice raised on the wall of a tense ureterocele may not admit reflux but is incompetent when the ureterocele is empty. When the orifice is normally placed, it lies back and implanted on the trigone and remains competent. Reflux resulting from moderate lateral ectopy of the LPU or from distortion of the orifice may recover after heminephrectomy, but those with very short or absent or amuscular submucosal segments may persist indefinitely.

Obstruction of the contralateral ureter

The fundus of a large ureterocele may overlap the midline, but because of the septum between the two halves of the trigone, it rarely invades or obstructs the

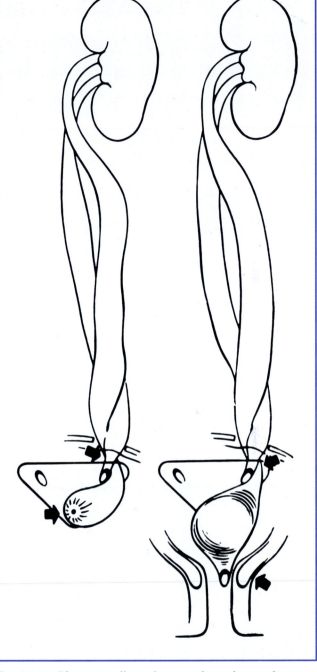

Fig. 24.11 Obstructive effects of ureteroceles on lower pole component of duplex ureters. (Left) Stenotic ureterocele compresses lower pole ureter in the hiatus. (Right) Giant ectopic ureterocele obstructed by the urethral sphincter (lower arrow) may compress both the orthotopic orifice and ureter in the bladder and hiatus respectively (upper arrow). (Reprinted, by permission, from Stephens, F.D. (1958), Ureterocele in infants and children. Aust. N.Z. J. Surg. 27: 288, Fig. 1.)

contralateral single ureteral meatus. Dilation of this ureter may be secondary to bladder-outlet obstruction caused by some ureteroceles, or may be a feature not of obstruction but of primary reflux.

Effect on the ipsilateral hiatus and bladder base

Defects in the musculature of the bladder base

Some ureteroceles are both intra- and extravesical, and the hiatus is correspondingly wide, as shown in a

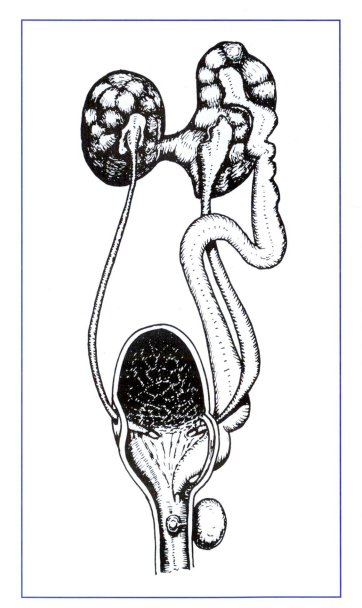

Fig. 24.12 *Intra-extravesical ectopic ureterocele of newborn male; diagram of specimen showing intra-extravesical ureterocele with wide hiatus and defective backing; eversion of the intravesical component through the muscular defect of the bladder base. Also present is a cyst of the utriculus masculinus, left duplex system and horseshoe kidney. (Reprinted, by permission, from Stephens, F.D. (1983), Congenital Malformations of the Urinary Tract, New York, Praeger, Fig. 21.12, p. 343.)*

newborn-male specimen (Fig. 24.12). The wide hiatus and long muscle defect in the gutter on the bladder base permit the ureterocele to evert posteriorly during voiding.

In another specimen from a newborn female, Baby M., with bilateral duplex systems (Fig. 24.7), the UPUs exhibited giant amuscular ureteroceles, the right being a cecoureterocele and the left a sphincteric type. The right hiatus was extremely large, accommodating the cranial extension of the ureterocele. The smooth muscle of the bladder base, internal sphincter and urethra was sparse underlying the floor of the amuscular ureterocele, and the voluntary muscle in the posterior quadrants of the urethra was totally deficient. It is likely in such circumstances that urinary continence would be impaired because of the defects in the sphincters. After excision of the ureterocele, it is necessary to bring together the stronger muscle from each side, thus restoring the sphincter complex of the trigone and bladder neck.

The everting ureterocele

When the hiatus is wide and the walls of the ureterocele are flaccid, the ureterocele may evert into its extravesical extension under the high pressure of voiding (Fig. 24.2). The tethering of the ureterocele at its orifice in the urethra and at some points in the circumference of the hiatus provides counterpressure and restraint on the extent of the eversion.

Koyanagi *et al.* (1980) studied the manner in which ureteroceles become everted extravesically by precise correlation of the alterations in shape and position of the ureterocele by both radiographical and endoscopic techniques. They demonstrated that eight of 24 ureteroceles everted into an extravesical position during the voiding phase of cystourethrography. The radiographic appearances of an everted ureterocele may resemble those of a paraureteral diverticulum, and endoscopy is required to differentiate the two conditions and to define the manner of eversion. Cystoscopic and endoureteral studies showed that the roof of the ureterocele, when subjected to increasing intravesical pressure, either 'refluxed' through a wide orifice into the lumen of the ureter (Type 1 eversion) or diverted along the craniolateral side of the ureter (Type 2, Fig 24.2). They claim that an abnormally wide hiatus is a prerequisite and integral component of the everting ureteroceles.

Radiological and cystoscopic clues to management of ureteroceles

Urinary infection, uraemia with failure to thrive, urethral obstruction with voiding difficulties, or sudden prolapse of the ureterocele at the external meatus bring the child with a ureterocele for examination.

Radiological investigation

The type and special properties of a ureterocele are elucidated in the course of comprehensive, routine urinary tract investigation. This includes examinations of urine, ultrasonography, micturition cystourethrography and intravenous pyelography when indicated. The image intensifier has been of great value in studying the dynamics and emptying of ureteroceles. In some, the type of ureterocele was diagnosed at cystoscopy and others only by surprise on direct examination at the time of suprapubic cystostomy.

The cystogram may show a large, rounded filling defect of the ureterocele distended by its non-opaque urine content at the bladder base. On fluoroscopy during voiding, the filling defect may remain unchanged if its orifice is stenotic, or disappear if its orifice is wide, as with sphincteric types. The ureterocele may prolapse into the urethra (Fig. 24.10) or fill with radiopaque medium by reflux (Fig. 22.11), or evert posteriorly, indicating a defect in the muscle backing on the bladder base (Fig. 24.2).

The intravenous pyeloureterogram depicts the renal segments of the kidneys. Characteristically, the upper segment is hydronephrotic with poor or inconspicuous function and together with its large ureter may displace the lower renal segment laterally and caudally (Fig. 24.13) sometimes creating the 'drooping lily' appearance of the calyces. The dilated upper pole calyx and ureter may become radiopaque, but usually late in the series of films, and the lower pole segment may show normal or reduced number of calyces or ureterocaliectasis. The LPU may be displaced or, if dilated, scalloped by the intertwining of the tortuous, tense radiolucent upper pole megaureter. Rarely, the UPU may end blindly in contact with the upper pole of the lower kidney.

In infants, the upper tracts on both sides are governed in their renal morphology primarily by the position of the orifice, but obstruction and infection may also complicate the radiological interpretations (Fig. 24.14).

Cystoscopy

Cystoscopy is important in determining the type and guiding the management of the ectopic ureterocele; the location and size of the orifices, and the dynamics of the ureterocele, serve as guides in management. If the ureterocele can be seen to contract actively and change its shape to that of a ureter lying invisible beneath the trigonal mucosa, surgical transposition of the orifice from urethra to trigone by minimal de-roofing, using the resectoscope for the purpose, is appropriate. This manoeuvre corrects the ureteral obstruction, cures the ureterocele and permits the ureteral musculature to maintain competence.

When the ureterocele on prolonged cystoscopic observation fails to show contractility but merely collapses, resection of the roof would exaggerate reflux, so

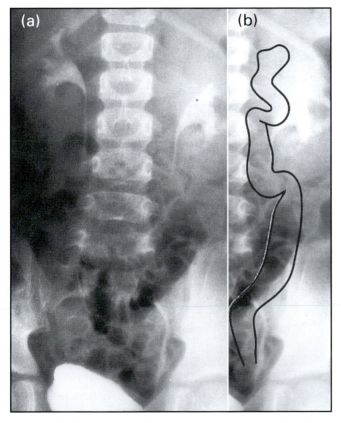

Fig. 24.13 *Displaced orthotopic component of left double kidney.* (**a**) *The upper pole and adjoining dilated urethral ectopic ureter displaced the lower pole caudally and laterally. Note lack of a minor calyx in pelvicalyceal system of orthotopic kidney compared with left pyelogram and curve in lower pole ureter caused by intertwining with the dilated ectopic ureter.* (**b**) *Overprint of ectopic ureter drawn from retrograde pyeloureterogram.* (*Reprinted, by permission, from Stephens, F.D. (1983),* Congenital Malformations of the Urinary Tract, *New York, Praeger, Fig. 21.13, p. 344.*)

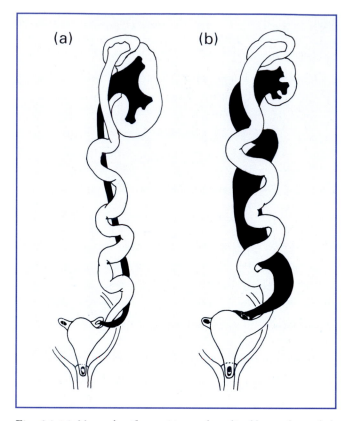

Fig. 24.14 *Ureteral orifice position and predictable renal morphology. (**a**) Lower-pole ureteric orifice in A position and kidney structure normal; ectopic ureterocele orifice in G position and kidney hypodysplastic. (**b**) Lower-pole ureteric orifice in C position and kidney segment hypoplastic; orifice of ectopic ureter in G position and kidney segment hypodysplastic. (Reprinted, by permission, from Stephens, F.D. (1979c), Bifid and double ureters, ureteroceles and fused kidneys, in Pediatric Surgery, 3rd edn, M.M. Ravitch et al. (eds). Chicago, Year Book, Fig. 108.6A,B, p. 1191.)*

resection alone is not adequate treatment in this situation, though together with catheter drainage of the bladder, it may serve to tide over an obstructive and infective crisis.

The renal segments of most ectopic ureteroceles are hypodysplastic and should usually be removed, together with the attached ureter, unless total renal function is so depleted that preservation of even a few nephrons in this poorly functioning segment is important.

Morphology

Cystoscopic examination of giant ureterocele gives evidence that some have the capacity to change shape under observation from a large, cystic swelling to a tubular ureter, and others are inert, merely collapsing the roof upon the floor. The writhing peristaltic activity of the former suggests healthy muscularization in the

submucosal ureter, whereas, in the latter, the walls are non-contractile and respond to intravesical pressures. Studies conducted on biopsy and necropsy specimens of ureteroceles confirm these *in vivo* obstructions.

The structure of the simple ureterocele upon the double system is similar to that upon the single ureter— some have full muscle coats with hypertrophy of muscle, and others exhibit varying degrees of muscle deficit more marked around the orifice and distal part of the ureterocele.

The remaining types of intravesical ureterocele and the less expanded urethral extension to the ectopic orifice showed a haphazard range of muscularization (Fig. 24.15):

1. Muscle throughout aligned in two or three layers equipping the structure for peristaltic activity as in ureterocele in Fig. 24.3.
2. Deficiency of the muscle distally (Fig. 24.16), and delicate attenuated muscle coats toward the vesical hiatus and in between some muscle in the floor. The walls were thick in some amuscular areas that were composed of collagen chiefly and some fibrocytes.
3. Deficiency of muscle throughout the ureterocele and extending into the juxtavesical ureter or even more cranially. In some hypomuscular ureteroceles, muscle strands could be seen in the floor, building up into thick bundles in the more cranial part of the uretero- cele toward the hiatus. In some amuscular areas, the epithelial linings of the bladder and ureterocele co- apted and lacked supporting tissue. These areas appeared macroscopically as bluish transparent blis- ters on the distended ureterocele.

The above findings are compatible with defects in the differentiation of the mesenchyme into smooth muscle resulting in hypoplasia or aplasia of myoblasts and excess of fibrocytes and collagen. Light and electron- microscopic examinations of ureteroceles by Tokunake *et al.* (1981) revealed absence of muscle in the roof of the majority of ureteroceles irrespective of type. Muscle cells, when present, were small. They contained only thin (actin) myofilaments and lacked the thick myosin myofilaments; the nexuses were attenuated. These authors considered that the myoblasts in the ureterocele were deficient in myosin and that the defective myogen- esis resulted in ballooning and ureterocele formation.

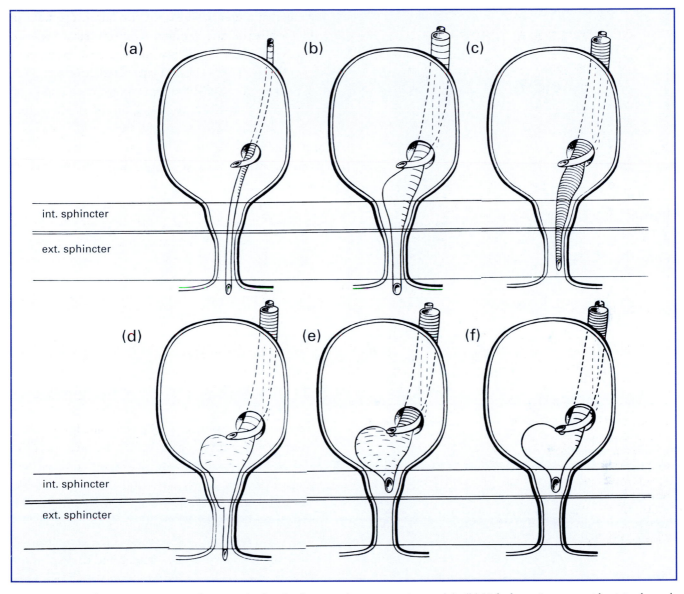

Fig. 24.15 *Muscle in ectopic ureters and ureteroceles found in biopsy and autopsy specimens. (**a**), (**b**) Vulval ectopic ureters with minimal muscle in floor and only in trigone zone. (**c**) Urethral ectopic ureter with circular and longitudinal muscle. (**d**) Sphincteric ureterocele devoid of muscle except in cranial part. (**e**) Sparse muscle especially distal. (**f**) Absence of muscle in the ureterocele. (Reprinted, by permission, after Stephens, F.D. (1963), Congenital Malformations of the Rectum, Anus and Genito-Urinary Tracts. Edinburgh, Livingstone, pp. 188, 190.)*

Necropsy specimens of cecoureterocele are rarely obtained, but one such has been restudied in detail by Gomez and Stephens (1983) and is described in full (Figs 24.7 and 24.17*). Deficiencies of the ureterocele and the musculature found in this specimen may explain some unusual urethrograms of two living patients and the occurrence of urinary incontinence which followed surgical excision of the cecoureterocele.

Autopsy of a female neonate, who died at age one day, revealed bilateral duplex kidneys and ureters, a right cecoureterocele and a left sphincteric ureterocele located on the upper pole ureters (Fig. 24.17). The urinary tracts were examined macroscopically, removed from the body and preserved in formalin. The entire length of the urethra, part of the bladder base and distal parts of both ureteroceles were blocked in paraffin wax.

* Reproduced by permission of The Williams and Wilkins Co from Gomez, F. and Stephens, F.D. 1983. Cecoureterocele: Morphology and Clinical Correlations. J. Urol. 129: 1017–19.

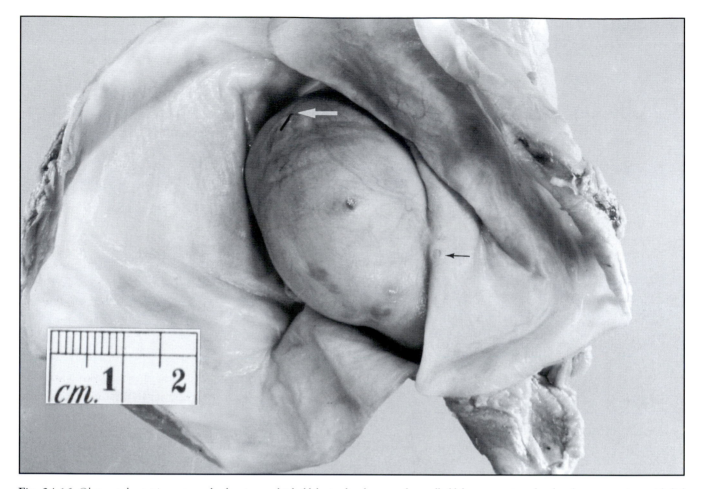

Fig. 24.16 *Obstructed ectopic ureterocele showing multiple blebs in distal amuscular wall; blebs are composed only of two co-apting epithelial walls; remainder of ureterocele is composed of a thick collagen layer between the epithelial linings of bladder and ureterocele. Note lower pole ureter (bristle and white arrow) and left contralateral single orifice (black arrow). (Reprinted, by permission, from Stephens, F.D. (1983), Congenital Malformations of the Urinary Tract, New York, Praeger, Fig. 21.16, p. 346.)*

The block was cut transversely in serial section of $10\,\mu m$ thickness from the external urethral orifice to include the urethra and bladder base. Every 100th and 101st sections were stained with haematoxylin & eosin and Masson stains, and studied by light microscopy. The urethra and trigone of two normal female newborns were cut in serial section and examined microscopically for comparison of the musculature with that of the urethra of the cecoureterocele specimen. The cecoureteroceles in both living patients (S.W. and N.W.) had been excised. S.W. was three years old and had infections traced to stasis caused by reflux of urine into the ureterocele. Voiding cystourethrography demonstrated that the cecum of the ureterocele became globular, expanded the muscular walls of the urethra, and compressed and obstructed the urethral lumen (Stephens, 1971). N.W. was three months old and had

septicaemia traced to urinary infection. Voiding cystourethrography demonstrated bilateral ectopic reflux cecoureteroceles that obstructed the urethral lumen, caused stasis and promoted infection. Opaque medium was trapped in the cecocele within the walls of the urethra (see Fig. 24.19). Surgical excision of the cecoureteroceles in these two patients was followed by urinary incontinence. Bladder-neck repair restored continence in patient S.W.

Autopsy specimen

The lower pole ureter on the right side was normal in dimensions but the renal segment was moderately hydronephrotic. The left lower-pole ureter was normal in dimensions and the renal parenchyma was well developed and not hydronephrotic. The ureters issued in the

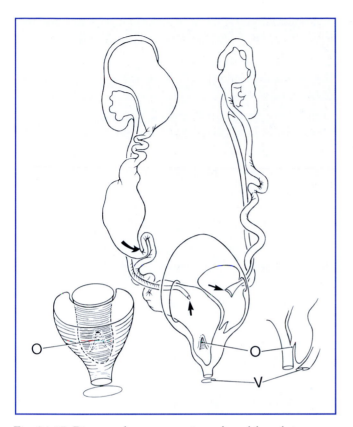

Fig. 24.17 *Diagram of necropsy specimen shows bilateral giant ureteroceles, bilateral duplex upper tracts, bladder and urethra. Right cecoureterocele with extravesical and urethral prolongations issued via rudimentary ureteral segment into upper urethra. Note potential obstructing flap valve (O) created by this rudimentary segment (insets): conjoined wall at outlet of ureteral aneurysm (curved arrow) and orifices of lower pole ureters (straight arrows). O, orifice of rudimentary ureter in urethra partially overlying junctional orifice of ureterocele and ureter creating flap valve. V, vagina. (Reprinted, with permission, from Gomez, F. and Stephens, F.D. (1983), Cecoureterocele: morphology and clinical correlations. J. Urol. 129: 1017–1019, Fig. 1.)*

bladder base on the cranial aspects of the ipsilateral upper pole ureteroceles.

Right upper pole ureter

The parenchyma of the right ectopic renal segment was uniformly thin (0.3 cm) and its one major calyx was hydronephrotic. The ureter had one aneurysmal segment, 2.5 cm in diameter, linked by slightly dilated tortuous ureteral segments above to the dilated pelvis and below to the ureterocele (Fig. 24.17). The distal ureter shared an angulated common wall with the aneurysm as shown in Fig. 24.17. This convolution did not obstruct the free orthograde flow of fluid into the distal ureter which, after a course of 6.5 cm, joined the

extravesical part of the ureterocele. The expanded ureterocele then entered the submucosal space of the bladder through a wide hiatal tunnel, and coursed through the bladder neck and urethra in this submucosal plane. The orifice of the ureterocele lay in the wide proximal urethra and the cecum of the ureterocele extended along the submucosal plane of the distal urethra. The orifice was wide and merged into the urethral lumen by an intervening, caudally directed, ultrashort segment of ureter (Fig. 24.17). The orifice in the urethra could be readily probed in a cranial direction but to enter the distal cecum the probe had to be tilted over the lip of the ascending posterior wall of this short segment of ureter. This lip was transparent and composed of apposing walls of the ureteral segment and the cecocele. This lip may act as a flap valve, permitting reflux but not efflux of urine.

Left upper pole ureter

The parenchyma of the left upper pole was thin (0.3 cm) and hydronephrotic, and the ureter was uniformly dilated to approximately 1.0 cm and slightly tortuous. The ureter expanded into a giant ureterocele that lay beneath the mucosa of the bladder neck, flush with the septum, between the two ureteroceles.

On each side the vesical hiatus was the common tunnel of entry for both ureters, the right hiatus being many times greater in dimension than normal to accommodate the extravesical extension of the ureterocele.

The bladder neck was expanded widely and the upper two-thirds of the urethra exhibited a prominent posterior bulge in which lay the cecocele. A distinct demarcation line between the main urethral wall and the bulging thinner wall could be seen.

Microscopic structure

The cecoureterocele was amuscular and its wall comprised two co-apting layers of vesicourethral and ureterocele epithelia on the roof, and a single epithelial wall on its floor supported by a thin fibrocollagen layer upon the muscular wall of the urethra (Fig. 24.18). The extravesical ureter became muscularized abruptly at its junction with the ureterocele but the dilated middle saccular segment of the ureter had a patchy distribution of muscle. The two co-apting walls (Fig. 24.17, curved arrow) were bound firmly together but each contained

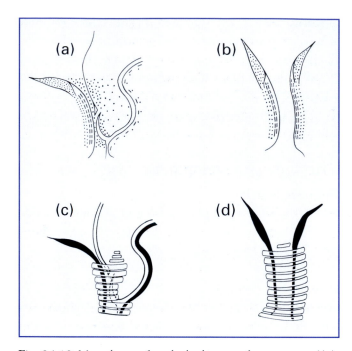

Fig. 24.18 *Musculature of urethral sphincters of autopsy case ((a), (c)) compared with normal newborn ((b), (d)). Diagrams depict lateral projections of bladder neck and urethra. (a) Widened bladder neck—internal sphincter (dots) strong in anterior but weak in posterior quadrants. Note outer circular muscle coat (dots) and inner longitudinal coats (cut lines) around anterior urethral quadrants and attenuated in posterior quadrants. (b) Normal distribution of involuntary muscle. (c) Distribution of voluntary muscle (transverse bands) forming strong coat in anterior quadrants of urethra and absence of voluntary muscle around posterior quadrants except for circumferential rung in most distal limit of urethra beneath cecocele. (d) Normal distribution of voluntary muscle. (Reprinted, with permission, from Gomez, F. and Stephens, F.D. (1983), Cecoureterocele: morphology and clinical correlations. J. Urol. 129: 1017–1019, Fig. 2.)*

muscle in the walls. The left ureterocele was an epithelial amuscular and thinly fibrocollagenous structure.

The mucosa of the bladder base was undermined and distended by the right and left intravesical ureteroceles. The level of the internal urinary meatus was identified by the muscle thickening of the internal sphincter noted on the anterior vesicourethral wall. The muscle of the internal sphincter diminished posterolaterally and hence the exact location of the internal urinary meatus could not be defined in this expanded bladder neck. In the bladder neck and the cranial two-thirds of the urethra, the muscle layers were intact and plainly visible anteriorly down to the external meatus but were much attenuated and intermingled with fibrocollagenous tissue over and around the posterior bulge (Fig. 24.18).

The voluntary muscle of the pelvic urethra was thin but extensive on the anterior wall, rising almost to the level of the internal urinary meatus and descending to the perineal membrane. The muscle swept posterocaudally around the expanded urethra only to the mid-lateral line that corresponded with the macroscopic demarcation of the base of the posterior bulge. The voluntary muscle coat from each side converged and met posteriorly only at one point, just beneath the overhanging bulge (Fig. 24.18). The arrangement of the voluntary muscle was such that a gap was present posteriorly, allowing the expanded amuscular tongue of the ureterocele, which was covered only by attenuated smooth muscle of the urethra, to protrude.

Normal female newborns

The involuntary sphincter was a well-marked circumferential thickening of the smooth muscle around the internal urinary meatus and upper quarter of the urethra. Between this sphincter and the external urethral meatus were two layers of involuntary muscle—inner longitudinal and outer circular—lying circumferentially beneath the urethral epithelium (Fig. 24.18b). The voluntary muscle of the external sphincter formed a thick and complete coat outside the smooth muscle, extending from the lower margin of the internal sphincter to the perineal membrane just short of the external meatus. The orientation of the muscle bundles was chiefly transverse (Fig. 24.18d). By contrast with the vesicourethral muscle of the ureterocele specimen, the normal muscle coats were of even thickness circumferentially and no gaps or areas of attenuation were present.

Discussion

The morphological findings, together with the observation that urinary incontinence occurred after surgical excision of the cecoceles in patients S.W. and N.W. indicate that: (1) a muscle deficit of the bladder neck and urethra may predispose to incontinence; (2) after excision of the vesical and bladder neck parts of the ureterocele, surgery to the distal tongue should be limited initially to division of the co-apting epithelial layers of the urethra and cecoureterocele; and (3) the hypomuscularity of the trigone; internal sphincter and adjoining urethra that backed the ureterocele should be repaired by co-aption of the thicker muscle bordering the weak wedge if incontinence persists.

Valvular orifice of the ureterocele and possible explanation

The orifice of the cecoureterocele in the urethra was different from that previously described in patient S.W., which was a simple side opening into the bladder. The ureterocele of the autopsy case communicated with the urethra through an ultrashort, obliquely directed segment of amuscular ureter. Its back wall co-apted the front wall of the cecum of the ureterocele, forming a flap valve that would close the outlet yet permit reverse flow from the urethra. If a similar valvular orifice was present in patient N.W. it would explain the retention of opaque medium in the cecocele (Fig. 24.19).

Defective muscle backing of ureteroceles in the trigone and bladder neck has been described by Williams *et al.* (1972). The absolute lack of voluntary muscle and the attenuated smooth muscle around the posterior half of the expanded urethra and bladder neck

found in the autopsy specimen suggest that the defect may be even more extensive with cecoureteroceles.

The cecoureterocele and the aneurysm have several features in common, which suggest a focal developmental enlargement. The near-normal calibre ureter above and below the aneurysm casts a shadow of doubt on the role of obstruction in this right upper tract.

Theories of development

Embryogenesis

In order to explain these curious developments we must first recapitulate some steps of the development of both single and double ureters.

Ureteric bud formation

The ureter begins at the 4-mm stage of development as a bud arising from the wolffian duct a short distance from its orifice in the cloaca; this bud elongates, expands and reaches out into the metanephric tissue which forms the renal parenchyma. This elongated bud is not a uniform-calibre tube, being narrow at the ureterovesical and pelvi-ureteric junctions, wide in mid-spindle, pelvis and

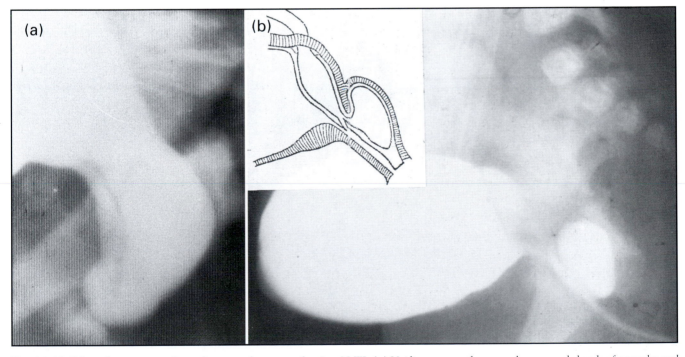

Fig. 24.19 *Bilateral cecoureteroceles and cystourethrograms of patient N.W.* (**a**) *Voiding cystourethrogram shows rounded ends of cecoceles and longitudinal filling defect caused by overlapping walls of two cecoceles.* (**b**) *Cystogram with opaque catheter in urethra and loculus of opaque medium locked in blind end of one cecocele by supposed flap valve across orifice, and contraction of internal sphincter. Inset: presumed orientation of anatomical structures.* (*Reprinted, with permission, from Gomez, F. and Stephens, F.D. (1983), Cecoureterocele: morphology and clinical correlations. J. Urol. 129: 1017–1019, Fig. 3.*)

calyces, and very small in the ducts of Bellini. This capacity for differential expansion and growth is a complex embryological feat, which may err and be responsible for some general or focal developmental irregularities in the size of some ureters or parts of ureters.

Cranial migration of the bud

Between the 4-mm and 10-mm stages, the terminal part of the wolffian duct distal to the ureteric bud (the common excretory duct) expands in trumpet form and is taken up into the vesicourethral canal. The orifice of the ureter in this way becomes separate and comes to lie craniolateral to the wolffian orifice. The wolffian duct is taken up into the vesicourethral canal for a further short distance cranial to the site of origin of the ureteric bud, thus incorporating extra buds arising cranial to the first bud into the bladder or urethra. Other, more ectopic buds arise beyond the expansile segment and remain attached to the wolffian duct (Figs 22.5 and 15.3). Ureteric migration is normally arrested on the lateral cornu of the trigone, thus ensuring a submucosal course of the intravesical ureter on the bladder base cranial and lateral to the trigone. Other ureters arising in close proximity to this bud either as junctional or separate buds follow the same migration pattern. Ectopic buds

arising from more cranial locations on the wolffian duct migrate part way to the bladder arresting in the bladder-neck region. Those buds arising from the wolffian duct beyond the zone of expansion issue into the urethra contiguous with the duct or remain attached to it and may become involved eventually with the müllerian migration.

Caudal migration in the female

At the 30-mm stage of development, the müllerian ducts issue into the urethra between the orifices of the wolffian ducts in the vicinity of the Müller's tubercle (verumontanum). In the female, they mature and incorporate the wolffian ducts in their walls, and then begin a distal müllerian migration, closely coordinated with elongation of the proximal urethra and broadening and shallowing of the urogenital sinus caudal to the site of entry of these ducts. Both the urethral and vaginal orifices shift from their hidden pelvic locations to exposed positions in the vestibule (Fig. 24.20) (Frazer, 1931).

The müllerian ducts at the site of union with the urogenital sinus undergo an almost cancer-like epithelial activity, expanding their walls and incorporating not only the wolffian ducts in their lateral walls, but also any stray ureters or parts of ureters that may be

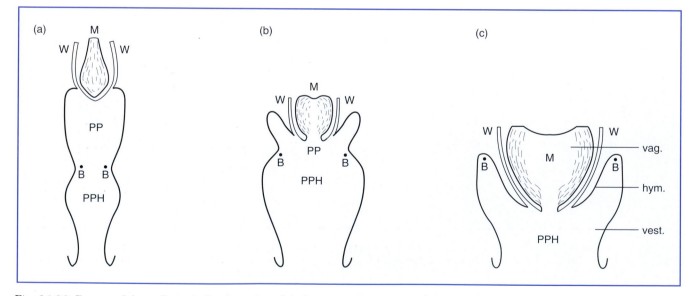

Fig. 24.20 *Descent of the müllerian bulbs, formation of the hymen, and conversion of the pars phallica of the urogenital sinus into vestibule. Openings of Bartholin's gland ducts (b) lie between pars pelvina (PP) and pars phallica (PPH) in (a) and come to issue at base of the hymen (Hym). (M = müllerian duct; W = wolffian duct; Vag = vagina). (Reprinted, by permission, from Frazer, J.E. (1931a), A Manual of Embryology. London, Baillière, Tindall & Cox, p. 438, Fig. 266.)*

abnormally present in the locality of Müller's hillock (Fig. 24.21).

Expansion of the vesicourethral canal from a tubular to a globular shape

At the time that the ureters are separating and migrating from the wolffian ducts, the anterior subdivision of the cloaca and the allantois is expanding to form the vesicourethral canal. This accelerated expansion occurs in embryos of 6–16 mm. It is considered that the bladder and bladder neck are formed from the cloaca and allantois, together with the gusset made from the expanded common excretory ducts. The terminal end of the ureter, though incorporated within the walls of the bladder, does not normally share in this rapid expansion of the vesicourethral anlage (Fig. 13.2). The later arrival of the urethral ectopic ureter may involve the submucosal ureterocele segment of this ureter in the same process that creates the globular shape of the bladder. The ureter, which arrives in mid-urethra later still, becomes involved with the distal migration of the müllerian ducts and rarely shares this expansion stimulus and the bud that remains attached to Gartner's duct is not so affected.

Atrophy of the wolffian ducts

The wolffian ducts are formed by the 4-mm stage and later act as the guidelines to the forming and migrating müllerian ducts. The müllerian ducts gain thick muscle coats in the female fetus, and incorporate the wolffian ducts in their lateral walls, where they wither and disappear in part or wholly. The remnants of the wolffian

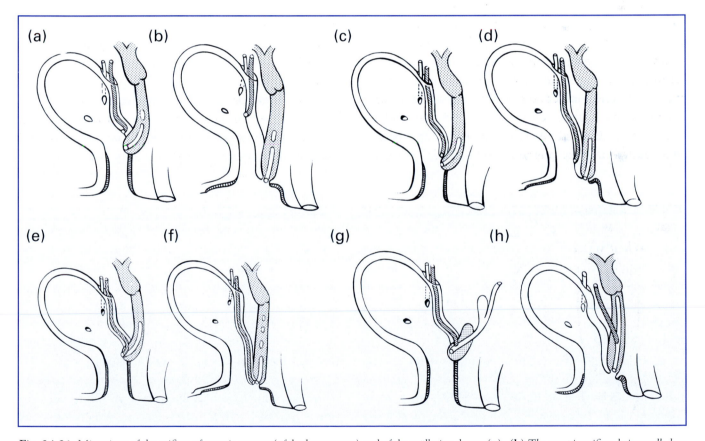

Fig. 24.21 *Migrations of the orifices of ectopic ureters (of duplex systems) and of the müllerian ducts. (**a**), (**b**) The ectopic orifice, being well clear of the wolffian duct orifice (**a**) at the time of arrival of the müllerian ducts, migrates cranially (**b**) uninfluenced by the müllerian ducts. (**c**), (**d**) When the ectopic orifice is adjacent to the wolffian orifices at the time of arrival of the müllerian ducts, it becomes involved in the caudal müllerian migration and is transposed part way along the urethra. (**e**), (**f**) If the ectopic orifice is contiguous with the wolffian orifice (**e**) it will 'hitchhike' with Gartner's ducts and müllerian ducts issuing on the hymen ((**f**), (**g**)). (**h**) The ectopic ureter, which retains its connection at a high level with the wolffian duct, takes a course posterior to the bladder to enter Gartner's duct in the lateral wall of the vagina at a higher level than the ureter that follows the submucosal course, and joins Garner's duct at the hymen ((**e**), (**f**)). (Reprinted, by permission, from Stephens, F.D. (1971), Cecoureterocele and concepts on the embryology and aetiology of ureteroceles. Aust. N.Z. J. Surg. 40: 239, Fig. 3.)*

ducts are called Gartner's ducts (Fig. 24.21). This process of atrophy may affect a 'stray' ectopic ureter that has retained its attachment to the wolffian duct. Hence a ureter may become blind in that part closely associated with the wolffian duct, and this may account for the rare blind-ending ureterocele (Figs 24.1g and 24.4).

The very rare ectopic ureter, which bypasses the bladder to enter the wolffian duct on the lateral wall of the vagina, does not undergo the focal terminal dilatation characteristic of ureteroceles. Presumably, the ureter lacks the stimulus derived from the expanding bladder.

Two-way migration of the ureter and cecoureterocele formation

It has been suggested that the ureter can be subjected to stimuli that are imposed on structures in which the ureter finds itself at different stages in development. First, the ureter and its orifice may be larger than normal as the result of an intrinsic growth stimulus of the bud. Second, if the ureteric orifice is in transit to its lateral trigonal site when the expansion stimulus strikes the vesicourethral canal, the ureter may also be affected by this stimulus. Third, the wolffian ducts, together with stray contiguous ectopic ureters, become incorporated in the highly activated müllerian bulbs, and so share the migration stimulus, which promotes the descent of all the structures toward the vestibular location.

It is postulated also that, on rare occasions, the distal wall of a terminal ureterocele may lap the müllerian duct, which then carries it caudally as a tongue along the submucosal plane of the urethra (Fig. 24.1f). Occasionally also, a ureteric orifice of a subterminal ureterocele may be engaged in the migration of the müllerian ducts, in which event the ureter distal to the ureterocele is drawn out as shown in Figs 24.1e and 24.8.

In explaining the complex embryology of the cecoureterocele, therefore, we must postulate the following: an intrinsically abnormal bud, an ectopic location of the orifice and a terminal ureterocele, the distal bulging wall of which laps the müllerian bulb and 'hitchhikes' on it toward the vestibule.

Aetiology
Ureteroceles without obstruction
Three examples of ureteroceles exhibiting large orifices in the bladder without obstruction of the ureter were found in the series of 60 ureteroceles (Fig. 24.1h). One of these three died from congenital anomalies of the heart, and the left ectopic ureter was found at postmortem examination to issue by a very large orifice onto the trigone proximal to the internal urethral meatus (Fig. 24.7). This ectopic ureter was part of a dilated duplex system, the LPU orifice being of normal dimensions and normally sited. Proximal to the ectopic orifice, the submucosal ureter was ballooned but collapsed. Serial sections were cut and prepared in paraffin for histological examination. Dr L. Cussen reported that the ureterocele was amuscular, the ureter acquiring a muscle coat where it emerged from the bladder wall to become extramural. On measurement, the muscle cells in the extravesical ureter were normal in dimensions, and there was no hyperplasia of muscle, indicating an absence of obstruction to the ureterocele. Two other similar examples were successfully treated surgically after careful checking that the wide orifice of the ureterocele issued on to the trigone, and after studying the radiographical appearance of the ureterocele and the dilated ureter. These three ureteroceles were formed in the absence of obstruction.

Role of obstruction in ureteroceles
There can be no doubt that many ureteroceles arise as dilations of the submucosal ureter secondary to stenosis of the ureteric orifice. Some ureteroceles may exhibit dilatation and muscle hypertrophy, both of which presumably are induced by the obstruction. The narrow orifice is possibly due to arrest of enlargement and failure to conform in size with the growth of the ureterovesical structures. Chwalla (1927) proposed that the ureteric bud is temporarily occluded at its origin during early embryogenesis by a membrane composed of apposing urogenital sinus and ureteric epithelium and that this membrane remains in part, causing stenosis.

Other ureteroceles, however, have large orifices, many times the normal calibre, lying within the bladder or urethra, and are often of very large dimensions, half filling the lumen of the bladder. Those ureteroceles, the orifices of which are abnormally large and lie within the squeeze of the internal sphincter, are subject to low-pressure obstruction, which may be conducive to focal expansion within the bladder, but there are many UPUs that issue in similar locations in the urethra without ureterocele formation (Stephens, 1963a). Some other factor besides obstruction operates in the formation of some ureteroceles, and in these, the muscle and collagen components in the walls are frequently abnormal (Uson, 1961; Stephens, 1963b; Tokunake et al., 1981).

Tanagho (1976) also questions the traditional obstructive concept of the aetiology of ectopic ureteroceles. He attributes ureterocele formation to the late arrival of the ectopic bud in the bladder. This delay allows the ampullary origin of the ureteric bud to overexpand and preform the ureterocele even before it has migrated to the bladder.

A very large orifice, a giant-sized ureterocele, a UPU location of the orifice, the duplex system so often present, and defects of muscle and renal parenchyma, all favour an embryological explanation of a ureterocele. The cecoureterocele, for all the reasons mentioned above with, in addition, the long tongue-like process under the floor of the urethra, is also most readily explained on the basis of a primary malformation influenced secondarily by the müllerian ducts. In many ureteroceles, however, some form of obstruction, such as that caused by the squeeze of the urethral sphincter upon the orifice, coexists and maintains the fullness of the ureterocele but is unlikely to be the primary or only factor in aetiology.

Treatment

Treatment of duplex intravesical ureter with ureterocele formation

Treatment of the ureterocele depends mainly on the relative value of the corresponding kidney to the patient. Other factors, such as the age of the patient and the presence of associated abnormalities of the other ureters and their corresponding kidneys, influence the timing and choice of operation.

When renal function is worth saving and the upper pole segment and ureterocele are isolated lesions
Stenotic type. The kidney associated with the single or duplex stenotic ureterocele, the orifice of which is in the trigone of the bladder, is usually of good quality in young children. It is, however, often symptomless until complications set in and, after many years, renal function undergoes deterioration from obstruction or infection. This type of ureterocele may pass unnoticed in childhood. Treatment is discussed in Chapter 16.

Sphincteric type. In the sphincteric ureterocele, in which the normal- or large-calibre orifice lies in the zone of the internal sphincter, the ureterocele may be partially de-roofed proximally from the orifice, in order that it may open freely into the bladder. Drainage of the bladder is indicated if the resection is undertaken in the presence of infection. This will circumvent the obstructive mechanism. Transurethral resection is indicated especially when cystoscopic examination reveals evidence of active peristalsis in the walls of the ureterocele. Vesicoureteral reflux is unlikely to ensue after minimum resection to recess the orifice into the bladder, and satisfactory results are obtained. For the non-propulsile ureterocele, recession of the orifice is much more likely to be followed by troublesome reflux. The procedure plus temporary catheter drainage alleviates the crisis of infection, and further surgery may be planned according to the results of further investigations.

In two patients, the ureterocele was sparingly deroofed by transurethral resection. Follow-up studies have shown that the ureterovesical valve mechanism was preserved and that the children were free from infection. In five others in whom the ectopic renal segment functioned sufficiently to cast a radiopaque shadow, free reflux followed the resection operation, which in all was more radical. Four of the children have now been followed for 8–10 years; two are free of infection, but the function of the renal segment is still minimal, and the two others have required excision of the ectopic segment of the kidney and ureter, not because of ill health but because of persisting bacilluria.

It seems that if the kidney function in the ectopic segment is initially poor by radiographical standards, no worthwhile improvement accrues subsequently.

Tank (pers. commun. 1981) advocates endoscopic deroofing of the ectopic ureterocele combined with temporary in-dwelling urethral catheter drainage of the bladder as a satisfactory method of internal–external drainage. Further surgery may be required subsequently, depending on the reflux status of all ureters and renal functions.

When renal function is not worth saving and the upper pole segment and ureterocele are isolated lesions
Total excision of the ectopic kidney, its ureter, the ureterocele, and the urethral extension is the ideal treatment for a defunct unit, but the great length of this

abnormal ureter imposes the necessity for two incisions. For this reason, excision of the ectopic kidney and the greater part of the extravesical ureter is performed as the primary measure. The caudal end of the ureter and ureterocele may be removed at this same operation, but may be deferred to a planned future date if a prolonged operation is contraindicated for other reasons.

Heminephrectomy combined with ureterectomy is adequate if the accompanying and contralateral ureters and kidneys are normal in size and function. To ensure that the blood supply to the remaining segment of the double kidney is not inadvertently impaired during the heminephrectomy procedure, the renal pedicle or the branches supplying the segment to be resected should be temporarily compressed with a gentle bulldog clamp. Then, after the capsule has been peeled back, the segment is separated by sharp and blunt dissection from lateral to medial sides, isolating, ligating, and dividing the hilar vessels of supply as they come free with the detached segment of the kidney. By this lateral-to-medial separation, the vessels to both parts of the double kidney are clearly identified before division, and the risks of ischaemia to the remaining segment are averted.

Some urologists (Belman et al., 1974) consider that the second operation on the ureterocele should not be undertaken unless troublesome symptoms or signs of infection, calculus formation, or prolapse persist or recur, or if the cecoureterocele obstructs the urethra. They advise that the stump of the ectopic ureter should be very short and the ureterocele drained through the stump via the flank for several days to allow infection to resolve.

At present, we cannot predict with certainty which ureteroceles remain benign after partial nephroureterectomy. For this reason, some surgeons prefer the total excision of the ectopic system, others prefer the nephroureterectomy and wait-and-see regimen, and yet others prefer primary endoscopic partial de-roofing and a planned regimen depending on the results of subsequent investigations including the status of reflux, response to medication of infection and status of renal function.

The ureteroceles that require excision or de-roofing as a planned immediate or planned secondary procedure after nephroureterectomy are those that (1) exhibit reflux, (2) obstruct the urethra such as the cecoureterocele or (3) are associated with wetting due to impairment of the bladder-neck muscle. A wait-and-see policy may be adopted after nephroureterectomy for other types such as the sphincteric (without reflux), sphincterostenotic and blind (after emptying by drainage) ureteroceles. A second operation would be indicated if infections recur in the ureterocele, reflux and infections occur in other ureters, the ureterocele fills by reflux and prolapses, a calculus forms in the ureterocele or posterior eversion of the ureterocele leads to incomplete emptying of the bladder and infection.

Treatment of the ureterocele and associated urinary anomalies

When the issue is complicated by associated anomalies of the remaining ipsilateral or contralateral ureters or of the lower urinary or genital tracts, priorities in the surgical management are planned to afford maximum protection of overall renal function. Suitable preliminary drainage of the upper tracts may precede specific management of the upper pole or poles depending on the total reflux status, infection and function in the duplex and contralateral kidneys.

Decisions concerning the treatment of the ureterocele are made when facts are assembled concerning the type, accompanying reflux in the other ureters and the status of the kidneys and ureters. In some patients it is safe to proceed forthwith, combining reimplantations with excision of the ureterocele and in others, heminephroureterectomy may precede surgical or non-surgical management of the ureterocele.

Ureteral triplication is an extreme rarity and may pass unnoticed or be found incidentally or may give rise to symptoms because of inherent defects in any one, or all, of the components. The case reports from past publications have been assembled from which the data concerning the orifice position and correlation of the renal morphology could be obtained. It was found that the orientation of ureteric orifice position to the segments of the kidney obeys the Weigert–Meyer law in only about half the number of patients under consideration. An embryological explanation for the mismatch of others is proposed.

Triplicate ureters
Classification of triplicate ureters

Smith (1946) classified the types of triplications based on his study of 10 previously reported cases and one of his own. This classification into four types has stood the test of time: Type I, complete triple ureters, that is, three separate ureters and three separate orifices; Type II, double ureter with one branch bifid; Type III, trifid ureter; and Type IV, two ureters emerging from the kidney, one of which bifurcates forming an inverse Y-junction resulting in ostial triplication. These types could be expressed numerically according to the numbers of ureters and orifices — 3 and 3, 3 and 2, 3 and 1, and 2 and 3. This classification fulfills the needs, but each type has anatomical variations; any of the triple ureters may exhibit one of many pathological complications, such as bifurcation, ectasia, vesicoureteral incompetence and reflux, ectopic orifices, obstruction, ureterocele formation, blind upper end or renal hypodysplasia. A very extensive urinary tract investigation is necessary to determine the anatomy and pathology in patients with symptomatic triple ureters in order to plan appropriate management.

Type I triplicate ureters: complete triple ureter (3 and 3)

Sixteen case reports were reviewed including the following new case report.

Case 9

In 1959, K.L.C., a six-year-old girl, complained of left loin pain of recent onset associated with an episode of urinary infection. Investigation revealed three separate normal calibre ureters on the left side and two on the right (Fig. 25.1). The function in all five renal segments was normal according to intravenous pyelography standards, the ureters were normal in calibre, and all five ureteric orifices lay on the trigone of the bladder. On the left side, the orifice in the 'F' position subserved the middle kidney, whereas the

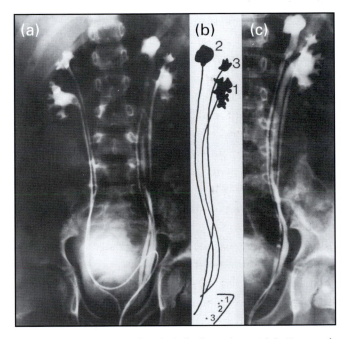

Fig. 25.1 *Type 1 triplex and duplex ureters.* (**a**) *Retrograde ureteropyelography showing (left) triple and (right) double ureters.* (**b**) *Course of left ureters as determined radiographically from all roentgenograms correlated with the positions of each ureteric orifice and corresponding kidney segments. The caudal ends of the ureters were defined after cystoscopic plotting of each orifice position (trigone 1, 2 and 3) and by injection of opaque medium, in turn, into each orifice of known location with immediate radiographic identification of each ureter and pelvis (lobes 1, 2 and 3). The orifices of the lower pole ureter lay in trigone position (1), the upper pole ureter in trigone position (2), close to position (1), and the intermediate pole in trigone position (3) lay near the internal urinary meatus.* (**c**) *Note that it is not possible to determine the course of the caudal ends of ureters relative to each other by radiography alone because of overlapping of ureters, opaque catheters and lack of information of exact sites of all orifices. (Small numerals and dots depict ureteric orifices in trigonal positions and large numerals indicate corresponding renal lobes.) (Reprinted, by permission, from Stephens, F.D. (1983), Congenital Malformations of the Urinary Tract, New York, Praeger, Fig. 22.1, p. 364.)*

'A' and 'E' orifices subserved the lower and upper poles respectively (Fig. 25.2, Case 9). On the right side, the orifice in the 'A' position subserved the lower two-thirds of the kidney, and that in the 'E' position subserved the upper pole. Vesicoureteral reflux was demonstrated in the left 'A'- and 'E'-position orifices, which subserved the lower and upper poles, respectively. The infection was treated appropriately and the reflux subsided spontaneously.

Clinical features

The case reports included in this chapter were obtained from journals published in the English language and were selected because sufficient detail was available concerning the positions of the ureteric orifices and the polarity of the renal segments they subtend. The analysis of the pertinent clinical data is shown on Tables 25.1 and 25.2 and Figs 25.2 and 25.3.

The female:male ratio was 13:3, the ages ranged from two to 74 years (average 21 years), and eight of the 16 patients were under eight years. The triplication occurred on the left side in nine and right side in seven. Duplex ureters occurred on the contralateral side in five of 16 (four double and one bifid). The Weigert–Meyer law was obeyed in seven. Six were non-conformers, and in three others, the combinations did not fit either pattern, were not known in some individual ureters, or the upper end of a member of the triplicated ureters was blind. It is occasionally bilateral (Kohri et al., 1978; Golomb and Ehrlich, 1989) and rarely inherited (Rich et al., 1987).

All three ureters and renal moieties may be structurally normal and cause no morbidity. Others, however, are intrinsically abnormal and give rise to symptoms and signs which are common to patients with duplex ureters (see Chapter 22). For example, relentless wetting in the periods between normal voidances in affected females, urinary-tract infection resulting from stasis due to

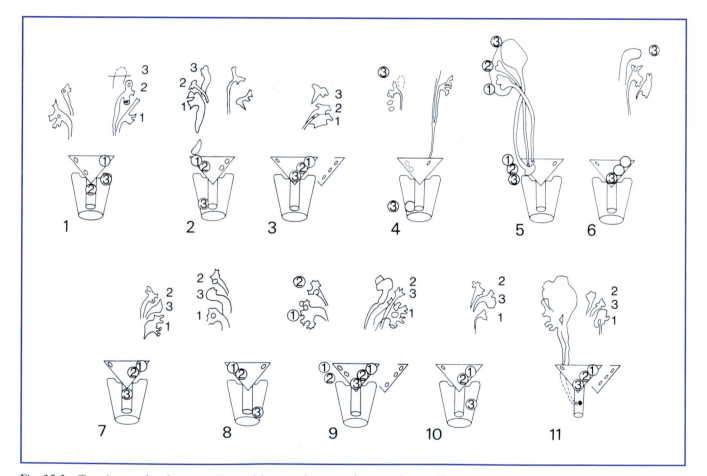

Fig. 25.2 *Type 1 ureteral triplication—Weigert–Meyer conformers and non-conformers. Drawings of radiographs or diagrams copied from radiographs in previously published articles with addition of orifice locations and corresponding renal segments where known and indicated by numerals. Cases 1–6 conformers and 7–11 (plus 13, Fig. 25.3) non-conformers. (References are to published articles itemized in Table 25.1.) (Reprinted, by permission, from Stephens, F.D. (1983), Congenital Malformations of the Urinary Tract, New York, Praeger, Fig. 22.2, p. 365.)*

Table 25.1 *Type 1 ureteral triplication: authors, years of publication of case reports and clinical details*

Authors	Year	Case number	Sex	Age	Side of triplication	Contralateral kidney	Weigert–Meyer law +†	Weigert–Meyer law −	Weigert–Meyer law Not known	Presenting feature§	Treatment Medication	Treatment Surgery of triplication
Parker et al.	1970	1	F	21	left	double	+	−	−	wet	−	+
Spangler	1963	2	F	7	right	double	+	−	−	wet	−	+
Wright and McFarlane	1955	3	F	38	left	single	+	−	−	UTI	+	−
Burt et al.	1970	4	F	17	right	bifid	+*	−	−	wet	−	+
Weinberg	1968	5	F	5	right	single	+	−	−	haematuria	−	+
Parvenin	1976	6	F	4	left	single	+*	−	−	UTI	−	+
Ringer and Macfarlan	1964	7	F	27	left	single	−	negative	−	UTI	−	+
Livaditus et al.	1964	8	F	2	right	single	−	negative	−	wet	−	+
Stephens	1961	9	F	4	left	double	−	negative	−	UTI	+	−
Perkins et al. (Case 5)	1973	10	F	7	left	single	−	negative	−	wet	−	+
Ireland and Chute	1955	11	M	45	left	double	−	negative***	−	incidental**	−	+***
Lau and Henline	1931	12	F	52	right	single	−	−	blind ureter	pain (no UTI)	+	−
Perkins et al. (Case 2)	1973	13	M	24	right	single	−	negative	−	BP	+	−
Woodruff	1941	14	M	74	right	single	−	−	+	incidental	+	−
Newman and Ditchek	1969	15	F	8	left	single	−	−	+	UTI	+	−
Blumberg	1976	16	F	6	left	single	+*	−	−	wet	−	+
Totals		16	F=13 M=3		L=9 R=6	double=5 single=11	7	6	3	−	6	9

*Only correlation reported was caudal-most orifice drains upper renal segment.

**Infection in contralateral ectopic ureter.

***Surgery to contralateral ectopic ureter.

§UTI = urinary tract infection; BP = blood pressure raised.

† + = obeys Weigert–Meyer law.

'negative' indicates non-conformity to Weigert–Meyer law.

Table 25-2 *Type I ureteral triplication: function, ureteric orifice positions of renal segments, and vesicoureteral reflux on side of triplication and contralateral side*

Authors	Case number	I.V.P. function			Ureteric orifice position			Vesicoureteral reflux			Contralateral ureter(s)		
		Upper-pole	Middle-pole	Lower-pole	Upper-pole ureter	Middle-pole ureter	Lower-pole ureter	Upper-pole ureter	Middle-pole ureter	Lower-pole ureter	Function	Ureteric orifice position	Vesico ureteral reflux
Parker *et al.*	1	none	good	good	H	G_1	A	nil	nil	nil	good	bl.**	nil
Spangler	2	none	good	good	G_2	bl.	bl.	nil	nil	R	good	bl.	nil
Wright and McFarlane	3	good	good	good	F	E	A	–	–	–	good	bl.	–
Burt *et al.*	4	poor	good	good	G_2	bl.	bl.	–	–	–	good	bl.	–
Weinberg	5	none	poor	none	F	A	A	–*	–	–*	poor	bl	–
Parvenin	6	poor	good	good	F	bl.	bl.	R	nil	nil	good	bl.	nil
Ringer and Macfarlan	7	good	none	good	E	G_1	A	–	–	–	good	bl.	–
Livaditus *et al.*	8	good	poor	good	E	G_3	A	–	–	–	good	bl.	–
Stephens	9	good	good	good	E	F	A	R	nil	R	good	bl.	nil
Perkins *et al.* (Case 5)	10	good	fair	good	bl.	H	bl.	–	–	–	good	bl.	–
Ireland and Chute	11	good	good	good	E	F	A	–	–	–	ortho good / ecto non good	bl. and G	–
Lau and Henline	12	good	–*	good	A'	A''	A	–	–	–	good	bl.	nil
Perkins *et al.* (Case 2)	13	good	good	good	bl.***	G_1	bl.***	nil	nil	nil	good	bl.	nil
Woodruff	14	good	good	good	A'	A'	A	–	–	–	good	bl.	–
Newman and Ditchek	15	good	good	good	bl.	bl.	bl.	–	–	–	good	bl.	–
Blumberg	16	poor	–*	good	–††	–††	A	R (post-operative)	R	R	good	bl.	nil

*Megaureters, not tested for reflux prior to nephroureterectomy. Reflux in contralateral megaureter tested postoperatively.
**bl. indicates location of ureteric orifice in bladder, but specific site not stated.
***Upper renal segment to upper ureteric orifice, middle segment to G orifice and lower segment to some point between.
†Ureter blind.
††Only two orifices seen and no correlations with renal segments established.
A' bunching of three orifices on cornu of trigone, correlation with renal segment.
A'' similar, but one ureter atretic.

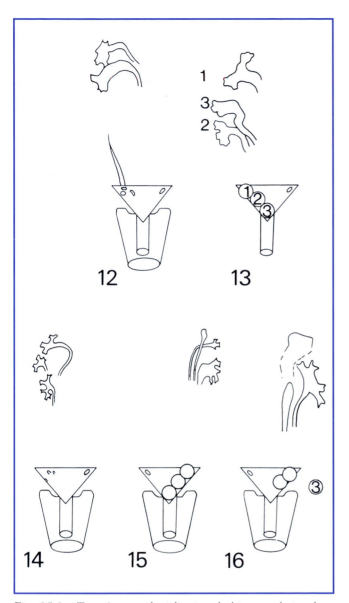

Fig. 25.3 *Type 1 ureteral triplications lacking correlation data. Case 12, bunched orifices and atresia of one ureter. Case 13, correlations unusual but data regarding possible bunching of orifices not available. Case 14, bunching of orifices and correlations not stated. Case 15, correlations not stated. Case 16, two of three orifices discovered and one ureter blind cranially and correlations lacking. (References are to published articles itemized in Table 25.1.) (Reprinted, by permission, from Stephens, F.D. (1983), Congenital Malformations of the Urinary Tract, New York, Praeger, Fig. 22.3, p. 366.)*

vesicoureteral and yo-yo reflux, ureteral obstruction, ureterocele (Weinberg, 1968; Gosalbez *et al.*, 1991) or megaureters.

The onset symptoms were urinary infection in six, wetting in six, haematuria following trauma in one, pain without infection in one, and raised blood pressure

found on routine check in one. Nine patients required surgery for the anomalies associated with the triple ureters, and one needed surgery for symptoms related to the contralateral ectopic double ureter. Operations such as partial nephrectomy prevailed for those triple ureters that conformed to the Weigert–Meyer law, and total nephroureterectomy, ureteral ligation, or ureteroureters that required surgery were either reflux megaureters, defunct kidney segments with orifices in the bladder, or non-reflux ureters issuing in the urethra or vagina.

Ureteric orifice locations
The orifice locations of the ureters were depicted in Figs 25.2 and 25.3. If the precise positions in the bladder were not stated but referred to as 'usual positions' or normal position, it has been presumed that the lower pole ureter issued most cranially as shown in Tables 25.1 and 25.2. Otherwise, the orifices are accurately shown according to the legends to the individual diagrams.

Case 13 is described both as a Weigert–Meyer non-conformer and as an example of junctional orifice locations and Case 15 is included because it is a documented triple ureter with three vesical orifices but without orifice–renal segment correlations.

Weigert–Meyer conformers (Cases 1–6 and 16). The lower-polar ureteric orifice in all seven patients was in the bladder and most cranially situated. The upper polar ureteric orifice was the most caudally located, three being in 'F', two in 'G2', one in 'H' position and one (Case 16) lay somewhere outside the bladder. The middle polar ureteric orifice was disposed somewhere between the other two, six being in the bladder and one in 'G1' position.

Weigert–Meyer non-conformers (Cases 7–11 and 13). The lower- and upper-polar ureteric orifices lay in the bladder in all six patients. The lower polar ureteric orifice was in 'A' position, and the upper pole orifice in 'E' position in four of the six. In all six instances, the orifices subtending the middle calyces were located caudal to both of the other two orifices in 'F' position (two cases), 'G1' (two cases) and 'G3' and 'H' (one each). In two patients, all three orifices were located in the bladder, but in Case 9, the orifices of the upper and lower renal segments were contiguous and removed from the middle segment orifice, and in Case 10, the orifices of the middle and upper segments were close together.

Junctional orifices (Cases 12, 13 and 14). In three patients, the grouping and location of the orifices were different from the conformers and non-conformers to the Weigert–Meyer law. All three orifices in two patients (Cases 12 and 14) lay bunched together on the lateral cornu of the trigone, and the segment-orifice correlations were not spelled out; in the third (Case 13), the grouping of orifices was not described, but the correlations were clearly defined (Fig. 25.3). The most cranial orifice on the trigone drained the upper renal segment, the middle orifice on the trigone the lower segment and the lower orifice in 'G1' position drained the middle segment. The exact spacing or grouping of these three orifices on the trigone was not stated, but the orifice locations of the upper and middle orifices suggest a junctional duplex relationship, whereas the lowest orifice is that of an independent third ureter from the middle renal segment. This independent ureter would obey the Weigert–Meyer law with respect to a duplex junctional 'unit' (see Fig. 25.7b).

In Case 12, the uppermost orifice subtended a blind ureter, and the other two orifices drained the lower and upper segments (correlations not stated). In Case 14, the three orifices lay together on a diagonal line across the narrow cornu of the trigone, but the correlations with renal segments were not stated.

The case of Livaditus, Maurseth and Skog (1964).

The position of the orifice of the ectopic ureter of this female child obeys the Weigert–Meyer law (Fig. 25.2, Case 8). The orifice lay, however, at the external urinary meatus on the contralateral side from the upper renal segment which it drained.

Two other patients with duplex systems, one under Stephens' care and one under the care of Dr Olaf Knutrud (pers. commun.) of Oslo, had similar crossover ureters. The ectopic orifice was situated in the vestibule on the side opposite that of its corresponding kidney segment. The embryogenesis of the crossover ectopic ureter in both the triplex and duplex ureters is not understood. The means by which an ectopic ureter in the female reaches the perineum has already been described. The müllerian ducts transpose the wolffian ducts, and any stray ureter contiguous with or joining them from the high position in the pelvis to the vestibule.

Two theories are proposed for the crossover orifice:

1. The müllerian ducts, after they meet in the pelvis, run a corkscrew course to the urogenital sinus and beyond, carrying with them the wolffian ducts (Stephens, 1966). In this way, the ectopic ureter and wolffian duct rotate around the sagittal axis. After dissolution of the septum between the two müllerian ducts, the vaginal orifice would exhibit no trace of the corkscrew course. An oblique orientation of the uterus, if found at the laparotomy, may support or refute this contention.

2. If only one müllerian duct developed, it may follow the ipsilateral wolffian duct without crossing it in the pelvis. Then both wolffian ducts would be incorporated in the same side wall of the vagina (Fig. 25.4). Any ectopic bud contiguous with the ipsilateral wolffian duct would hop over the midline to issue in the vestibule on the contralateral side of the vagina. The external appearance of the vagina would not reveal any clues, though ultrasonography, hysterography or laparotomy would determine the state of the müllerian system and refute or support the theory.

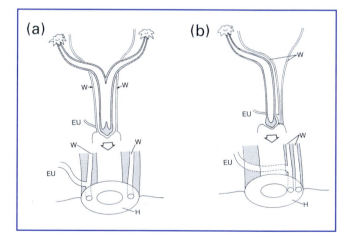

Fig. 25.4 *Pathoembryology of ipsilateral and 'crossover' ectopic ureters. (**a**) An ipsilateral ectopic ureter (EU) located on wolffian duct (W) descends with the vaginal bulbs to the perineum on the ipsilateral side of the renal segment. Upper part of diagram represents relative positions in the pelvis and lower half in the vestibule. (**b**) Crossover ectopic ureter (EU) presupposes a single vaginal bulb remaining lateral to the ipsilateral wolffian duct (W), which carries the ectopic ureter with it to the opposite side. Upper diagram shows bulb in urogenital sinus high in the pelvis and lower diagram vagina in vestibule. (H = hymen.) (Reprinted, by permission, from Stephens, F.D. (1983), Congenital Malformations of the Urinary Tract, New York, Praeger, Fig. 22.4, p. 366.)*

Comparison of renal-segment function in Weigert–Meyer conformers and non-conformers and other combinations

Renal function in Weigert–Meyer conformers. In six of the seven patients, the function in the upper segment was poor or absent. The orifice was abnormal intrinsically (either stenotic with ureterocele or incompetent) or in positions 'G' or 'H'. In the sixth patient, the function in the upper segment was normal and the ureteric orifice was trigonal in position. In the seventh patient, the orifice was outside the bladder.

Renal function in Weigert–Meyer non-conformers. In three middle segments the function was absent, poor, or exhibited caliectasis with brisk function, respectively. All three orifices were external to the bladder. The function in the three remaining middle segments was good, and two of the orifices were trigonal and one was located at the 'bladder neck' (Case 13).

Renal function in other combinations. Four triplications are lumped together because the specifics of some of the ureteric orifices were not entirely clear. The correlation of Cases 12, 14, 15 and 16 was not stated fully, and though the correlations were accurately stated in Case 13, grouping of the orifices is by inference only. These records, however, provide enough information upon which to base some deductions concerning embryological explanations for correlations of orifice position and renal segment and to accent the occurrence of two blind ureters in 16 triplications.

Correlation of renal function and ureteric orifice position. In these three groups, which include 46 renal segments and 48 ureteric orifices, 33 orifices were located on the trigone and intrinsically normal subtending normal functioning renal segments. Four orifices located in the bladder subtended renal segments with poor or absent function. All four ureters were ectatic with intrinsic defects of the orifice (ureterocele in one and mega-ureters in three of unknown cause). Of nine ureteric orifices located outside the bladder, seven subtended poor or non-functioning renal segments and two (Case 1 and Case 13) subtended segments with good function. Two of the 48 ureteric orifices, one trigonal (Case 12) and one not identified (Case 16) subtended blind ureters. It appears that if the ureteric orifice is located in near-normal position, the corresponding renal segments of the triplications develop normally unless the ureter itself is pathological.

Type II triplicate ureters: double ureter with one bifid (3 and 2)

Gill (1952) compiled two Type II case reports and McKelvie (1955) reported a third example. In all three, the bifid ureter was derived from the middle and lower pelves; the single ureter in each kidney emerged from the upper pelvis. The ureters in McKelvie's patient issued onto the trigone; the stem of the bifid ureter issued in the normal site, and the orifice of the ureter from the upper pelvis was positioned in accordance with Weigert–Meyer law. Axelrod (1954) recorded a case of triplication of the ureter also with bifid common stem draining the lower and middle calyces and with the most distal orifice on the trigone draining the upper pole in accordance with the Weigert–Meyer law.

Type III triplicate ureters: trifid ureters with a single ureteric orifice (3 and 1)

Gill (1952) collected seven case reports, including one of his own. In six of the trifid kidneys, two of the ureters met to form one ureter, which then joined the third to form a single ureter that issued into the bladder by one orifice. In one, which was a small, pelvic UPU kidney, all three ureters converged separately on a small, common chamber, which drained directly into the bladder. This juxtavesical expansion may represent a triple junction of stems and compound orifice, or a diverticulum of the bladder with ureteric orifices closely located (Fig. 25.5).

The Y-junctions were high or low, and the bifid and trifid stems were correspondingly short or long.

Type IV triplicate ureters: three ureters becoming two cranially with double kidney (2 and 3)

In this variant of triplication, three ipsilateral ureters emerge from the bladder from three separate orifices. Two of the ureters join to form one, thus converting triplication caudally into duplication cranially. Though 11 examples of ureters that were single cranially and split to form an inverted Y have been reported (Klauber

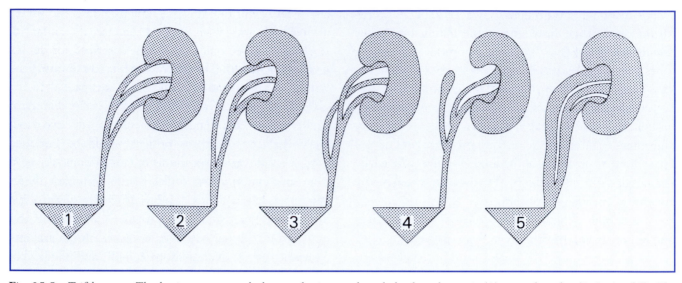

Fig. 25.5 *Trifid ureters. The dominant ureter to the lower pole gives one branch that branches again (1) or two branches (2, 3, 4 and 5). The branches subtend the middle and upper renal segments in a fortuitous manner. Note the megasystems in (5), indicating possible lateral ureteral ectopy. (Reprinted, by permission, from Stephens, F.D. (1983), Congenital Malformations of the Urinary Tract, New York, Praeger, Fig. 22.5, p. 367.)*

and Reid, 1972), it is very rare for an authentic example of this Type IV triplication to be reported, apart from that of Chwalla and cited by Smith (1946).

Embryogenesis of triplicated ureters

Trifid ureters

In the Type III triplications recorded by Gill (1952), the ureters were single caudally, bifid centrally and trifid cranially (Fig. 25.5). The common stem to the lower pole either gave off two branches in series to the upper or middle segments, or one branch that branched again. Further branchings would lead to quadruplication (Soderdahl *et al.*, 1976). If the common stem and the continuation of it to the lower pole is regarded as the mother or dominant ureter, it can spawn two daughter branches in series or one daughter that generates granddaughter ureters to the remaining segments.

Taking this family concept to Type II, the mother ureter to the lower pole can spawn a daughter branch. A sister ureter, having budded separately from the wolffian duct, subtends the left-over renal segment. Alternatively, the mother or dominant ureter may remain unbranched to the lower pole; the sister ureter branches a niece, and each subtends the upper or middle pole. The Type II triplication series of four including three from Gill's (1952) series and Axelrod's (1954) case had a mother-and-daughter- and a sister-ureter relationship.

Triple ureters

The next step in the family tree analogy is Type I, comprising three maiden-sister ureters, the dominant one arising from the cornu of the trigone and subtending the lower pole. Her sister ureter to the middle or upper segment has an orifice more caudal on the UPU pathway, and her next sister to the vacant remaining segment has another orifice still further down the pathway. It seems to be a matter of chance whether the first sister or second sister ureters subtend the middle or upper pole, and hence a matter of chance whether the triplication combination obeys or disobeys the Weigert–Meyer law.

The Weigert–Meyer budding arrangement
Separate ureteric buds in line

Three independent ureters draining the lower, middle and upper poles with orifices sited in reverse order along the UPU pathway can be explained readily by independent budding of three metanephric buds in line from the wolffian duct. Each bud arises from the posteromedial aspect of the duct and penetrates directly the adjacent and corresponding segment of the metanephros. Each bud rotates around the wolffian duct to achieve an anterolateral relationship and is absorbed sequentially with the terminal wolffian duct into the urinary tract.

The second and third buds, however, have an option of inducing either the whole of the middle and upper segments of the kidney or just the anterior or posterior lobes or lobules. Furthermore, the calyces of the anterior or posterior middle and upper lobules sometimes normally combine longitudinally and exhibit irregular groupings (Figs 25.1 and 25.2). Hence, under such circumstances, the ureters subserving these anterior or posterior lobular groupings cross as they grow to reach to the target calyces (Fig. 25.6). The crossing accounts for the non-conforming triplications in which the orifice of the ureter subserving the middle calyces issues caudal to and remote from, the other two.

Bunching of buds

There is also the 'bunch combination' of orifice-to-segment relationship, which occurred in one (Case 13) and possibly three (Cases 12 and 14) of the 16 examples of Type I. In Case 13, the most caudal orifice subtended the middle pole, the cranial orifice subtended the upper pole and the middle orifice of the dominant ureter drained the lower pole. The dominant ureter (analogous to the mother ureter) had its orifice on the trigone, and the sister ureter draining the upper pole had an orifice cranial to it and presumably on the cranial quadrant of the arc of the ectopic pathway as described for duplex ureters (Fig. 22.6). The second sister ureter draining the middle segment had an orifice that was caudal to the other two (Fig. 25.7a). Theoretically, if the dominant ureter has two contiguous sister orifices with two junctional orifices, all three orifices would be bunched together. The orifices of the sister ureters would array on the arcway around the orifice of the dominant ureter (Fig. 25.3, Cases 12 and 14; Fig. 25.7b,c). It is possible also that the orifice of the dominant ureter may be normally sited together with a sister orifice on the arc, and a second sister orifice may be remote and caudal but also with a junctional orifice related to her arcway (Fig. 25.7d). Embryologically, therefore, multiple orifice positions may be arranged in an orderly but complex manner, though to the clinician they may appear capricious and in disarray.

Junctional budding

With junctional budding, the three metanephric ducts bud contiguously; they rotate as a unit from the postero-

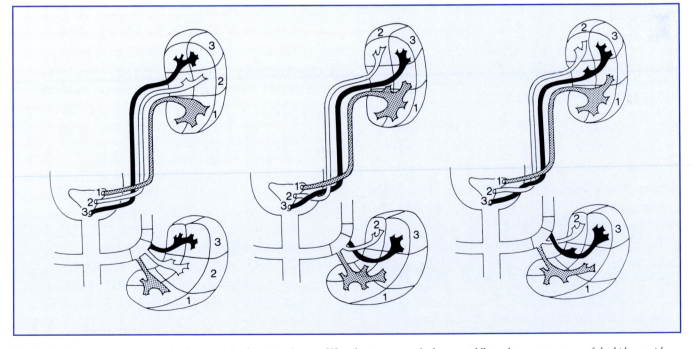

Fig. 25.6 *Course of the ureteral buds. (Left) Buds arising from wolffian duct target on the lower middle and upper segments of the kidney without crossing (lower half of diagram), but cross subsequently (upper half). (Right) Buds from wolffian duct target on lower segment, anterior lobules of middle and upper segments, and remaining lobules of upper segment. The upper two ureteric buds presumably cross at their origin (lower half of diagram) and cross again (upper half of diagram). (Middle) Variations on the theme. (Reprinted, by permission, from Stephens, F.D. (1983),* Congenital Malformations of the Urinary Tract, *New York, Praeger, Fig. 22.6, p. 367.)*

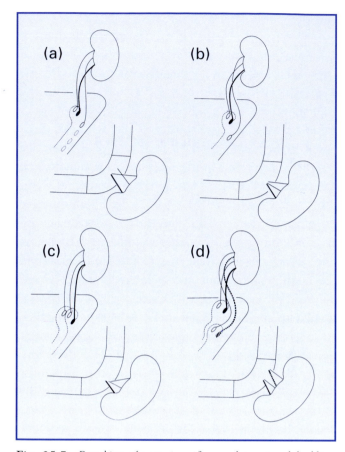

Fig. 25.7 *Bunching of ureteric orifices and junctional budding. (a) Dominant ureter (heavy black line) arising in apposition with junctional bud and separate from the third bud (lower half of diagram) and arranged finally on ectopic pathway. (b), (c) Variants. (d) Quadruplicate budding and double bunching. (Reprinted by permission, from Stephens F.D. (1983), Congenital Malformations of the Urinary Tract, New York, Praeger, Fig. 22.7, p. 368.)*

medial to the anterolateral aspects of the wolffian duct, pivoting on the composite origin. The origins of three buds rotate not only on the wolffian duct, but on themselves, maintaining their contiguous relationships throughout their migration to the trigone. The orifices on the trigone become disposed about the dominant ureter on the arc of the ectopic pathway.

Variations in distribution of renal lobes to triplicate ureters

The dominant ureter penetrates the lower pole of the metanephros and the others home in on the upper and middle poles. As was observed in Types II and III triplications, it seems to be a matter of chance as to which segments these two branches penetrate. With Type I triplication, the ureters are all completely independent,

the dominant ureter arising most distally from the wolffian duct and regularly penetrating the lower pole. Sometimes the upper pole ureter subtends only one or two minor calyces and only a small slice of mesenchyme, whereas the middle ureter combines middle calyces and several of the upper pole as well. Sometimes the lower pole ureter takes over some of the infundibulae of the middle segment. The upper pole ureter may also be aggressive and embrace infundibula of the anterior or posterior lobes of the middle segment.

When the Weigert–Meyer law was obeyed, the upper polar segment and ureter had fewer minor calyces, and the middle segment correspondingly more, whereas the non-conformers exhibited the reverse.

The middle segment of the kidney is normally divided sharply into anterior and posterior lobes, each with its own anterior and posterior calyces. Furthermore, the normal independent infundibulae of these middle calyces usually join the lower major calyx independently or join together with the infundibulum of the upper calyx, or they enter the pelvis of the kidney independently (see Figs 27.1 and 27.2). It is likely that the ureter and its calyces and lobules of the middle segment of a triplicate system would reflect the variations seen in the undivided kidney and pelvis.

Correlations between orifice position and renal segment in triplicate systems

Pathoembryology

The ureteric buds arise either from the wolffian duct separately, contiguously or as a single stem that divides. The ureteric bud to the lower major moiety is transposed first to the lateral corner of the trigone by a process of expansion and incorporation of the terminal segment of the wolffian (common excretory) duct into trigone on the bladder base and urethra. In Type 1 the two other separate ureters follow in succession from duct to bladder or urethra or genital tracts on the ectopic pathway. If two of the three buds are contiguous, the two orifices remain contiguous in the urinary tract. If all three buds are contiguous, the two junctional ureteric orifices crowd around the master orifice in the lateral corner of the trigone on the medial arc of the ectopic pathway. In Type II ureters, one of the two buds bifurcates but the process of absorption of the terminal end of the wolffian duct and its buds is similar to that of Type 1. Trifid ureters (Type III) arise from the wolffian duct by a single master bud, its orifice being transposed to the lateral corner of the trigone. The common stem of the master ureter may be short or long. The bud may trifurcate forming a common chamber or extrarenal 'ureteropelvis', or give off one or two branches in series forming bifurcate ureteropelves, or one branch may bifurcate into two sub-branches. The main stem or master ureter subtends the lower renal moiety and branches and sub-branches subserve either the middle or upper moieties.

Treatment

The principles of management of duplications of the ureterorenal systems apply also to triplications (see Chapter 22) with few exceptions.

Defunct kidney and upper pole defective segments or combined upper and middle defective moieties may require total or partial nephrourecterectomy, respectively. A defective middle moiety only may pose difficult excisional surgery and if ablation is required it may be safer to remove the upper moiety as well. Uretero-ureterostomy is, however, a simple alternative. Further surgery at the same time or later to excise the distal ectopic ureter or ureterocele may be necessary. Lower pole ablation is indicated if this moiety alone is defective. Vesicoureteral reflux of urine causing infection may require medication and in certain instances an appropriate form of antireflux surgery. Ureteroureterostomy may be indicated if the bifid or trifid ureters are ectatic in order to switch the junction or junctions from a low to high level in order to reduce the volume of static urine and yo-yo reflux and prevent recurrences of infection.

Type IV triplication: Inverted Y junction

A bud that fails to reach metanephric mesenchyme may either remain blind, usually with a saccular upper end, as occurred in two reported cases, or the bud may impact into an adjoining ureter. The likely explanation for the inverted-Y deformity is the meeting and fusion of two buds, the third remaining single. They join to form a single stem, as they approach the metanephros, the anomaly being a double ureter below and a single ureter above the junction. This, together with the third ureter, creates a vicarious form of triplication. Though authentic examples of inverted-Y duplications of the ureter have been recorded, it is doubtful whether any such anomalies have been discovered with triplication.

Quadruplicate ureters

Begg (1953) described the pyelograms of a woman with two ureters to the right kidney and four to the left. The right kidney was unique in that the master ureter entered from the medial aspect, and the smaller, independent ureter from the lateral side. The left kidney was even more unique; it had two medial separate ureters which drained the upper and lower portions of the kidney in the usual manner of duplex systems. However, the two lateral independent ureters, which ran together but in a lateral course, removed from the medial couplet joined the lower and middle segments of the same kidney from the lateral side. All the ureters from both sides were of normal calibre and could be traced radiographically into the true pelvis and presumably to the bladder. Being untroubled before and since an attack of abdominal pain, the patient declined further investigation, so no information is available concerning ureteric orifice positions. Begg (1953) gave four theoretical explanations for this unique arrangement, which he labelled 'sextuplicitas renum'.

1. There were two mesonephric ducts, from which arose two ureteric buds from the right and four from the left.
2. The lateral ureters on each side represent mesonephric systems, which persisted and continued to function. He postulated a single mesonephric duct on the left side and double on the right.
3. There were four mesonephric ducts; the two on the right side gave rise to one ureteric bud each, and the two on the left gave rise to two separate ureteric buds.
4. The extra kidneys and ureters were teratomatous.

Soderdahl et al. (1976) describe the upper urinary tracts of a male patient aged 21 years with bilateral reflux megaureters. The right ureter had four branches to the kidney, and on the left side, there were three long branches to the kidney, and one extra branch ended blindly.

Quintuplicate kidney and ureters

One specimen of quintuplicate ureters was available for dissection. The common stem bifurcated in the upper quarter of its length. The upper branch promptly divided into two ureters, one of which entered the upper pole, and the other the posterior part of the middle segment. The lower branch of the main stem divided into four short extrarenal infundibula; the longest infundibulum or 'ureter' subserving the anterior middle segment and the other three the lower pole. Thus the anterior and posterior middle segment calyces were subserved by ureters branching from the upper and lower main bifurcations.

A study was undertaken to examine the mechanism of obstruction caused by angulation of the ureter over the so-called 'aberrant' renal vessels and to explain the aetiology of this ureterovascular tangle. Obstruction undoubtedly accompanied the ureterovascular tangle, but whether the vessel, the ureter, or the bulging pelvis is the primary obstruction agent, is controversial. The term 'aberrant' favours the vessel as the primary cause, though this term in this context proved to be a misnomer.

Renal vessels: terminology

The terms used here to describe the renal arteries are those of Graves (1971) who demonstrated the extra- and intrarenal vascular trees of normal kidneys by means of coloured resin casts. He defined the normal segmental vessels and the normal variants, the 'aberrant' renal artery and the accessory artery. The renal artery arises from the aorta and divides into anterior and posterior branches. The anterior branch divides into upper and middle segmental branches to the corresponding anterior segments, and a lower segmental branch, which gives anterior and posterior divisions to the lower pole. The posterior branch arches over the pelvis and supplies the smaller posterior upper and middle segments and a small part of the lower pole. Most often these vessels enter the hilum of the kidney (Fig. 26.1).

The lower hilar segmental vessel, however, may arise from any point along the course of the main renal artery or from the aorta, and all are variants of the normal. When an artery enters the lower pole directly, it has been termed an 'accessory' or 'aberrant' vessel, but Graves (1971) found that these vessels were the main segmental vessels to the lower pole and were therefore neither accessory nor aberrant. This polar vessel may arise precociously from the renal artery, aorta, or

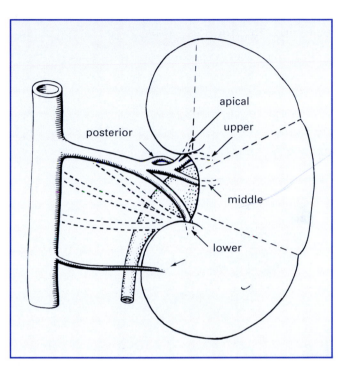

Fig. 26.1 *The renal artery and its main branches: variations in origin (dashed lines) of the lower segmental artery with its hilar insertion; alternate lower pole artery entering lower pole directly. (Reprinted, by permission, from Barnett, J.S. and Stephens, F.D. (1962), The role of the lower segmental vessel in the aetiology of hydronephrosis. Aust. N.Z. J. Surg. 31: 201, Fig. 1.)*

common or internal iliac arteries, but does not err from its intrarenal destination. In the following study of hydronephrosis caused by ureteropelvic obstruction and the ureterovascular tangle, the vessel implicated was the lower anterior hilar segmental artery.

Here we will present evidence, based on the normal intrarenal and extrarenal vascular anatomy described by Graves (1954), the implication of the lower hilar segmental vessels in nine patients and a specimen of horseshoe kidney with ureteropelvic obstructions, that the terms 'aberrant' and 'accessory' are misnomers.

*Reprinted, with changes, by permission of the Williams and Wilkins Co., from Stephens, F.D. (1982), Ureterovascular hydronephrosis and the 'aberrant' renal vessels. J. Urol. 128: 984. (The original study was undertaken by Barnett, J.S. and Stephens, F.D. (1962), Aust. N.Z. J. Surg. 31: 201.)

Ureterovascular hydronephrosis and the lie of renal vessels in other renal anomalies

Nine examples of ureterovascular hydronephrosis were studied in children at the time of operation. Two of the kidneys were excised and subjected to further examinations. One postmortem specimen of horseshoe kidney exhibiting bilateral nonrotated pelves and bilateral obstruction of the upper ureters by lower segmental vessels was also available.

The extrarenal vessels and pelviureteric junctions of 25 normal kidneys were examined for comparison by Barnett and Stephens (1962) and the anatomical rela-

tionships were found to concur with those of Graves (1971). In addition, the ureterovascular relations were observed in 47 specimens of hydronephrosis due to other causes, five specimens of non-rotated kidneys, and 35 horseshoe kidneys with and without non-rotated or incompletely rotated pelves.

The vascular tangle

Of 37 consecutive childhood patients with uretero-pelvic junction obstruction (UPJ) and hydronephrosis, the lower anterior hilar segmental vessels were implicated in nine (Barnett and Stephens, 1962). The anomaly was left-sided in all nine in this series, though

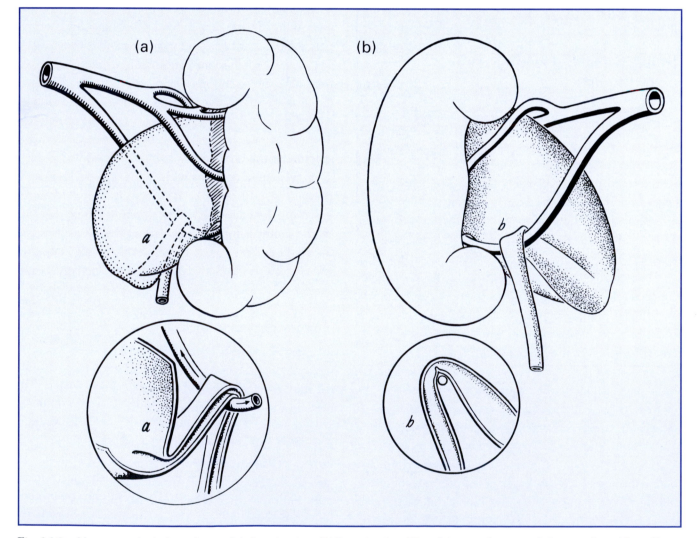

Fig. 26.2   *Ureterovascular hydronephroses. (a) Anterior view. (b) Posterior view. The pelvis protrudes anteriorly between the middle and lower segmental vessels angulating the UPJ and hooking the upper ureter over the vessel. Insets show the flattening and obstructive mechanisms at both the UPJ and the upper ureter. (Reprinted, by permission, from Barnett, J.S. and Stephens, F.D. (1962), The role of the lower segmental vessel in the aetiology of hydronephrosis. Aust. N.Z. J. Surg. 31: 201, Fig. 3.)*

it occurs rarely on the right side. In all, the vessels entered the hilum in the normal situation and in all, the pelvis bulged anteriorly between the lower and middle hilar segmental vessels (Figs 26.2 and 26.3). Since this series was analysed, other such patients have

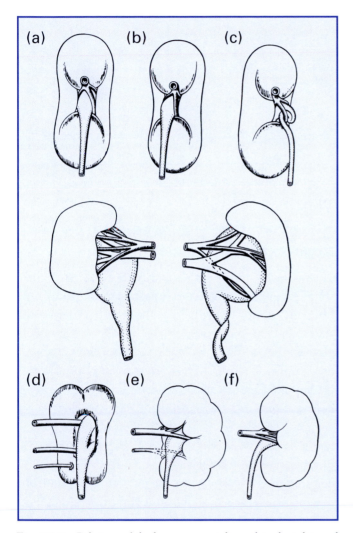

Fig. 26.3 *Relations of the lower segmental vessel to the pelvis and UPJ. (Upper row) (a), (b) The pelvis in normal mid- and posterior position and the artery resting anteriorly on the pelvis. (c) The pelvis anterior and the artery crosses in front of the UPJ to reach the hilum. (Middle row) The segmental vessels in hydronephroses associated with other urinary tract obstructions and with vesicoureteric reflux. The vessels arch over the anterior aspect of the enlarged pelvis cranial to the UPJ. (Lower row) Lower segmental vessels in unrotated (d), partially rotated (e) and fully rotated (f) kidneys and pelves. Note the abnormal medial entry into the hilum and lower pole in (d) and the normal lateral entry in (f). The vessel in (e) may gain harmless abnormal medial fixation or normal fixation with ureteral obstruction. (Reprinted, by permission, from Barnett, J.S. and Stephens, F.D. (1962), The role of the lower segmental vessel in the aetiology of hydronephrosis. Aust. N.Z. J. Surg. 31: 201 Figs 7, 9, and 10.)*

been treated surgically and the subsequent observations confirm these findings.

In bulging between the hilar segmental vessels, the expanding pelvis angulates the adjoining ureter at the UPJ and hooks the ureter over the lower segmental vessels, creating partial obstructions at both sites (Fig. 26.2). At the time of surgical exploration, the angulated ureter was found to be bound loosely by fascial adhesions to the pelvis. On manual compression of the pelvis or by topping up the pelvis with saline from a syringe, urine flowed into, and expanded, the segment of ureter between the UPJ and the vessel that demarcated the site of the second obstruction. Calibration at these sites revealed an elastic narrowing of the ureter at the site of crossing of the vessels in two, but normal or generous calibres in the remainder. Lifting the vessels off the pelvis and ureter and opening out the angulations by separation of the adhesions permitted free flow of urine and peristalsis along the ureter. In two patients, the near-functionless kidneys were removed and the ureters were examined microscopically. Hypertrophy of muscle was apparent above the vessels but no evidence of fibrosis or stricture at the UPJ or the site of the vessels was found.

It was concluded that with filling and bulging of the pelvis, the UPJ becomes flattened and hitched to the adjoining distended pelvis; with further filling, the slack in the ureter is further taken up as the ureter becomes taut and arches over the vessel, creating a second obstruction at the hook. Overfilling of the pelvis exaggerates the hook, which causes the painful crises.

The ureterovascular relationships in normal kidneys, in other hydronephroses and in non-rotated and horseshoe kidneys

The course of the lower hilar segmental vessels with respect to the UPJ was determined in specimens of normal kidneys, hydronephroses from other causes, malrotated kidneys and horseshoe kidneys.

1. In normal postmortem kidneys, the pelvis faced medially in 14, slightly anteromedially in one and posteromedially in nine, and was directed away from the vessels, which lay on a more anterior plane (Fig. 26.3).
2. The relationship of the lower hilar vessels to enlargements of the pelvis was studied in 47 examples of hydronephros associated with other intrinsic lesions

at the UPJ, lower ureteric or urethral obstructions and vesicoureteral reflux. In none did the vessels implicate the UPJ or ureter; the lower segmental vessels traversed an arc over the cranial aspect of the enlarged pelvis (Fig. 26.3).

3. Dissection of five specimens exhibiting non-rotation of the kidney revealed that the lower hilar segmental vessels entered the lower pole medial to the pelvis and that the UPJ was in no way disturbed by any of the vessels (Fig. 26.3).

4. The vessels to the lower pole in 34 of 35 horseshoe kidneys were found to enter the hilum or renal substance medial, inferior or superior to the UPJ (Cook and Stephens, 1977). Other vessels were also present entering the renal substance from the posterior aspect. The UPJ and upper ureters were not fouled by ureterovascular hooks or hitches in these 34 kidneys, which exhibited midline or lateral fusion with medial rotation or degrees of non-rotation or lateral rotation of the pelves. In one horseshoe kidney specimen, however, obtained from a boy of seven years who died from renal failure, the upper ends of the ureters were obstructed by the lower segmental vessels (Fig. 26.4). In this specimen, both

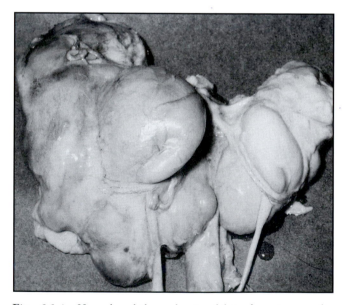

Fig. 26.4 *Horseshoe kidney showing bilateral ureterovascular hydronephroses and malrotated pelves; the lower segmental vessels compress the upper ureter against the lower pole and angulate the UPJ on each side. Note the distension of the segment of the ureter above the vessels. (Reprinted, by permission, from Stephens, F.D. (1983), Congenital Malformations of the Urinary Tract, New York, Praeger, Fig. 23.4, p. 376.)*

pelves faced anteriorly; the lower segmental vessels to each kidney crossed in front of the upper ends of the ureters to reach the lateral and embryologically normal sites of entry into the hila of the kidneys. The pelves, ureters, and UPJs above the sites of compression by the vessels were much dilated. The combination of non-rotation of the pelvis with a normal anatomical site of entry of the anterior lower segmental vessels into the hilum created a ureterovascular tangle, and a mortal danger to this child. Figure 26.4 shows clearly the obstructive hook at the vessels and hitch of the upper ureter to the pelvis. The confluence of the lumen of the pelvis with upper ureter at the UPJ consequent on long-standing hyperdilatation in this extreme state of fullness of the tract above the hook can also be seen.

An embryologic explanation of the ureterovascular tangle

During development and migration of the kidney at the time it is approaching its loin position, the pelvis turns from an anterior to medial orientation. It is during this stage of ascent and rotation that the kidney achieves its permanent blood supply developed from the network of mesonephric vessels. These vessels are arranged in ladder pattern from aorta to the mesonephros, and the kidney tunnels its way posterior to the vessels to reach the loin (Fig. 26.5). As the kidney climbs, it derives its blood supply seriatim from the higher and sheds the lower step of the vascular ladder. That which forms the definitive renal artery, traverses the upper anterior aspect of the pelvis to divide and enter the hilum of the kidney. If the definitive artery forms after rotation, it usually enters medially, and becomes posterior if rotation occurs. The ureteropelvic junction is not vulnerable to compression by the lower segmental artery in either case. However, if the definitive artery forms before or during rotation and gains entry into the hilus anterior to the pelvis, then the lower segmental vessel may lie across the UPJ. If then rotation is arrested as with the horseshoe kidney specimen (Fig. 26.4), or is retarded or incomplete, the pelvis remains fixed in its anterior orientation with respect to the renal vessels and the UPJ is vulnerable to compression against solid renal substance by the lower segmental branch. This anterior

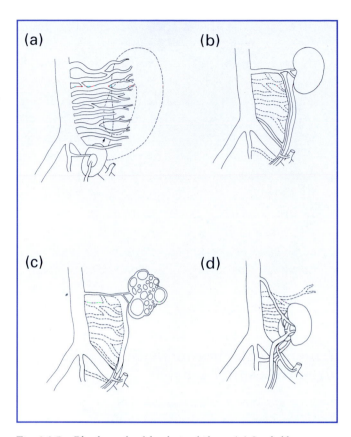

Fig. 26.5 *Blood vessels of developing kidney. (**a**) Stepladder arrangement of mesonephric vessels; kidney ascends behind the vessels and mesonephros (after Felix, 1912). (**b**) Definitive renal artery after stepwise takeover of higher mesonephric vessels and disappearance of most of lower vessels and persistence of marginal vessels on ureter. (**c**) Atresia of ureter and multicystic kidney, ischaemia of ureter and bud components of kidney resulting from presumed defective takeover or premature shutdown of mesonephric vessels. (**d**) Arrested migration and ectopic kidney with irregular anastomotic channels derived from the mesonephric vessels. (Reprinted, by permission, from Stephens, F.D. (1983), Congenital Malformations of the Urinary Tract, New York, Praeger, Fig. 23.5, p. 376.)*

pelvis then bulges between the middle and lower vessels, hooks up and acutely angulates the ureter over the artery, and causes ureteropelvic obstruction.

Though the anterior orientation of the pelvis occurs early in development of the embryo, the obstruction induced by the vessel being partial usually causes serious obstructive crises only when sufficient time has elapsed to permit severe pelvic ballooning. Hence the onset of the chief symptom of pain denoting intermittent obstructive crises may be delayed into school age or even later.

Since it was found that the ureterovascular tangle did not develop in other forms of hydronephrosis in which the pelvis was medially directed, it is reasonable to

attribute the primary aetiology of this condition to defective rotation of the renal pelvis. The lower hilar segmental vessels, which compressed the ureter, were not aberrant but were in the right place at the wrong time.

Diagnosis and treatment

In the preoperative search for the diagnosis of the ureterovascular tangle, the spherical anterior pelvis and the filling of the smaller proximal segment of ureter hitched to it, without filling of the ureter beyond, creates on pyelography a 'double-bubble' appearance, which is diagnostic of this double trouble (Fig. 26.6). This may be visible on the excretion urograph if the kidney function is brisk and good. Trap films taken following retrograde pyelography exhibit this same appearance if the pelvis is well opacified; if however, the ureter caudal to the hook is also opacified, the appearances are not necessarily diagnostic of the double obstruction so typical of the ureterovascular obstructions (Fig. 26.6). Aortography has been used effectively to demonstrate the lower segmental vessel winding around the anteriorly directed pelvis and ureter, but since exploration is the final measure for diagnosis and cure of symptoms, the patient may be spared this procedure.

In one specimen obtained from an elderly patient, the kidney was hydronephrotic and functionless, and the ureter at the site of the hook by the vessels was totally obstructed (Fig. 26.7). The lumen was occluded. This finding, together with the two ureters, which exhibited 'elastic' narrowings on calibration, may indicate that with time and recurrent tension on the ureter, the mucosa may become ischaemic and fibrose, stenose and finally close the lumen.

Graves (1956) found that the blood supply to the lower pole sometimes comes through an extrahilar lower polar vessel, in which case the hilar segmental vessel is not present. Because the segmental arteries are end arteries, the lower segmental vessel, wherever it enters the kidney, should not be divided as a means of undoing the tangle. The Anderson–Hynes dismembered pyeloplasty permits trimming of the ureteropelvic redundancy, eliminates any suspected intrinsic stenosis, preserves the viability of the lower pole, and allows the segmental vessels to lie harmlessly posterior to the reconstructed UPJ.

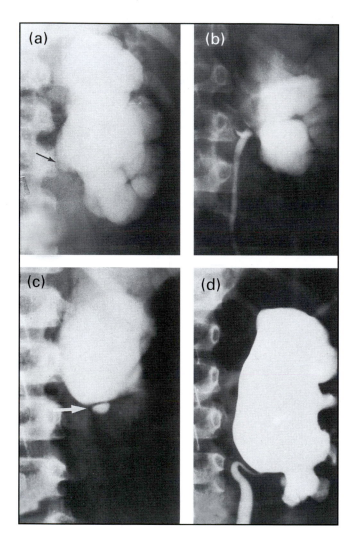

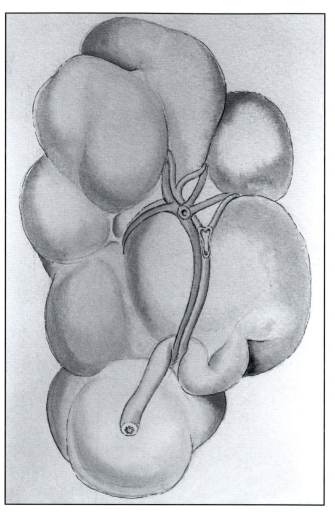

Fig. 26.6 *Retrograde pyelograms showing radiographic appearances of ureterovascular hydronephrosis and hydronephrosis caused by ureteropelvic fascial bands. (a) A three-hour trap film of P.L., aged eight years, showing globule of opaque medium held up between the UPJ (arrow) and the site of obstruction caused by the lower segmental vessels. (b) Infusion ureteropyelogram showing angulation at the site of crossing by the vessel and medium in the upper segment of the ureter. (c) A 30-minute trap film of W.B, aged eight years, with ureterovascular hydronephrosis, showing the outline of the anterior pelvis, filling defect at UPJ (arrow) and medium in the upper segment of the ureter, but not below it, and denoting the second obstruction caused by the vessel. (d) Infusion ureteropyelogram showing angulation and eccentric insertion of the upper ureter and obstruction at UPJ caused by fascial banding of ureter to pelvis. Note that the 'double bubble' with an empty ureter distal to it, as demonstrated on delayed trap films, is diagnostic of ureterovascular tangle, but the angulation seen during retrograde infusion ureterograms is non-specific. ((a), (b), (d), Reprinted, by permission, from Stephens, F.D. (1983), Congenital Malformations of the Urinary Tract, New York, Praeger, Fig. 23.6, p. 337. (c) reprinted, by permission, from Barnett, J.S. and Stephens, F.D. (1962), The role of the lower segmental vessel in the aetiology of hydronephrosis. Aust. N.Z. J. Surg. 31: 201, Fig. 2.)*

Fig. 26.7 *Medial aspect of a ureterovascular hydronephrosis removed from an elderly patient, demonstrating the anterior pelvis bulging between the middle and lower segmental vessels, with ureter hooked (and totally occluded) at the site of angulation by the vessels. (Reprinted, by permission, from Stephens, F.D. (1983), Congenital Malformations of the Urinary Tract, New York, Praeger, Fig. 23.7, p. 378.)*

The kidney

V

The normal development of the kidney was described in detail by Felix (1912b) and more recently by Potter (1972b) using data derived from microdissection of fetal kidneys. These authors have clarified many controversial issues concerning the nephron attachments to the collecting ducts, the formation of the capillary tufts and cystic dysplasia in the kidney. Those features of normal development, drawn mainly from the descriptions by Potter (1972b) that are pertinent to the particular renal anomalies will be described here.

The wolffian duct forms in the intermediate mesoderm of the embryo by the longitudinal linking of the nephron vesicles of the pronephros and mesonephros in the thoracolumbar regions. Its solid end grows caudally to enter the undivided cloaca at the 4-mm stage and then canalizes. At the same time that the cloaca is subdividing, the caudal segment of the wolffian duct, called the common mesonephric duct, is being incorporated into the posterior wall of the urogenital compartment. The ureteric bud arises from this segment where the duct turns to cross over the nephrogenic cord from its lateral to medial side. This common duct widens in a trumpet shape and exstrophies into the urinary tract where it becomes the urethrovesical trigone (Fig. 13.2a). In so doing, it achieves separate entry for the wolffian duct into the urethra and for the ureter into the bladder.

The hollow ureteric bud and the adjacent metanephric blastema gain contact, interact and combine in the formation of the kidney (Fig. 19.10). From the bud develop the ureter, calyces and the collecting ducts, and from the blastema, the nephronogenic and stromagenic structures. The bud contacts the terminal segment of the nephrogenic cord at the level of the future first sacral segment, elongates as the kidney migrates to the region of the second lumbar segment, and forms the calyces and collecting ducts. The metanephric blastema covers the primitive pelvis of the bud like a cap, and disconnects itself from the nephrogenic cord while in the sacral site and interacts with the bud during migration.

When settled in the lumbar region, it combines with the bud and differentiates into cortical structures. Contact between bud and metanephros occurs at four weeks' gestation (crown–rump length, 4 mm); migration of the kidney takes place between four and six weeks (16 mm) and nephronogenesis from six weeks to 34 weeks (see Fig. 27.3). The migratory path follows the cleavage plane behind the still-large mesonephros (and gonad) and the umbilical artery and in front of the iliac vessels. The kidney indents and arrests against the embryonic relatively massive suprarenal gland.

Architecture of the kidney and pelvis

Renal lobes

The architecture of the kidneys runs to a regular pattern. Upper, middle (hilar) and lower divisions are divided longitudinally into anterior and posterior lobes subserved by anterior and posterior calyces. The papillae in these calyces and their pyramids subserve lobules within the lobes. Interlobar and interlobular boundary lines are apparent as grooves on the surface of the fetal kidney, but are rarely visible in the mature kidney.

Calyces and lobules

The primary branchings of the ureteric bud determine the eventual pelvicalyceal patterns and their corresponding renal lobules. The bud may divide forming the double major calyx type or expand to form a pelvis. The double calyceal pattern is arranged as lower and upper major calyces with two middle or hilar calyces arising from either the lower or upper calyx (Fig. 27.1). More commonly, the bud dilates to form the pelvic type with multiple infundibulae communicating with minor calyces (Fig. 27.2) (Sykes, 1964).

The minor calyces in the fetal stage outnumber those in adult kidneys though the number of renal lobes and lobules stays much the same in the young and old. The reduction in number of minor calyces is brought about by fusion of some of the fetal calyces and papillae.

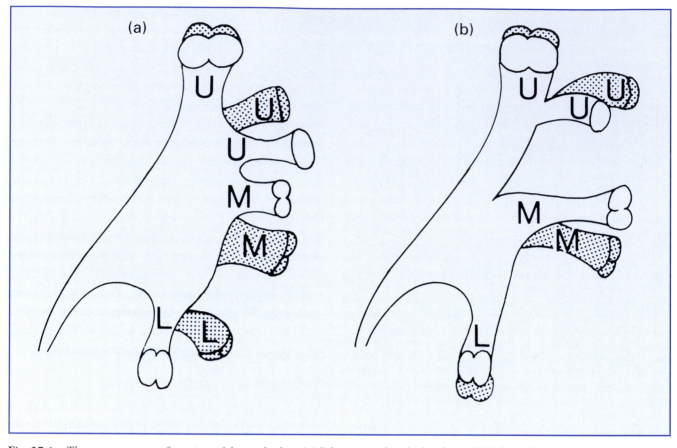

Fig. 27.1 *The two common configurations of the renal pelvis. (**a**) Pelvic type with multiple calyces. (**b**) Pelvis with double calyceal pattern (posterior calyces stippled; U, M and L denote upper, middle and lower calyces). (Reprinted, by permission, after Sykes, D. (1964), The morphology of renal lobulations and calyces: their relationship to partial nephrectomy. Br. J. Surg. 51: 294, Figs 13a and 14.)*

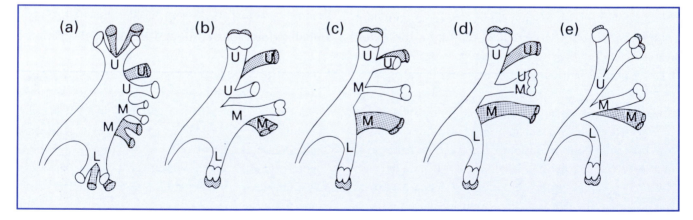

Fig. 27.2 *Variants in configuration and fusion of the minor calyces. (**a**) Pelvic type with non-fusion. (**b**) Wandering upper minor calyx and anteroposterior side-to-side fusions of minor calyces of upper and lower pole calyces, and longitudinal fusions of only the two anterior and two posterior calyces of the middle segment. (**c**) Stray middle calyces. (**d**) Linkage of upper and middle calyces. (**e**) Trifid pelvis. (Posterior calyces stippled; U, M and L denote upper, middle and lower calyces.) (Reprinted, by permission, from Stephens, F.D. (1983), Congenital Malformations of the Urinary Tract, New York, Praeger, Fig. 24.2, p. 387.)*

Usually the branchings of the polar and hilar calyces create approximately 14 minor calyces, around which are arranged 14 pyramids with their papillae. These 14 minor calyces subserve seven anterior and the corresponding seven smaller posterior lobules; three pairs in the upper pole, one pair each for the lobules of the hilar lobes and two pairs for the lower pole. In late fetal and early postnatal development, the calyceal number is reduced to eight, and the papillae to 10 or 11 by fusion. In the upper and lower poles, fusion occurs generally between anterior and posterior minor calyces, whereas in the middle lobes, the fusion occurs most frequently between anterior or posterior pairs of minor calyces (Sykes, 1964) (Fig. 27.2). Though the regular adult lobular pattern comprises about eight calyces and pyramids, sometimes there are many more.

The extreme complexity of the modelling and branching of the ampullae of the ureteric bud in the formation of its pelvis and calyces is conducive to variations of the normal shape and size of the pelvis and multiplicity of the minor calyces.

Extrarenal branchings of the bud

During the migratory period, the primitive pelvis of the ureteric bud dichotomizes into upper and lower poles and also forms anterior and posterior projections in the interpolar regions around which the upper middle and lower renal lobes develop. The pelvis flattens, and the polar and interpolar projections elongate and undergo repetitive dichotomous divisions. The first five such branchings in the poles and the first three in the interpolar projections dilate and coalesce into the renal pelvis and major calyces (Fig. 27.3).

A similar series of dichotomous branchings from the ends of those before takes place though even more rapidly, so that the dilating lumens become confluent concurrently with the branchings and form the minor calyces (Fig. 27.4). The linking branches between the first and second series remain relatively unexpanded as the infundibula between the major and minor calyces. The branchings peripheral to the calyx are the papillary ducts. Their orifices honeycomb the calyceal wall, which is known as the cribriform plate, and the ducts themselves being the third series of dichotomous branchings into the substance of the blastema. The cribriform plate is, at first, convex, but with proliferation of the nephric structures particularly the concentric growth of the loops of Henle, the plate flattens and finally inverts into the lumen of the calyx as the papilla. The pelvis and minor calyces undergo expansion contemporaneous with the appearance of the first nephrons, possibly in response to urine secretion (Potter, 1972c).

From here on, the papillary and collecting ducts and their ampullae react intimately with the nephronogenic and stromagenic mesenchyme to create functioning nephrons in continuity with the collecting systems.

Intrarenal branchings of the bud

The differentiation of the structures of the kidney, according to Potter (1972), can be considered in four stages of ampullary activity.

Stage I

This is the period of dichotomy, from the fifth week (4 mm) to the 14th or 15th week. The dichotomous ampullary divisions up to and including the period of

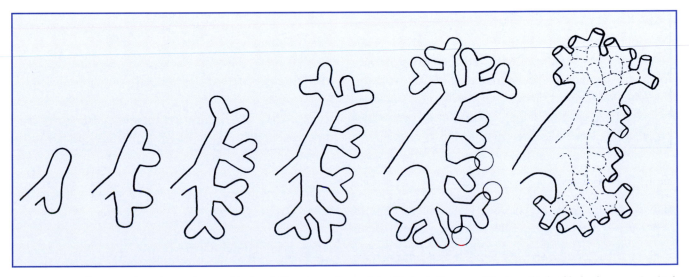

Fig. 27.3 *Dichotomous branchings of ureteral bud and dilatation to form pelvis. Circles indicate possible sites of infundibulae between the third, fourth or fifth generations and the next series of branchings and expansions that give rise to the minor calyces. (Reprinted, by permission, from Potter, E.L. (1972),* Normal and Abnormal Development of the Kidney. *Chicago: Year Book, Fig. 1.15, p. 15.)*

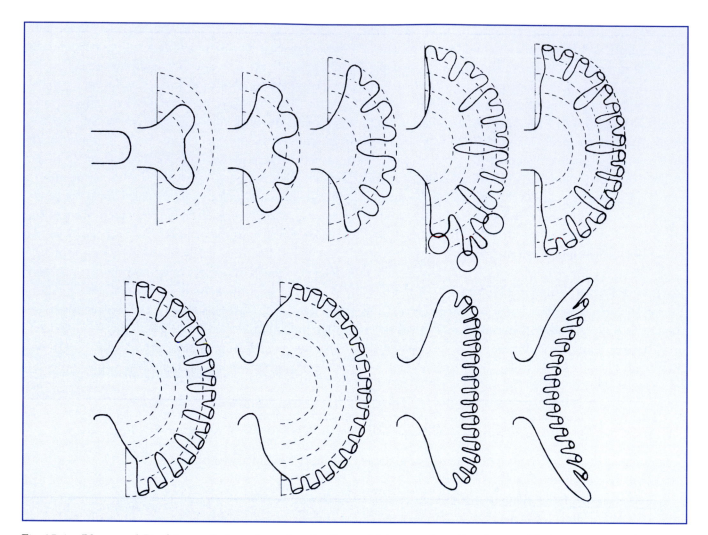

Fig. 27.4 *(Upper row) Development of minor calyx and papilla. Repeated dichotomous branchings for several further generations with resorption of septa forming the minor calyx. The circles indicate the generation at which the branch may remain unexpanded, forming a papillary duct. (Lower row) Multiplication and growth of nephrons in the parenchyma cause inversion of calyx and the papilla. (Reprinted, by permission, from Potter, E.L.(1972), Normal and Abnormal Development of the Kidney. Chicago: Year Book, Fig. 1.21, p. 20.)*

the migration of the kidney to the lumbar region (approximately sixth week) give rise to pelvis, calyces and papillary ducts, and from then to the 15th week, the ampullae undergo further dichotomous divisions forming the collecting ducts. The characteristic of the ampullae of Stage I is dichotomy into two new ampullae, each of which induces a nephron and, after linkage of the nephrons to it, grows a new stem and divides again into two more ampullae (Fig. 27.5). This performance repeats for seven or eight generations of nephrons, which link to collecting ducts that radiate fanwise from the papillae. The nephrons in Stage I rarely remain as functioning nephrons and usually degenerate.

Stage II of arcades

From 14–15 to 20–22 weeks, the ampullae no longer dichotomize, but grow peripherally, sequentially inducing arcades of four to six permanent nephrons (Fig. 27.6). The connecting tubules of these nephrons become successively linked together and linked to the advancing ampulla by a common channel. This complex changeover linkage creates the arcade from which several (two to eight) nephrons hang like catkins from a twig.

Stage III of straight stems

The ampulla, which formed the arcade in Stage II, stops arcading and grows peripherally. It induces nephrons,

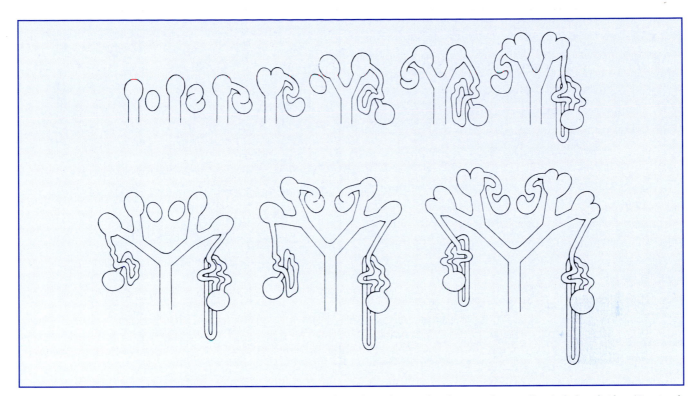

Fig. 27.5 *Stage I of ampullary activity: formation of collecting tubules and attachment of nephrons to the ampulla which then divides. (Reprinted, by permission, from Potter, E.L. (1972),* Normal and Abnormal Development of the Kidney. *Chicago: Year Book, Fig. 1.39, p. 32.)*

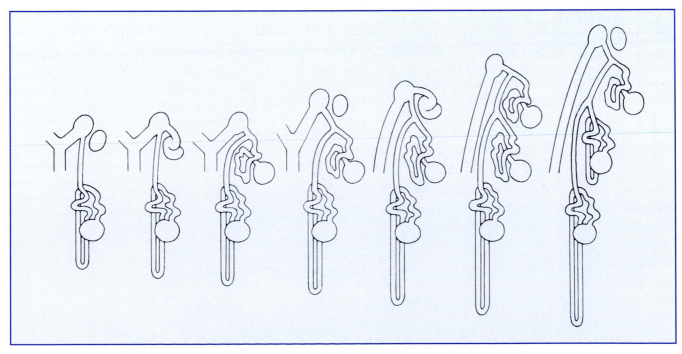

Fig. 27.6 *Stage II of ampullary activity: formation of arcades of nephrons attaching to ampulla by a linked composite connecting piece. (Reprinted, by permission, from Potter, E.L. (1972),* Normal and Abnormal Development of the Kidney. *Chicago: Year Book, Fig. 1.46, p. 36.)*

which connect seriatim with the newly formed collecting duct and drop behind as the ampulla advances. In this period from 20–22 to 32–36 weeks, four to six more nephrons are formed, and these lie nearest the capsule of the kidney and are the youngest and latest to form (Fig. 27.7). The method of ampullary division and connection of the nephron in all three periods is depicted in Fig. 27.8.

Stage IV of quiescence

Ampullary activity ceases and the kidney growth in the last six weeks of fetal life and during childhood is by maturation of those tubules and nephrons already present at the beginning of this period.

The nephron

The nephron vesicle

The metanephric blastema is at first a cap of metanephric mesoderm surrounding the ureteric bud. The nephrogenic constituents polarize in the upper, lower and mid-lobes around the primitive pelvis and major and middle calyces. When the collecting ducts and their ampullae penetrate the blastema, the nephrogenic cells palisade around each ampulla, and the lobes become partitioned into lobules. These cells undergo intense mitotic activity around each ampulla, and in the midst of each clump of cells, a lumen forms creating a vesicle. The development of the nephron from this stage, together with its manner of linkage to the connecting duct of the ampulla, runs to a standard pattern generation after generation.

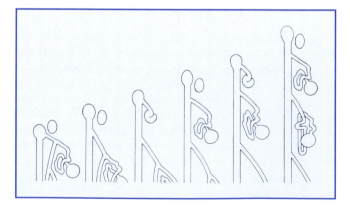

Fig. 27.7 *Stage III of ampullary activity: repeated direct attachments of nephrons to head of ampulla, receding along the collecting duct as ampulla advances peripherally. (Reprinted, by permission, from Potter, E.L. (1972), Normal and Abnormal Development of the Kidney. Chicago: Year Book, Fig. 1.55, p. 41.)*

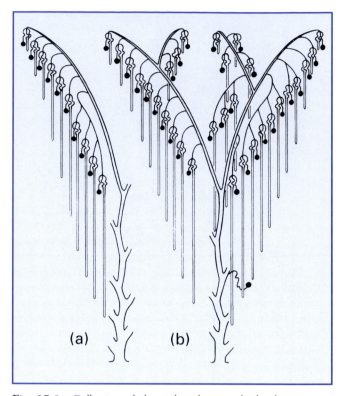

Fig. 27.8 *Collecting tubules and nephrons at birth, showing most common arrangement (a), with possible variations (b). (Reprinted, by permission, from Potter, E.L. (1972), Normal and Abnormal Development of the Kidney. Chicago: Year Book, Fig. 1.59, p. 43.)*

The vesicle indents from two sides, converting the lumen into the form of an 'S', one end of which attaches and canalizes in continuity with the ampullary connecting piece. The other end of the vesicle becomes cupped and is invaded by vascular mesenchyme, in which a capillary lake develops (Fig. 27.9). This capillary network of glomerulus is capped by the cells of the vesicle, which form Bowman's capsule, the lumen of which is Bowman's space. Together they form the malpighian corpuscle. The vesicle hangs from the connecting piece and grows lengthwise. The first part to elongate is the connecting piece, followed by Henle's loop, which grows centrally toward the pelvis, followed by the distal convoluted tubule, and finally the proximal convoluted tubule, which eventually becomes much longer relatively than the distal convolutions.

Differentiation

Differentiation of the components of the nephron from the first appearance of the vesicle to the stage when all its components are recognizable takes approximately

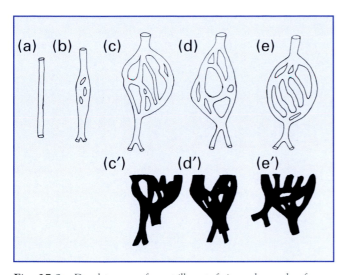

Fig. 27.9 *Development of a capillary tuft in a glomerulus from a simple capillary (**a**), which broadens and fenestrates (**b**), progressively to various patterns (**c**), (**d**) and (**e**), as shown by microdissection. (**c′**), (**d′**) and (**e′**) indicate the vascular network as it would appear if filled with India ink after the afferent and efferent vessels were approximated. (Reprinted, by permission, from Potter, E.L. (1972), Normal and Abnormal Development of the Kidney. Chicago: Year Book, Fig. 1.81, p. 54.)*

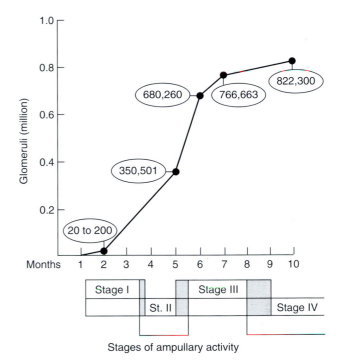

Fig. 27.10 *Rate curve showing increases in glomerular populations during fetal life. Total numbers of glomeruli in six fetal kidneys are shown in ellipses. Also shown are the four stages of ampullary activity in relation to glomerular population. (By permission, after Potter, E.L. (1972), quoting Osathanondh, V., in Normal and Abnormal Development of the Kidney. Chicago: Year Book, p. 73.)*

five weeks. As from about the stage of eight weeks (25-mm crown–rump length), the first vesicles appear and, from then on, until 34 weeks, new generations keep forming. After 34 weeks, new nephrons rarely appear, but those that are present continue to grow, elongate and mature during pre- and postnatal periods. The combined bulk of the loops of Henle and the proximal convoluted tubules contribute predominantly to the growth of the kidney in the postnatal period.

The absolute numbers of glomeruli (nephrons) counted in six kidneys by Osathanondh (quoted by Potter, 1972d), at eight weeks' gestation was 20 and 200 renal vesicles; at 20 weeks 350 501 glomeruli; at 24 weeks, 680 260; at 28 weeks, 766 663; and at 40 weeks, 822 300 nephrons (Fig. 27.10). Each mature kidney contains approximately one million nephrons.

Malformations of the renal ducts and nephrons

The extremely complex ampullary branchings and expansions that model the calyces and collecting ducts are conducive to variants, either normal or abnormal, of the pattern and structure of the collecting system. In addition, the intricate nature of the development and connection of the nephrons to the collecting ducts also contributes to parenchymal imperfections and cyst formations. It is possible that the primary embryologic error occurring in the ureteric bud may set in train a chain reaction affecting development of the ureter, pelvis, calyces and intrarenal structures (Fig. 27.11). Small programming errors could upset the pattern of development creating small or large pelves and calyces; too many of the dichotomous branchings could be taken up to form large calyces at the expense of the nephron-bearing ampullae, resulting in calyceal clubbing; collecting tubules and loops of Henle may be out of proportion, being too short, too long, or too wide; intrarenal cysts of Bowman's capsules or of tubules may result from unrestrained developmental expansions; the intricate capillaries that differentiate in the tuft may remain rudimentary; very rapid lengthening of the limb of the nephron tubules and loops of Henle and gaps in the accompanying network of vessels may result in ischaemia and isolated obstructive cyst formation.

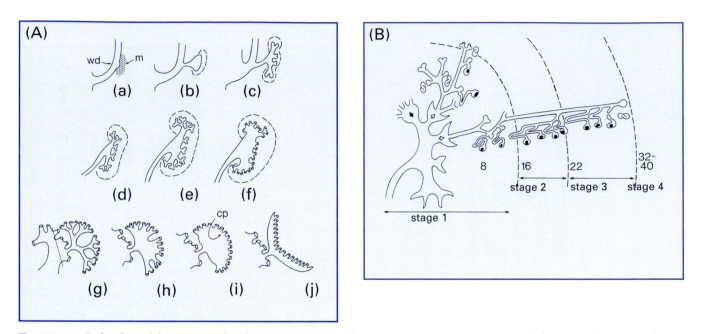

Fig. 27.11 *Embryology of the ureteric and nephronic components of the upper urinary tract. **A**, programmed the ureteric bud. (**a**) Bud arises from wolffian duct (wd) and penetrates metanephric mesenchyme (m). (**b**) Mesenchyme caps the expanded end of the bud. (**c**) Bud develops polar, hilar, and ampullary projections, which dichotomize. (**d**, **e**) More dichotomous divisions. (**f**) Confluence of the lumens of the divisions forming pelvis and major calyces. (**g**) Second series of ampullary divisions forming minor calyx (shown in one only). (**h**) Confluence of lumens except first division, which forms the infundibulum. (**i**) Expansion of the lumen to form rounded minor calyx with orifices of the papillary ducts in the convex cribriform plate (cp). (**j**) Inversion of the plate to form the papilla. **B**, The nephronic components. The minor calyces are shown in their early spherical shape with cribriform plate (black arrow) and later indented, forming papilla (open arrow). Nephrons develop in periods according to the nature of ampullary activity. Stage I. 5 to 15 weeks—nephrons induced by dichotomizing ampullae of branching collecting ducts. Stage II. 16 to 21 weeks—the ampulla induces nephrons, which are linked by a common duct to a collecting duct, the so-called arcades in the inner cortex. Stage III. 22 to 32 weeks—the ampulla advances toward the capsule, inducing nephrons, which connect independently to its newly formed collecting duct in the outer cortex. Stage IV. 32 to 40 weeks—the ampullae rarely divide, and the already established nephrons mature. (**A**, reprinted from Cook, W.A. and Stephens, F.D., after Potter, E.L. (1972), In Normal and Abnormal Development of the Kidney. Chicago: Year Book, Figs 1.15 and 1.21, pp. 15 and 21. **B**, reprinted from Cook, W.A. and Stephens, F.D. (1988), Urologic anomalies. In Diseases of the Kidneys, R.W. Schrier and C.W. Gottschalk (eds). Boston: Little, Brown, Fig. 22.10B, p. 706.)*

The nephrogenic cord being mesoblastic in origin and derived from the primitive streak, contains multipotential mesodermal cells. Most cells differentiate into nephronic or regular stromal tissue. Some, however, fail to differentiate and form fibrous tissue, collagen, muscle, cartilage, or even bone. Undifferentiated mesodermal structures may appear as isolated clumps or plaques of cells in an otherwise normal kidney or replace nephronic structures forming, in the extreme example, the mesoblastic nephroma.

In the absence of a ureteric bud, the kidney does not form. With ureteral atresia, the kidneys may be multicystic and hypodysplastic. If ectopic locations of the ureteric orifices are expressions of abnormal origins of ureteric buds, then the abnormal collecting systems and intrarenal parenchymal defects associated with them may also be components of a panbud deformity.

Nephron hypoplasia and dysplasia are not infrequent accompaniments of reflux megaureters with or without lower tract obstruction (Fig. 27.12). Abnormal urodynamics of reflux and partial obstruction occurring at highly active developmental phases of embryonic and fetal growth may cause dysgenesis of the collecting or parenchymal structures. The familiar association of renal lesions with vesicoureteral reflux and partial obstruction of the urethra has led to the assumption that the renal disturbances and upper-tract dilatation result from the effects of the abnormal urodynamics *in utero* upon the developing structures. Kidneys, however, can develop normally in the presence of reflux or incomplete obstruction, and numerous studies have been undertaken on kidneys of babies to evaluate the primary or secondary nature of these renal lesions.

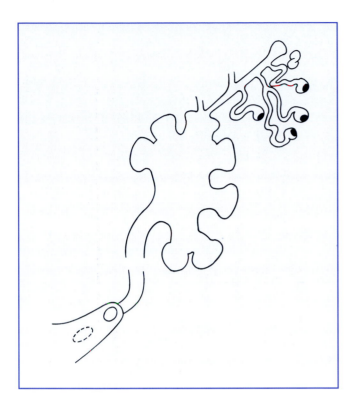

Fig. 27.12 *Development of upper urinary tract associated with lateral ectopic ureteric orifice. Note ureterocaliectasis, irregular inductions of nephrons and oligonephronia. (Reprinted, by permission, from Stephens, F.D. (1995), Embryology of the upper genitourinary tract. In Paediatric Urology, 3rd edn, S. Koff and B. O'Donnell (eds). London: Butterworth Heinemann, Fig. 5A.)*

Mackie and Stephens (1975) and Mackie *et al.* (1975) found that renal morphology depended on the normal or abnormal position of the ureteric orifices in patients with duplex ureters (Fig. 30.2). Henneberry and Stephens (1980) correlated renal hypodysplasia with lateral ureteric ectopy in urethral valve patients (Chapter 33 page 341). Schwarz *et al.* (1981) compared the abnormal renal morphology of infants' kidneys associated with vesicoureteral reflux, partial urethral obstruction, and ureteral obstruction complete and incomplete, to determine whether the abnormal morphology resulted from abnormal urodynamics acting initially upon normally developing kidneys or whether the ureteric bud and metanephric blastema were malformed *ab initio.*

Correlations obtained by W.F. Heale (pers. comm. (F.D.S.)) of ureteric orifice shape and position with shape and size of calyces and overall ureteric dimensions in patients with vesicoureteral reflux and reflux nephropathy implicate the ureteric bud as the primary defect

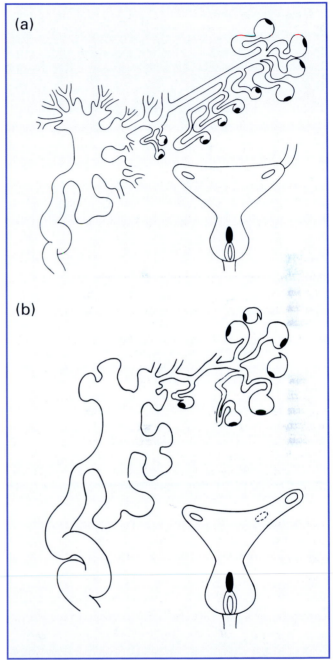

Fig. 27.13 *Development of the upper tract associated with partial urethral obstruction caused by urethral valve. (**a**) With ureteric orifice in normal position, ureterocaliectasis, glomerular cysts and normal array of nephrons (cf. Fig. 27.10). (**b**) With ureteric orifice laterally situated, maximum ureterocaliectasis and derangement of collecting tubules and nephrons and cystic glomeruli. Inset, trigone denoting orifice positions and prostatic urethra with verumontanum (black) and valve cusps of Type 1 valves. (Reprinted, by permission, from Stephens, F.D. (1995), Embryology of the upper genitourinary tract. In Paediatric Urology, 3rd edn, S. Koff and B. O'Donnell (eds). London: Butterworth Heinemann, Fig. 5B, C.)*

and the combined megaureteronephropathy as the consequence of its intrinsic maldevelopment.

Renal development in the presence of incomplete obstruction such as stenosis of the ureter at any level occurs along normal lines but back pressure causes general dilatation of pelvis, calyces, ducts and tubules, and cystic dilatation of Bowman's capsules. The ureteric orifice position is normally located in these lesions. Development in the presence of complete obstruction in the ureter causes extreme disruption of the kidney (see Fig. 14.2). The atretic process is ischaemic in origin and may result in an imperforate diaphragm in the ureter with obstructive hydronephrosis and intercommunicating dilated ducts and cysts and arrest of nephron induction or it may extend through ureter and pelvis, through ducts and tubules causing obstructive cysts of ampullae and nephrons or extreme hypodysplasia or a mixture of both. The ischaemic process continues in some kidneys after birth accounting for gradual diminution in size or even disappearance of the kidney.

The effects of partial urethral obstruction or renal development are similar to those caused by partial obstruction of the ureter if the ureteric orifice position on the trigone is normal (Fig. 27.13a). If, however, the ureteric orifice is laterally ectopic the defective ectopic bud lacks full inductive properties resulting in disorganization of ampullae and nephrons and oligonephronia (Fig. 27.13b). Those nephrons that are formed early undergo general changes caused by back pressure. Complete urethral obstruction causes back pressure on any functioning nephrons and arrest of all subsequent inductions whatever the position of the ureteric orifice.

It should be noted that fistula formation between bladder and amnion or dialysis of urine from renal duct system or vesical diverticula into the peritoneal cavity may in some foetuses with urethral obstruction partially eliminate the effects of back pressure.

28

Fused kidneys: morphologic study and a theory of embryogenesis*

A study was made of 50 fused kidneys, a fused kidney being a conglomerate of renal tissue, the ureters of which issue into both sides of the bladder. The observed morphologic renal patterns were correlated with co-existing anomalies in the genitourinary and other organ systems. A theory of embryogenesis was developed to explain asymmetric patterns of renal fusion.

Though two types of renal fusion have been generally recognized—horseshoe kidney and crossed renal ectopia—there is a rich diversity in the gross configuration of fused kidneys. The L-shaped kidney, in particular, has seemed to be a transition form between horseshoe kidney and crossed renal ectopia (Wilmer, 1938). In this chapter, a horseshoe kidney is defined as a fused kidney that occupies space on both sides of the vertebral column, the ureters of which do not cross the midline before entering the renal sinuses. A crossed fused ectopic kidney is one that lies almost entirely on one side of the midline, the contralateral ureter of which crosses the midline before entering the renal sinus. The former was originally described by da Carpi in 1522 and the latter by Panarolus in 1654 (quoted by Wilmer, 1938).

Campbell (1951f) found the incidence of horseshoe kidney to be 1 in 405 autopsies and that of crossed fused ectopia to be 1 in 1300 in his autopsy series, with males predominating in both instances. The studies of Gutierrez (1931), Abeshouse (1947), Glenn (1959), Kolln et al. (1972), Kelalis et al. (1973) and Hendren et al. (1976), have illustrated the morbidity associated with these anomalies, which makes their recognition important to the urologist. Understanding the embryologic basis of renal fusion and the associated hydronephrosis and renal dysfunction enhances awareness and promotes effective therapy.

Forty-one specimens were collected at postmortem examination—35 horseshoe and six crossed renal ectopic kidneys. Thirty-nine of the specimens were obtained from stillborn babies or neonates, and two were from older individuals. The specimens were subjected to careful gross dissection and radiographic study. The records and X-rays of eight patients with crossed renal ectopia and one with horseshoe kidney were also reviewed. Males predominated with ratios of 25:11 and 12:2 in individuals with horseshoe kidney and crossed renal ectopia, respectively (Table 28.1).

Two of the 41 deaths were attributable to urinary tract disease. Renal failure was the cause of death in one neonate with crossed renal ectopia, bilateral megaureter and hypoplastic renal tissue. A seven-year-old child with horseshoe kidney and bilateral vascular ureteropelvic junction obstruction died from septicaemia associated with urinary tract infection. The remaining deaths were due chiefly to prematurity or cardiopulmonary anomalies. Seven of the nine living patients presented with urological complaints; the remaining two had abdominal pain.

Table 28.1 *Fused kidneys*

Horseshoe kidneys[*]		Crossed renal ectopia[**]	
Postmortem specimens	35	Postmortem specimens	8
Stillborns	9	Living patients	8
Neonates	24		
Other	2		
Living patients	1		
Total numbers of cases	36[*]		14[**]

[*](25 males, 11 females). [**](12 males, 2 females).
Source: Adapted from Cook, W.A. and Stephens, F.D. (1977), Fused kidneys: morphologic study and theory of embryogenesis, in *Urinary System Malformations in Children*. Bergsma, D. and Duckett, J.W. (eds) *Birth Defects*, Original Article Series XIII(5), New York, Alan R. Liss, for National Foundation, March of Dimes, BD:OAS XIII(5): 328, Table 1.

*Reprinted with changes, by permission of the publisher, from Cook, W.A. and Stephens, F.D. (1977), Fused kidneys: morphologic study and theory of embryogenesis, in Urinary System Malformations in Children. D. Bergsma and J.W. Duckett (eds). New York: Alan R. Liss for the National Foundation, March of Dimes, BD:OAS XIII(5): 327–340.

Horseshoe kidney

Horseshoe kidneys were categorized on the basis of their relationship to the vertebral column. Two patterns were recognized: midline fusion and lateral fusion of the renal units. In the lateral fusion one of the pelvicalyceal systems drained a portion of renal tissue, which extended across the midline.

The orientation of the renal pelves was correlated with the craniocaudal width of the isthmus in the midline fused group. When the width of the isthmus was less than one-third renal length, the pelves were medially or antero-medially oriented to their respective renal units. When the isthmus was equal to or greater than one-third renal length, the pelves were anteriorly or laterally oriented. In the laterally fused group, which included the majority of L-shaped kidneys, the pelvis of the upright unit generally exhibited a medial orientation, whereas that of the trans-verse unit exhibited a lateral orientation (Fig. 28.1).

Crossed fused ectopic kidneys

Among the 14 crossed fused ectopic kidneys, the con-tralateral ureter served the lower renal unit in 12 instances, and the upper unit in one. There was one example of fusion in which the pelves were side-by-side. The orientation of the pelves of the contralateral and ipsilateral ureters varied. In some instances, both pelves faced the same direction, either medial, anterior, or lateral, but in other instances, the pelves were oriented in different directions with respect to each other.

Associated anomalies

A wide variety of coexisting genitourinary anomalies were identified (Table 28.2). Hydronephrosis occurred most frequently (46 of 103 ureters) and was categorized as reflux (27 ureters), obstruction (eight ureters) and megaureter, the aetiology of which was indeterminate (11 ureters). These conditions were correlated with the types of fused kidneys in which they were found (Table 28.3). The occurrence of hydronephrosis in midline fused kidneys (6 of 31 ureters) was much less frequent than in laterally fused kidneys (22 of 43 ureters) and crossed fused upper pole ureter kidneys (18 of 29 ureters). Only three instances of hydronephrosis due to extrinsic ureteral compression occurred—two vascular ureteropelvic junction obstructions associated with anteriorly oriented renal pelves and a third ureter,

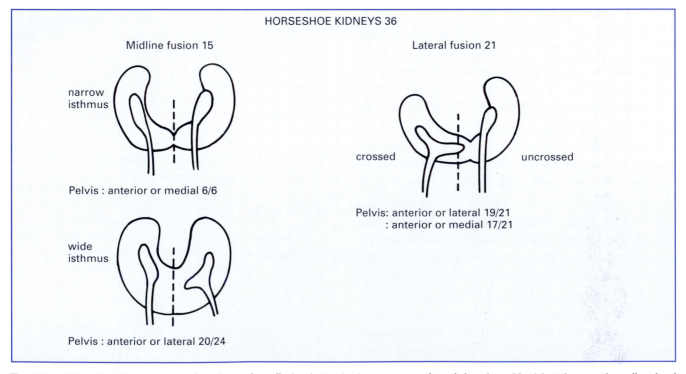

Fig. 28.1 *Horseshoe kidneys were either midline or laterally fused. Renal pelvis orientation depended on the width of the isthmus in the midline fused groups and on the position of the individual renal components in the laterally fused group. (Reprinted, by permission, from Cook, W.A. and Stephens, F.D. (1977), Fused kidneys: morphologic study and theory of embryogenesis, in Urinary System Malformations in Children, D. Bergsma and J.W. Duckett (eds) New York: Alan R. Liss for the National Foundation, March of Dimes, BD:OAS XII(5): 329, Fig. 1, p. 329.)*

Table 28.2 *Associated genitourinary abnormalities*

Abnormalities	Horseshoe (n = 36)	Crossed renal ectopia (n = 14)
Hydronephrosis	28/74 ureters	18/29 ureters
Genital	5	3
Duplication	2	4
Renal cystic disease	1	1
Exstrophy	1	0
Urethral valves	0	1

Source: Cook, W.A. and Stephens, F.D. (1977), Fused kidneys: morphologic study and theory of embryogenesis, in *Urinary System Malformations in Children*. Bergsma, D. and Duckett, J.W. (eds) *Birth defects*, Original Article Series XIII(5), New York, Alan R. Liss, for National Foundation, March of Dimes, BD:OAS XIII(5): 330, Table 2.

Table 28.3 *Correlation of fused kidney type with aetiology of hydronephrosis*

Aetiology	Midline fusion (n = 15)	Lateral fusion (n = 21)	Crossed renal ectopia (n = 14)
Reflux	2/31 ureters	12/43 ureters	13/29 ureters
Obstruction		6/43 ureters	2/29 ureters
Megaureter (? aetiology)	4/31 ureters	4/43 ureters	3/29 ureters

Source: Cook, W.A. and Stephens, F.D. (1977), Fused kidneys: morphologic study and theory of embryogenesis, in *Urinary System Malformations in Children*. Bergsma, D. and Duckett, J.W. (eds) *Birth defects*, Original Article Series XIII(5), New York, Alan R. Liss, for National Foundation, March of Dimes, BD:OAS XIII(5): 330, Table 3.

which was embedded in the isthmus of a laterally fused horseshoe kidney.

In the present series, comprised mainly of single ureters, the precise location of 45 ureteral orifices was correlated with the radiographical and the morphological character of the corresponding ureters and renal segments (Mackie and Stephens, 1975) (Chapter 30). Twelve of 14 ureteral orifices located in the 'A' position had normal upper tracts. All 19 lateral ectopic orifices ('B', 'C' and 'D' positions) were associated with reflux hydronephrosis. Eleven of 12 orifices in positions 'E', 'F', 'G' and 'H' were associated with hydronephrosis of varied aetiology (Table 28.4). It was apparent that a normally located orifice presaged normal parenchymal development, whereas abnormal locations portended deformities of the ureter and pelvis.

There was an appreciable incidence of anomalies in other organ systems (Table 28.5). Considered note-

Table 28.4 *Correlation of ureteral orifice position with appearance of upper tract*

Ureteral orifice position (n = 45)	Upper tract appearance	n
A (14)	Normal	12
	Reflux	1
	Cystic	1
B (4)	Reflux	4
C (14)	Reflux	1
D (1)	Reflux	1
E (3)	Reflux	1
	Cystic	1
	Megaureter (? aetiology)	1
F (4)	Reflux	2
	Megaureter (? aetiology)	2
G (3)	Megaureter (? aetiology)	3
H (2)	Obstruction	2

Source: Cook, W.A. and Stephens, F.D. (1977), Fused kidneys: morphologic study and theory of embryogenesis, in *Urinary System Malformations in Children*. Bergsma, D. and Duckett, J.W. (eds) *Birth Defects*, Original Article Series XIII(5), New York, Alan R. Liss, for the National Foundation, March of Dimes BD:OAS XIII(5): 332, Table 4.

Table 28.5 *Anomalies in other organ systems*

System	Midline fusion (n =15)	Lateral fusion (n =21)	Crossed ectopic (n =14)
Cardiopulmonary	8	13	4
Gastrointestinal (high anorectal agenesis)	2	8 (4)	9 (5)
Neurologic (vertebral)	3 (2)	7 (5)	5 (5)
Peripheral skeletal	5	6	3
Facial	1	4	0
Chromosomal	2	2	1
Omphalocele	2	1	0
Total:	23	41	22

Source: Cook, W.A. and Stephens, F.D. (1977), Fused kidneys: morphologic study and theory of embryogenesis, in *Urinary System Malformations in Children*. Bergsma, D. and Duckett, J.W. (eds) *Birth Defects*, Original Article Series XIII(5), New York, Alan R. Liss, for the National Foundation, March of Dimes, BD:OAS XIII(5): 332, Table 5.

worthy with respect to embryogenesis were the anorectal and the vertebral malformations, which included scoliosis, spina bifida with myelomeningocele, hemivertebrae and sacral agenesis. Nine examples of high anorectal agenesis were recorded among the laterally fused horseshoe kidneys and the crossed fused ectopic kidneys, whereas none was found in the midline fused horseshoe kidneys. Eight examples were noted of co-existing vertebral and anorectal anomalies, four each in the laterally fused and crossed fused groups.

Embryogenesis

The development of the kidneys depends upon the union of the ureteric buds and nephrogenic cords in the embryo of four weeks' gestation (Kiebel and Mall, 1912). The embryo at this age is approximately 5 mm (crown–rump length) and exhibits a marked degree of anterior flexion of the hind end (Arey, 1974d). The nephrogenic cords are the caudal ends of the mesonephric ridges, which hug the posterolateral body wall following the curvature of the spine. The wolffian ducts cling to their lateral aspects on the posterior body wall, except at their caudal ends, where the ducts lift off the back wall and cross anteriorly and medially over the nephrogenic cords to meet the cloaca (Figs 28.2 and 28.3). A ureteric bud arises from the posterior aspect of the 'knee' or point of angulation of the wolffian duct, which floats over the anterior aspect of the nephrogenic cord (Meyer, 1946). This occurs at the approximate level of the first or second sacral segment.

Subsequent growth and straightening of the hind end together with differential growth of the developing pelvic structures including the kidneys leads to relative ascent of the kidneys to the dorsolumbar region. By the seventh week (17-mm stage), the kidneys have emerged from the pelvis, and by the ninth week (30-mm stage), they have assumed their near-final position, far removed from their initial position adjacent to the orifice of the ureteric bud (Gruenwald, 1943).

Two embryological explanations of renal fusion are feasible: fusion of parenchymal elements from both nephrogenic bodies or development of a fused kidney from a single nephrogenic cord that has been met by the

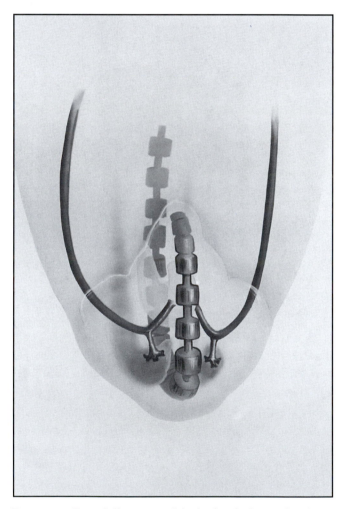

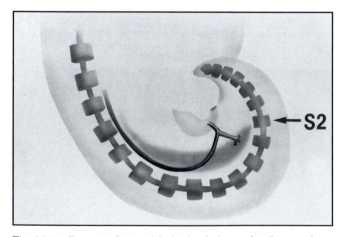

Fig. 28.2 *Parasagittal view of the hind end of normal 4–5-mm embryo, demonstrating the anterior flexion of the 'tail' and the relationship of the terminal wolffian duct to the nephrogenic body and to the second sacral vertebra (S2). (Reprinted, by permission, from Cook, W.A. and Stephens, F.D. (1977), Fused kidneys: morphologic study and theory of embryogenesis, in D. Bergsma and J.W. Duckett (eds) Urinary System Malformations in Children. New York: Alan R. Liss for the National Foundation, March of Dimes, BD:OAS XII(5): Fig. 3, p. 333.)*

Fig. 28.3 *Frontal illustration of the hind end of normal 4–5-mm embryo, demonstrating the anterior flexion of the 'tail' of the trunk and the relationship of the terminal wolffian duct and body to the 'tail'. (Reprinted, by permission, from Cook, W.A. and Stephens, F.D. (1977), Fused kidneys: morphologic study and theory of embryogenesis, in D. Bergsma and J.W. Duckett (eds) Urinary System Malformations in Children. New York: Alan R. Liss for the National Foundation, March of Dimes, BD:OAS XII(5): Fig. 4, p. 334.)*

ureteric buds arising from both wolffian ducts. In the first instance, the morphological pattern corresponds to a horseshoe kidney, whereas, in the second, the resultant kidney exemplifies crossed renal ectopia.

Symmetric renal fusion

Renal fusion, presumably, occurs during the early stages (5–12 mm) of renal genesis before the enlarging kidneys have migrated from their points of origin in the relatively confined true pelvis and before the renal capsule has matured (Friedland and De Vries, 1975). Midline fusion is a symmetric phenomenon and thus results from aberrations that influence the relative positions of both renal masses equally with respect to the midline. Abnormal variations in growth or ventral flexion of the hind end, for example, may limit the

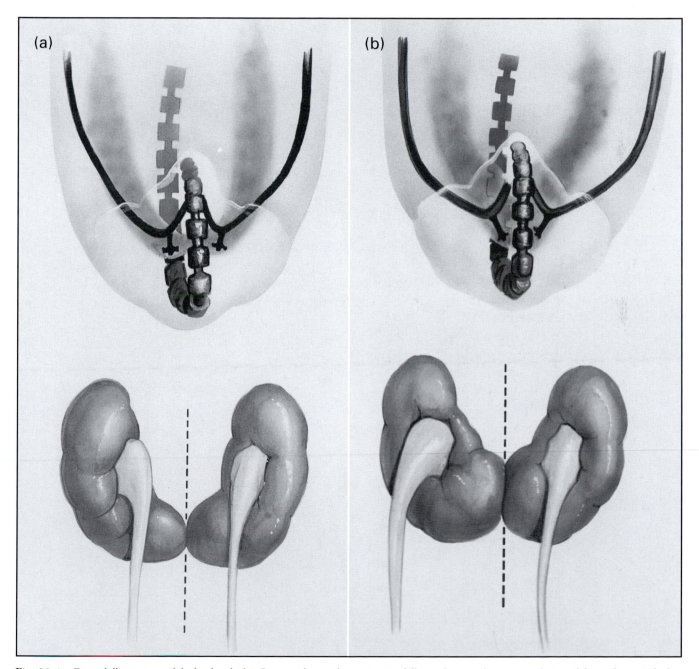

Fig. 28.4 *Frontal illustrations of the hind end of 4–5-mm embryos, demonstrating different degrees of symmetric fusion of the nephrogenic bodies* **(a)**, **(b)**. *(Reprinted, by permission, from Cook, W.A. and Stephens, F.D. (1977), Fused kidneys: morphologic study and theory of embryogenesis, in D. Bergsma and J.W. Duckett (eds) Urinary System Malformations in Children. New York: Alan R. Liss for National Foundation, March of Dimes, BD:OAS XII(5): Fig. 5, p. 335.)*

space available in the pelvis or cause caudal or medial prolongation of the nephrogenic cords. Delayed straightening of the hind end may defer renal ascent long enough that midline fusion of the enlarging kidney occurs (Fig. 28.4).

Asymmetric renal fusion

Laterally fused horseshoe kidneys and crossed renal ectopia are asymmetric conditions requiring a theory of embryogenesis that dictates differential placement of the paired primordial structures with respect to the

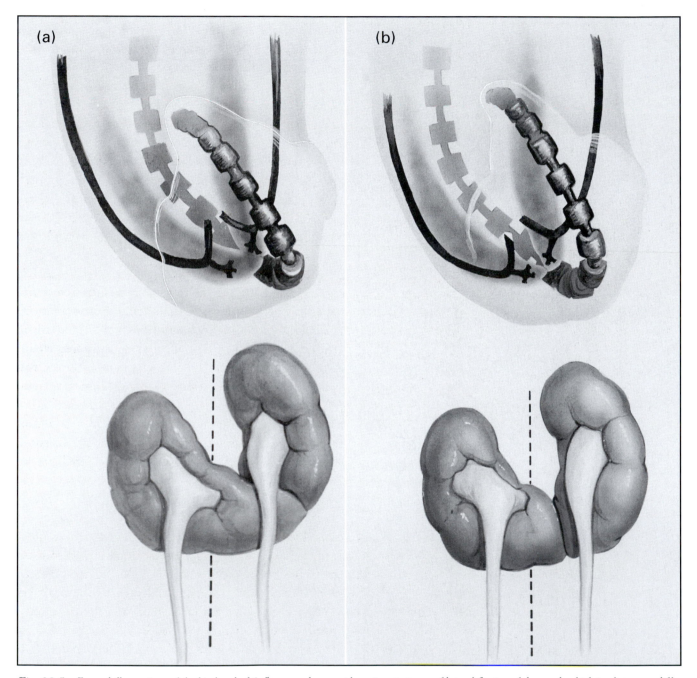

Fig. 28.5 *Frontal illustrations of the hind end of 4–5-mm embryos with various patterns of lateral flexion of the trunk which predispose to different configurations of renal fusion* (**a**), (**b**), (**c**), *all of which assume an asymmetric location with respect to the midline with renal ascent, exemplifying laterally fused horseshoe kidneys. (Reprinted, by permission, from Cook, W.A. and Stephens, F.D. (1977), Fused kidneys: morphologic study and theory of embryogenesis, in D. Bergsma and J.W. Duckett (eds) Urinary System Malformations in Children. New York: Alan R. Liss for the National Foundation, March of Dimes, BD:OAS XII(5): Fig. 6, p. 336.)*

midline. Asymmetric renal fusion can be explained by the effects lateral flexion of the trunk and rotation of the hind end may exert on the developing nephrogenic cords and wolffian ducts.

Lateral fusion

The nephrogenic cords occupy a posterior position behind the body cavity and run parallel with the spine of the embryo. Assuming that the developing lumbosacral spine undergoes exaggerated lateral flexion, the distal portion of the nephrogenic cord on the convex side of the spine may be deviated toward the midline (Brown, 1931; Meyer, 1946). The nephrogenic cord on the concave side may be deviated laterally but

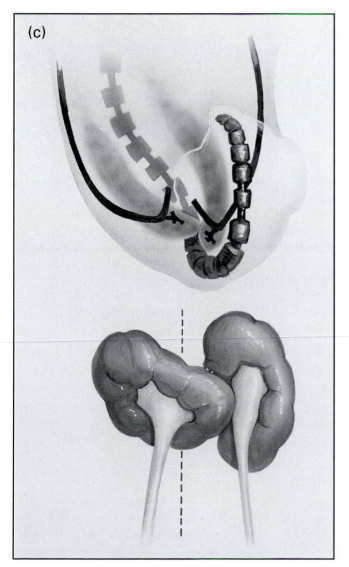

(c)

Fig. 28.5 *(continued)*

is hemmed in by the pelvic side wall. If this relative crowding occurs at the time of renal genesis, it may predispose to fusion of the developing kidneys. The point of fusion is initially close to the midline with respect to the primitive sacral vertebrae, but, as the hind end straightens and the fused kidneys ascend cranially, the point of fusion comes to lie on the concave side of the spine. Thus, the resultant horse-shoe kidney is asymmetric with respect to the midline (Fig. 28.5a,b,c).

Crossed fusion

The ureteral buds arise from points on the wolffian ducts that are anterior to the nephrogenic cords in the ventrally flexed hind end. Lateral flexion and rotation of the 'tail' may carry the cloaca and its attached wolffian ducts across the midline over to either side of the trunk. Thus, the position of the ureteric buds relative to the midline may be affected by abnormal orientation of the 'tail' relative to the trunk.

In the extreme, this may allow both right and left ureteric buds to overlie and induce either one of the nephrogenic bodies, thus inducing crossed renal ectopia. The gross configuration of the involved nephrogenic cord may be affected by associated lateral flexion of the trunk. The orientation of the ureters to the future kidney depends on the relative positions of the ureteral buds and the involved nephrogenic cord. Thus, the crossed ureter and its pelvis may be either superiorly or inferiorly located, and pelvis-oriented medially, laterally, or anteriorly to the renal parenchyma (Fig. 28.6a,b,c).

Fusions associated with vertebral, cloacal and bud anomalies

Other authors have noted an association between renal and both vertebral and anorectal anomalies (Roberts, 1961; Smith, 1968; Belman and King, 1972; Vitko *et al.*, 1972). The association of asymmetric patterns of renal fusion in this series with high-level anorectal defects and vertebral anomalies, including hemivertebra, scoliosis, vertebral agenesis and spina bifida, tends to link them embryologically. Faulty partition of the cloaca by the urorectal septum may be caused by exaggerated flexion and rotation of the hind end (Piekarski and Stephens, 1976). However, the normal range of flexion

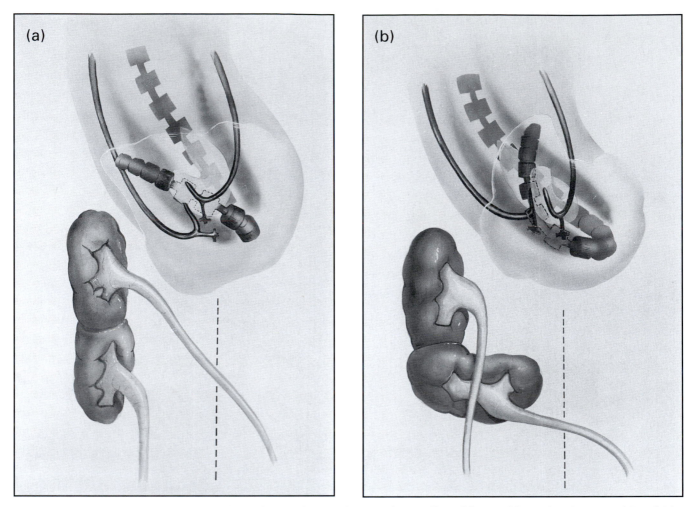

Fig. 28.6 *Frontal illustrations of the hind end of 4–5-mm embryos with various degrees of lateral flexion of the trunk and rotation of the tail (**a**), (**b**) and (**c**) which cause the ureteral buds to induce a single nephrogenic body, thus producing different patterns of crossed renal ectopia. (Reprinted, by permission, from Cook, W.A. and Stephens, F.D. (1977), Fused kidneys: morphologic study and theory of embryogenesis, in D. Bergsma and J.W. Duckett (eds) Urinary System Malformations in Children. New York: Alan R. Liss for the National Foundation, March of Dimes, BD:OAS XII(5): Fig. 7, p. 337.)*

and rotation of the hind end at this critical period of fetal development seems sufficient to support the theory even in the absence of recognizable abnormal vertebral curvature or defect at birth.

Finally, the common occurrence of aberrant ureteral orifices and their associated anomalous upper tracts in asymmetric patterns of renal fusion may also reflect the effects of abnormal flexion and rotation of the hind end. The ureteric bud arises from a knee-like bend in the terminal wolffian duct. The position of this critical point on a wolffian duct may be altered by variation in the configuration of the hind end, thus leading to an aberrantly located ureteral orifice subserving an abnormal upper tract (Meyer, 1946).

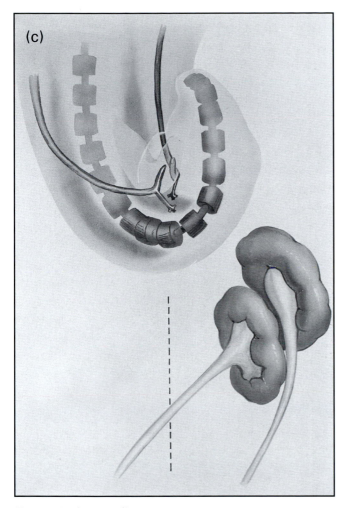

Fig. 28.6 (*continued*)

29

Embryogenesis of anterior and lateral renal pelvis and extraordinary renal fusion

The pelves of horseshoe kidneys are frequently anterior, anteromedial, or anterolateral in orientation (see Fig. 28.1). A single kidney lying in the loin may exhibit an anterior pelvis or various grades of medial or lateral positioning of the pelvis (Fig. 29.1a,b).

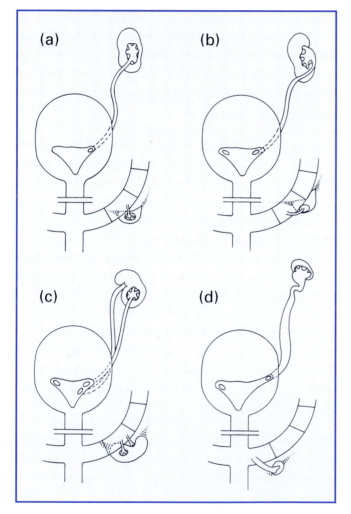

Fig. 29.1 *Non-rotation of the kidney and malposition of the pelvis.* (**a**) *Implantation of ureteric bud onto front of twisted metanephros, which migrates cranially, retaining this abnormal orientation.* (**b**) *Lateral implantation and lateral pelvis.* (**c**) *Medial and frontal implantations of duplex system, retaining medial and anterior orientations after migration of the kidney.* (**d**) *End-on implantation of caudal bud and consequent reflux megaureter, and angulated, sometimes valvular, ureteropelvic junction, cranially directed calyces and hypoplastic kidney.* (Reprinted, by permission, from Stephens, F.D. (1983), Congenital Malformations of the Urinary Tract, New York, Praeger, Fig. 26.1, p. 409.)

Duplex kidneys nearly always have the normal medial pelvic orientation, but sometimes the lower pelvis is disposed anteriorly and the upper one medially (Fig. 29.1c). Rarely, a solitary ureter provides an anterior common pelvis to both right and left kidneys (Fig. 29.2a,b,c).

The embryogenesis of the anterior pelvis of horseshoes, the common pelvis, crossed renal ectopy, double, and laterally rotated single kidneys is somewhat controversial. First, does fusion of horseshoe kidneys take place by collision or wandering of migrating kidneys, or is the fusion and laterality established at the time of induction of the metanephric blastema? Second, does fusion halt rotation in horseshoe kidneys; and third, what makes a pelvis turn laterally instead of medially?

Morphology

Some clues to the embryogenesis were obtained from the study of postmortem specimens and from case reports of fused, misplaced double, and malrotated kidneys and pelves.

Transverse fusion of horseshoe kidneys

Horseshoe kidneys were found to exhibit medial or anterior pelves or one medial and the other anterior (Chapter 28). The greater the width of the bridge in symmetrical horseshoes, the more anterior were the pelves. The kidneys that overlapped the midline in the asymmetrical horseshoes exhibited the most anterior or anterolaterally disposed pelves. Upright kidneys with a slender bridge, however, exhibited medially disposed pelves. It follows that it was not the bridge or its anchoring effect that prevented rotation or ascent, but some other factor or factors. Some rare variants of horseshoes associated with solitary ureters also provided evidence as to the nature of these factors (Fig. 29.2).

Transverse fusions of the renal pelves
Renal pelves in series
One rare specimen was available for personal examination at the Children's Memorial Hospital, Chicago. Case C.A. (aged four hours) died from hypoxia and

transverse pelvic fusions with extreme renal hypodysplasia. Autopsy revealed additional multiple anomalies, including a rectourethral fistula, penile stricture, vertebral anomalies and features of the Potter syndrome. The transversely lying fused pelvis was formed in two parts, the right-sided pelvis being connected to the left-sided pelvis by a narrow, short, transverse infundibulum (Fig. 29.2a,b,c). The left pelvis led to a solitary reflux megaureter, which issued into the left side of the bladder. Both large, cup-like pelves had cranially oriented dilated and rounded minor calyces, upon which lay a thin, dysplastic and hypoplastic covering of parenchyma which joined in the midline of the body.

T-type ureter

Two other rare examples of transverse intercommunicating pelves were reported. In one, a single ureter branched into separate right and left renal pelves (Fig. 29.2e; Rose and Vaughan, 1975) and in the other, a fused 'cake' kidney was drained by a solitary divided ureter (Kandzari et al., 1972). This combination termed here the T-type ureter distinguishes it from the 'Y'-type of bifid ureters. Both babies exhibited anorectal and vaginal malformations and one had sacral agenesis also.

Petrovcić and Milić (1956) and Potampa et al. (1949) described examples of crossed renal ectopy with an intercommunicating infundibulum from the right pelvis of the crossed kidney back to a renal parenchyma on the same side from which the ureter arose. The ureteric bud, which subtended the two kidneys in these patients, crisscrossed the midline and is herein referred to as the 'criss-cross' bud and kidney. The pyeloureterograms have appearances that suggest the ureteropelvic junctions are anteriorly disposed, and in one (Petrovcić and Milić's case), the kidney was explored and the relationship is indicated in Fig. 29.2d. Cass and Vitco (1972) reported a similar case (Fig. 29.2f).

The common pelvis of the T-type may join separate kidneys (Fig. 29.2e) or fused kidneys (Kandzari et al., 1972), whereas the common pelvis with infundibula arranged 'in series' to the contralateral kidney naturally joins fused kidneys (Fig. 29.2d).

Duplex kidneys

Most kidneys with bifid or double ureters undergo normal rotation with medially disposed pelves. However, in two of 15 specimens of duplex systems dissected, the pelvis of the lower moiety was anterior and that of the upper was medial in one, and in the other, the pelves to both moieties were anterior. This suggests that as far as disposition of the pelves of duplex kidneys is concerned, each moiety and its pelvis develops autonomously (Fig. 29.1c).

Kidneys with lateral pelves

Some kidneys that are well formed and located in the loin exhibit anterolateral or lateral dispositions of the pelvis and ureter. Whereas anterior or anteromedial positions may be arrests of normal rotation of the kidney, lateral positions invoke either malrotation or some other factor to explain the morphology.

Embryogenesis of abnormalities of fusion and rotation

All these abnormalities may be explained by one all-embracing error of development, namely the initial abnormal anatomical relationships of bud to metanephros.

'Implantation' theory
Duplex and triplex kidneys
Multiple buds arising in line from the wolffian duct induce metanephric mesoderm of the contiguous parallel metanephros.

Symmetrical and asymmetrical horseshoe kidneys
Ureteric buds from each wolffian duct induce metanephroi, which are located at the caudal ends of abnormally prolonged nephrogenic bodies which meet or overlap the midline (Chapter 28).

T-type and transverse pelvic fusions
A single ureteric bud divides and induces contiguous ends of both metanephroi, forming a T-type pelvic fusion; or the bud induces the ipsilateral metanephros and sprouts an exogenous infundibulum, which jumps to the contralateral contiguous metanephros. The bud dichotomizes to form the pelvis in the transverse instead of the longitudinal axis (Figs 29.2e).

Crossed renal ectopy
The ureteric bud and wolffian duct are shifted medially to overlie the end of the opposite metanephros, which it

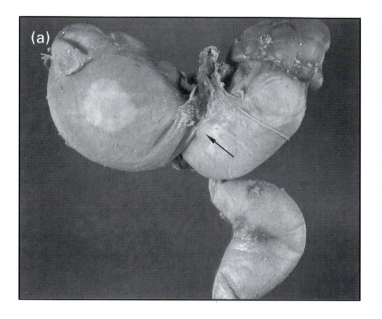

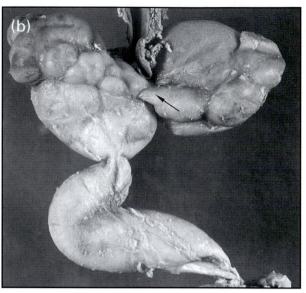

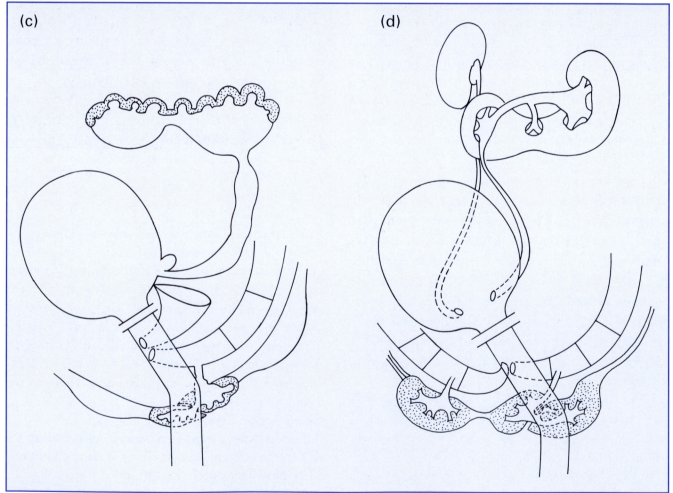

Fig. 29.2   *(continued)*

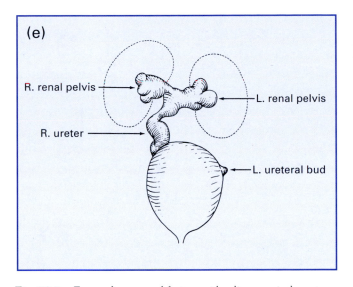

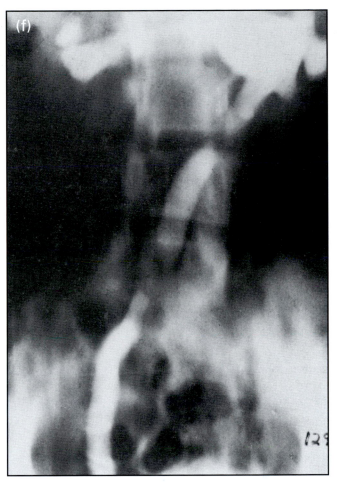

Fig. 29.2 *Extraordinary renal fusions with solitary or single ureters.
(a) Baby C.A., showing solitary megaureter, common pelvis joined in
midline (arrow) in anteroposterior view. (b) In posteroanterior view
(arrow denotes the point of fusion of the two kidneys). (c) Diagram of
Baby A., showing presumed implantation of solitary bud arising from
wolffian duct, deviated by rectourethral and sacral malformations, and
implanting into overlapping tail ends of the nephrogenic bodies, resulting in a transverse fused kidney and common pelvis. (d) Criss-cross
kidney and single ureter; lower part shows presumed implantation of
single bud into overlapping nephrogenic cords, resulting in crossed renal
ectopy linked to uncrossed fused kidney. (e) Rare T-type pelvis and
separate kidneys, resulting from implantation of the solitary bud into
ends of both nephrogenic cords. (f) Tomogram of criss-cross kidney
and solitary ureter. (a), (b), (c) Reprinted, by permission, from
Stephens, F.D. (1983), Congenital Malformations of the Urinary
Tract, New York, Praeger, Fig. 26.A, B, C, p. 410. (d) Reprinted,
by permission, after Petrovcić, F. and Milić, N. (1956), Horseshoe
kidney with crossed ureter condition after right nephrectomy. Br. J.
Radiol. 29: 114, Fig. 3. (e) Reprinted, by permission, from Rose, G.
and Vaughan, E.D., Jr. (1975), Common renal pelvis: a case report.
J. Urol. 113: 234, Fig. 2. (f) Reprinted, by permission, from Cass,
A.S. and Vitco, R.J. (1972), An unusual variety of crossed renal
ectopy with only one ureter. J. Urol. 107: 1056, Fig. 1.)*

induces. The kidney so formed ascends on its own side
of the embryo, the ureter crosses the midline, forming
crossed renal ectopy (Fig. 28.6). If a major infundibulum of such a bud jumps back over the midline to
induce also the metanephros of the same side, then
the criss-cross deformity develops. These cross-over
ureterorenal malformations may arise from solitary
ureters or together with others (Fig. 29.2d).

The long infundibulum, which recrosses the midline, is
a strong indicator that fusions can and probably do occur
at the moment of ureteral budding from the wolffian duct
when both metanephroi are overlapping. It is unlikely for

two reasons that the long infundibulum would contact
the metanephros of the opposite side after the ipsilateral
kidney had begun its migration. First, the ipsilateral
kidney diverges from the midline and the opposite
metanephros, and second, the contralateral metanephros
would not migrate and keep pace with the ipsilateral
kidney if it were not induced by the bud at the same time.

Anterior and lateral pelves

If the wolffian duct and nephrogenic cords diverge, the
implantation site of the bud upon the metanephros may
be tangential, creating anterolateral or lateral pelvic dispositions (Fig. 29.1b).

The lower pole ureter of a double kidney may strike
tangentially the lower moiety of the metanephros, which

is twisted caudally out of alignment with the upper moiety, resulting in different pelvic orientations (Fig. 29.1c).

End-on kidney

If the ureteric bud arises caudal to the end of the metanephros, it may induce the formation of a kidney end-on to the pelvis. The deformity is apparent in some reflux megaureters, which presumably arise from the most distal reach of the wolffian duct (common excretory duct) and implant into the stub end of the metanephros (Fig. 29.1d). The ureteropelvic junction folds on itself and, in some instances, is held tightly against the pelvis by the pelviureteric fascia causing a valve-like obstruction.

Associated local malformations

It was found that other malformations of the pelvic organs, partial sacral agenesis, or scoliosis coexisted with the extraordinary ureteric-bud anomalies. It is well established from specimens that the wolffian ducts are cranially displaced in rectovesical, rectourethral and some rectogenital-fistula anomalies (see Fig. 2.5). In all probability, the nephrogenic bodies are also initially displaced, skewed and ill-developed, accounting for the parenchymal dysmorphologies.

Other theories of embryogenesis

Horseshoe kidneys and crossed renal ectopy may also be explained on the basis of wandering kidneys during ascent from the pelvis to the loin. At one stage of migration, when the kidneys are negotiating the barrier made by the umbilical arteries (Kelly and Burnam, 1914), or before the kidneys reach the arteries (Friedland and De Vries, 1975), their lower poles turn medially and collide, and one kidney may be diverted to the opposite side if the kidneys ascend at levels different from one another.

Rotational abnormalities may derive from lack of the normal rotation of the kidney pelvis from anterior to medial orientation or malrotation toward a lateral disposition. These theories are simple and plausible for single kidneys, but the duplex kidney, with the upper pelvis medial and the lower pelvis anterior and also perhaps the lateral pelvis of a single kidney may be better explained by the 'implantation' theory. Some forms of crossed renal ectopy are also more readily explained by abnormal ureteral implantation than by extraordinary transpositions and somersaults of one kidney, pelvis and ureter over the other during the migration from pelvis towards the loin.

Ureteral orifices located in the bladder have been described according to their position, shape and correlation with the occurrence of vesicoureteral reflux. Abnormally located orifices in the urethra and genital tracts are commonly associated with large ureters and abnormal renal parenchyma. Furthermore, the ureterocaliectasis and nephropathy associated with reflux and obstruction are commonly attributed to the abnormal dynamic effects on the renal parenchyma in the fetus or later.

Resulting from a study of 51 postmortem specimens of duplex kidneys, an embryological explanation is proposed for these changes in the ureter and kidney based on abnormal wolffian duct sitings of the ureteral buds, which grow out and penetrate adjacent abnormal zones on the nephrogenic ridges. Thus, the position of the ureteral orifices in the urogenital tracts provides the clue to the embryogenesis of the kidney structure and the characteristic nephropathy so often associated with double ureters.

Duplex kidneys with bifid and double ureters

A study was made of 51 specimens of duplex kidneys, bladders and urethras of 36 infants dying of various causes in the neonatal period. In addition, seven specimens from children as old as six years were also studied. Of these 51 duplex systems, there were 40 double ureters and 11 bifid ureters with a distal common stem.

Each specimen was described according to kidney size, macroscopic and microscopic appearance (double kidney plus contralateral kidney), diameter of ureters at mid-spindle, course of the ureters and the relation of one to other, position of orifices of the ureters, and histological appearance of the upper-pole ureter and lower-pole ureter renal segments and opposite kidneys. An objective assessment was also made of the glomerular population and thickness of the cortex and medulla.

Measurements of the width of the cortex and medulla were taken with a measuring grid placed over the stained section on the slide. The number of glomeruli per unit area of cortex was calculated by counting all glomeruli within a 1-mm width for the full thickness of the cortex.

Paraffin sections of 7-μm thickness were prepared with haematoxylin-eosin and Masson stains. They were described by a pathologist unfamiliar with the specimens in order to obtain unbiased diagnoses of renal parenchyma hypoplasia, dysplasia or pyelonephritis, for example.

Location and identification of duplex structures

The ureters of the cranial and caudal segments of the duplex kidney and its ureters are termed upper-pole ureter (UPU) and lower-pole ureter (LPU), respectively. It was soon apparent that most of the duplex-kidney segments had a macroscopically normal appearance when the orifices issued within the normal limits of the trigone of the bladder. It was also apparent that the kidney segments were most often abnormal when the orifices issued elsewhere. The locations of the orifices of the duplex ureters were grouped into three zones: (1) normal trigonal, (2) caudo-displaced and (3) craniodisplaced. They were further subdivided into eight specific situations within these zones: A, E and F in the normal zone; G and H in the caudal zone; B and C, as described by Lyon et al. (1969); and D, more laterally in a diverticulum, in the cranial zone. The G and H locations in the male subject occupy the upper third of the posterior urethra and vas. However, in the female subject, the G orifice may occur at any level in the whole length of the urethra or on the perineal bridge between the urethra and vagina, and the H orifice issues into the Gartner's duct in the wall of the vagina (Fig. 30.1).

*Reprinted, with modifications, from Mackie, G.G. and Stephens, F.D. (1975), Duplex kidneys: a correlation of renal dysplasia with position of ureteral orifice. J. Urol. 114: 274.

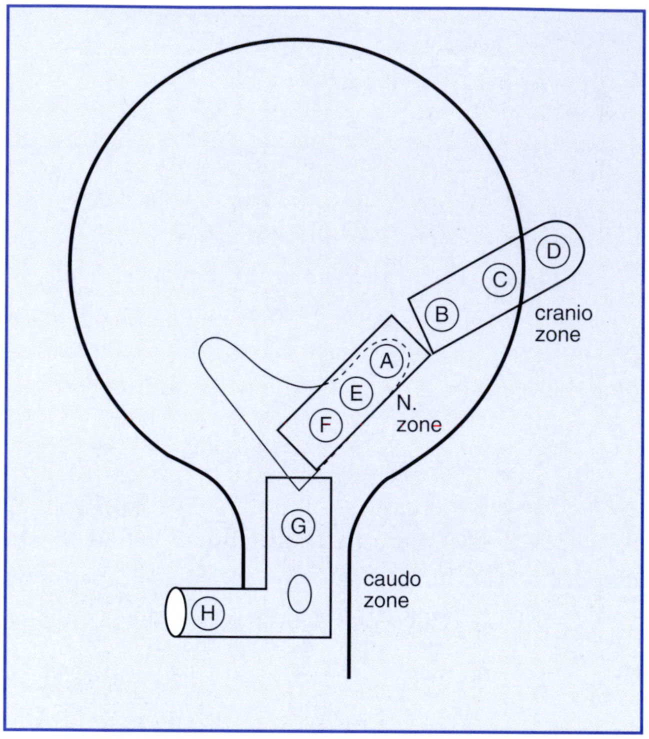

Fig. 30.1 *Diagram of bladder and urethra, showing three zones of ureteral orifices: normal N zone A, E, and F; lateral in cranio zone B, C, and D in diverticulum; and caudo zone G in urethra and H in sex ducts. (Reprinted, by permission, from Mackie, G.G. and Stephens, F.D. (1975), Duplex kidneys: a correlation of renal dysplasia with position of ureteral orifice. J. Urol. 114: 274, Fig. 1.)*

Renal morphology associated with ureteric orifice position

In duplex kidneys, the orifice of the ureter of the UPU renal segment lay caudal and medial to the orifice of the LPU in conformity with the Weigert–Meyer law (see page 222). Uncommon exceptions are those orifices of the UPU that lay in close proximity but cranial and medial to the normally sited orifice of the LPU on the cornu of the otherwise normal trigone (Stephens, 1958).

We found that the ureteral orifices of both ureters of the duplex kidney or the single ureter of a bifid kidney issued onto the normal trigonal zone in 16 double and seven bifid kidneys. The ureteral orifices of 28 duplex kidneys lay elsewhere as follows: caudal and normal zones (seven), cranial and normal (seven) and cranial and cranial zones (eight) and cranial and caudal zones (six) (Fig. 30.2).

Correlation of renal structure and ureteral size with the position of the orifice was directed to individual kidney segments rather than to the double kidneys because of the confusion caused by orifices of duplex segments arising from more than one zone. All of the kidney segments associated with the orifices in each of the three zones were considered together. Fifty-six renal segments issued on the normal zone, 14 on the caudal zone and 32 on the cranial zone (Table 30.1).

Table 30.1 *Statistical analysis of renal segments and ureters*

Orifice zone	Orifices	Segments (n)	Mean ureteral diameter (cm)	Cortical thickness (mm)[*]	Medullary thickness (mm)	Glomeruli[*]	Histology Normal	Histology Dysplasia
Normal	A, E, F	56	0.3	2.4 (1.09)	3.9 (1.23)	18.0 (6.22)	56	0
Caudo zone	G, H	14	1.5	0.7 (0.59)[†]	1.4 (1.36)[†]	6.6 (9.27)[†]	0	14
Cranio zone	B, C, D	32	0.33	1.7 (1.43)[‡]	2.3 (1.64)[†]	11.9 (7.99)[†]	24	8
	B	23	0.35	2.3 (1.35)	3.2 (1.25)	16.0 (4.54)	23	0
	C							
	D	9	1.2	0.4 (0.26)[†]	0.5 (0.56)[†]	1.1 (2.60)[†]	1	8

[*]Numbers in parentheses are standard deviations.
[†]Difference from normal significant ($p = 0.002$).
[‡]Difference from normal significant ($p = 0.05$).
Source: Mackie, G.G. and Stephens, F.D. (1975), Duplex kidneys: A correlation of renal dysplasia with position of the ureteral orifice. J. Urol. 114: 274, Table 1.

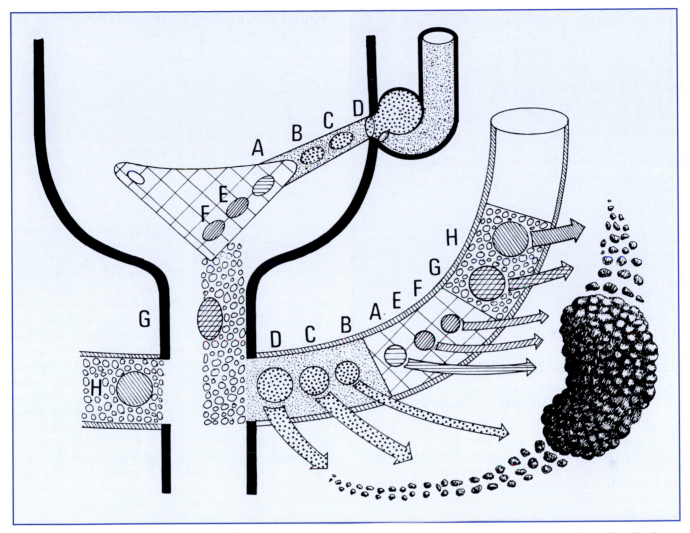

Fig. 30.2 *Relationship of orifice zones in bladder and urethra to points of origin from wolffian duct is shown, as well as relationship of bud positions on wolffian duct to nephrogenic blastema. (Reprinted, by permission, from Mackie, G.G. and Stephens, F.D. (1975), Duplex kidneys: a correlation of renal dysplasia with position of the ureteral orifice. J. Urol. 114: 274, Fig. 2.)*

Normal zone segments (A, E and F orifices)

There were 30 UPU and 26 LPU segments of duplex kidneys, 42 of which had double ureters and 14 of which had bifid ureters. These 56 kidney segments exhibited normal-looking markings, substance and calices, and the microstructure was that of normal, compact nephrons. None showed more than minor variants commonly occurring in the kidney of a normal newborn or premature baby.

An objective assessment of the numbers of glomeruli in the cortex and of the thickness of cortex and medulla was made by the technique described. Mean values were found of 18 glomeruli per unit area, a cortical thickness of 2.4 mm and medullary thickness of 3.9 mm. These measurements provide baseline figures for statistical comparison of the segments from other zones.

The ureters of these duplex kidneys were not enlarged, the mean mid-spindle measurement being 0.3 cm (normal 0.35 cm) (Cussen, 1967a). The ectopic ureter was 0.29 cm compared with orthotopic 0.33 cm.

In these 56 segments, four showed mild hydronephrosis and large ureters, two resulting from obstruction by stenotic ureteroceles and two associated with ureteroceles issuing into the bladder in the F position. The renal architecture was normal in all four segments. One kidney segment from a premature baby showed excessive areas of rudimentary, subcapsular nephrogenic structures.

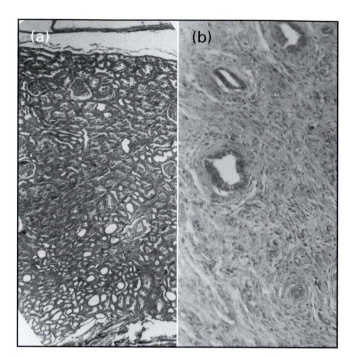

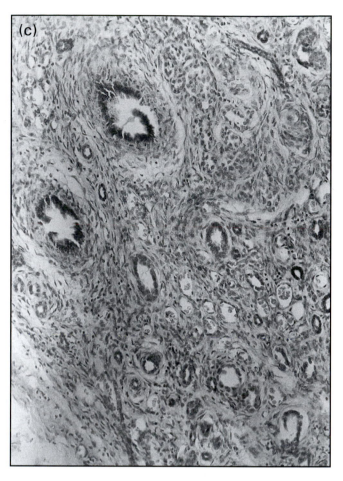

Fig. 30.3 *Hypoplasia and dysplasia of kidneys with ureteric orifices in C and G positions. (**a**) Baby H.B. Area of thin cortex (×25). (**b**)Fibrocellular medulla in one area with whorling around primitive ducts in kidney with ureteric orifice in C position (×225). (**c**) Baby B.H. Area of nubbin of kidney with G position ureteric orifice showing disorganized parenchyma with sparse glomeruli, tubules, ductules, primitive ducts and mesenchymal tissue. (Reproduced, by permission, from Mackie, G.G. and Stephens, F.D. (1975), Duplex kidneys: a correlation of renal dysplasia with position of the ureteral orifice. J. Urol. 114: 274, Fig. 3.)*

Caudal zone segments (G and H orifices)

The group of caudal zone segments included 14 renal segments, all of which were ectopic segments of duplex kidneys. All of the renal segments were small nubbins and lobulated or flat plaques upon a large, bulbous ureter. The microstructure in all segments showed areas of dysplasia, characterized by prominent, large ductules lined by cuboidal cells with pyknotic nuclei areas of whorled or loose mesenchymal connective tissue, and cysts in the subcortical and interlobular areas. It also showed glomerulotubular disproportion seen as closely packed glomerular clusters around ductules but lacking convoluted tubules and loops of Henle, cartilage plaques, and, in some areas, thickened vessels.

In these newborn specimens, there was complete absence of lymphocytic or polymorphic aggregations and fibrosis of past inflammation.

The assessment of the glomerular population revealed a mean value of 6.6 glomeruli per unit area of cortex

(p = 0.002). The mean values for cortical and medullary thickness were 0.7 and 1.4 mm (p = 0.002).

The ureters of these segments showed dilatation and tortuosity, and the mean mid-spindle diameter was 1.5 cm. Of the ureters, six issued in the G position, four of which exhibited ureteroceles, and one issued in the H position.

Cranial zone segments (B, C and D orifices)

Of the 32 kidney segments in the cranial zone, eight were UPU and 24 were LPU segments of the duplex kidney. In 21 of these 32 renal segments, the macroscopic appearance and microarchitecture were normal. These segments corresponded with the B orifice location, and the ureters were normal in appearance and size. Measurements revealed a near-normal mean value of 16 glomeruli, and cortical and medullary thicknesses of 2.3 and 3.2 mm, respectively.

In 11 renal segments, the kidneys were abnormal to the naked eye, the orifices were located in the C and D positions. The mean values of the glomerular counts in these renal segments were 1.1 glomeruli per unit area of cortex and the thicknesses of the cortex and medulla were 0.43 and 0.51 mm, respectively, indicating a severity of renal abnormality as gross as in the caudal zone renal segments (Fig. 30.3).

The ureters of these renal segments were abnormally large and tortuous, with a mean diameter of 1.2 cm.

The microstructure of the segments associated with C and D orifices was abnormal in architecture of parenchyma. The appearance of the dysplasia differed from that in the renal segments of the caudal zone in some features, although many were similar. The abnormality of the C and D orifices was more of hypoplasia, with dysplastic areas alternating with normal zones. Wedges of ductules with whorled mesenchyme abutted thin normal areas. Cysts were less common, and the medulla was narrowed, owing to absence of loops of Henle and short or absent proximal and distal convoluted tubules. The histological results are indicated in Table 30.1.

Renal dysplasias

Renal dysplasia and ureteric orifice position

The results of this study of neonatal duplex kidneys have demonstrated a strong association between ureteral orifice position and renal abnormality. Orifices opening in the normal zone resulted in normal ureters and kidney segments, macroscopically and microscopically. Displacement of orifices laterally onto the lateral bladder base or wall or caudally into the urethra, perineum, or sex ducts resulted in abnormalities of the associated renal segment. The abnormality worsened the farther the orifice was displaced. The extreme in either direction was severe renal dysplasia and hypoplasia.

The pattern of dysplasia differed in appearance at either end of the spectrum of displacement.

The features of dysplasia in these specimens have been enumerated and correspond to previous descriptions of dysplasia (Baggenstoss, 1951; Ericsson and Ivemark, 1958a, b; Bialestock, 1963; Pathak and Williams, 1964; Persky et al., 1967; Bernstein, 1968).

Renal dysplasia with orifice position in the cranial zone

The C and D orifices in some instances had no renal tissue draped over a dilated ureteral bud. The majority had a thin rim of renal tissue alternating with areas of ductules surrounded by mesenchymal tissue. The pattern of dysplasia suggests normal outgrowth of the straight ducts from the calyx of the ureteral bud contacting the patchy tail end of the metanephric blastema. Where the straight ducts contact normal islands of blastema, normal renal structures form and, where they fail to find blastema, only ductules appear.

Renal dysplasia with orifice position in the caudal zone

The ureters issuing in the G and H positions occasionally had dilated cranial ends capped by lobulated nubbins of dysplastic tissue. More often, the segments showed thick areas of renal tissue comprising normal structures interposed with wedge areas of cysts and sparse cortical and medullary tubules, as described previously. The architecture suggests that the dysplastic areas are caused by contact of the developing straight ducts with nests of involuting mesonephric tissue, resulting in cystic dilatations of the duct systems and failure of development of glomeruli, proximal and distal convoluted tubules and loops of Henle.

Most explanations of the abnormalities seen in duplex kidneys have referred to a functional cause. The abnormalities of the ectopic segment are derived from the effects of obstruction by urethral sphincter squeeze on the ureter or ureterocele on the sensitive developing renal blastema, while those of the orthotopic segments result from damage of these embryonic tissues by the dynamic effects of reflux or infection.

Our findings regarding this neonatal population of virtually no infection and those of others suggest that areas of dysplasia are prima facie, and may predispose to development of pyelonephritis (Marshall, 1953; Ericsson et al., 1958a,b; Bialestock, 1963; Persky et al., 1967).

Relation of obstruction and vesicoureteral reflux to renal dysplasia

Obstruction as a cause of dysplasia is refuted by Tanagho (1972) in his observations of kidneys subjected to ureteral obstruction in the fetal lamb. Also, none of the four single kidneys additional to the bifid kidneys described herein, all of which were associated with stenotic ureteroceles issuing on the normal orifice zone, showed dysplasia.

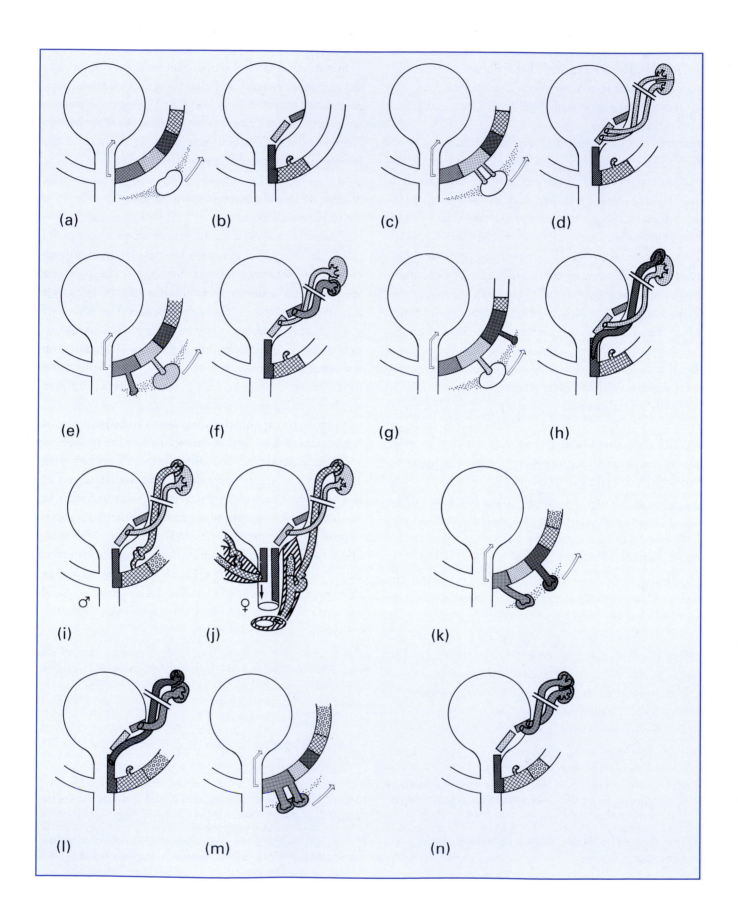

The case for reflux is more difficult to disprove but certainly dysplasia was not found in any of the 21 renal segments corresponding with B position orifices in the cranial zone, many of which would be expected to have exhibited reflux (Lyon et al., 1969).

Embryological explanation of dysplasia

At the 4-mm stage (four weeks) of development of the normal embryo, the primitive endodermal cloaca is undivided. Between the 4- and 16-mm stages (six weeks), the urorectal septum divides the cloaca in the coronal plane into the urinary and rectal compartments. The wolffian (mesonephric) ducts issue first in the undivided cloaca near the anterior part of the cloacal membrane at the 4-mm stage but recede to the level of the Müller's tubercle (verumontanum) in the anterior urinary compartment of the newly divided cloaca of the 16-mm embryo. The terminal part of the wolffian duct is called the 'common excretory duct', and it is that part of the duct distal to the ureteral bud or buds.

The common excretory duct together with a small additional contiguous segment cranial to it is taken up into the enlarging vesicourinary canal by a process of tubular dilatation affecting predominantly the upper lip (Brockis, 1952; Hamilton et al., 1978b). The opened-out walls of the wolffian duct form the trigone, and the ureteral bud comes to lie characteristically in the cornu of the trigone (Figs 30.4 and 30.5).

If the ureteral bud arises more medially or laterally from the wolffian duct, migration of the ureters in the bladder would result in its position being either too far lateral on the bladder base or in the urethra or genital tracts, respectively.

In duplex kidneys, the two segments are co-apted, but the excretory systems and blood supply are entirely separated. The ureters may be bifid, joining to form a common stem, or may remain separate, issuing by two separate orifices. The LPU nearly always contributes the two major calyces to the lower major segment of the double kidney, and its orifice is situated cranial to that of the UPU. Bifid ureters presumably arise from the common excretory duct as a single bud that divides prematurely, forming a ureteropelvis and two elongated major calyces. Double ureters presumably arise as two buds. The locations of the ureteral orifices of the ureteral buds undergo a switch in relationships when migrating into the urethra and bladder. The orifice of the caudal ureteral bud attains a more cranial final location in the bladder than that of the cranial bud. In the reshuffle, the distal end of the UPU crosses behind the LPU. It is this switch and crossing that explains the Weigert–Meyer law.

In order to explain the variations in the positions of the orifices as described in this analysis of the specimens and the characteristic nephropathy corresponding with each orifice zone, it is postulated that the distal end of the wolffian duct in the vicinity of the ureteral buds may be demarcated into three short equal sections, which expand and become incorporated seriatim into the vesicourethral canal. The terminal section is taken up to form the cranial zone in the bladder base, the second or middle section is taken up to form the normal trigonal

Fig. 30.4 *Correlations of positions of orifices of duplex ureteric buds and ureters with renal morphology. (a) Wolffian duct sections are shown in relation to nephrogenic mass. Note direction of migration of kidney cranially and wolffian duct into developing bladder. (b) Migration of wolffian duct sections transposed into urinary tract. (c) Double ureteral buds arising from normal sections strike nephrogenic mass and migration occurs in direction of arrows. (d) Duplex kidney with both ureteric orifices on normal zone in bladder. Kidney morphology is normal. (e) Upper-pole ureter (UPU) bud arises from normal section and strikes normal nephrogenic mass. Lower-pole ureter (LPU) arises from caudal section and strikes hypoplastic blastema. (f) After migration, UPU orifice on normal zone and kidney normal. Orifice of LPU is laterally ectopic and kidney is oligonephronic. (g) LPU bud arises from normal section and strikes normal nephrogenic mass; UPU bud arises too far cranially on wolffian duct and strikes abnormal nephrogenic section. (h) After migration, UPU orifice located in caudal urethral zone and LPU orifice in normal zone. (i) LPU arises even further laterally than in (g) on wolffian duct at site of seminal vesicle and strikes abnormal nephrogenic mass; LPU bud arises from normal section and kidney is normal. After migration UPU remains attached to seminal vesicle; LPU orifice on trigone. (j) Female counterpart showing müllerian duct (heavy hatch) having engulfed the wolffian duct and attachment of the UPU before (left side of diagram) and after (right side of diagram) migration of the vaginal plate to the vestibule. (k) UPU arises from the cranial section of the wolffian duct and LPU from the medial section; both meet abnormal nephrogenic mesoderm. (l) After migration the UPU orifice is urethral and LPU orifice is lateral in position. (m) UPU and LPU buds arise from caudal section of the wolffian duct, both meet depleted nephrogenic mesoderm. (n) Both migrate to laterally ectopic positions in the bladder. (Reprinted, after Mackie, G.G. and Stephens, F.D. (1975), Duplex kidneys: a correlation of renal dysplasia with position of the ureteral orifice. J. Urol. 114: 274, Fig. 5.)*

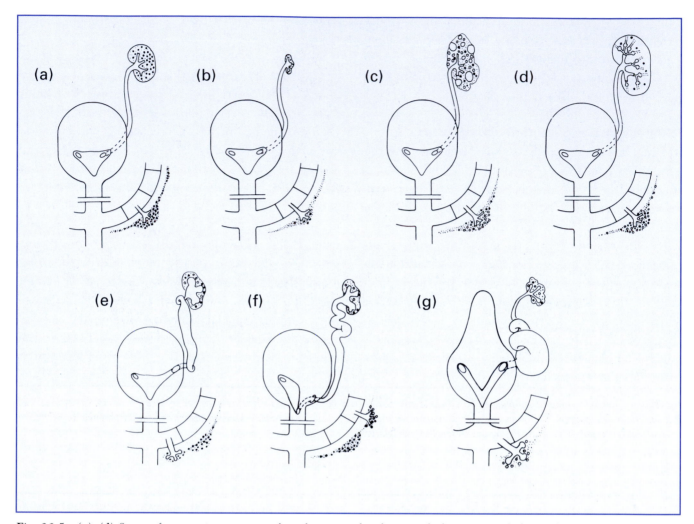

Fig. 30.5 (*a*)–(*d*) *Status of upper urinary tract resulting from normal and ureteric bud positions and abnormal metanephros.* (*a*) *Normal metanephros.* (*b*) *Teratogenic or chromosomal renal dysgenesis.* (*c*) *Heritable polycystic metanephros.* (*d*) *Infantile polycystic metanephros.* (*e*)–(*f*) *The bud theory of the relation of abnormal renal morphology to abnormal ureteric orifice position.* (*e*) *Ectopic bud induces sparce nephrogenic blastema in the tail of the nephrogenic cord resulting in ureteronephric dysgenesis.* (*f*) *Ectopic bud induces involuting zone of nephrogenic cord creating renal hypodysplasia.* (*g*) *Abnormal renal morphology and ureteric orifice position in prune belly syndrome—abnormal bud and ureteronephric dysgenesis.*

zone in the bladder, and the third and most cranial section of the duct is incorporated into the caudal zone. The orifices of ureteral buds emerging from any of these three sections migrate to the corresponding zone in the vesicourethral canal.

The orifices of abnormal buds arising from the third part are projected into the urethra or may remain attached to the wolffian duct. In the female subject, those ureters issuing contiguous with or into the wolffian duct are carried caudally in the müllerian ducts to the distal urethra and the perineum, or maintained a connection with Gartner's duct in the vaginal wall (Stephens, 1971).

It is further postulated that the metanephrogenic body, which is located in the mesenchyme adjacent to the wolffian duct, is also divided into three parts, corresponding closely with the terminal three sections of the wolffian duct. The middle section represents the main mass of metanephric tissue and, when contacted by a ureteral bud or buds from the middle section of the wolffian duct, normal renal structures develop. Renal segments derived from either end of the normal part of the renal blastema may be expected to show evidence of involuting changes, atrophy or dystrophy. Under such circumstances, it could be presumed that the site of origin of the ureteral bud not only determines the point

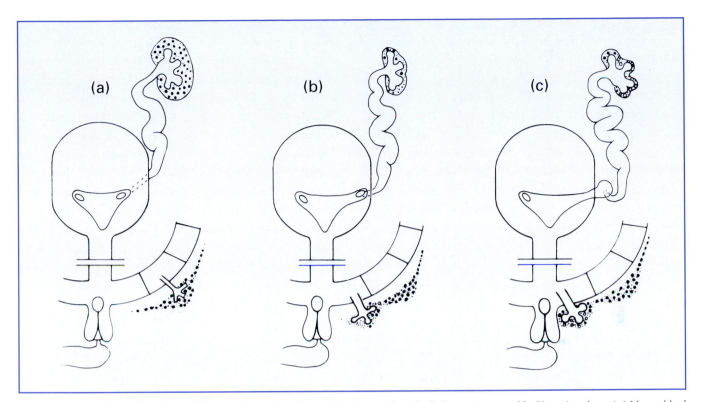

Fig. 30.6 *Correlation of renal morphology with ureteric orifice position in partial urethral obstruction caused by Young's valves. (**a**) Normal bud and ureteric orifice position and obstructive renal morphology only. (**b**) Ectopic bud, lateral ureteric ectopy and oligonephronia. (**c**) Extreme ectopy of bud, ureteral orifice in diverticulum and renal hypodysplasia.*

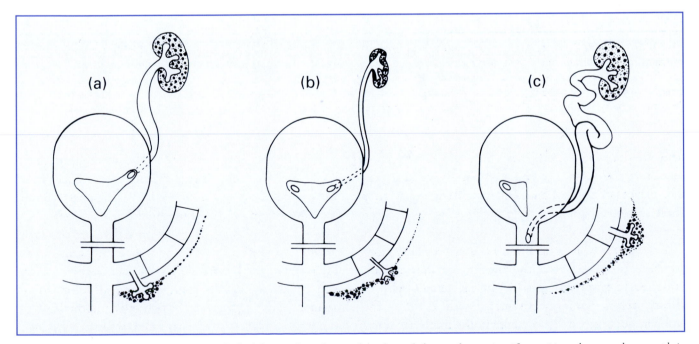

Fig. 30.7 *An explanation of exceptions to the bud theory of correlation of renal morphology and ureteric orifice position: the normal metanephric mesoblast shifts longitudinally with or without a corresponding shift of bud orifice position. (**a**) Normal renal morphogenesis with ectopic bud position. (**b**) Abnormal morphogenesis with normal orifice position. (**c**) Normal renal morphology with ectopia of ureteric orifice in urethra.*

of issue into the vesicourethral canal at one end of the ureter, but also the nature of the kidney at the other end and its intervening ureter (Fig. 30.5).

Permutations of the bud theory theme

The correlations between ureteric orifice location and the morphology of the kidney hold true in most instances of double and single ureters. However, errors in the formation and location of the metanephros may cause renal malformations when the ureteric bud arises from a normal or abnormal section of the wolffian duct. The metanephros may be abnormal or absent, or poly-cystic in the presence of a normal ureteric bud and oligonephronic if the orifice location is ectopic (Fig. 30.5 e,f,g). Similar metanephric variations occur with lateral ectopia of the ureteric orifice in patients with Young's valves of the urethra though back pressure causes impairment of nephrons (Fig. 30.6). In some instances, the metanephros is well induced by an ectopic ureter and this may occur because the metanephric mesenchyme is also ectopically placed (Fig. 30.7a,c). Occasionally, the metanephric mesenchyme is oligonephronic adjacent to a normal bud and perhaps in this instance the main mass of mesenchyme is caudal or cranial to the bud or defective (Fig. 30.7b).

Varieties of horseshoe kidneys arise because of excessive medial location of the metanephros. The mesenchyme impacts symmetrically from each side in the midline or that from one side overlaps the midline to impact asymmetrically. Bud location may be normal or abnormal and the metanephric mesenchyme may be hyper- or oligonephronic or dysplastic (Fig. 30.8).

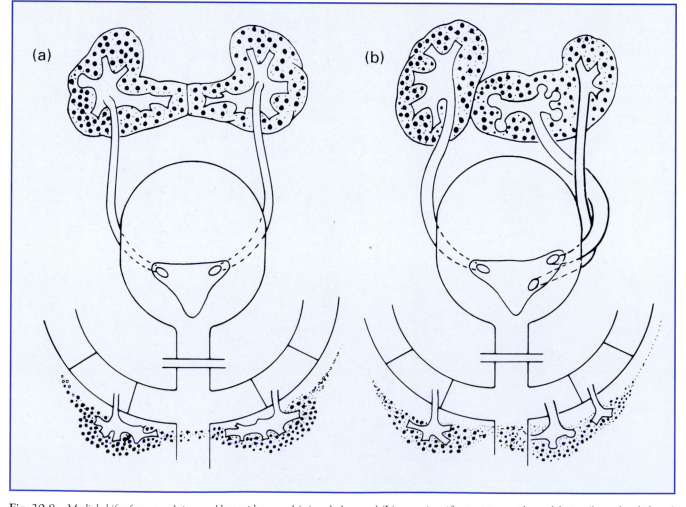

Fig. 30.8 *Medial shift of metanephric mesoblast with normal (**a**) and abnormal (**b**) ureteric orifice positions with renal fusion (horseshoe kidneys) and normal renal morphogenesis. Metanephric blastema is prolonged medially and normal and ectopic ureteric buds induce healthy blastema.*

The ureteric orifice: the embryological key to radiological status of duplex kidneys*

In this study, the ureteric orifice position of duplex ureters in the bladder or urethra of children was correlated with the kidney configuration as determined by X-ray examination and, in some, by surgical excision and biopsy.

The previous study of 51 necropsy specimens of duplex kidneys, ureters, and bladders of neonates revealed a close correlation between ureteric orifice position and kidney morphology (Chapter 30).

This clinical study of children further confirms that the position and type of ureteral orifices act as guides to renal order and disorder in duplex kidneys. A radiographical classification of kidney configurations was invoked to match and correlate form with orifice position. From this cystoradiographical study, it appears that renal abnormalities occur when ureteric buds arise from faulty locations in the wolffian duct during embryogenesis.

Clinical study of patients with bifid and double ureters

Children who had been examined for various reasons, such as pain and dysuria, wetting, or urinary infection, and found to have duplex kidneys, formed the basis of this study. Fifty-seven children with a total of 61 duplex kidneys and 122 upper-pole ureter (UPU) and lower pole ureter (LPU) segments were studied. X-ray studies consisted of intravenous pyelography, voiding cystourethrography (VCU), and, sometimes, retrograde pyelography at the time of cystoscopy.

Reflux has been graded in a standard manner as described by Rolleston et al. (1970) (see Appendix 1, No. 18). Reflux was 'slight' when dye passed up the ureter but did not fill the pelvis and calyces, 'moderate' when the dye reached the pelvis but the calyces were not clubbed and 'gross' when the calyces were abnormally expanded.

Duplex in preference to single kidneys were studied because of the much wider range in variation of ureteral orifice positions issuing from the two renal segments, thus providing a higher yield of abnormality.

Cystoscopy was performed by two of the authors, often both being present at the study to individually examine and describe the ureteral orifices and their positions. When studies were complete, the tracing of kidney inlines and outlines were made from the intravenous pyelograms, VCU and retrograde pyelograms, and were compounded into a diagram together with a plot of the cystoscopic findings.

Ureters were classed as megaureter when the ureterogram diameter was ≥ 1 cm. Cussen (1967a) quantified ureter diameter for age, and our choice of ≥ 1 cm, measured on X-ray, regarded as abnormal, allowed for the magnification error.

In all 61 duplex kidneys, the lower pole segment contributed the lower and middle major calyces, while the upper pole segment was drained by the upper major calyx. Variations in the number of minor calyces opening from the middle and upper major calyces were seen.

The Weigert–Meyer rule (page 222) governed orifice position of the UPU and LPU and renal segments, namely, the cranial renal segment ureter issued medial or distal to that of the caudal segment in the urinary tract.

Terminology

Ureteral orifices were classified according to the description of Lyon et al. (1969), with the addition of extra letters to designate other sites found with duplex kidneys; these specific sites were grouped into three zones, normal ('A', 'E', 'F' orifices), caudal zone ('G' and 'H' orifices), and cranial zone ('B', 'C', 'D' orifices) (see Fig. 30.1).

*Reprinted, with changes, from Mackie, G.G., Awang, H. and Stephens, F.D. (1975), The ureteric orifice: The embryologic key to radiologic status of duplex kidneys. J. Pediatr. Surg. 10: 473.

In this chapter the ureters of the duplex kidneys were called double when each issued separately into the lower urinary tract and bifid when the ureters met in a Y-junction to form a common stem issuing by one orifice. The letters 'A' to 'H' (see Figs 14.5 and 30.1) were used to designate orifice positions and the descriptive appearances of the orifices were those defined by Lyon *et al.* (1969), namely, normal, stadium, horseshoe and golf-hole (see Fig. 19.1).

For the purposes of correlation of kidney segment type with ureteric position, the kidney segments were first classified into α, β and γ types according to radiographical criteria. Then, every designated orifice position in each of the three zones was allocated either an α-, β- or γ-type renal segment. The tally provided the data for analysis and validity of the hypothesis.

The radiographical criteria of the α, β and γ segments were as follows. The α-kidney segments were smooth in contour with thick nephrograms, cupped, normal calyces and exhibited prompt excretion; β segments were thin, smooth or irregular in outline, the calyces were clubbed or closely clustered, and function

was impaired; γ segments had irregular or invisible outlines with minimal, absent, or cystic renal parenchyma exhibiting very poor or absent function on intravenous pyelograms (Fig. 31.1). VCU or retrograde pyelography was needed in γ segments to show the calyces as large, clubbed, and merging with one another and the pelvis.

Radiological types of renal segments associated with ureteric-orifice position

Figure 31.2 provides the correlation between renal segment types and the positions in zones of the corresponding ureteric orifices.

Normal zone: orifice positions 'A', 'E', 'F'

The orifices in the normal zone lay within the confines of the trigonal zone. The most lateral normal position corresponds with the 'A' position. There were 57 orifices in position 'A', five in 'E' and four in 'F'.

Examination of the X-rays of all 66 kidney segments associated with orifices in this normal trigonal zone revealed that 63 were normal kidney segments, and three were β segments. All three β segments had orifices situated in the 'F' position, which may be considered as a junctional group of orifices bordering on the caudal zone.

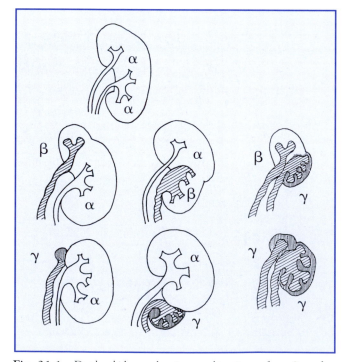

Fig. 31.1 *Duplex kidneys showing combinations of α, β, and γ radiological segments. (Reprinted, by permission, from Mackie, G.G., Awang, H. and Stephens, F.D. (1975), The ureteric orifice: The embryologic key to radiologic status of duplex kidneys. J. Pediatr. Surg. 10: 473, Fig. 2.)*

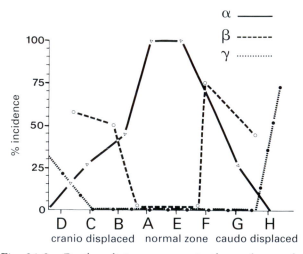

Fig. 31.2 *Graph outlining percentage incidence of types of renal segments to the zones of orifice positions; α segments are found mainly in the normal zone, β segments in the borderlands between zones and γ segments exclusively in the farthest reaches of the cranial and caudal zones. (Reprinted, by permission, from Mackie, G.G., Awang, H. and Stephens F.D. (1975), The ureteric orifice: The embryologic key to radiologic status of duplex kidneys. J. Pediatr. Surg. 10: 473, Fig. 3.)*

The associated ureters to these segments in all but one were < 1 cm in diameter. The appearance of the orifices was predominantly cone or stadium, and the mean submucosal ureteral tunnel length was 10.3 mm (10 mm is considered normal). Reflux was found in 16 ureters (29 per cent) of this group. The reflux was 'moderate' in 12 and 'slight' in four. The close correlation of type of renal segment with endoscopic position of the orifice on the trigone is shown in Fig. 31.2.

Cranial zone: orifice positions 'B', 'C', 'D'

The cranial-zone group comprised 37 orifices of ureters from the LPU or UPU segments issuing on the bladder base in a lateral extension of the cornu of the trigone. Orifices in the 'B' position lay lateral but adjacent to 'A', with 'D' position orifices located within a diverticulum on the bladder wall. 'C' position lay between 'B' and 'D'. There were 19 and 17 orifices in the 'B' and 'C' positions, respectively, and one in the 'D' position.

The X-ray findings of these 37 associated renal segments revealed that 14 had normal appearances, and 23 were abnormal, 20 showing β segments and three γ segments.

Seventeen of 37 ureters of the segments in this zone were normal (< 1 cm in diameter). Twelve showed megaureters, 10 being associated with orifices in the 'C' or 'D' position. The orifice appearance in 19 was abnormal; 14 were described as horseshoe and five as golf-hole. The mean tunnel length measurement was 7.6 mm for the 'B' position and 2.7 mm for the 'C' and 'D' positions.

Reflux occurred in 80 per cent of ureters in this zone. It was moderate in 19 and gross in nine. The 'C'- and 'D'-position orifices were associated with reflux in 17 of 18 ureters, or 94 per cent, while 'B'-orifice ureters showed reflux in 11 of 17, or 65 per cent.

None of the β kidney segments was available for histological examination, and the one γ segment showed dysplastic change of the renal parenchyma according to the criteria previously outlined.

Caudal zone: orifice positions 'G' and 'H'

The caudal zone group of 19 urethral positioned orifices was associated with abnormalities of the ectopic renal segment of the duplex kidney. The 'G'-position orifice was accompanied by a ureterocele in 13 of 17. The 'G' position ranged from the bladder neck to the verumon-

tanum in the male, or along the whole length of the urethra and the urethrovaginal perineal bridge in the female. The 'H'-position orifice may lie in the ejaculatory duct or seminal vesicle in the male, or Gartner's duct and hymen in the female. Examination of the renal segments associated with 'G' and 'H' orifices showed all 19 to have abnormal appearances; eight were β type, and 11 were γ. Seventeen of the 19 ureters were > 1 cm in diameter, and 13 of these measured $\geq$ 2 cm. Tunnel lengths were considerably elongated, but were not measured in this group, and reflux occurred in 26 per cent. It was slight in one, moderate in two, and gross in two.

Eleven of 15 excised ectopic segments showed histologic changes of renal dysplasia and hypoplasia. Intravenous or retrograde pyelograms showing representative types of renal segments are shown in Figs 31.3, 31.4 and 31.5.

Eleven of the 61 duplex kidneys (22 renal segments) were of bifid variety, eight having orifices in the 'A' position, one in the 'B' position and two in the 'C' position. All the renal segments were α types. Nineteen of the 20 ureters were normal in dimensions; only one LPU with

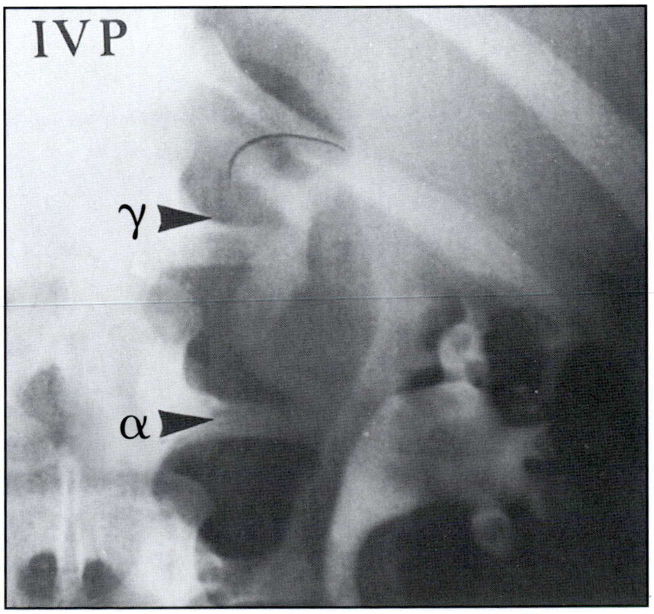

Fig. 31.3 *Left duplex kidney with ectopic segment γ ('H'-position orifice) and renal segment; orthotopic segment α ('A'-position orifice) on intravenous pyelogram with renal segment. (Reprinted, by permission, from Mackie, G.G., Awang, H. and Stephens, F.D. (1975), The ureteric orifice: The embryologic key to radiologic status of duplex kidneys. J. Pediatr. Surg. 10: 473, Fig. 4.)*

Table 31.1 *Correlation of orifice zone to ureteric and renal abnormality and incidence of reflux*

| Zone | Number of renal segments | Orifice type | | | | Mean tunnel length (cm) | Reflux (%) | Megaureter (>1 cm) | Kidney type | | | Morphology | | Not excised |
		Normal	Stadium	Horseshoe	Golf-hole				a	β	γ	Dysplasia	Normal	
Normal (A,E,F)	66	27	9	6	0	1.3	29% 4 slight 12 moderate	3%	63	3	0	N/A*	N/A*	66
Craniozone (B,C,D)	37	2	6	14	5	0.5	80% 12 moderate 9 gross	27.1%	14	20	3	1	1	36
Caudozone (G,H)	19		13 (Ureteroceles)			†	26% 1 slight 2 moderate 2 gross	89%	0	8	11	11	4	4

*Not measured.
†N/A = not available.
Source: Mackie, G.G., Awang, H. and Stephens, F.D. (1975), The ureteric orifice: The embryologic key to radiologic status of duplex kidneys. *J. Pediatr. Surg.* 10: 473, Table 1.

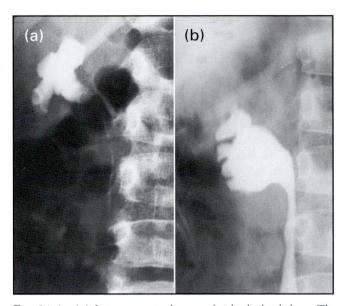

Fig. 31.4 (*a*) *Intravenous pyelogram of right duplex kidney. The upper segment is hypertrophic with 'A'-positioned orifice; the lower segment does not visualize on intravenous pyelogram.* (**b**) *Retrograde pyelogram (and micturition cystoureterogram). The non-functioning segment with 'C' orifice is visualized. (Reprinted, by permission, from Mackie, G.G. Awang, H. and Stephens, F.D. (1975), The ureteric orifice: The embryologic key to radiologic status of duplex kidneys. J. Pediatr. Surg. 10: 473, Fig. 5.)*

common stem issuing in the 'C' position measured 1 cm in diameter. The above data are shown in Table 31.1.

Correlation of radiological type with orifice location

This study demonstrates the correlation between normal or abnormal ureteral-orifice positions and corresponding renal segment type. It was found that when one or both ureteric orifices arose from the normal zone of the trigone, the orifice appearance and tunnel length were normal; reflux occurred infrequently, and the ureter and renal segment appeared normal. When one or both orifices were sited in the cranial zone, then the orifice appearance was abnormal, tunnel length short, reflux common and the ureteral diameter was larger. The associated renal segment assumed an abnormal appearance, being either β or γ type.

Orifices located in the caudal zone were associated with ureteroceles, which may permit both reflux and obstruction. The ureters were also abnormally widened, and the renal segments were abnormal, being γ or less

frequently β in type. These radiological abnormalities corresponded in 12 of 16 segments removed with dysplasia of the renal segments. This corroborates the previous findings in an infection-free series of specimens of neonatal duplex kidneys where renal segments of the displaced ureter were found to have a high incidence of dysplasia. 'B' and 'F' sites can be regarded as borderland areas between the zones and, as such, could be expected to be associated with normal and mildly abnormal renal segments. In fact, half were normal and half were β kidneys. If these borderland areas were ignored on the basis that they represent transition types, then it becomes clear that the normal-zone orifices beget normal renal segments, and abnormal zone orifices beget abnormal segments.

Embryological explanation

This close correlation of orifice position with renal type is reasonably explained by defective embryogenesis, which, though more commonly seen with duplex units, also applied equally with single-ureter systems. The fact that bifid ureters, which represent very late splitting of the ureteral bud, always had the same appearance in each segment, further supports this view.

This theory postulates a very close approximation of the zone of the nephrogenic ridge, which gives rise to the normal renal parenchyma to that section of the wolffian duct from which normal ureters arise. When both ureteric buds arise from this site, both kidney segments exhibit normal parenchymal development. If ureteric buds arise from the wolffian duct caudal or cranial to this section, they will contact either the depleted tail end of the nephrogenic ridge or the area destined to atrophy or transformation to gonadal structures, respectively. Thus, the thin parenchyma of the orthotopic kidney, which can be detected sonographically or radiographically, may be correctly interpreted as hypoplasia, and the small, poorly functioning or cystic nubbins of ectopic segments may be hypodysplastic renal structures.

Hitherto, these radiographically abnormal kidney segments have often been attributed to infection or the dynamic effects of reflux or obstruction on the developing kidney, which results in areas of dysplasia (Bialestock, 1963; Hartman and Hodson, 1969; Cussen, 1971b; Johnston, 1972). Analyses of the kidneys and

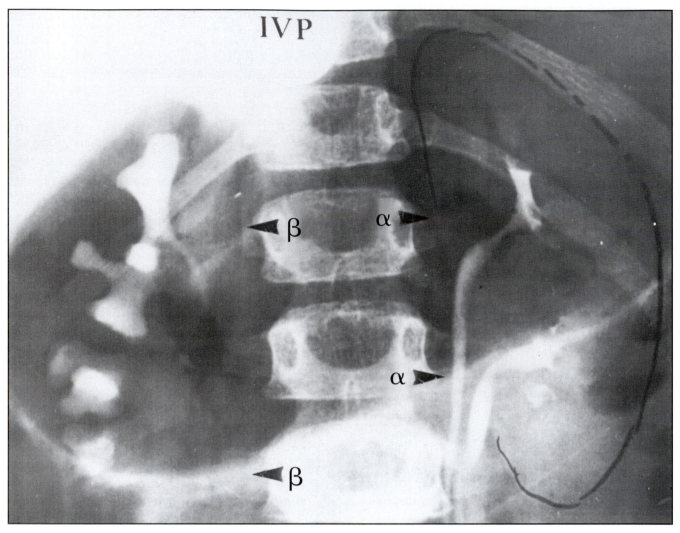

Fig. 31.5 *Bilateral duplex kidneys. The left kidney shows both upper and lower segments. (This kidney has a bifid ureter in the 'A' position.) The right kidney shows both upper and lower segments (the UPU orifice in 'G' position and associated with a ureterocele; LPU orifice in 'B' position). (Reprinted, by permission, from Mackie, G.G., Awang, H. and Stephens, F.D. (1975), The ureteric orifice: The embryologic key to radiologic status of duplex kidneys. J. Pediatr. Surg. 10: 473, Fig. 6.)*

ureters in this series suggest that the dysplastic segments arise *ab initio* owing to the abnormal site of origin of the bud. Infection, when it occurs at some later stage in childhood, may merely bring to notice a pre-existing abnormal state of the kidney. On radiological grounds, however, the aetiology remains unresolved unless the ureteric orifices can be shown to be abnormal in position and correlated with the renal changes.

Abnormal positioning of the kidney may be caused by a number of factors:

1. Arrest of development on the normal path of migration (pelvic or lumbar kidney).
2. Migration beyond the normal limit (superior ectopic thoracic kidney).
3. Ectopia of the metanephros (horseshoe kidney) impacting, overlapping and overriding.
4. Induction of contralateral metanephros by wandering ureteric bud (crossed renal ectopia).
5. Duplex wolffian ducts, each with its own ureteric bud and kidney (supernumerary kidney).

Pelvic and lumbar renal ectopy

Arrest of the normal path of renal ascent occurs. The ureteric bud and metanephros may set out along the normal embryological path and arrest at any level. The step-by step takeover of renal blood vessels, which initially are pelvic in origin but subsequently low and then high lumbar, is also arrested. The pelvis of the ectopic kidney is typically anterior and the vessels are generally multiple, hilar and cortical. The ureteric orifice is sometimes ectopic, indicating likely defective inducer capacity in such instances.

Congenital superior ectopic (thoracic) kidney*

Renal ectopia cranial to the normal lumbar location is a rare entity which bears many names including superior and thoracic kidney. The cranially located kidney may lie above or below or partly through the diaphragm and is usually normal in size and function. The pelvis may be anterior and the ureter considerably longer than normal. It has been clinically significant chiefly because of frequent misdiagnosis and unnecessary exploratory surgery.

The purpose of this section and the review of previous publications is to describe the anatomy and diagnostic criteria and terminology of types of superior kidneys with respect to the diaphragm, the vertebral levels of the upper poles, the renal arteries and the adrenal glands. A distinction is made between the high kidney which migrates beyond its normal location and that which is swept cranially with other organs into the foramen of Bochdalek. The intrinsic migratory capability of the kidney is apparent from the nature of the embryology of the structures in the pathway of the high kidney. Newer diagnostic modalities serve the clinician well in elucidating the nature of the mass in the vicinity of the diaphragm seen on radiographs of the chest.

Nomenclature

The term 'superior kidney' pertains to a kidney which according to vertebral levels is located more cranially than normal. 'Superior' is preferred to such terms as 'thoracic' or 'intrathoracic' kidney because the latter terms do not include high kidneys which lie below or partly above and partly below the diaphragm. The superior kidney may lie entirely above the hemidiaphragm, partly through it, under it, or with other abdominal viscera in a Bochdalek defect of the diaphragm. These sub-types are herein designated (1) supra-, (2) trans-, (3) infradiaphragmatic and (4) Bochdalek ectopic kidneys.

Eventration is a congenital smooth elevation of the thinned out hemidiaphragm, and the kidney may be located in a superior though infradiaphragmatic position.

Three illustrative examples of sub-types 2, 3 and 4 superior kidneys showing typical radiographic or anatomic features are reported. Seven case reports of Bochdalek defects are included to provide evidence as to the influence of the developing diaphragm on the embryogenesis of superior kidneys. Selected case reports

*This section is reproduced in part, with modifications, with permission of Excerpta Medica. From N'Guessen, G., Stephens, F.D. and Pick J. (1984), Congenital superior ectopic (thoracic) kidney. Urology, 24(3), 219–228.

of superior kidneys, together with our interpretations of vertebral levels obtained from the illustrations of the chest X-ray films were collated with respect to radio-graphical and anatomical evidence as to the locations of the kidneys and their relationship to the diaphragm and vertebral bodies. Case reports of superior kidneys with a history of trauma or a suspicion of trauma were excluded.

Case reports

Case 1

A mentally retarded female, aged six months, had a trans-diaphragmatic left kidney. She died of pneumonic consolidation of the right lung. Previous chest X-ray film revealed a soft-tissue mass projecting posteromedially above the left hemidiaphragm. Gastrointestinal radiography showed that the viscera lay below the diaphragm. Intravenous pyelography proved that the mass consisted of the upper half of the left good kidney with its upper

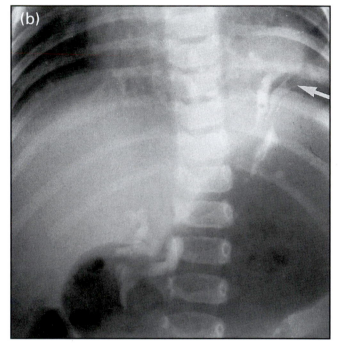

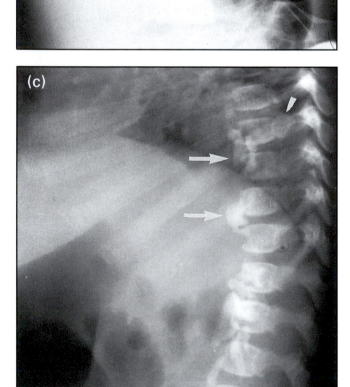

Fig. 32.1 *Transdiaphragmatic superior kidney (Case 1). (**a**) Chest X-ray film: soft tissue density behind heart (arrows). (**b**), (**c**) Radiopaque medium in calyces of left kidney above and below diaphragm on anteroposterior and lateral radiographs (arrows) and in calyces of right kidney in normal location. (Reprinted, with permission, from N'Guessen, G., Stephens, F.D. and Pick, J. (1984), Congenital superior ectopic (thoracic) kidney. Urology 24(3): 220, Fig. 1.)*

border at the level of the intervertebral disk between the seventh and eighth thoracic vertebrae. The right kidney pelvis lay in normal location beside the second and third lumbar vertebrae. The dome of the left hemidiaphragm lay at the level of the ninth thoracic (T9) vertebra (Fig. 32.1).

Case 2

This premature male baby, birth weight 2100 g, died aged 23 days of multiple anomalies including bilateral diaphragmatic eventrations, cloacal exstrophy and a closed sacral meningocele (Fig. 32.2). The chromosomes were normal. Chest X-ray film revealed a narrow bell-shaped thoracic cage and left hemidiaphragm at level of T9 verte-bra, and on fluoroscopy the hemidiaphragm was immobile. The right diaphragm lay at level of T12 and was immobile. 'Butterfly' anomalies of T8, T9 and T11 vertebrae were present.

Nuclide scaning showed good function in the left kidney and absence of function on the right side. Necropsy revealed the typical features of cloacal exstrophy. In addition, a thin see-through membrane with pleura attached formed the cupola which capped the upper half of the left kidney. This kidney was normal in size and structure and reached to the seventh vertebral level. This membrane was sparsely muscularized peripherally. The ureter was elongated and the vessels arose in the lumbar region and coursed cranially to the hilus. On the right side, the diaphragm formed a similar translucent cupola covering over the right very small hypodysplastic kidney. Its vessels also coursed cranially from a lumbar origin. The cap of diaphragm over the small kidney lay at T12 vertebral level, and the remainder of the diaphragm was on the level of the first lumbar vertebra. The right kidney was dysplastic and weighed only 4 g. The right ureter was not identified and was believed to be atretic.

The left adrenal gland lay in its normal location but caudal to and contiguous with the lower pole of the superior kidney. It was oval in shape, flat, longitudinally oriented, and weighed 4 g. It was normal microscopically. The right adrenal was pyramidal, weighed 4 g, and was draped over the anterior surface of the kidney.

Case 3

A female, aged 27 months, had a Bochdalek defect of the diaphragm on the right side. A respiratory infection developed

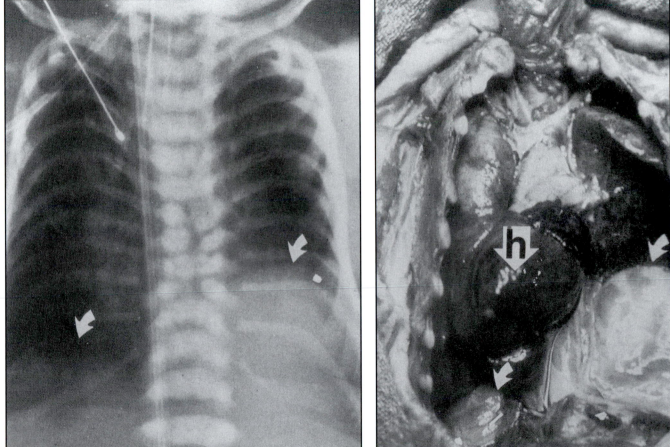

Fig. 32.2 *Infradiaphragmatic superior kidney (Case 2). (a) Chest X-ray film: soft-tissue density below cupola of left diaphragm at level of T9 vertebra; right cupola at T12; note also 'butterfly' vertebrae and bell-shaped chest. (b) At necropsy, anterior aspect of thoracic cavity and translu-cent left cupola overlying left kidney and other viscera, and also translucent right cupola capping right mini-kidney and viscera. (h = heart; arrows = thinned-out cupolas.) (Reprinted, with permission, from N'Guessen, G., Stephens, F.D. and Pick, J. (1984), Congenital superior ectopic (thoracic) kidney. Urology 24(3): 220, Fig. 2.)*

warranting a chest X-ray film at 21 months which showed an irregular outline of diaphragm and viscera at the T8 vertebral level. A barium enema revealed colon and small intestine above the liver and diaphragm on the right side to the level of the fifth vertebral body.

Because of respiratory distress, surgical repair of the diaphragm was undertaken. On withdrawing the viscera through the defect in the diaphragm the pleura was found to be intact. The posterior half of the diaphragm was deficient, and the anterior half had no attachment to the posterior wall of the right thoracic cage. The right kidney, which was mobile, and part of the liver lay in this retropleural space. The free posterior edge of the diaphragm was tacked to the posterior body wall, and the kidney and viscera were placed below the line of repair. The renal vessels and adrenal gland were not seen. Recovery was uneventful, and the child remains well.

Cases 4 to 10
The diaphragms of eight babies who died soon after birth of the effects of Bochdalek defects were dissected and described to determine whether or not any of the defects were conducive to superior locations of the kidney. The kidneys in seven of the eight babies were normally placed, but in one the right kidney lay above the defect of the diaphragm. The findings are described in case reports in the section on embryogenesis and in Table 32.1.

Orientation of diaphragms and kidneys to bodies of vertebrae

The diaphragm gains attachment anteriorly to the xyphoid process which lies approximately level with the body of T10 vertebra. Posteriorly it arises on each side from the lumbocostal arches which attach to the body and transverse processes of the first lumbar vertebra and the tips of the twelfth ribs, and the crura which have a longitudinal origin from the bodies of L1, L2 and L3 (Fig. 32.3). The diaphragm is level with the eighth rib in the mid-axillary line on each side corresponding approximately with the level of the tenth vertebral body. The diaphragm also arises from the costochondral junctions of T6 to T10, and muscle bundles converge radially to insert into the right and left aponeurotic leaflets of the central tendon. The levels of the domes of the right and left hemidiaphragms in the adult rise to approximately T8 and T9, respectively, on forced expiration with the patient in the erect position (Williams and Warwick, 1980). Avery (1964) put the level of the domes of the diaphragm in the newborn infant at the seventh rib posteriorly or a little lower. This corresponds to the body of the T7 vertebra. She found that the excursion during crying was slightly more than one interspace (Fig. 32.3).

The central segment of the diaphragm is perforated by major structures passing between the thorax and the abdomen. The aortic hiatus lies at level of body of L1, the oesophageal hiatus at T10 and the vena caval foramen at T8.

Table 32.1 *Clinical features, types of defect of diaphragm, and organ situations in Bochdalek hernias*

Case No.	Sex	Side	Type of diaphragm defect*	Sac	Ribs	Positions of organs		Liver in diaphragm defect	Remarks
						Kidney	Adrenal		
4	M	L	C	+	12	Normal	Normal	Lobule constricted at base	Pericardial defect
5	F	L	C	0	12	Normal	Normal	Lobule (congested)	
6	M	L	A,B	0	11	Normal	Normal	Lobule constricted at base	
7	F	L	A,B	0	11	Normal	Normal	Lobe with abnormal contour	
8	M	L	A,B,C	0	12	Normal	Normal	Lobe tightly constricted almost amputated	Cardiac anomaly
9	F	L	A,B,C,D	0	12+ cervical rib	Normal	Normal	Lobule deeply constricted	Cardiac anomaly
10	M	R	A,B,C	0	12	Superior	With kidney	Part of lobe	Renal artery origin normal, sequestered lobe of lung

*See Fig. 32.4.
Source: N'Guessen, G., Stephens, F. D. and Pick, J. (1984), Congenital superior ectopic (thoracic) kidney. *Urology* 24(3), Table 1.

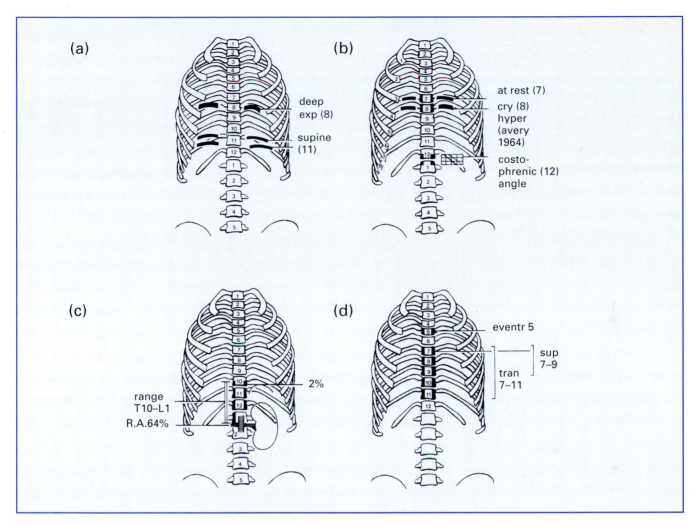

Fig. 32.3 *Vertebral body levels of cupolas of diaphragm and of normal and superior kidneys. (**a**) Levels of cupolas in adult when supine, T11, and erect, T12 and on deep inspiration, T8. (**b**) In newborn baby cupola at T7 at rest and T8 when crying or hyperventilating. (**c**) Kidney normally lies beside T12–L3; superior border ranges between L1 and T10. Renal artery arises from aorta at level of L1–2 disk in 64 per cent of normal individuals and between upper and lower borders of L1 and L2, respectively, in remainder. (**d**) Upper borders of superior kidneys range between T7 and T11 with transdiaphragmatic, T7–T9 with supradiaphragmatic; cupola in eventration may rise to T5 with kidney high but beneath diaphragm. (Reprinted, with permission, from N'Guessen, G., Stephens, F.D. and Pick, J. (1984), Congenital superior ectopic (thoracic) kidney. Urology 24(3): 222, Fig. 3.)*

Of special interest regarding superior kidneys is the lumbocostal trigone of the diaphragm. The posteromedial sheet of muscle bundles arising from lateral lumbocostal arches courses craniolaterally to insert into the lateral leaflet of the central tendon. The posterolateral sheet of muscle bundles arising from the tips of the twelfth and eleventh ribs is directed craniomedially also to insert into the lateral leaflet. Between the origins of these two sheets of muscle is a small, thin lumbocostal triangle. The upper pole of the normal kidney and adrenal gland lie on the posteromedial muscle sheet. The fused anterior and posterior layers of the perirenal fascia of Gerota gain fibrous attachment to the fascia of this sheet just cranial to the lumbocostal arches.

Normal kidney and its orientation to vertebrae

The kidney usually lies opposite the twelfth thoracic and first three lumbar vertebrae, the pelvis being at the level of the bodies of the L2 and L3 vertebrae but may lie at a slightly higher level (Fig. 32.3c).

Currarino and Pinckney (1981) found radiographically on routine intravenous pyelogram (IVP) studies of patients in supine position that the upper border of the kidney lay at the T11/T12 intervertebral disk and slightly above or below but occasionally lying as high as T10. Other studies have shown that the renal artery most often arises from the aorta at the level of the disk between L1 and L2 but may arise as high as L1 (Anson and McVay, 1936) and that the hilum and pelvis are situated opposite the bodies of L2 and L3 vertebrae.

Diaphragm, transdiaphragmatic kidneys and vertebral levels

The data were obtained from 41 case reports and the accompanying X-ray photographs (42 kidneys) including one bilateral and our Case 1. The vertebral levels of the domes of the diaphragms of 28 subjects as measured on anteroposterior projections was T8 in two (Wolfromm, 1940; Hill and Bunts, 1960), T9 in four (Barloon et al., 1957; Reboud and Bernard, 1958; Bernard et al., 1959; Moazzenzadeh et al., 1977), T10 in 11 (Paul et al., 1960; Rognon, 1960; Burke et al., 1967; DeCastro and Schumacher, 1969; Hertz and Schahn, 1969; Lundius, 1975; Kangarloo et al., 1977; Nakala and Sakaguchi, 1977; Ramos et al., 1979; Kirschenbaum et al., 1981) and in Case 1, T11 in five (Cruickshank, 1952; Berlin et al., 1957; Pescione, 1957; Gwinn and Fletcher, 1968) and T12 in six (Bugden, 1950; Schwartz and Frankel, 1952; Berlin et al., 1957; Hill and Bunts, 1960; Lozano and Rodriguez, 1975).

Twenty-six of the 42 transdiaphragmatic kidneys were diagnosed by one or more of the following modalities: chest radiography, excretory or retrograde pyelography, contrast studies, pneumography, renography, and latterly, computed tomography scans and sonography. The vertebral levels of the upper poles were T8 in 11 cases (Wolfromm, 1940; Barloon et al., 1957; Schapira et al., 1965; Burke et al., 1967; Hertz and Schahn, 1969; Lundius, 1975; Lozano and Rodriguez, 1975; Moazzenzadeh et al., 1977; Kangarloo et al., 1977; Kirschenbaum et al., 1981; Ramos et al., 1979), T9 in 10 cases (Berlin et al., 1957; Pescione, 1957; Hill and Bunts; 1960; DeCastro and Schumacher, 1969; Moazzenzadeh et al., 1977; Nakala and Sakaguchi, 1977; Ramos et al., 1979; Elkin, 1980), T10 in one case (Fleischner et al., 1950), T11 in three cases (Schwartz and Frankel, 1952; Reboud and Bernard, 1958; Gwinn and Fletcher, 1968) and T12 in one case (Berlin et al., 1957). The domes of the diaphragms were most commonly at the T10 and T11 levels, whereas the upper poles of the kidneys were predominantly at T8 and T9. The renal opacity was seen on the lateral chest film to protrude through a defect in the sloping posterior part of the diaphragm.

Thirteen of the 42 transdiaphragmatic kidneys were proved to be protruding through the diaphragm by thoracotomy or necropsy examinations. The vertebral levels were obtained from the case reports and X-ray films. The upper poles of nine of these kidneys lay at the level of T7 in one patient (Kumar De et al., 1968), T8 in three (Barloon et al., 1957; Bernard et al., 1959; Hill and Bunts, 1960), T9 in three (Cruickshank, 1952; Paul et al., 1960; Rognon, 1960), T10 in one (Reboud and Bernard, 1958) and T11 in one (Bugden, 1950). Twelve of the kidneys penetrated the sloping posterior wall of the diaphragm in the costovertebral gutter and ranged between one-quarter and three-quarters through the diaphragm. The thin cap overlying the protruding kidney was described as fibrous in five (Barloon et al., 1957; Paul et al., 1960; Rognon, 1960; Hertz and Schahn, 1969; Moazzenzadeh et al., 1977), pleural in five (Bugden, 1950; Cruickshank, 1952; Reboud and Bernard, 1958; Bernard et al., 1959; Hill and Bunts, 1960), thin fascia and relaxed diaphragm in one (Williams and Warwick, 1980) and in one (Campbell, 1951) the kidney was described as plugging a hole in the diaphragm. Two kidneys were constricted by the diaphragm (Bernard et al., 1959; Rognon, 1960).

The lateral chest X-ray film on deep inspiration showed the rounded radiopacity of the high kidney protruding in the paravertebral gutter and clear confirmation of the nature of the mass was obtained in 32 by excretory urography (Fig. 32.1). Pneumography was advocated by Pescione (1957) and Veran et al. (1958) to determine the relationship of the kidney to the diaphragm. They showed by pneumoretroperitoneography that a confined sickle-like crescent of gas straddled the upper pole of the protruding kidney.

Diaphragm with supradiaphragmatic kidney

The hemidiaphragm was described in the case reports of six patients who had supradiaphragmatic kidneys confirmed by thoracotomy (Daroczi, 1956; Laumonier et al., 1957; Franciskovic and Marincic, 1959; Nini, 1961; Noordijk, 1967; Emmett, 1977). Four were on the right side and two on the left. The kidneys lay entirely above the diaphragm in the paravertebral gutter and were extrapleural. The vertebral level of the dome of the diaphragm was T10 in one patient whose superior kidney rose to the level of T8 (Noordijk, 1967) and was not available in the other five. The diaphragm was observed at thoracotomy to be normal in three (Laumonier *et al.*, 1957; Franciskovic and Marincic, 1959; Noordijk, 1967), adherent to the lower pole of the kidney in one (Nini, 1961) and had a small aperture posteromedially which accommodated the descending ureter and ascending renal vessels in two (Daroczi, 1956; Franciskovic and Marincic, 1959). The vertebral levels of the upper poles, read from illustrations of chest radiographs, were T7 (Laumoniet *et al.*, 1957), T8 (Franciskovic and Marincic, 1959; Nordijk, 1967; Emmett, 1977), T9 (Daroczi, 1956) and in one case the level was not available (Nini, 1961). Renal artery was lumbar in origin in three (Daroczi, 1956; Franciskovic and Marincic, 1959; Noordijk, 1967), double with the vessel to the upper pole arising from the thoracic aorta in one (Laumonier *et al.*, 1957) and the origins were not stated in two (Nini, 1961; Emmett, 1977). The adrenal gland was found to be above the kidney in one case (Daroczi, 1956), and was not mentioned in the others. From the case descriptions, it is clear that the supradiaphragmatic kidney can be an extrapleural organ with a lumbar blood supply and lodged totally above the well-formed and muscularized hemidiaphragm.

Diaphragm with infradiaphragmatic superior kidney

With eventration, a condition in which the hemidiaphragm is mainly fibrous, the vertebral level of the dome may be as high as T4.

From the descriptions and illustrations in five case reports of patients with eventration described in urologic journals, and our Case 2 (bilateral eventration), the vertebral levels of the upper borders of the six right and left kidneys which lay under the eventrated hemidiaphragms were defined by pneumography, contrast radiography, thoracotomy or necropsy. These levels were T5 in two cases (Bulgrin and Holmes, 1955; Tamura *et al.*, 1970), T8 in two cases (Baurys and Servosa, 1949; Spillane and Prather, 1952), and in our necropsy Case 2. The superior kidneys in three of the patients were on the right side, in two patients on the left side, and in one, bilateral.

The hemidiaphragms in our Case 2 were so thin that the kidneys when viewed from the thorax could be clearly seen through the fine translucent membrane and overlying pleura (Fig. 32.2). The diaphragm was described as a thin translucent white membrane in one patient (Spillane and Prather, 1952), and intact and fibrous in a necropsy case (Bulgrin and Holmes, 1955).

The superior kidneys in all but the necropsy case had been shown to be otherwise near normal in shape and function and with elongated ureters. The kidneys of the necropsy subject (Case 2) were both superior; the left was normal in size and structure with normal but elongated ureter and hilar vessels which were derived from a normal lumbar origin; the right kidney was small and dysplastic with ureteral atresia. The origins of the renal vessels were also lumbar. The adrenal gland on the left side was discoid in shape and caudal to the superior kidney. The position of the adrenal glands in the other five patients was not known.

Bochdalek defects of diaphragm and kidney position

The diaphragms of seven newborn babies with Bochdalek hernias were studied pre- and postmortem (Table 32.1, Fig. 32.4). The documented operative findings of a right superior kidney and Bochdalek defect of Case 3 and a review of pertinent features of superior kidneys from 13 previous case reports are also described.

The kidney position relative to the Bochdalek defect in the seven newborn necropsy subjects was determined by dissection. Of the seven, four were male and three female. Six were on the left side and one on the right. The kidneys and adrenal glands were in normal position in all six subjects with defects on the left side. The right kidney with the adrenal in normal location relative to the kidney was rotated through the defect in the diaphragm and could be readily transposed on its pedicle to the abdomen. The level of origin from the aorta of the renal arteries was normal in all subjects.

On the left side, the defects of the diaphragm occurred in the left leaf of the central tendon and pleuroperitoneal membrane in two (Cases 4 and 5), and in both the muscular diaphragm in the periphery was intact (Fig. 32.4). A sac was present in one (Case 4). The posterolateral and posterior quadrants were defective in two (Cases 6 and 7), and in another the defect

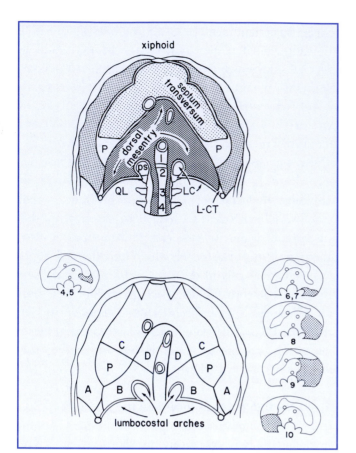

Fig. 32.4 (Upper diagram) *Embryologic components of diaphragm represented as two horseshoes and two crescents. Upper horseshoe is central tendon (light stipple) derived from septum transversum; lower horseshoe or hoof (hatched) is mediastinal and derived from dorsal mesentery, and crescents (heavy stipple) represent body wall or transversus abdominus components (ps = psoas muscle; QL = quadratus lumborum muscle; LC = lumbocostal arches; L-CT = lumbocostal trigone; P = pleuroperitoneal membrane; numerals 1–4 = lumbar vertebrae). (Lower diagram) Embryologic areas of diaphragm affected in association with superior kidney and Bochdalek defects. Case 1 (trans-diaphragmatic kidney) B defect of dorsal mesentery component. Cases 4 and 5 (inset) P defect of pleuroperitoneal membrane. Cases 6 and 7, A and B defects of components derived from lateral body wall and dorsal mesentery. Case 8, A and B defects plus defects of pleuroperitoneal P and part of septum transversum C. Case 9, A, B, P and C defects plus defect of dorsal mesentery component D adjoining oesophagus. Case 10, right defects of A, B, P and part of C components. (Reprinted, with permission, from N'Guessen, G., Stephens, F.D. and Pick, J. (1984), Congenital superior ectopic (thoracic) kidney. Urology 24(3): 224, Fig. 4.)*

comprised part of the left leaf of the central tendon and the posterolateral and posterior quadrants (Case 8). In the sixth baby (Case 9), the posterior half of the diaphragm which included the greater part of the left lateral leaf of the central tendon, the posterolateral and

posterior parts and the medial area adjacent to the oesophagus, was absent. In these four babies (Cases 6 to 9) the periphery of the diaphragm was defective around the trigone, and no posterior rim or cuff of diaphragm was present. In two, the twelfth rib was absent (Fig. 32.4 and Table 32.1). In these babies (Cases 4 and 9), most often the intestines, spleen, and stomach herniated through the defect. A lobe or lobule of liver indented by the edge of the diaphragm jammed the defect in five subjects, and in two others the left lobe was distorted or congested indicating that it too had herniated.

On the right side (Case 10), the wide defect involved the greater part of the right leaf of the central tendon and both the posterolateral and posterior quadrants (Fig. 32.4). The twelfth rib was present, but no cuff or diaphragm was found around the defect posteriorly. The kidney and adrenal gland together with a large right liver lobe and intestines and a sequestered lung lobe lay in and above the defect.

One living patient (Case 3) aged two years was found at operation to have on the right side posterolateral and posterior defects of the diaphragm and a superior kidney. The pleura was intact in this patient, and a large retro-pleural space was filled with colon, intestines, a constricted lobule of the right lobe of the liver and the kidney. The adrenal gland and renal vessels were not identified at operation. The edge of the anterior half of the diaphragm was sutured to the posterior abdominal wall and the mobile kidney with adrenal was readily placed caudal to the level of repair. The right diaphragmatic defect in this patient was similar in many respects to that of the necropsy subject except for the intact pleura and a presumed ultra-thin and invisible 'pleuroperitoneal' sac lining and retropleural space above the diaphragm.

A review of 13 other case reports of subjects with Bochdalek hernia in whom the superior location of the kidney was documented at operation, necropsy, computed tomography scan or pneumography revealed:

1. Six (Veran *et al.*, 1958; Fuzione and Molnar, 1966; Neuhauser, 1970; Boulesteix *et al.*, 1971; Kadowaki *et al.*, 1983) were on the right side with kidney and part of liver herniated, including one patient (Neuhauser, 1970), in whom the defect was repaired

leaving the high kidney above the diaphragm and returning the liver component to the abdomen; the renal vessels were lumbar in origin in three, higher than normal in one, and not stated in two.

2. Seven (Campbell 1930, 1951; Paul and Kanageruntheram, 1957; Latarjet et al., 1970; Ramos et al., 1979) were on the left side with herniation of kidney, stomach intestines, and in some, part of the liver or spleen; the upper poles of the kidneys lay approximately at T7 in two (Ramos et al., 1979), T9 in one (Kadowaki et al., 1983), T8 in one (Veran et al., 1958) and T10 in one (Fuzione and Molnar, 1966).

The origin of the renal vessels was recorded in five of the 13 subjects, being lumbar in three and higher than normal in two.

From all the data obtained from our observations and the records of case histories of subjects with Bochdalek defects and detailed descriptions of the kidneys, we found that the kidney location may be normal even when the posterior half of the diaphragm was entirely lacking; that uncommonly the kidney may be mobile and lying cranially with other viscera on an elongated lumbar vessel; that rarely the kidney may have a vessel of higher origin than normal indicating a superior ectopic location of the kidney (Neuhauser, 1970; Kadowaki et al., 1983), and that the kidneys were normal in structure whether normally placed or higher than normal.

Adrenal glands associated with superior kidneys

These organs were recognized only in patients subjected to thoracotomy or laparotomy or necropsy examinations of the diaphragms and superior kidneys.

Infradiaphragmatic superior kidneys and adrenal glands

Of the six case reports of superior kidneys with eventration, the adrenal glands were described only in our Case 2 in whom both hemidiaphragms were eventrated. The left normal kidney rose in the thorax below the diaphragm to the level of the T9 vertebral body, and the small right dysplastic kidney lay at level of T12. The left adrenal gland was flat, oval, and discoid and normal in location with respect to the vertebral bodies but lay entirely caudal to the kidney. On the right side the adrenal gland was normal in size, shape, and structure and lay on the anteromedial aspect enveloping the upper two-thirds of the kidney.

Transdiaphragmatic kidneys and adrenal glands

The transdiaphragmatic kidneys were explored by thoracotomy in 13 patients and by autopsy in one subject (Mikulicz-Radecki, 1922). The location of the adrenal gland was described in seven as being above the kidney in three (Barloon et al., 1957; Hill and Bunts, 1960; Rognon, 1960), behind in one (Bernard et al., 1959), below in one (Mikulicz-Radecki, 1922), high with the kidney in one (Campbell, 1951) and 'not above the kidney' in one (Campbell, 1951). The gland was not mentioned in six. Five of the seven adrenal glands so described were on the right and two were on the left side.

Supradiaphragmatic kidneys and the adrenal

Of six case reports of exploration of the supradiaphragmatic kidney by thoracotomy the adrenal gland was not mentioned in five and was described as being with the kidney and above the diaphragm in one case (Daroczi, 1956).

Adrenal glands and Bochdalek hernias

Of the 13 subjects with superior kidneys and Bochdalek hernias, the diaphragms were explored surgically in 12 and at autopsy in one. The adrenal glands were found to be above the left kidney in one (Latarjet et al., 1970), rotated to a higher than normal position with the right kidney in one (Reboud and Bernard, 1958), in two the adrenal gland was stated to be 'not above the kidney', (Boulesteix et al., 1971) and information was lacking in nine. Of seven other necropsy subjects with Bochdalek defects examined by us (Table 32.1), the kidneys and the adrenal glands were normal in position of six even though in three the diaphragm deficiency extended posteromedially and hence would offer no barrier to ascent of either kidney or adrenal. In the seventh baby, the right kidney rotated cranially into the defect but the adrenal remained in normal position relative to the upper pole of the kidney (Case 10).

The position of the adrenal gland in a few recorded examples was either above, behind, or below the superior kidney and when below, its shape was flattened and oval.

Embryogenesis of superior ectopic kidney and defects of diaphragm

Ascent of the kidney to a superior ectopic location is intimately associated with the development of other organs in and beyond its normal path of ascent. Under normal circumstances at the crown–rump 16–20 mm stage (6–7 weeks) embryo the kidney has translocated from S2 level to the loin at future vertebral levels T12 to L3. The kidney then laps the inferior surface of the diaphragm and impacts into the developing adrenal gland.

The developing diaphragm begins as the transverse septum, an infold of mesoderm from the anterior body wall of the embryo. This septum impinges on the foregut, and together with the dorsal mesentery completes the separation of the thorax from the abdomen in the midline. To either side lie the narrow pleuroperitoneal canals joining the pleural cavities with the abdominal coelom. The right and left lung buds grow rapidly into the pleural canals above the septum and excavate the inner layer of mesoderm of the body wall forming peripheral rims which edge medially toward the septum. These rims together with the septum and dorsal mesentery reduce the lumina of the pleuroperitoneal canals. The small lumens remaining become occluded at the 20-mm stage (eight weeks) by a thin pleuroperitoneal membrane which forms at the meeting point of all the components of the diaphragm and subsequently becomes muscularized (Fig. 32.4).

The components of the fully formed diaphragm are the central tendon which is derived from the septum transversum, the central muscle mass around the oesophagus, the great vessels and the posteromedial segment forms from the dorsal mesentery, and the peripheral muscle is added in from the mesoderm of the body wall representing the inturned thoracic continuation of the transversus abdominus muscle.

When viewed from the abdominal aspect, these embryological derivatives of the diaphragm can be depicted as two horseshoes and two crescents (Fig. 32.4). The anterior horseshoe originates from the transverse septum, the posterior from the dorsal mesentery and the crescents from the body wall. It is possible that the lumbocostal trigone represents the cleavage line between the contributions from the dorsal mesentery and the body wall (Cases 6–10, Table 32.1 and Fig. 32.4) and more centrally placed foramen in the hemidiaphragm is caused by failure of formation of the pleuroperitoneal membrane (Cases 4 and 5, Table 32.1 and Fig. 32.4).

If the kidney overshoots its mark continuing in the retroperitoneal plane before the posterior components of the diaphragm have come together, it will ascend in a plane posteromedial to the pleuroperitoneal canal and medial to the lumbocostal trigone. The diaphragm may then thinly and closely envelop the renal protrusion and form normally elsewhere as with the transdiaphragmatic kidney, or develop into a completely normal diaphragm caudal to the supradiaphragmatic kidney. In either instance, the kidney or the protruding part of the kidney is also enveloped by pleura and is firmly and irreducibly fixed in the high situation. If, however, the kidney overshoots its resting place after the components of the diaphragm have united, the superior kidney remains retroperitoneal and infradiaphragmatic. That the kidney actually migrates to its superior position is demonstrated by the occasional thoracic origin of the renal artery (Campbell, 1930; Laumonier et al., 1957), and the hitchhiking of the adrenal gland on the kidney or the bypassing of it by the kidney (Case 2).

The superior kidney in association with Bochdalek hernias is a rarity and is different from other superior kidneys in that it rarely has an enveloping cap of thinned out diaphragm, is retroperitoneal, rides through a wide deficit in company with other viscera, is mobile and can be withdrawn with other viscera from the thorax.

The position of the kidney, however, is usually normal with the upper pole at T11 or T12 either under or in the foramen of Bochdalek; the cupola of the diaphragm sinks somewhat caudally and the 'high' position of the kidney is more apparent than real.

Rarely, the kidney may be superior with its artery arising from an abnormally high origin (Kadowaki et al., 1983), indicating that the kidney had actually migrated through the foramen of Bochdalek to a permanently superior position.

Adrenal gland and liver in association with superior kidney

Another phenomenon of interest in the theory of embryogenesis of superior kidneys is the influence of the developing adrenal gland and liver on renal position.

Normally, the adrenal gland is forming at the 12-mm stage prior to arrival of the kidney in the loin. The left adrenal assumes a pyramidal shape fitting over the upper pole of the kidney. It was noted that the adrenal in subjects with superior kidneys may lie (1) above a supra-diaphragmatic kidney (Daroczi, 1956), or below (Nini, 1961) and (2) in transdiaphragmatic kidneys above (Barloon et al., 1957; Hill and Bunts, 1960; Rognon, 1960), or posterior (Bernard et al., 1959). Hence the kidney can meet the adrenal in a superior position, carry the adrenal with it or glide past it leaving the adrenal flattened in shape at its normal location. When the kidney was sufficiently mobile to encroach on the Bochdalek defect, the adrenal retained its polar location with regard to the kidney (Laterjet et al., 1970). With eventration of the diaphragm, the left kidney was superior and infradiaphragmatic and the adrenal gland was caudal to the kidney (Case 2).

In all the specimens (Cases 4 to 10) of Bochdalek hernias a part of the liver was protruding into the defect; in four it was the major part of a lobe and in three a lobule of a lobe. In four the protruding part was deeply constricted by the free edge of the diaphragm and in one almost to the point of amputation of the lobe. Presumably the liver, developing very early in the septum transversum proliferates abnormally in a cranial direction as well as caudally. Liver formation precedes closure of the pleuroperitoneal canal, and it, like the transdiaphragmatic superior kidney, may expand cranially preventing fusion of the components of the diaphragm.

We conclude that the mechanism of migration to superior locations is intrinsic in the kidney, the kidney migration is independent of and precedes the development of the diaphragm and adrenal gland, the migration is active rather than a passive rearrangement of structures in the growing organism, and that the transdiaphragmatic kidney and the liver impair fusion of the components of the diaphragm.

Horseshoe kidney

Ectopia of the metanephros. Caudomedial displacement of the tail end of one or both metanephroi may cause end-on, end-to-side or side-by-side contiguity with so-called horseshoe kidney malformation. The impaction of the metanephroi occurs in the future true pelvic site and the conglomerate migrates cranially to either near the normal level or short of it. Midline impactions lead to symmetric horseshoes, whereas others eventuate into the wide varieties of asymmetric forms. Predisposing causes of asymmetric metanephric impactions are agenesis of sacral segments and high cloacal defects.

Crossed renal ectopia

Induction of contralateral metanephros by the ureteric bud from the opposite side. If the ureteric bud arises from a wolffian duct that leans towards the opposite side, this bud may find itself in close association with the opposite metanephros which it then induces to form crossed renal ectopia. Such a kidney may be the sole kidney, a fused kidney with two ureters (one ipsi- and one contralateral) or more than two ureters may arise from one or both sides. A predisposing cause is hemivertebra of the lower lumbar or sacral vertebra with consequent scoliosis and deviation of the paraxial mesoderm and wolffian duct.

Supernumerary kidney*

Fifty-eight case reports of patients with supernumerary kidneys have been studied to determine the morphology, vagaries and embryogenesis of this rare and poorly documented anomaly. The supernumerary kidney usually was located caudal to the ipsilateral kidney when subserved by a bifid ureter and cranially when the ureters were separate. The Weigert–Meyer law (page 222) for duplex fused kidneys was obeyed by the supernumerary ureter in most fully documented cases of double ureters. Pathological conditions of the upper urinary tract occurred in more than 50 per cent of the patients with a bifid system, who were prone to have hydronephrosis and calculous disease, and with a double system, who were prone to have complications resulting from supernumerary ureteral ectopia. Double tails to the

---

*Reproduced in part, with the permission of The Williams and Wilkins Co. (1983) from N' Guessan, G. and Stepehens, F.D. Supernumerary Kidney J. Urol. 130: 649–653.

nephrogenic cords, each induced by a branch of a bifid bud or by one of two separate buds as opposed to tandem inductions of a single metanephros, were regarded as the probable embryogenesis.

Fusion of portions of kidneys with bifid or double ureters is a common and well documented duplex type of anomaly. Supernumerary kidneys are separate from the ipsilateral kidney and are subserved by a branch of a bifid ureter or a separate (double) ureter. These kidneys are documented poorly and are extremely rare.

Geisinger (1937) aptly defined a supernumerary kidney as 'the "free" accessory organ, which is a distinct, encapsulated, large or small parenchymatous mass topographically related to the usual kidney by a loose, cellular attachment at most and often by no attachment whatsoever.'

Herein is described in detail a necropsy specimen of the urinary tract with a supernumerary kidney. Data from case reports concerning the location and morphology of supernumerary kidney, and the orientation of the kidney, ureter and ureteral orifice to that of the ipsilateral kidney and ureter are reviewed. The natural history and mode of embryogenesis are compared with those of fused kidneys.

A specimen of a supernumerary kidney from a newborn with cloacal exstrophy was available for study. The kidneys, ureters, bladder, cloacal structures and vessels were dissected and histological examinations were made.

A total of 58 cases were reviewed, including 9 necropsy specimens examined by Stephens. Of these cases 29 were reported by Kretschmer (1929), seven by Geisinger (1937) and the remainder by other investigators (Hanley, 1942; Shane, 1942; Bacon, 1947; Exley and Hotchkiss, 1944; Rubin, 1948; Carlson, 1950; Campbell, 1970; Browne and Glashan, 1971; Wulfekuhler and Dube, 1971; Hicks et al., 1976; Sasidharan et al., 1976; Antony, 1977; Assayer, 1870 cited by Campbell 1930; Fourie, 1981; Tada et al., 1981; Pinter et al., 1982). One patient had bilateral supernumerary kidneys. In many instances the details were scanty but sufficient data were extracted to make some firm proposals.

The supernumerary kidney generally was distinguished from the ipsilateral kidney by its small size and/or abnormal position. The kidney was either a component of a bifid ureteral system or a completely duplicated system. Of 59 kidneys (58 patients), 21 were associated with bifid ureters and 19 with double ureters. Of the latter 19 kidneys the ureteral orifice-kidney correlations were shown clearly in 12, while the correlations were not available in seven. It was not known whether the ureters were bifid or completely separate in 18 patients.

There were 25 male and 27 female patients, while the sex was not stated in six. The supernumerary kidney lay on the right side in 19 patients and the left side in 37, while the side was not stated in two. Average patient age at the time the supernumerary kidney was discovered was 36 years (25 years for patients with double ureters, 36 years for those with bifid ureters and 33 years for those in the undetermined group). Six patients were ≤ 20 years old, while the age was not recorded in 15.

Case report

A 12-day old male newborn, with a weight of 1975g and crown–rump length of 31 cm, died of a left supernumerary kidney, exomphalos, cloacal exstrophy and multiple other malformations and deformities.

An autopsy specimen consisted of two left kidneys, one right kidney, cloacal exstrophy with small segments of ileum and large intestine, and the aorta and inferior vena cava (Fig. 32.5). The testes were not present in the specimen but the nuclear chromatin pattern was male.

The left ipsilateral kidney was bulky, low and placed transversely with the hilus facing left. The kidney measured $5.5 \times 1.5 \times 1.8$ cm and was grooved deeply by the common iliac artery posteriorly. The pelvis was intrarenal. The ureter was normal in calibre and issued from the hilus, traversing the wall of the exstrophic bladder. The aorta had two arteries that entered the cortex posteriorly and the hilus posterolaterally. The renal vein emerged from the parenchyma in a groove on the anterior surface. Histologically, the kidney was normal in structure, did not exhibit infection and had a radial glomerular count (Schwarz et al., 1981) of six.

The supernumerary kidney was small ($2 \times 0.6 \times 0.6$ cm) and reniform but lay transversely in the left loin with the hilus directed caudally. The ureter was 1.5–2.0 cm in diameter and highly tortuous, coursed anterior to and grooved the upper pole of the ipsilateral kidney, and entered the back of the exstrophied bladder contiguous with the ipsilateral ureter.

The supernumerary kidney was hypoplastic and the radial count of glomeruli was three to four. The medulla contained large-calibre collecting ducts, some of which were necrosed within small abscesses. Cortical vessels showed perivascular collections of white cells.

The contralateral right kidney was disk-shaped, flattened anteroposteriorly and small (3.0×1.5 cm). The kidney lay in the right loin at a level slightly caudal to the supernumerary kidney. The pelvis was intrarenal and the hilus was anteromedial. The dilated, moderately tortuous ureter measured ≤ 1.5 cm in diameter and traversed the wall of the right exstrophic bladder.

The right and left parts of the exstrophied bladder were separated by a sagittal segment of alimentary structures, which extended from the splayed umbilicus to the perineum. A short

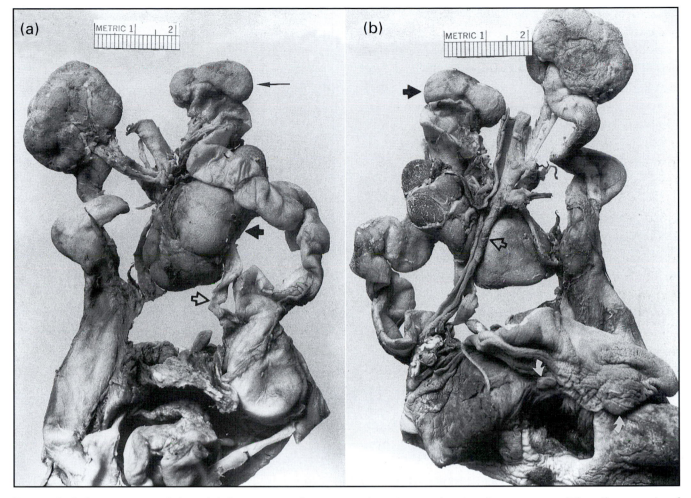

Fig. 32.5 *Left supernumerary kidney. (**a**) Anterior view of upper tracts shows transversely oriented supernumerary kidney (long arrow) and megaureter crossing caudally located left kidney (heavy black arrow) with normal calibre ureter (open arrow) and small right kidney with mega-ureter. (**b**) Posterior view of supernumerary kidney (black arrow), left and right kidneys with megaureters, and aorta and left common iliac artery (open arrow). Cloacal exstrophic bladder and central cecal stoma are flipped over to show perineum, and right and left phallus (white arrows). (Reprinted, with permission, from N'Guessan, G. and Stephens, F.D. (1983), Supernumerary kidney. J. Urol. 130: 649, Fig. 1.)*

stubby cecum issued by a wide orifice, 2.0 cm in diameter, occupied most of this central alimentary segment. The terminal ileum, and two long and slightly tortuous vermiform appendices entered the sac of the caecum. There was no hindgut apart from the caecum.

The perineum was smooth and the anus was absent. On each side of the perineum was a small buried penis that lay contiguous with the caudal margins of the split trigone. The scrota were wide, flat and lacking testes.

Vertebral anomalies associated with the myelomeningocele and multiple hemivertebrae were reported by the radiologist.

Morphology of the supernumerary and ipsilateral kidneys

The supernumerary kidney was cranial to the ipsilateral kidney in 19 patients, caudal in 32, posterior in three and not known in five. In two instances one bifid and

one double supernumerary ureteral systems were associated with structurally normal horseshoe kidney malformations. The separate supernumerary kidney in each instance was cranial to the smaller left component of the horseshoe kidney. The ureters formed a Y-junction in one patient (Hicks *et al.*, 1976), and were completely separate in one case in which the supernumerary ureter issued caudally on the trigone (Hanley, 1942).

Of the 59 supernumerary kidneys 17 (29 per cent) were small, 10 (17 per cent) had no pathological condition and no information was given in 14 (24 per cent). The remaining 18 kidneys (31 per cent) exhibited some form of pathologic condition: seven had hydronephrosis, three had carcinoma, one had papillary cyst adenoma, four had pyonephrosis or pyelonephritis, two had cysts and one had marked lobulation. Of 13 ipsilateral kidneys two had hydronephrosis, three had carcinoma, two had pyonephrosis, four had calculi and two were horseshoe kidneys, while of the contralateral kidneys three had hydronephrosis and two were horseshoe kidneys (one also had hydronephrosis).

Of the 58 patients, pathological conditions of the supernumerary and ipsilateral kidneys occurred in six with bifid ureters, two with carcinomas and two with hydronephrosis. In two patients the supernumerary kidney was small and the ipsilateral kidney had calculous disease. Of the patients with double ureters two had similar pathologic lesions in the supernumerary and ipsilateral kidneys: one had carcinoma and one had pyonephrosis.

Bifid supernumerary combinations

When the urinary systems of the supernumerary and ipsilateral kidneys were confluent the supernumerary kidney was cranial in five patients, caudal in 15 and behind in one. The supernumerary kidney was smaller than the ipsilateral kidney in five patients and the size was not stated in 10. The six supernumerary systems with pathological conditions are excluded.

The confluence of the ureters took several forms. The ureters converged to form a Y-junction in 15 of 21 bifid combinations. In two cases the ureter from the caudal supernumerary kidney coursed cranially, forming an inverted Y-junction (Dixon, 1910; Thielman, 1914). In the case reported by Linberg the ipsilateral ureter joined the anterior pelvis of the supernumerary kidney on the pelvic brim and emerged caudally as the common stem ureter for both kidneys (Linberg, 1924). Browne and Glashan (1971) described a triple junction at the pelvic brim of the ipsilateral ureter with the supernumerary kidney pelvis, which had its own ureter coursing distally, and also the exiting caudal portion of the ipsilateral ureter (Browne and Glashan, 1971). Pinter and associates (1982) described a specimen in which two cranially located supernumerary rudimentary hydronephrotic kidneys were joined by their ureters to a large hydronephrotic pelvis from which a dilated ureter emerged that became atretic more caudally (Fig. 32.6) (Von Hansemann, 1897; McArthur, 1908; Dixon, 1910; Debierre, 1911; Thielman, 1914; Isaja, 1921; Linberg, 1924; Maximovitch, 1927; Kretschmer, 1929,

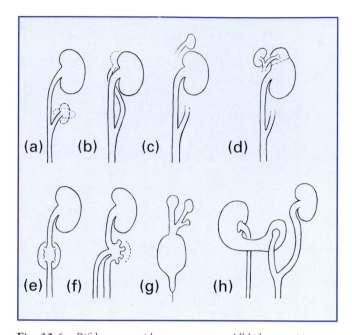

Fig. 32.6 *Bifid ureters with common stem. All kidney positions are relative only and are depicted on left side for ease of interpretation. Dashed lines indicate that detail was not defined. Supernumerary kidneys may be caudal, behind and cranial to ipsilateral kidney. (**a**) Supernumerary ureter beside (or inverted Y with) ipsilateral ureter. (**b**) Supernumerary ureter posterior to ureteropelvic junction. (**c**) Course of supernumerary ureter is not known. (**d**) Supernumerary and duplex kidneys with supernumerary and upper pole ureters forming Y-junction. Common stem joins ipsilateral ureter or remains separate. (**e**)–(**g**) Extraordinary junctions of supernumerary systems with ipsilateral ureter. (**h**) Supernumerary ureter and ureter from separate horseshoe kidney form Y-junction. Note that contralateral ureter runs posterior to isthmus. (**a**) Von Hansemann, (1897) cited by Geisinger; McArthur, L.L. (1908) cited by Geisinger; Dixon, A.F. (1910) cited by Geisinger and Thielman, cited by Neckarsulmer, K. (1914). Isaja, A. (1921); Maximovitch, A.S. (1927) cited by Geisinger; Kretschmer, H.L. (1929); Saccone, A. and Hendler, H.B. (1934); Geisinger, J.F. (1937); Bacon, S.K. (1947); Campbell, M.F. (1970); Fourie, T. (1981). (**b**) Kretschmer, H.L. (1929). (**c**) Debierre, cited by Cobb, F. and Giddings, H.G. (1911). (**d**) Geisinger, J.F. (1937). (**e**)–(**g**) Browne, M.K. et al. (1971); Pinter et al. (1982); Linberg, B.E. (1924) cited by Geisinger. (**h**) Hicks et al. (1976). (See References.) (Reprinted, with permission, from, N'Guessan, G. and Stephens, F.D. (1983), Supernumerary kidney. J. Urol. 130: 649, Fig. 2.)*

1933; Saccone and Hendler, 1934; Geisinger, 1937; Bacon, 1947; Campbell, 1970; Browne and Glashan, 1971; Hicks et al., 1976; Fourie, 1981; Pinter et al., 1982).

Of the 21 bifid systems reported the supernumerary kidney was small in five, hydronephrotic in four and carcinomatous in two. The ipsilateral kidney was small in three cases, hydronephrotic in two and carcinomatous in two, while calculous disease was present in three and one was a horseshoe kidney. Of the 21 supernumerary and ipsilateral kidneys (including small kidneys) pathologic conditions occurred in one kidney in 52 per cent and in both kidneys in 29 per cent.

Supernumerary and ipsilateral kidneys with double ureters

Of the 19 patients in this group the position and correlation of the kidneys and both ureteral orifices were determined accurately in 12, while in seven the supernumerary and ipsilateral orifices opened on the trigone but the correlation of orifice positions with the corresponding kidney and ureter was lacking. The supernumerary kidney was cranial to the ipsilateral kidney in 11 patients, caudal in seven and unknown in one. The kidneys were small in six patients, hydronephrotic in two, carcinomatous in one, infected in three, cystic in one, normal in two and not described in four. Pathological conditions of the supernumerary kidney (including small kidneys) occurred in 13 of the 19 patients (68 per cent).

Of the 19 ipsilateral kidneys in this group one was small, one was pyonephrotic, one was carcinomatous and one was a horseshoe kidney. Excluding the horseshoe kidney, three ipsilateral kidneys (16 per cent) had pathological conditions. The contralateral kidneys were hydronephrotic in two patients, horseshoe shaped and hydronephrotic in one and duplex in one.

Double ureters and the Weigert–Meyer principle

Although this law pertains to duplex (fused) kidneys and their ureters it was found that of the 12 double ureters with known ureteral orifice-kidney correlations nine obeyed the law, including eight with supernumerary kidneys cranial and one caudal to the ipsilateral kidney (Fig. 32.7) (Clifford, 1908; Mills, 1911; Israel, 1918; Samuels *et al.*, 1922; Fischer and Rosenloecher, 1925; Hanley, 1942; Shane, 1942; Antony, 1977; Tada *et al.*, 1981). In two patients the ureter of the caudal supernumerary kidney did not follow the rule and issued on the trigone below the ipsilateral ureter. In our postmortem specimen the ureters co-apted in the wall of the split left half of the trigone of the cloacal exstrophic bladder.

Of the nine cases that obeyed the law the orifice of the supernumerary kidney lay on the trigone in the bladder in five and on the urethrovaginal bridge or vagina in four. The position of the ipsilateral ureteral

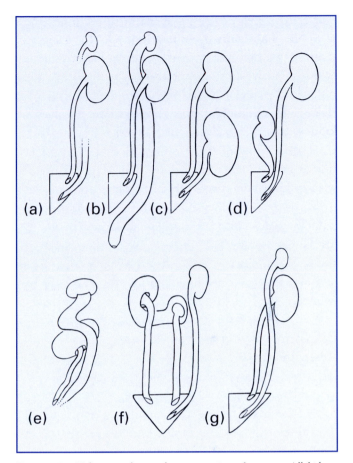

Fig. 32.7 *Kidneys with complete separation of ureters. All kidney positions are relative only and are depicted on left side for ease of interpretation. Dashed lines indicate that detail was not defined. (**a**) Cranial location of supernumerary kidney and ureteral relationship to ureteropelvic junction of ipsilateral kidney are not known. (**b**) Cranial location of supernumerary kidney and ureter was posterior. Ureteral orifice positions are caudal to ipsilateral ureteral orifice. (**c**) Supernumerary kidney and ureteral orifice are caudal to ipsilateral system. (**d**) Supernumerary kidney is caudal and ureteral orifice is cranial to ipsilateral system. (**e**) Supernumerary kidney of present case is cranial. Ureter grooved anterior surface of ipsilateral kidney and intramural ureter coapted ipsilateral orifice. (**f**) Supernumerary kidney is cranial and ureteral orifice is caudal to ureter of left horseshoe kidney. (**g**) Supernumerary kidney is cranial and its ureter is anterior to ureteropelvic junction of ipsilateral kidney with orifice caudal to ipsilateral orifice. (**a**) Antony, J. (1977); Clifford, A.B. (1908) cited by Geisinger; Mills, W.M. (1911). (**b**) Shane, J.H. (1942); Samuels et al. (1922) cited by Geisinger; Israel, I. (1918) cited by Geisinger. (**c**) Tada, et al. (1981). (**d**) Fischer and Rosenloecher (1925) cited by Geisinger. (**f**) Hanley, H.G. (1942). G. Rubin, J.S. (1948). (See References.) (Reprinted, with permission, from N'Guessan, (**g**) and Stephens, F.D. (1983), Supernumerary kidney. J. Urol. 130: 649, Fig. 1.)*

orifice was trigonal in all nine cases. In one patient with a vaginal supernumerary orifice the contralateral kidney was of the conventional duplex type, obeying the law and with the two ureteral orifices on the trigone.

Supernumerary kidneys with bifid or double ureters (indeterminate findings)

In these 18 patients the supernumerary and ipsilateral kidneys had two ureters, neither of which was traced far enough to determine whether they joined together or remained independent. Of the supernumerary kidneys 10 were caudal, three cranial and two behind or beside the ipsilateral kidney. The location of four kidneys was not known. There were four male and 11 female patients, while the sex was not stated in three. The supernumerary kidney was on the right side in seven patients and on the left side in 11, while the side was not known in one. The supernumerary kidney was small in six cases, equal in size to the normal left kidney in one, pathological in four, normal in one and not recorded in seven.

In one patient the ureter of the supernumerary kidney formed a Y-junction with a ureter from an upper pole of a fused duplex kidney (Geisinger, 1937). The stem of the Y was separate from the pelvis and adjoining ureter of the lower portion of the duplex kidney (Fig. 32.6d). Neither ureter was traced to its destination caudally. This arrangement provides a link in embryogenesis between supernumerary and duplex fused kidneys.

Comparison of supernumerary and duplex systems

The anatomical differences between the upper tracts of supernumerary and duplex systems are shown in Table 32.2. The supernumerary kidney and ureter of the 21 patients with bifid systems lay posterior to the ipsilateral ureter in six and in front in one (Bacon, 1947), while no clear statement was given in the remaining 14. Of the 19 patients with double systems the supernumerary kidney or juxtaposed ureter lay behind the ipsilateral kidney in three and in front in two (Rubin, 1948) (including our study), while no information was available concerning the remaining 14. In patients with duplex, double or bifid systems the ureter from the cranial portion passed anterior to the ureteropelvic junction of the caudal portion (Stephens, 1958).

In 15 patients the bifid supernumerary ureters formed a Y-junction with the ipsilateral ureter similar to bifid duplex ureters. However, in two patients the supernumerary ureters coursed cranially from the caudally located supernumerary kidney to meet in a reverse Y-junction, one having short infundibular connections with the passing ipsilateral ureter and one having a three-way junction. Finally, two patients had horseshoe kidneys in association with separate supernumerary kidneys whereas those with bifid duplex horseshoe kidneys had parenchymal continuity, although with separate collecting systems.

Embryogenesis of supernumerary kidneys

The differences between the rare supernumerary kidney and ureters, and the common fused duplex system suggest that there may be a fundamental difference in embryogenesis (Geisinger, 1937).

In fused duplex bifid kidneys with bifid ureters, one bud bifurcates and each branch penetrates independently a composite metanephric mass of mesenchyme. When two buds arise separately from the wolffian duct and penetrate the same metanephric mass, two independent renal urinary collecting systems form but the parenchymas remain fused. But the wider apart or the more ectopic the location of the ureteral bud the more likely the renal parenchyma will exhibit hypoplasia or dysplasia. However, the renal parenchymas remain fused. The intrarenal collecting systems of each ureter are integral although separate components of one entire kidney.

In supernumerary kidneys with bifid ureters one bud bifurcates and each branch penetrates independently a metanephric mass, which develops into separate reniform kidneys: one usually is the larger ipsilateral kidney, and one is the smaller and usually caudally located supernumerary kidney. When separate buds arise from the wolffian duct in close proximity to each other or wide apart the independent supernumerary kidneys usually are cranial and close to the ipsilateral kidney. In other words, the location of the origin of the buds from the wolffian duct does not determine whether the kidneys were fused or separate. However, when the two buds arise separately the ureteral orifice of the cranially located supernumerary kidney usually lies caudal to the orifice of the caudally located kidney, indicating that the budding sites are similar to those of the duplex fused kidneys. Therefore, it seems that the difference lies not in the origin of the bud but in the form or topography of the nephrogenic cord.

Table 32.2 *Comparison of anatomy of supernumerary and duplex upper urinary tracts*

Tissue	Supernumerary kidney	Upper pole of duplex kidney
Parenchyma and calices	Detached	Attached
Capsules	Separate	Attached
Shape*	Reniform	Polar
Size*	Smaller or occasionally equal to or larger	Smaller
Y-junction of bifid systems	Y, Y reversed or Y with one short arm	Y
Calices	Extra in supernumerary kidney and full set in ipsilateral kidney	Upper pole major (or minor) calix only and missing major (or minor) calix only and remainder of duplex kidney
Vascular supply	Separate	Separate

Relationship of supernumerary kidney to ipsilateral kidney:

In sagittal plane	Total no.	Bifid	Double	Intermediate	
Cranial	19	5	11	3	All cranial
Level	3	1	0	2	
Caudal	32	15	7	10	
Unknown	5	0	1	4	
Totals:	59	21	19	19	

In coronal plane	Total no.	Posterior	Anterior	Unknown	
Bifid	21	3	1	17	Ureteropelvic junction anterior
Double	19	3	2	14	Ureteropelvic junction anterior

*When kidney is non-pathologic.
Source: N'Guessan, G. and Stephens, F.D. (1983), Supernumerary kidney. *J. Urol.* 130: 652.

When all of the anatomical relationships of the supernumerary kidney, pelvis and ureter are combined to those of the ipsilateral kidney and ureter the embryogenesis conforms rationally to a theory that invokes separate metanephroi, one lying behind the other, rather than a single metanephros divided longitudinally. The caudal end of the nephrogenic cord may divide into two metanephric tails. These tails separate entirely when the natural involution of the nephrogenic connection with the mesonephros is complete. When induced by separate or bifid ureteral buds they form separate renoblasts. Alternatively, a single bud may roam up or down across one tail to get to the other, inducing a juxtaureteral kidney at the crossing (Fig. 32.6e) (Linberg, 1924) or one branch of a bifid bud may induce a duplex segment in one tail and the other branch may divide, inducing one pole of the duplex kidney and a supernumerary kidney (Fig. 32.6d) (Geisinger, 1937). One bud may induce a renoblast in one tail and the other bud may impact into that pelvis but continue beyond to induce an ipsilateral kidney in the other tail (Fig. 32.6f) (Browne and Glashan, 1971).

Another explanation for complete separation of the supernumerary from the ipsilateral kidney may be fragmentation of a metanephros. Fragmentation possibly may occur from linear infarction with the separated viable fragments being induced by separate or bifid ureteral buds. Geisinger proposed that the gap may be caused by a wide break in the vascularization between two independently vascularized and developing parts of the metanephros (Geisinger, 1937).

Clinical significance

Supernumerary kidneys with leaking ectopic orifices, pathological changes and accompanying symptoms, or stasis and infection or calculous formations in bifid ureters should be removed. However, if the condition is found incidentally without any untoward symptoms or pathological condition what should be the management?

If the unsuspected condition is found at the time of an operation, the kidney is small or abnormal in appearance and the renal function of the ipsilateral and contralateral kidneys is satisfactory the supernumerary kidney and its ureter should be excised. However, if the discovery is made incidentally during examination of a patient, elective excision of a small and abnormal kidney is indicated and if the kidney is healthy, long-term careful observation with regular follow-up is advisable in view of the risks of infection, calculous disease and neoplastic transformation.

Renal hypoplasia and dysplasia in infants with posterior urethral valves*

The existence of renal dysplasia with posterior urethral valves and other congenital urinary anomalies has been documented frequently (Rattner *et al.*, 1963; Bialestock, 1965; Perksy *et al.*, 1967; Cussen, 1971b; Risdon, 1971; Milliken and Hodgson, 1972; Filmer *et al.*, 1974; Newman *et al.*, 1974; Mackie and Stephens, 1975). When discussing the pathogenesis of renal dysplasia, many authors have questioned the role of urinary tract obstruction in its aetiology (Rattner *et al.*, 1963; Pathnak and Williams, 1964; Persky *et al.*, 1967; Bernstein, 1971; Risdon, 1971; Stecker *et al.*, 1973; Newman *et al.*, 1974; Potter and Craig, 1975). Beck states that complete urinary tract obstruction, surgically induced in fetal lambs *in utero* before the 70-mm stage, can result in cystic dysplasia of the kidney (Beck, 1971). In our present autopsy series of 19 patients with severe but incomplete urinary obstruction from posterior urethral valves, some exhibited asymmetric renal morphology, that is, a dysplastic kidney on one side and normal architecture in the contralateral kidney. Bialestock (1965) had previously made this same observation in a group of children with congenital urethral obstruction. She referred to 'built-in controls', which were renal units without reflux in patients with contralateral vesicoureteral reflux. In such patients, it seems reasonable to assume that factors other than urethral obstruction also contribute to the determination of renal morphology. Mackie and Stephens (1975) and Wickramasinghe and Stephens (1977) have demonstrated correlations between ureteral orifice position and renal morphology in children with paraureteral diverticula and duplex kidneys, respectively. The present study was undertaken to test whether ureteral orifice position may be the primary determinant of upper tract morphology in infants with posterior urethral valves and to ascertain whether vesicoureteral reflux or incomplete obstruction or both contribute to the development of renal dysplasia *in utero*.

Necropsy specimens of kidneys in patients with urethral valves

The study consisted of 19 patients with urethral valves, comprising a total of 34 renal units, in the postmortem state. The lower tracts had been studied radiographically in 11 patients during life to determine the presence or absence of vesicoureteral reflux and urethral obstruction. An additional four patients had cystograms performed at necropsy, and the remaining four patients were not tested for reflux. The autopsy specimens were collected from 1950 to 1975. The ages of the patients at the time of death ranged from 10 days to six years; nine patients were less than three months old, and an additional five were between three and six months old at the time of death. Of the 19 patients, three represent previously unreported cases of posterior urethral valves. All others have been reported by Cussen (1971b), and Wickramasinghe and Stephens (1977).

The specimens comprised not only the kidneys but also the ureters, bladder and urethra. While in the fresh state, these organs were filled with 10 per cent formalin, allowed to fix in the distended state, and then dissected. Representative areas of renal parenchyma were selected, and four blocks were cut through the papilla or calyx, medulla and cortex to the capsule. The blocks were embedded in paraffin, sectioned and stained with haematoxylin & eosin for histological examination.

Upper tracts of patients with posterior urethral valves

All of the patients exhibited incomplete urethral obstruction secondary to posterior urethral valves. Based on Young's classification, there were 10 Type I and nine Type III valves.

*Reprinted with changes, by permission of the Williams and Wilkins Co., from Henneberry, M.O. and Stephens, F.D. (1980), Renal hypoplasia and dysplasia in infants with posterior urethral valves. J. Urol. 123: 912.

Ureteral orifice position

The position of the ureteral orifices was designated 'A', 'B' or 'C' as originally described by Lyon et al. (1969). Orifices that were lateral to the 'C' position entered the bladder within a diverticulum. These were classified as 'D1', 'D2' or 'D3', depending on whether the orifice was located on the neck, the side wall, or the dome of the diverticulum, respectively (Fig. 33.1). There were 10 orifices in the 'B' positions, eight in the 'C' position, one in the 'D1' position, 13 in the 'D2' position and two in the 'D3' position.

Reflux

Voiding cystourethrograms were performed in 15 of the 19 patients. Vesicoureteral reflux was present in only one of 10 ureters tested with 'B'-position orifices, and three of seven ureters in the 'C'-position. All but one of the 13 ureters that entered a diverticulum and were studied radiographically exhibited reflux.

Morphological classification of kidneys

Each of the 34 kidneys was classified into one of three groups, according to the gross morphological criteria described by Wickramasinghe and Stephens (1977). Based on the data of Hodson et al. (1962), the mean renal length of a full-term infant at birth is 5.5 cm. The criteria for Group 1 kidneys were absence of caliectasis, length in the distended state > 6 cm, and an average parenchymal thickness, measured along the columns of Bertin, >2 cm. The parenchymal thickness usually was narrower over the calyx and papilla than over the

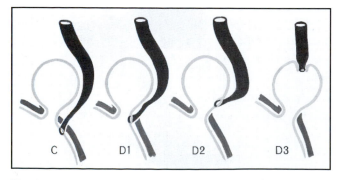

Fig. 33.1 Locations of 'C'- and 'D'- position ureteral orifices associated with hiatal diverticulum. 'C' orifice is separate. 'D1' on neck, 'D2' on side wall and 'D3' on dome. (Reprinted, by permission, from Henneberry, M.O. and Stephens, F.D. (1980), Renal hypoplasia and dysplasia in infants with posterior urethral valves. J. Urol. 123: 912, Fig. 1.)

columns of Bertin. Group 2 kidneys exhibited mild caliectasis, length > 6 cm, and parenchymal thickness of 1.5–2 cm along the columns of Bertin. Group 3a kidneys were < 6 cm in length, 0.5–1.5 cm in thickness, and had moderate to severe caliectasis. The kidneys of group 3b were bizarre, ranging from 2 to 6 cm in length with gross hydronephrosis and a thin shell or broken rim of parenchyma < 0.5 cm in thickness.

Measurement of renal hypoplasia and dysplasia

Owing to availability, only 12 of the 19 patients had kidneys that were examined histologically, accounting for a total of 22 renal units. An estimate of the number of glomerular counts in each kidney was made by counting the glomeruli along more than 10 parallel medullary rays from medulla to capsule and computing a mean for each kidney. By this technique, the glomerular counts in normal kidneys was estimated to vary from 7 to 9. This figure is smaller than that determined by Potter and Craig (1975) who found 12–18 generations by microdissection. However, for the purposes of this study, the histological assessment of glomerular counts proved to be simple and reproducible, and could be standardized for comparison of kidney substance (Fig. 33.2).

An index of dysplasia was obtained for each renal unit by assigning points. Two points each were awarded for the presence of primitive ducts, embryonic stroma, cartilage and periductal whorling or one point each if the aforementioned structures were present in sparse quantity (Fig. 33.3). Two points each were assigned for the presence of microscopic subcapsular cysts or an irregular distribution of nephrons in the form of islands surrounded by dysplastic tissue. None of the kidneys exhibited macroscopic cysts.

Correlation of renal morphology with orifice position

Gross renal morphology

Of the 10 'B'-position ureters, nine had Group 2 kidneys and one had a Group 3a kidney. Of eight 'C'-position ureters, six had Group 2 kidneys and two had Group 3a kidneys. The one 'D1' orifice had a Group 3a kidney. Of the 13 'D2' ureters, there was one Group 2 kidney, five Group 3a and seven Group 3b. Both 'D3' ureters were associated with Group 3b kidneys (Table 33.1).

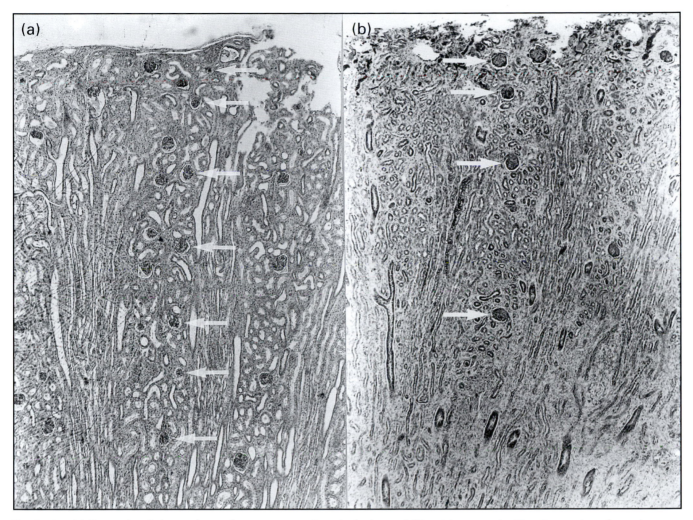

Fig. 33.2 *(a) Section from kidney without reflux in neonate with urethral valves and 'B'-position ureteral orifice. Arrows show glomerular count of seven along parallel medullary ray. (b) Glomerular count of four in kidney with reflux and ureteral orifice in 'D3' position. (Reprinted, by permission, from Henneberry, M.O. and Stephens, F.D. (1980), Renal hypoplasia and dysplasia in infants with posterior urethral valves. J. Urol. 123: 912, Fig. 2.)*

Table 33.1 *Correlation of gross renal morphology with ureteral orifice position in 34 renal units*

Ureteral orifice position	Gross renal morphology		
	Group 2	Group 3a	Group 3b
B	9	1	–
C	6	2	–
D1	–	1	–
D2	1	6	6
D3	–	–	2
Totals	16	10	8

Source: Henneberry, M.O. and Stephens, F.D. (1980), Renal hypoplasia and dysplasia in infants with posterior urethral valves. *J. Urol.* 123: 912, Table 1.

Glomerular population

For those 11 patients who had histological evaluation, the number of glomerular counts was calculated for each kidney and compared with ureteral orifice positions (Table 33.2). The number of glomerular counts in the kidneys with uniform gross appearance is an indication of the relative glomerular population within that kidney; that is, the fewer the number of generations, the smaller the population. The mean number of glomerular counts in the 'B' group was 6, and in the 'C' group, it was 5. The values for 'D2' and 'D3' groups were 3.1 and 1, respectively. For purposes of statistical analysis, the 'B' and 'C' orifices were combined as well as the 'D2' and 'D3' orifices. The difference between the glomerular

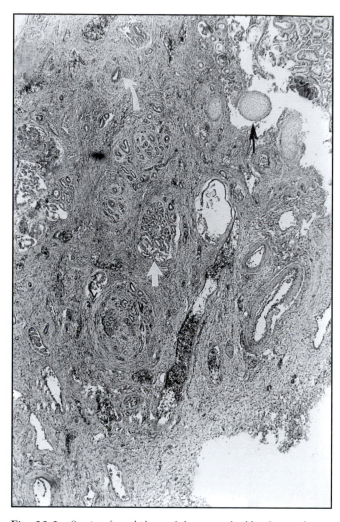

Fig. 33.3 *Section from kidney of three-month-old infant with urethral valves and 'D3' ureteral orifice. Black arrow shows cartilage plaque, white arrow demonstrates tubules surrounded by embryonic stroma, and curved white arrow points to primitive ductule.(Reprinted, by permission, from Henneberry, M.O. and Stephens, F.D. (1980), Renal hypoplasia and dysplasia in infants with posterior urethral valves. J. Urol. 123: 912, Fig. 3.)*

Table 33.2 *Correlation of glomerular counts and renal dysplasia index with ureteral orifice position*

Ureteral orifice position	No. renal units	Mean glomerular count[*]	Mean dysplasia index[†]
B	4	6.0	4.7
C	7	5.0	3.3
D2	10	3.1	6.1
D3	1	1.0	12.0
Total	22		

[*]When groups B and C are combined and compared to Group D2 plus D3 value is 0.02 (Student's test).
[†]When groups B and C are combined and compared to Group D2 plus D3 value is 0.05 (Student's test).
Source: Henneberry, M.O. and Stephens, F.D. (1980), Renal hypoplasia and dysplasia in infants with posterior urethral valves. J. Urol. 123: 912, Table 2.

comparing them to all the 'D' orifices, the difference in the mean index of dysplasia was significant, with a *p* value of 0.05 (Student's test).

Thus, 'B' and 'C' ureteral orifices were associated with kidneys that were more hypoplastic than normal, the architecture of which was otherwise relatively normal. However, kidneys with 'D' orifices were markedly dysplastic, and the degree of hypoplasia was significantly greater as seen by the lower glomerular counts.

Pathogenesis of renal hypoplasia and dysplasia associated with posterior urethral valves

Incomplete urethral obstruction of severe degree, sufficient to cause enlargement and hypertrophy of the bladders, trigones, and ureters of the specimens described regardless of the presence of vesicoureteral reflux, may account for all the structural changes in these kidneys. However, the kidneys with near normal orifice positions were near normal in structure, those with extreme lateral position orifices were highly dysplastic, and those with intermediate grades of lateral displacement exhibited thin parenchyma with fewer than normal nephrons but minimal dysplasia.

Incomplete but severe urethral obstruction causes impairment of function and eventual destruction of renal parenchyma, but it also may induce malformation of the developing nephrons *in utero*. These changes may be enhanced further by additional urodynamic effects of

counts in these two groups was highly significant, with a *p* value of 0.02 (Student's test).

Dysplasia

The index of dysplasia for the four kidneys with ureters in the 'B' position ranged from 3 to 7, with a mean of 4.7. The dysplasia indexes for the seven kidneys with 'C'-position ureters ranged from 0 to 6, with a mean of 3.3. The mean index of dysplasia for the 10 kidneys with 'D2'-ureters was 6.1 with a range of 3 to 10. The one kidney with a 'D3' ureteral orifice had an index of dysplasia of 12, the highest for all kidneys studied (Table 33.2). Again, combining the 'B' group and 'C' group and vesicoureteral reflux. In this study of kidneys in infants subjected to severe urethral obstruction with overflow and dilated upper tracts, the following observations were not readily explained on the basis of back pressure alone and cast doubt on the concept of deformation of the fetal nephrons by incomplete urinary obstruction: (1) parenchymal development was normal or nearly so as confirmed by histological examinations in four of the 22 kidneys with gross dilatation and tortuosity of the ureters, and (2) there was a spectrum of glomerular deficit and renal dysplasia that was progressively more severe the more lateral the ureteral orifice was sited.

In this study, the ureteral orifice position was plotted carefully to determine whether it reflected the changes in renal morphology as proposed by Mackie and Stephens (1975), who studied the correlation in double-ureter anomalies in infants and children. The findings indicate that their 'bud theory' applies equally well to non-duplicated ureters in patients with partial urethral obstruction with or without vesicoureteral reflux, and explains more readily the renal morphology in the two aforementioned itemized circumstances. They postulated that the position of origin of the ureteral bud from the wolffian duct determined not only the final position of the ureteral orifice in the bladder or urogenital tracts, but also the quality of the renal parenchyma. The bud arising from the normal position on the duct gains a normal position on the trigone and penetrates the normal metanephric mesenchyme, forming a normal kidney. The buds arising more caudally from the duct acquire orifices in the 'B', 'C' or 'D' positions, and penetrate and induce the mesenchyme of the tail end of the nephrogenic ridge, producing renal morphologies that show increasing degrees of hypoplasia and dysplasia cor-

responding with the 'B', 'C' and 'D' ureteral orifice positions, respectively. In this study of kidneys in infants with incomplete urethral obstruction, the same correlation between kidney structure and ureteral orifice position applied.

The parenchyma of kidneys with a normal ureteral orifice position had the potential for excellent renal function. Kidneys with ureteral orifices located in diverticula were severely dysplastic, whereas those with ureteral orifices located laterally in the bladder were thin, with low glomerular counts, and non-dysplastic. In most instances, these dysplastic and non-dysplastic thin kidneys had dilated ureters that were shown to exhibit reflux in addition to obstruction, and yet the renal morphologies were different. We attribute the differences in morphologies primarily to UPU origins of the ureteral buds from the most caudal part of the wolffian duct. This leads to induction of defective or sparse mesenchyme of the tail end of the nephrogenic cord with resultant dysplasia and hypoplasia, respectively. The key to the potential quality of the renal parenchyma is the ureteral orifice position.

The occurrence of near-normal kidneys with normal or high glomerular counts in patients with severe partial urethral obstruction indicates that the fetal kidney develops normally irrespective of the so-called back-pressure effect of obstruction. The thin, non-dysplastic kidneys associated with lateral ectopy and reflux are attributed chiefly to the sparseness of the mesenchyme in the tail of the nephrogenic ridge, but some atrophy from back pressure may contribute to the thinness, although the kidney in the newborn period lacked evidence of atrophy of the parenchyma on histological examination.

Quantification of renal hypoplasia and dysplasia

Congenital renal malformations have been classified hitherto on the basis of nephron microdissection studies (Potter, 1972e), the surgical aspects of cysts and dysplasia (Spence *et al.*, 1957) and a broad overview of the generally available clinical, radiological and morphological data (Ericsson and Ivemark, 1958a,b; Bialestock, 1963; Pathak and Williams, 1964; Bernstein, 1973; Filmer *et al.*, 1974; Mackie and Stephens, 1975; Risdon, *et al.*, 1975). In these classifications, most agreement was found in the heritable polycystic conditions and these are described in Chapter 35. Controversy remains concerning the role of the abnormal urodynamics of obstruction and ectopia of the ureteric orifice in the genesis of hypoplasia and dysplasia of the renal parenchyma. In this study, methods of quantifying renal hypoplasia and dysplasia were devised in order to compare and contrast the structure of individual kidneys and to determine whether hypoplasia and dysplasia were due to primary malformation or to acquired deformation of fetal and neonatal nephrons.

The abnormal kidneys were obtained from infants and children exhibiting ectopy of the ureteric orifices, congenital obstructions in the urinary tract and vesico-ureteral reflux.

Definitions

Renal hypoplasia means, for the purpose of this study, a deficiency in total nephron population as compared with that of normal kidneys. Renal dysplasia means the formation of abnormal nephrons and mesenchymal stroma but excludes inflammation or tumours. Renal hypodysplasia is the combination of hypoplasia and dysplasia.

In order to quantify hypoplasia and dysplasia, a scale (the HD scale) was devised from radial glomerular counts, dysplasia scores and the ratio of normal nephrons to dysplastic structures. A radial glomerular count means the average number of glomeruli arrayed alongside a straight medullary ray cut in section from calyx to capsule and perpendicular to the capsule of the kidney (Fig. 34.1). The dysplasia score means the total number of points allotted to any one kidney according to the types of abnormal structures present that met the criteria of dysplasia. The ratio of normal to abnormal structures was judged from low-power microscopy surveys of areas of renal tissue expressed as a percentage of nephrons.

The unit of hypodysplasia is one-eighth of the average normal radial glomerular count of 8 ± 0.5 in some kidneys in which the dysplasia score or ratio of normal to abnormal parenchyma was at variance with the count.

Grading of renal hypodysplasia

For this study, 70 kidneys or segments of duplex kidneys were prepared for histological examination. All except eight were obtained from babies under six months of age. The kidneys, together with ureters, bladder, and urethra in most instances, were collected from subjects exhibiting obstruction of the urinary tract and lateral or medial ectopy of the ipsilateral ureteric orifice (Table 34.1). Vesicoureteral reflux was demonstrated by voiding cystourethrography during life in only 11 patients. In some duplex kidneys one or both segments were appropriate for the study.

Hypoplasia

Hypoplasia was a feature of these kidneys with or without dysplasia and was graded histologically. The kidneys were sectioned from the middle of the papilla or calyx straight through the centre of the overlying parenchyma to the

Reprinted, with changes, by permission of the Williams and Wilkins Co., from Schwarz, R.D., Stephens, F.D. and Cussen, L.J. (1981), The pathogenesis of renal dysplasia, parts 1, 2, 3. Invest. Urol. 19: 94–101.

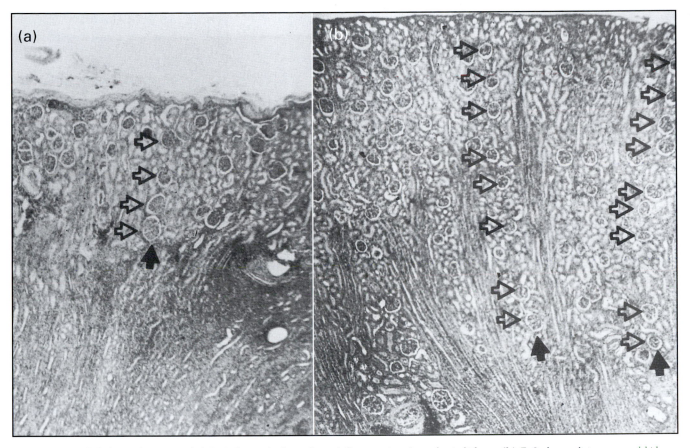

Fig. 34.1 *Radial glomerular count.* (*a*) *3–4 glomeruli alongside medullary ray in a hypoplastic kidney.* (*b*) *7–8 glomeruli in a normal kidney.* (*Reprinted, by permission, from Schwarz, R.D., Stephens, F.D. and Cussen, L.J. (1981), The pathogenesis of renal dysplasia. I. Quantification of hypoplasia and dysplasia.* J. Invest. Urol. 19: 94, *Fig. 1.*)

Table 34.1 *Urinary tract state associated with hypoplasia and dysplasia of the kidney*

State of the urinary tract	Hypodysplastic kidneys (n)
Complete urinary obstructions	19
Lateral ectopy of the ureteric orifice	10
Lateral ectopy of the ureteric orifice with partial urethral obstruction	18
Caudal ectopy of ureteric orifice (including two with complete obstruction of vas distal to 'H' junction)	12
Prune-belly syndrome	9
Non-obstructed normal calibre ureter	3
Total	71

Source: Schwarz, R.D., Stephens, F.D. and Cussen L.J. (1981), The pathogenesis of renal dysplasia. I. Quantification of hypoplasia and dysplasia. J. Urol. 19: 94, Table 1.

capsule, so that radial glomerular counts could be made of the nephrons alongside the few straight medullary rays (Fig. 34.1). It was necessary to obtain serial sections in order to select several that exhibited appropriate orientation of the medullary rays for the assessment. The radial glomerular count was an average of several counts, and there was striking consistency in multiple sections from a given renal segment. In duplex kidneys, the counts for each segment were calculated independently and in those few kidneys exhibiting focal infection, the counts were made in non-infected parts. A range of 7 to 9 glomeruli lying alongside straight rays was found in 23 normal kidneys of full-term neonates using this two-dimensional technique. These counts were reproducible by independent observers.

Radial glomerular counts

Counts were recorded in the 70 kidneys and segments of kidneys, whether or not they were hydronephrotic, cystic, or dysplastic, and whether there was a rim of renal parenchyma or only 'islands' of nephrons surrounded by dysplastic tissue (Fig. 34.2). The term 'hypoplasia' included all kidneys with radial glomerular counts of < 7.

Histologically, the dysplastic structures were clearly demarcated from the normally formed nephrons (Fig. 34.2). In extreme degrees of dysplasia, the nephrons were clustered together surrounded by dysplastic tissue.

Ratio of nephrons to dysplastic structures

By low-power scanning of many sections, the approximate proportion of normal to abnormal structures could be judged. For each kidney or renal segment, the ratio

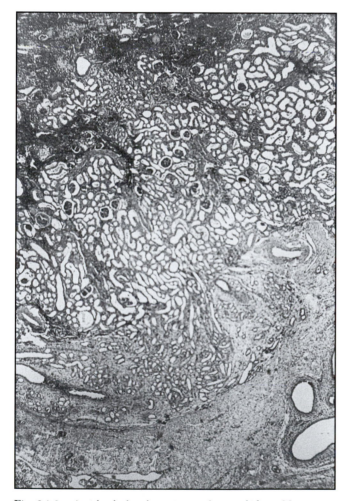

Fig. 34.2 *An island of nephrons in a multicystic kidney. Note sparse glomeruli, dilated tubules and ductules, and sharp demarcation from fibrous and cystic dysplastic structures. (Reprinted, by permission, from Schwarz, R.D., Stephens, F.D. and Cussen, L.J. (1981), The pathogenesis of renal dysplasia. I. Quantification of hypoplasia and dysplasia. J. Invest. Urol. 19: 94, Fig. 2.)*

was expressed as 'percent nephrons'. Some small islands of nephrons exhibited higher radial glomerular counts than dysplasia scores. In these circumstances, the ratio was used to modify the count, whereas in most kidneys, all three parameters could be correlated.

Grading of dysplasia

The degree of dysplasia was assessed semiquantitatively for each kidney, based on a subjective assessment of the histological features of dysplasia that have been previously defined (Ericsson and Ivemark, 1958a,b; Pathak and Williams, 1964; Potter, 1972e; Bernstein, 1973; Risdon *et al.*, 1975). A score of up to 4 points was given for each of five histological features. The total point count then represented the dysplasia score. The five histological categories in order of importance were: I, primitive ducts; II, ductules with low cuboidal epithelium and mesenchymal collars; III, cartilage; IV, areas of loose mesenchymal and fibrous tissues; V, cysts and heterotopic erythropoiesis. While cysts and heterotopic erythropoiesis might be non-specific changes in kidneys of older children, they appear to be expressions of malformations in neonatal kidneys; because they are dubious criteria, they are coupled to reduce their value.

In assigning a point count to the primitive ducts and ductules, the quantity and quality were considered. The more common ductules with low cuboidal epithelium, which were considered to be a less specific criterion of dysplasia, were scored lower (1 point) than occasional dilated primitive ducts lined by distinctly abnormal high columnar ciliated epithelium with large, pale nuclei (4 points), which are regarded as the hallmark. The score allotted to primitive ducts was multiplied by a factor of 1.5 to accentuate the importance of this diagnostic criterion. The assessment of other features was quantitative. The presence of a solitary cartilage plaque (1 point) was less significant than several large plaques in different situations (3 or 4 points).

The sum was then considered a dysplasia score. The minimum score for a dysplastic kidney was 1.5 and the maximum was 15.5 out of a mathematically possible total of 22, which represented the most severe dysplasia.

These three parameters were plotted one against the other and analysed statistically to determine the degrees of association. The correlations formed the basis of the hypodysplasia scale upon which each kidney was given a rating for the comparisons of morphologies associated with obstruction and malformations in the urinary tract.

Correlation of parameters of hypoplasia and dysplasia

The extent of hypoplasia found in the kidneys in this series was graded by radial glomerular counts and the percentage of normal nephrons. The two parameters of hypoplasia showed close correlation ($r = -0.94$, $p < 0.001$) (Fig. 34.3). The dysplasia score was found to correlate with the extent of hypoplasia measured by both the above-mentioned techniques ($r = -0.862$ and $r = -0.765$, $p < 0.001$) (Fig. 34.4a,b). It was found that the more dysplastic kidneys (scores < 8) had less hypoplasia and more normal structures. These correlations support the semiquantitative techniques of measurement, and were reproducible by independent observers.

The histological data and the correlations provided the basis for construction of the HD scale for measurement of hypodysplasia and for use as a tool for comparison of individual kidneys. A base figure was given to each kidney initially according to the radial count, the normal being 7 to 9, and the counts for abnormal kidneys ranging between 7 and 0. In some of the

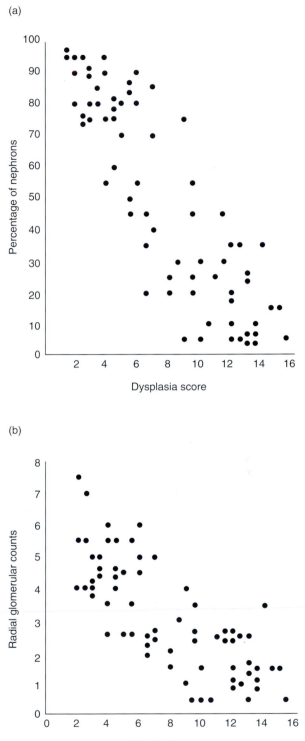

(a)

(b)

Fig. 34.4 *Correlation of dysplasia with hypoplasia. (**a**) Estimated percentage of nephrons correlates with dysplasia score ($r = -0.862$, $p < 0.001$). (**b**) Radial glomerular counts correlate with dysplasia score ($r = -0.765$, $p < 0.001$) in 70 kidneys. (Reprinted, by permission, from Schwarz, R.D., Stephens, F.D. and Cussen, L.J. (1981), The pathogenesis of renal dysplasia. I. Quantification of hypoplasia and dysplasia. J. Invest. Urol. 19: 94, Fig. 4.)*

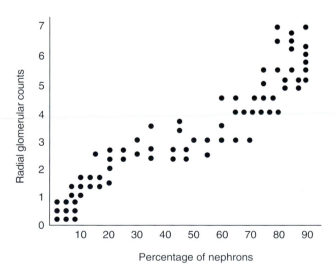

Fig. 34.3 *Correlation of radial glomerular counts with the estimated percentage of normal nephric tissue present ($r = -0.94$, $p < 0.001$) in 68 kidneys. (Reprinted, by permission, from Schwarz, R.D., Stephens, F.D. and Cussen, L.J. (1981), The pathogenesis of renal dysplasia. I. Quantification of hypoplasia and dysplasia. J. Invest. Urol. 19: 94, Fig. 3.)*

kidneys, plots of the radial counts and dysplasia scores represented in Fig. 34.4b scatter at some distance from a line of best-fit drawn through the centre of the dots, indicating a somewhat less-distinct correlation. Such kidneys contained localized areas of either severe dysplasia or more structures that were atypical of the kidney as a whole. When assigning a hypodysplasia rating to any one kidney, therefore, the radial glomerular count was unmodified when the count and dysplasia scores correlated closely, but was modified up or down the scale to the extent of half a unit toward the predominating general morphology if the dysplasia score was at variance with the radial count. The ratio of normal to abnormal structures helped in the decision to upgrade or downgrade the base figure. With familiarity of the methods of evaluating these parameters, the final hypodysplasia rating or index of each kidney was reproducible by different observers to within 0.5 of a unit on the scale.

Parameters for renal hypodysplasia quantification

The scheme outlined for quantifying hypoplasia and dysplasia was made possible when it was shown that the correlations between radial glomerular counts, percentage of normal nephrons and dysplasia scores were valid. With the appropriate selection and sectioning of a region that most nearly represented the general morphological character of the kidney, an accurate grading could be made on the hypodysplasia scale on the basis of radial glomerular counts for kidneys with hypoplasia alone and with minimal but clearly present dysplasia. When the hypoplasia was more severe and dysplasia more conspicuous and when nephron areas became localized to clumps surrounded by dysplasia, then the dysplasia score became an important correlate of the radial glomerular count.

The majority of the kidneys studied were from neonates or infants under three months of age before the long-term urodynamic effects of obstruction or reflux and inflammation had destroyed the original morphology. By the use of this hypodysplasia scale, it was then possible to compare and contrast the renal morphologies of babies with upper pole ureteric orifices and urinary obstructions, and to determine the aetiologic agents that were most significant in the pathogenesis of hypoplasia and dysplasia.

The significance of lateral and medial ectopy of the ureteric orifice

The relative importance of ureteric bud defects and abnormal urodynamics such as urinary-tract obstruction or vesicoureteral reflux in the genesis of renal hypoplasia and dysplasia remains controversial. A histological technique that provided a reproducible method of quantifying and grading renal hypodysplasia is described in Chapter 33. Recent studies by Mackie and Stephens (1975) have produced evidence in support of an embryological association between renal morphology and ureteric orifice position in babies and children with double ureters. Degrees of hypoplasia and dysplasia also correlated with degrees of lateral ectopy of single ureters in postmortem specimens from babies with urethral obstruction caused by congenital urethral valves (Chapter 33). In the present study, kidneys were graded to compare degrees of hypodysplasia associated with lateral ureteric orifice positions with and without urethral obstruction and with caudal ectopy of the orifice.

The degree of hypodysplasia was graded using the HD scale. Normal kidneys had 7–9 HD units, while progressively more severe hypoplasia and dysplasia had progressively lower HD values.

The position of the ureteral orifice was categorized by the method of Mackie et al. (1975). The normal trigonal orifice with a normal submucosal tunnel was labelled 'A' position. A 'C'-position orifice verged on the position of the hiatus, a 'B' orifice was sited halfway between the 'A' and 'C' positions; a 'D'-position orifice lay in a hiatal diverticulum.

Ureteral orifices issuing in the posterior urethra at or cranial to the verumontanum were labelled 'G' while those joining the male genital tract were labelled 'H'. In the female, the 'G'-position orifices were labelled 'G1' if located in the proximal half of the urethra and 'G2' in the distal urethra and urethrovaginal bridge. When the ureter issued on to the hymen or into Gartner's duct in the vaginal wall, it was labelled 'H' (see Figs 14.3 and 34.5).

Kidneys associated with the following groups of ectopic-orifice positions were analysed for hypodyspla-

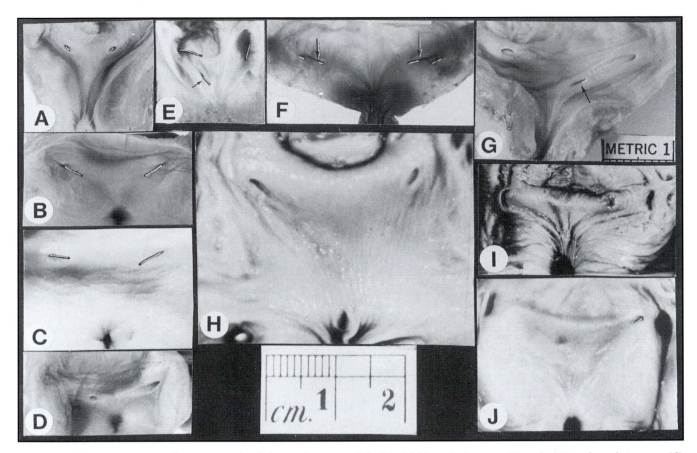

Fig. 34.5 *Necropsy specimens showing normal and abnormal positions. (**a**), (**b**), (**c**) Normal trigones at 12 weeks, 40 weeks and six years. (**d**) Newborn baby's trigone with left orifice in 'C' position. (**e**) Right ureteric orifices in 'C' and 'E' (arrow) and left in 'D' position (bristle). (**f**) Bilateral duplex ureters, 'A' orifices (arrows) of upper pole ureters and 'B' orifices of lower pole ureters. (**g**) Left, 'B'- and 'E'-orifice positions; right 'A' position. (**h**) Baby of six weeks with urethral valves, orifices in 'B' position. (**i**) Baby of five weeks, urethral valves and (right) orifice in 'D' position and (left) in 'B' position. (**j**) Baby of eight weeks, with urethral valves and (right) orifice in 'D' position and (left) in 'C' position. Scale applies to all trigones. (Reprinted, by permission, from Schwarz, R.D., Stephens, F.D. and Cussen, L.J. (1981), The pathogenesis of renal dysplasia. II. The significance of lateral and medial ectopy of the ureteric orifice. J. Invest. Urol. 19: 97, Fig. 2.)*

sia: (I) Non-obstructed lateral ectopy 'B'-, 'C'- and 'D'-positions; (II) lateral ectopy associated with posterior urethral valves; and (III) caudal ectopy ('G' and 'H' positions). No difference was found in the histological quality of kidneys with single ectopic ureters and renal segments of double systems with the same ectopic ureteric orifice position, so single and duplex systems were put together for this analysis.

Renal morphology and ureteric orifice position

Non-obstructed lateral ectopy

This group of 30 kidneys or segments of kidneys comprised five with 'B' ureteric orifices, 18 with 'C' orifices and seven with 'D' orifices. Four kidneys from three older children (ages $7\frac{1}{2}$ years, 13 years and a third whose age was not recorded) were included in this series because the renal parenchyma was well preserved and suitable for the study.

The kidneys associated with 'B'-position ureteral orifices showed normal or near normal HD gradings (mean = 7.6 HD units, S.D. ± 0.9). Those kidneys associated with 'C'-position orifice showed moderate hypodysplastic malformations (mean = 5.2 HD units, S.D. ± 1.8) while those with 'D'-position orifices were severely malformed (mean = 2.8 HD units, S.D. ± 1.2) (Table 34.2) (Fig. 34.6).

Macroscopic cysts were present in four of the seven kidneys with 'D'-position ureteral orifices. These cysts

Table 34.2 *Comparison of mean hypodysplasia values of kidneys with 'B', 'C', and 'D' ureteric orifice positions with and without urethral obstruction*

Kidney status[*]	'B'	'C'	'D'
Kidneys non-obstructed	7.6 ± 0.86	5.2 ± 1.84	2.8 ± 1.22
Kidneys partially obstructed by urethral valves	6.9 ± 4.2	5.7 ± 1.84	2.8 ± 1.97
Total	7.27 ± 0.75	5.37 ± 1.81	2.8 ± 1.61

[*]The non-obstructed kidneys were not distinguishable from partially obstructed kidneys ($p > 0.1$), whereas kidneys of 'B'-orifice ureters had higher HD grades than those with 'C'-orifice ureters ($p < 0.01$) and those with C position orifices had higher grades than those with 'D'-position orifices ($p < 0.01$). Values are expressed as the mean ± S.D.
Source: Schwarz, R.D., Stephens, F.D. and Cussen, L.J. (1981), The pathogenesis of renal dysplasia, II. The significance of lateral and medial ectopy of the ureteric orifice. *J. Urol.* 19: 97, Table 1.

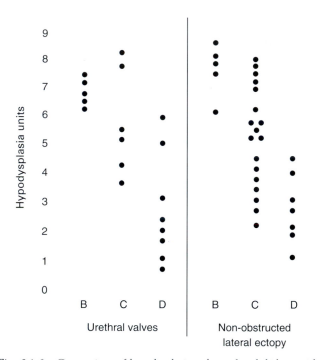

Fig. 34.6 *Comparison of hypodysplasia values of each kidney with 'B', 'C', or 'D' ureteric orifice position from babies with or without urinary obstruction. Note similar distribution of values of 'B', 'C' and 'D' columns of obstructed and non-obstructed kidneys. (Reprinted, by permission, from Schwarz, R.D., Stephens, F.D. and Cussen, L.J. (1981), The pathogenesis of renal dysplasia. II. The significance of lateral and medial ectopy of the ureteric orifice.* J. Invest. Urol. *19: 97, Fig. 3.)*

were subcapsular and thick-walled and some exhibited a glomerular tuft. Microscopic cysts with thick walls were found more commonly among the dysplastic structures. Hydroureteronephrosis occurred in many specimens and was especially pronounced in those with extreme lateral ectopy of the ureteric orifice. These kidneys showed no general dilatation of the convoluted tubules or Bowman spaces nor a layer of microscopic glomerular subcapsular cysts, such as were observed in kidneys subjected to back pressure of urinary obstruction (Potter, 1972d).

Lateral ectopy associated with posterior urethral valves

Nineteen specimens of kidneys, ureters and bladders associated with urethral valves, from 12 babies under six months of age (mean = 1.3 months) and from one child of five years were studied. Although they all showed hydronephrotic dilatation, the histology of the kidneys ranged from a normally formed cortex to extreme cystic hypodysplasia with a corresponding wide range on the HD scale.

To determine whether correlations of hypodysplasia and ureteric orifice position applied to kidneys of babies with posterior urethral valves, the obstructed kidneys were grouped according to ureteral orifice position ('B', 'C', 'D') and each kidney was then graded on the HD scale. None of the ureteral orifices was found to lie in the 'A'-position. The five kidneys associated with 'B' ureteral orifices were graded between 6 and 8 HD units

(mean = 6.9, S.D. ± 0.4). The six kidneys associated with 'C'-position ureteral orifices showed a mean of 5.75 HD units (S.D. ± 1.8), while the eight kidneys associated with 'D'-position orifices had a mean of 2.8 HD units (S.D. ± 2.0) (Table 34.2) (Fig. 34.6). Henneberry and Stephens (1980), using a different grading system, found a similar correlation between orifice position and renal morphology in babies with urinary obstruction caused by urethral valves.

All of the kidneys showed moderate to gross degrees of hydroureteronephrosis. Generalized nephron dilatation was a common microscopic feature, presumably related to the obstructions, as it was a feature seen only in obstructed kidneys.

Macroscopic cysts were found in seven kidneys, five of them associated with 'D'-position orifices, and most of those kidneys showed extreme hypodysplasia. One of the kidneys associated with a 'B' position had a normal HD rating but showed glomerular subcapsular cysts that were only just visible macroscopically. These orderly subcapsular cysts of uniform size appeared similar to those described by Potter (1972g) in specimens associated with urethral valves, while the cysts of the 'D' kidneys were like those found in the non-obstructed dysplastic kidneys with 'D'-position orifices.

In both the obstructed and non-obstructed groups, increasing lateral ectopy was associated with increasingly severe hypodysplasia. When analysed, no statistical difference was found between the HD grades of obstructed and non-obstructed groups for each ureteral orifice position ($p > 0.1$). A statistically significant difference was found in the HD ratings of the kidneys in both groups with different orifice positions ($p < 0.01$) (Table 34.2).

Caudal ectopy

In this group of 21 kidneys, three, seven and 11 of the corresponding ureters had 'F'-, 'G'-, and 'H'-position orifices respectively. All three of the 'F'-position ureters were associated with upper pole segments of duplex systems with the orifice in the trigone at or near the bladder neck. Two of them exhibited ureteroceles. When plotted on the hypodysplasia scale, two kidneys fell within the normal range, while one with ureteric orifice on the 'F–G' boundary showed HD grade between 4 and 4.5 units (Fig. 34.7).

Five of the seven kidneys with 'G'-position ureteric orifices were from duplex systems, and included three with non-stenotic ureteroceles. The ureters and pelvis were abnormally dilated presumably because of the obstruction caused by the squeeze of the urethral sphincter on the ureters within its grasp. When plotted on the hypodysplasia scale, this group showed an even scatter ranging from near normal to major hypodysplasia (mean = 3.9 HD units, S.D. ± 1.6).

No unique pattern could be attributed to single or double systems, to the presence or absence of ureteroceles, or to the high or low 'G' positions of the orifices within the urethra or on the urethrovaginal bridge ('G1' and 'G2').

Nine of the 11 'H'-position kidneys were from males (Schwarz and Stephens, 1978). Two of the kidneys were subjected to complete urinary obstruction and were excluded from this part of the study. The remaining seven kidneys had ureters attached to the vas deferens.

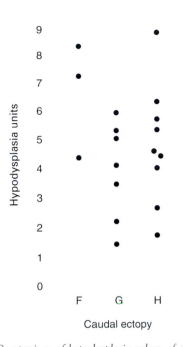

Fig. 34.7 *Comparison of hypodysplasia values of each kidney with caudal ectopy of the ureteric orifice. Note the wide scatter in the low range in 'G' and 'H' columns, but also some unexpected high values in the 'H' column. (Reprinted, by permission, from Schwarz, R.D., Stephens, F.D. and Cussen, L.J. (1981), The pathogenesis of renal dysplasia. II. The significance of lateral and medial ectopy of the ureteric orifice.* J. Invest. Urol. 19: 97, Fig. 4.)

In four of these specimens, the vas issued at its normal position in the urethra, and in three, the vas entered ectopically at the bladder neck or on the trigone. The kidneys varied in morphology from normal to extreme hypodysplasia with a mean of 4.3 HD units (S.D. ± 2.2). The range and the mean grades of the kidneys with 'H'-position ureters were similar to those of the 'G' kidneys.

Aetiology of renal hypodysplasia

Most of the specimens of non-obstructed ureters with lateral ectopy of the ureteric orifices would be expected to exhibit reflux. Only 11 of the 34 specimens with lateral ectopic orifices had previously been tested for reflux by voiding cystourethrography during the short life of the patients. Reflux was primary in five, and in six it was associated with obstruction by valves in the posterior urethra. The HD grades of those kidneys of the 'B' and 'C' ureteric positions showed no statistical difference between the reflux and non-reflux groups, indicating that the effects of reflux on the developing kidney may be less significant than the dysgenetic effects of abnormal orifice position (Table 34.3). In both the non-obstructed and obstructed urinary tracts, degrees of lateral ectopy and grades of renal hypodysplasia could be correlated. In this study of cystic dysplasia in association with congenital urethral obstruction, Cussen (1971b) found that 18 of 33 kidneys associated with reflux and obstructed by urethral valves showed cystic dysplasia, but that in the remaining 15 kidneys, cystic dysplasia was not present. He concluded that reflux and obstruction were not necessarily essential to the pathogenesis of the renal lesion, and that some other factor or factors might contribute to the abnormal morphology of the kidneys.

Orifice position—the missing link

It is proposed that ectopic orifice position is the missing link that associates ectopic budding of the ureter with ureteral induction of ectopic and defective nephrogenic mesenchyme peripheral in the wolffian body to that of the predestined metanephros.

Ectopy of the ureteric orifice, whether lateral or caudal, denotes an abnormality of the bud and the adjacent segment of the nephrogenic cord. Correlation between degree of lateral ectopy and grade of hypodysplasia may occur because the more ectopic buds arising from the wolffian duct are more abnormal and meet progressively deteriorating grades of mesenchyme peripheral to the predestined zone of the metanephros.

For normal development, the kidney depends on both the normal inducer capability of the bud and normal mesenchyme. A defect of one or both leads to a range of renal abnormalities. In the context of ectopic buds and hypodysplasia, the bud may lack inducer qualities, and

Table 34.3 *Mean HD values of reflux and non-reflux renal units with 'B' or 'C' orifice*

Orifice	Reflux units	Non-reflux units
'B' orifice	1	1
'C' orifice	5	4
Hypodysplasia values*	5.9 ± 1.4	5.5 + 2.1 (*p* > 0.5)

*Values are expressed as the mean ± S.D.
Source: Schwarz, R.D., Stephens, F.D. and Cussen, L.J. (1981), The pathogenesis of renal dysplasia, II. The significance of lateral and medial ectopy of the ureteric orifice. *J. Urol.* 19: 97, Table 2.

the adjacent nephrogenic cord may be unreceptive or defective. The pinpoint origin of the bud compared with the relatively broad body of the normal metanephros accounts for near-normal kidneys associated with moderate degrees of ureteral ectopy. However, with more extreme ectopic sites of origin, the defective bud is more likely to unite with patchy or involuting nephrogenic or stromagenic mesenchyme distant from the body of the metanephros, leading to both hypoplasia and dysplasia.

Lateral and medial ectopy, acquired or congenital in origin

Tanagho et al. (1965) related lateral ectopy to defective trigonal muscle and defective ureteric muscular attachments of the terminal ureter to it. They postulated that lateral displacement of the ureteric orifice in patients with primary reflux resulted from the weakly opposed pull of the ureter causing elongation of the trigone. Lateral displacement with saccule formation was considered by Hutch and Amar (1972) to be secondary to infravesical obstruction or neurological disease; the hiatus expands, a saccule of vesical mucosa protrudes, and the ureteric orifice is drawn toward or into it. Two different theories were thus proposed to explain the lateral displacement with the implications that the orifice position was originally normal. An alternative explanation of lateral ectopy of the ureteric orifice is that the submucosal ureter is absent in part or totally, owing to initial dystopic budding of the ureter from the wolffian duct (Ambrose and Nicholson, 1962). This theory explains the array of both lateral and medial ectopic positions of double ureters, and the theory can readily be extended to incorporate non-duplicated ureters. It may apply also to lateral ectopic ureters occurring with congenital urethral obstructions. 'D'-position orifices may form in the paraureteral diverticulum, which may be an extension of the wolffian duct component of the trigone beyond the limits of the bladder wall. The diverticulum and the extreme lateral orifice position may arise as primary malformations rather than as secondarily acquired defects (Stephens, 1979a).

The renal morphology correlated generally with medial ectopy of the ureteric orifice, but some kidneys did not conform and tended to undermine the bud theory. These ureters arise as buds from positions cranial to the metanephric zone and enter the nephrogenic cord more cranially where it comprises a mixture of meta- and mesonephric mesenchyme. The inducer capability of the bud and the relative proportions of inducible versus involuting mesenchyme may account for some unpredictable renal developments. On the other hand, the lateral ectopic ureters, which arise as buds from the distal reaches of the wolffian duct, are more likely to meet the progressively more depleted mesenchyme of the withering tail of the nephrogenic cord, and the resulting kidneys conform to a pattern. Though bud position may determine the morphology in the majority of these kidneys, the nature and stage of development of the nephrogenic cord where ectopic buds penetrate it also plays an important role in the formation of the renal parenchyma.

The effect of complete and incomplete urinary obstruction on the developing kidney

Hypoplastic and dysplastic renal malformations have been previously studied and classified according to clinical, pathological, radiological, and embryological criteria (Spence et al., 1957; Ericsson and Ivemark, 1958a,b; Bialestock, 1963; Pathak and Williams, 1964; Potter, 1972g; Bernstein, 1973; Filmer et al., 1974; Risdon et al., 1975). Studies by Mackie, Awang and Stephens (1975) have produced evidence in support of an embryological association between renal morphology and the position of the ureteral orifices in the urogenital tracts of children with single and double ureters. Controversy persists concerning the effects of abnormal urodynamics on fetal renal development, including cyst formation and the production of dysplasia.

Bernstein (1973) has shown that complete obstruction caused by ureteral atresia was associated with multicystic hypodysplasia. He also demonstrated dysplastic changes adjacent to infarcts and biopsy sites (Bernstein, 1968), and suggested that hypodysplasia may be a nonspecific entity with many aetiologies. Babies with incomplete obstruction from posterior urethral valves have a high incidence of renal hypodysplasia, which was shown to correlate closely with ureteric orifice position. Quantitative analyses of the microstructure of the kidneys of babies with complete and incomplete obstructions of the urinary tract and ectopic locations

of the ureteric orifices provide data from which the effects of abnormal urodynamics on the developing kidney can be deduced.

The HD scale based on a histological grading of hypoplasia and dysplasia was again used as a tool to study the relative effects on the fetal kidney of abnormal urodynamics. A study was undertaken to evaluate the relative effects of complete and incomplete urinary obstruction on the developing kidney.

The 54 kidneys analysed in this study were, with two exceptions, obtained from babies under six months of age. All the kidneys had been subjected to ureteral or urethral obstruction during fetal life and infancy. Each kidney was assessed histologically and assigned an HD value. In order to avoid bias, identification of the slides of the sections from kidneys of infants with ectopic ureteric orifices and complete and incomplete obstructions of the ureter and urethra was not made during these determinations.

In addition to identifying the type of obstruction present, the position of the ureteral orifice was documented and categorized according to the scheme devised by Mackie and Stephens (1975).

Kidneys with complete and incomplete obstructions of the ureter or urethra were studied.

Morphology of kidneys with complete urinary obstruction

There were 21 specimens of kidneys with complete urinary obstruction. At the time of diagnosis, the infants were under six months of age, with a mean age of less than one month; the oldest child was $1\frac{1}{2}$ years of age. The obstructing lesion was atresia in 14 ureters, of which the orifice position was 'A' in seven, 'B' in one, and not known in six. Of the remaining seven specimens, the ureter in two joined an atretic vas in 'H' position; the urethra was atretic in one prune-belly baby and the two ureteric orifices were laterally located. In three, an obstruction in the ureters when perfused permitted retrograde but not antegrade flow, the orifice positions were not known.

Sixteen of the 22 kidneys were multicystic resembling a bunch of grapes. Three were 'shell' kidneys around a hydronephrotic sac, and three were macroscopically small, solid and dysplastic. In three of the multicystic kidneys in which a patency was found in the pelvis or calyces cranial to the atretic segment, the lumen, when filled with fluid, communicated by narrow ducts with peripheral cysts.

In this group of multicystic kidneys, the origin of the cysts could only rarely be identified histologically as glomerular or tubular. Some cysts contained rudimentary glomeruli and had thin walls lined by flattened cuboidal epithelium. Other cysts had flattened epithelium, but with thick, fibrocollagenous walls possibly of ampullary and collecting-duct origin. Nephrons with normal appearances exhibited dilatation of the convoluted tubules, presumably related to the urinary obstruction. In 10 multicystic kidneys, the diameter of the convoluted tubules was much enlarged, averaging 60 μm, and the tubular wall was thin, averaging 9 μm. This finding compares with the normal tubular diameter of 31 μm and epithelial cell-wall thickness of 12.5 μm, as determined in 14 normal neonatal kidneys measured by the same microscopic technique.

All of the kidneys associated with complete obstruction of the urinary tract were hypoplastic and dysplastic. In three of the kidneys with relatively mild degrees of hypoplasia, associated with atresia of the ureter, a continuous layer of well-formed cortex lay deep to an outer rim of small, subcapsular cysts. In those kidneys with severest degrees of hypodysplasia, the few near-normal nephrons lay in clumps surrounded by dysplastic structures.

When plotted on the HD scale, the kidney grades ranged from 0 to 4 with a mean of 1.8 units (S.D. ± 1.0) (Fig. 34.8). No differences could be found between the ranges of the HD values of cystic or solid kidneys, the kidneys with high or low ureteral atresias, or those with urethral atresia or the functionally complete valve-like ureteral obstructions.

Morphology of kidneys with incomplete urinary obstruction

Of 32 kidneys studied, 13 had ureteral obstructions with normal orifice position, while all 19 kidneys and ureters accompanying posterior urethral valves showed lateral ectopy of the ureteral orifice.

Incomplete ureteral obstruction

This group of 13 kidneys and ureters included seven examples of ureteropelvic obstructions and six with

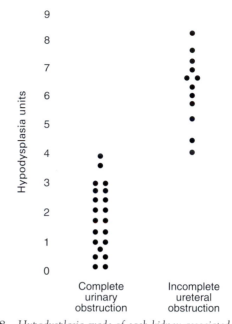

Fig. 34.8 *Hypodysplasia grade of each kidney associated with complete obstruction of ureter or urethra and incomplete obstruction of ureter. Note the low and high grades with complete and incomplete obstructions, respectively. (Reprinted, by permission, from Schwarz, R.D., Stephens, F.D. and Cussen, L.J. (1981), The pathogenesis of renal dysplasia. III. Complete and incomplete urinary obstruction. J. Invest. Urol. 19: 101, Fig. 1.)*

primary obstructive megaureters (Maizels and Stephens, 1980). Each kidney demonstrated hydronephrotic dilatation. The ureteric orifices were normally located on the trigone. All of the partially obstructed kidneys showed normal to near normal cortices (mean HD value = 6.3 units) (S.D. ± 1.2). One hydronephrotic kidney of a one-week-old baby showed subcapsular glomerular cysts at autopsy but demonstrated 5–7 radial glomerular counts. Dysplasia was minimal or absent in all others.

Hydronephrosis was sometimes associated with thinning of the parenchyma, predominantly the medulla, and with clubbing or dilatation of the calyces.

Incomplete urethral obstruction with lateral ectopy of the ureteric orifice

It has already been shown in the 19 kidneys associated with partial urinary obstruction caused by posterior urethral valves that the gradings of hypodysplasia correlated with positions 'B', 'C', and 'D' of the ureteric orifices. Although all the kidneys exhibited hydronephrotic dilatation, the histology of the kidneys ranged from a normally formed cortex to extreme cystic hypodysplasia with corresponding gradings on the HD scale. The correlation was similar to that found between grades of renal hypodysplasia with non-obstructive lateral ectopy of the ureteric orifices (Table 34.4). While there was a consistent difference between the HD values of kidneys for each orifice position in each group ($p < 0.01$), there was no significant difference between the HD grades of the obstructed and non-obstructed groups for each orifice position ($p > 0.1$).

Correlation of renal morphology with urinary obstruction

The clinical relationship between complete urinary obstruction and hypodysplasia has been documented (Spence et al., 1957; Pathak and Williams, 1964; Bernstein, 1968; Cussen, 1976). The association of hypodysplasia with posterior urethral valves (Henneberry and Stephens, 1980) and ureteral ectopy (Mackie and Stephens, 1975; Schwarz et al., 1981) has also been made.

Aetiology of renal dysplasia with complete urinary obstruction

The renal malformation associated with complete urinary obstruction occurs early in organogenesis of the kidney. Beck (1971) considered that complete obstruction produced by ligation of the ureters of lambs prior to 70 days' gestation caused dysplasia. The present study indicates that complete urinary obstruction anywhere in the urinary tract of the embryo results in severe grades of hypodysplasia.

The hypodysplastic malformation associated with complete urinary obstruction showed no distinguishing histological features compared with hypodysplasias from other causes, except for the nephron dilatation, which was presumably related to raised urodynamic back pressures.

Complete obstruction may occur *ab initio*, for example a blind persisting mesonephric duct with ureter attached or impermeable urethra, or may be acquired as with ureteral atresia. The fibrous structure of the attenuated atretic ureter is compatible with ischaemia occurring during the phase of rapid elongation of the ureter when the kidney is migrating to the loin. Multicystic and dysplastic kidneys associated with ureteral atresia exhibit features that may result from a combination of obstructive and ischaemic impairment of ampullary and metanephric development. Renal structures already formed at the onset of the ureteral obstruction or ischaemia remain as a deep zone of nephrons or as islands amidst dysplastic structure (Bialestock, 1960b). Those ampullae and nephron vesicles in the active processes of induction, formation, and junction either arrest, degenerate, or develop in dysplastic fashion into grape-like cysts and microcysts, and rudimentary ducts and tubules supported in abundant mesenchymal stroma.

Ischaemia due either to the effects of obstructive back pressure in the kidney or to the ischaemic involvement of both ureter and kidney may contribute to the renal state. Ljungqvist (1965) found in similar dysplastic kidneys a characteristic microangiographic arrangement denoting a renal lobular distribution of extremely small vessels. The disparity of degrees of hypodysplasia found in multicystic kidneys may be due to the time of onset of complete obstruction or ischaemia in relation to the stage of development of the nephrons.

Aetiology of renal morphology with incomplete ureteral and urethral obstruction

Tanagho (1972) induced partial obstruction of the ureter of fetal lambs at 75–80 days' gestation causing obstructive changes in the kidney but not dysplasia. In the present study, kidneys of infants with incomplete ureteral obstruction exhibited hydronephrosis, but they

Table 34.4 *Mean hypodysplasia values of kidneys with lateral ectopy of the ureteric orifices ('B', 'C', and 'D' positions) without urinary tract obstruction and with partial obstruction of the urethra by posterior urethral valves*

Kidney status	'B'	'C'	'D'
Kidneys non-obstructed	7.6 ± 0.86 ($p > 0.1$)	5.2 ± 1.84 ($p > 0.1$)	2.8 ± 1.22 ($p > 0.1$)
Kidneys partially obstructed by urethral valves	6.9 ± 0.42	5.7 ± 1.84	2.8 ± 1.97
Total	7.27 ± 0.75 ($p < 0.01$)	5.37 ± 1.84 ($p < 0.01$)	2.8 ± 1.61 ($p < 0.01$)

Source: Schwarz, R.D., Stephens, F.D. and Cussen, L.J. (1981), the pathogenesis of renal dysplasia, III. Complete and incomplete urinary obstruction. *J. Urol.* 19: 101, Table 1.

rarely showed hypodysplastic malformation. The medulla was usually thin, but the cortex exhibited orderly formation of glomeruli. The presence of a subcapsular layer of small glomerular cysts in four of these kidneys may indicate a special response of the youngest developing nephrons to the effects of obstruction. Further, the presence of dilated thin-walled convoluted tubules in obstructed kidneys may reflect the effects of chronic dynamic back pressures. Though the malformations of the ureter that gave rise to incomplete obstruction occurred at a very early stage, nephron development must have proceeded in an orderly manner more or less unimpaired. The onset of hydronephrotic changes brought about by obstruction presumably occurred later in fetal life and early infancy but the back pressure did not give rise to dysplasia. This concept is supported by the lack of dysplasia noted in kidneys of babies whose ureters exhibited simple intra vesical stenotic ureteroceles (Chapter 16).

The development of kidneys associated with partial obstruction due to posterior urethral valves varied from near normal to frank dysplasia. Severe renal dysplasia occurred in the kidneys with extremely lateral orifice position and was rare in those with near-normal orifice position. The HD gradings of these kidneys correlated with orifice position and matched also those of nonobstructed kidneys with ureters having equivalent orifice positions.

Cussen (1971b) noted that cystic dysplasia was associated with 18 of 33 reflux ureters with urethral valves, but that the remaining 15 kidneys did not exhibit cystic dysplasia. He concluded that neither the obstruction nor the reflux was necessarily a determinant of the cystic dysplasia.

Ureteric orifice position was not taken into account in the study by Cussen (1971b). This feature may be significant in the explanation of the renal hypodysplasia. Malposition of the ureteric orifice denotes an abnormal site of origin of the ureteric bud from the wolffian duct and consequent entry of the bud into the tail end of the nephrogenic cord peripheral to the metanephros. With more marked degrees of ectopy, both the inducer capability of the bud and the mesenchymal quality of the nephrogenic cord may be at fault, resulting in hypodysplasia.

On the basis of the observations in the studies, abnormal orifice position correlates with renal dysplasia, and the bud theory is invoked to explain the correlation. The question arises, however, as to whether partial obstruction of the urethra causes lateral displacement of the orifices as a secondary phenomenon reflecting the degree of obstruction with or without superimposed reflux. This argument cannot presently be refuted, but the findings of unilateral or bilateral lateral ectopy of different degrees with urethral valves, the similarity of the grades of kidneys associated with lateral ectopy with and without urethral obstruction, and the relative lack of dysplasia in kidneys accompanying partial ureteral or urethral obstructions with near-normal orifice locations argue against obstruction or reflux being the initiators of the abnormalities. However, bud dysgenesis, which was found originally to explain the renal dysmorphism with double ureters and subsequently with obstructions due to urethral valves, provides a comprehensive and logical explanation of the correlation of the renal morphology and abnormal orifice position in babies with urethral obstruction.

In this chapter, a 'urologic' schema of intrarenal dysgenesis is arranged in order to subdivide and define the congenital hypoplasias (oligonephronias) and dysplasias from the genetic and non-genetic parenchymal cystic diseases. Renal hypoplasia and dysplasia have been described more fully in Chapters 33 and 34. Emphasis in this classification of hypoplasia and dysplasia is laid upon the ureteric orifice position as a guide to the understanding of the renal morphology, a key observation and entity that have been omitted in previous classifications. Except for inclusion in the classification and a few explanatory notes and illustrations of the morphology, the lesions will not be further described here. For the renal cystic diseases that have not been described elsewhere in this book, an annotation, together with illustrations, and where appropriate, a concept of the pathologic embryology, follows. Syndromes involving the kidney and urinary system, as annotated by Chantler (1975) are appended with genetic and chromosomal characteristics (Appendix 2).

The classification is based on deductive embryology and pathological characteristics including simple hypoplasia (oligonephronia) which cannot always be assessed by routine microscopic examination alone. Furthermore, the pathological status may not be truly assessed by radiological or macroscopic criteria, in which event the more suitable descriptive term to use is renal dysmorphia. However, dysmorphia can be qualified by additional terms such as 'dwarf', 'thin', 'triad', 'sponge' or 'polycystic', when appropriate non-pathological criteria are forthcoming from radiological or ultrasonic observations or studies of renal function.

It should be noted that a Committee representing the Section of Urology, American Academy of Pediatrics (on which the author was a member) developed a paper defining a Classification, Nomenclature and Terminology of Renal Dysgenesis and Cystic Disease of the Kidney (Glassberg et al., 1987). This paper should be consulted as the classification differs in some minor details from that described below. In this chapter the author and co-author have retained their own classification as it is a record of their own observations. However, the Committee's paper contains considerably more detail on certain lesions beyond the brief annotations described in this chapter.

Classification

1. Renal hypoplasia (oligonephronia)
   A. Hypoplasia (oligonephronia) with normal ureteric orifice position—the 'dwarf' kidney
   B. Hypoplasia (oligonephronia) with abnormal ureteric orifice position—the 'thin' kidney
2. Renal dysplasia
   A. Renal hypodysplasia with single or double systems
      (i) Hypodysplastic kidney with ureteric orifice in normal position
         (a) without obstruction
         (b) with partial obstruction of ureter or ureteropelvic junction
      (ii) Hypodysplastic thin kidney or nubbin with extreme medial and distal or lateral ectopia of ureteric orifice respectively
      (iii) Hypodysplastic thin kidney with lateral ectopy of ureteric orifice and partial urethral obstruction
      (iv) Hypodysplastic triad (prune belly) kidney with dysmorphia and dysplasia of ureter and lateral ectopy of the ureteric orifice
   B. Multicystic dysplastic kidney with complete obstruction of the ureter or urinary tract as with ureteral atresia or blind ureterocele or urethral atresia. The kidney may be enlarged and deformed by grape-like cysts, or small with dysplasia and microcysts. The ureteric orifice may be in a normal or abnormal position

*This chapter is jointly authored by F.D. Stephens and L.J. Cussen.

3. Renal cystic dysgenesis with normal ureters and orifices in normal position or in positions not hitherto recorded

A. Genetic

   (i)   Autosomal dominant (adult type) polycystic kidneys
         (a) Type 1
         (b) Type 2

   (ii) Autosomal recessive (infantile type) polycystic kidneys
         (a) perinatal
         (b) congenital hepatic fibrosis
         (c) intermediate types

   (iii) Medullary cystic kidneys (including nephronophthisis)
         (a) autosomal dominant
         (b) autosomal recessive
         (c) ? sporadic

   (iv) Microcystic kidneys (congenital nephrosis)

   (v)   Cysts associated with multiple malformation syndromes
         (a) chromosomal anomalies
         (b) mutant-gene syndromes

   (vi) Glomerulocystic kidneys (some cases acquired)
         (a) autosomal dominant
         (b) familial hypoplastic
         (c) others (overlap with (v))

B. Non-genetic

   (i)   Simple cysts, single or multiple
   (ii)   Medullary sponge kidney
   (iii) Glomerulocystic kidneys (overlap with A (vi))
   (iv)   Neoplasms with cystic changes
          (a) multilocular cystic kidneys (cystic adenoma)
          (b) cysts in intrarenal teratoma, mesoblastic nephroma, nephroblastoma, and carcinoma of kidney
   (v)   Pyelogenic cysts (pelvic and calyceal diverticula)
   (vi)   Parapelvic cysts
   (vii) Perinephric cysts
   (viii) Acquired renal cystic disease (chronic renal failure)

Renal hypoplasia (oligonephronia)

Hypoplasia with normal ureteric orifice position

This is the compact 'dwarf' kidney with normal morphology of smaller-than-normal number of functioning nephrons. The condition may be uni- or bilateral, and the location of the kidney may be normal or abnormal. The dwarf kidney is rare, affects males and females equally, and is sporadic. The term 'hypoplastic kidney' has been used traditionally to denote this form of kidney and may be the best term under the circumstances. However, 'oligonephronia' would be suitable, denoting a quantitative deficiency in the metanephric primordia.

Hypoplasia with abnormal ureteric orifice position

This is represented by the 'thin' kidney with ectatic calyces and collecting system and moderate departure of the ureteric orifice positions from the normal trigone in either lateral or medial directions.

Because of the common association of the thin parenchyma with vesicoureteral reflux, the thinness has been considered to be secondary to the back-pressure effects of either primary or secondary reflux. The thinness, however, may derive predominantly from an initial oligonephronia resulting from abnormal interaction of an abnormally sited bud with the metanephros.

This thin ectatic kidney with ureteral ectopia is common in single and duplex ureters and is usually accompanied by vesicoureteral reflux. Lateral ureteric ectopia is more common in females, and may be inherited either as an autosomal recessive or dominant with variable penetrance (Burger and Smith, 1971; Dwoskin, 1976; Bailey, 1979; Heale et al., 1979). Hence the accompanying renal hypoplasia may be heritable.

Embryogenesis of 'dwarf' and 'thin' kidneys with ureteric orifices in normal position

Intrarenal branchings of normal ampullae or collecting ducts arising from normal ureteric buds may arrest because of quantitatively deficient metanephrogenic mesenchyme, resulting in an otherwise normal though dwarf kidney.

It may not be generally realized that the calyces of the embryonic kidney are at first rounded in shape, and it is not until the nephrons proliferate and the loops of Henle grow centrally from cortex into the medulla that the papillae form. Hence deficiency in numbers of nephrons in association with a normal ureteric bud determines the size of the compact dwarf kidney, whereas the bud anomaly associated with lateral ectopia determines the degree of ureterectasis, the configuration of the calyces, the number of nephrons and the thinness of the kidney. The compact dwarf kidney arising from a normal bud exhibits a miniature pelvis and calyces in proportion to renal size, whereas the 'thin' kidney arising from a megabud may have calyces that are large, blunt, clubbed or spherical (Sommer and Stephens, 1981) (Fig. 35.1).

Pathology of the dwarf and thin ectatic kidneys
The nephrons and calyces are well formed but fewer than normal, accounting for the dwarf kidney. Boissonnat (1962) has stressed also the importance of small numbers of minor calyces and pyramids in the thin ectatic kidneys. If the condition is bilateral, hypertrophy of the nephrons may become so marked that the condition is referred to as 'oligomeganephronia'.

Sometimes a sharply demarcated segment of an undersized kidney exhibits a deep circumferential groove overlying an elongated calyx. The intervening tissue is fibrotic with sparse, thyroid-like, or atrophic tubules that lack functioning glomeruli, and occasionally dysplastic ducts (Habib, 1979) (Fig. 35.2). The blood vessels are thick-walled with accompanying endarteritis. Ask-Upmark (1929) described this lesion in seven patients with hypertension. He attributed the demarcated zone to a developmental hypoplasia. In more recent studies that include routine use of cysto-urethrography, similar lesions, sometimes multiple, have been found in association with vesicoureteral reflux. Tests for reflux were not undertaken in the patients described by Ask-Upmark, so the alternative view that the 'hypoplastic' segment in such patients is a 'scar' derived from infection and reflux is more soundly based (Arant et al., 1979).

Renal dysplasia
Renal hypodysplasia
The combination of renal hypoplasia and dysplasia has also been elaborated extensively in Chapter 34, giving the view of the author and colleagues on this somewhat controversial pathogenesis. Renal dysplasia is a developmental anomaly of nephrogenic and stromagenic structures

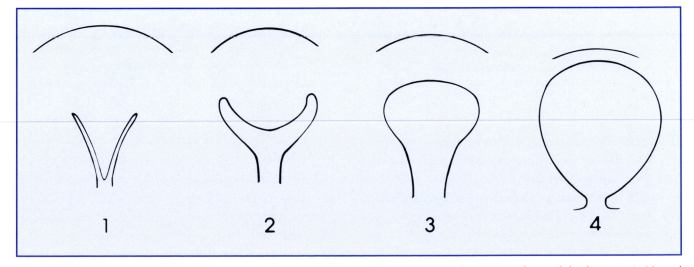

Fig. 35.1 *Schematic representation of macroscopic shapes of papillae and calyces as seen in obstruction and normal development. 1. Normal papilla. 2. Blunt papilla. 3. Clubbed calyx. 4. Globular calyx. Figures read from 1 to 4 show advance of papillary and calyceal changes resulting from chronic partial obstruction of the urinary tract. Figures read in reverse order, from 4 to 1, indicate the shapes and stages of development of the minor calyx and papilla from the initial single cavity formed by coalescence of multiple divisions of the ureteric bud. (Reprinted, by permission, from Sommer, J.T. and Stephens, F.D. (1981), Morphogenesis of nephropathy with partial ureteral obstruction and vesicoureteral reflux. J. Urol. 125: 67, Fig. 1.)*

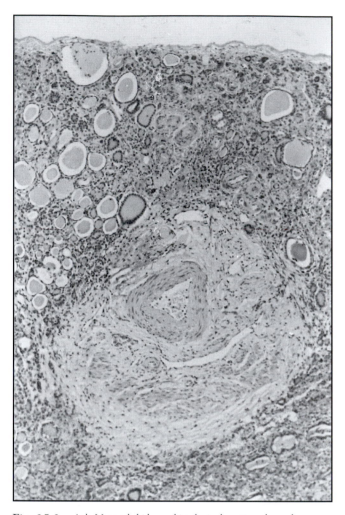

Fig. 35.2 *Ask-Upmark kidney: histological section through narrow corticomedullary segment. Note colloid-filled thyroid-like tubules, fibrosis in cortex, thick-walled blood vessel and absence of glomeruli. (Reprinted, with permission, from Stephens, F.D. and Cussen, L.J. (1983), Congenital Malformations of the Urinary Tract, F.D. Stephens (ed.), Fig. 31.2, p. 476. New York: Praeger.)*

characterized by the presence of abnormal primitive ducts and ductules in embryonic mesenchymal connective tissue and, commonly, with cysts and cartilage. These structures lie amidst normal nephrons in varying proportions in different kidneys. The degree of nephron hypoplasia is usually proportional to the degree of dysplasia; hence the term 'hypodysplasia' is appropriate. The kidney may be large, with macrocysts, or small, with sparse microcysts. 'Dysplasia' is a term that should be used when the abnormal structure of the kidney is identified pathologically.

Renal hypodysplasia may occur in association with the following:

(i) Hypodysplastic compact dwarf kidney with normal ureters and collecting systems with some functional nephrons. The metanephric mesenchyme may be primarily at fault, and lacking in response to induction by the normal ureteric bud.

Hydronephrotic kidneys associated with partial ureteropelvic junction or ureteral obstruction rarely exhibit evidence of dysplasia. The renal parenchyma is uniformly thin as a result of obstructive atrophy or oligonephronia. Sometimes the parenchyma is extremely thin, sometimes patchy in distribution, and occasionally absent. Such kidneys in infants may exhibit excess of fibrous tissue and abnormal ducts and nephrons. In these extreme examples, the morphology may result not only from obstructive atrophy but also an initial hypoplastic or dysplastic metanephros.

(ii) The hypodysplastic thin kidney occurs typically with extreme lateral ectopia of the ureteric orifice with its reflux megaureter. The small hypodysplastic nubbin is commonly associated with ectopic orifices that issue in the urethra, vagina or vas, with or without an accompanying ureterocele. Both types of kidney exhibit a mixture of functional and dysfunctional nephrons and other stromal dysplasias.

(iii) Hypodysplastic thin kidney with megaureter and lateral ectopy of the ureteral orifice occurs commonly with partial urethral obstruction by Young's valves. Obstructive cysts of Bowman's capsules may be present in the subcapsular cortex (Chapter 33). They may enlarge and become barely visible to the naked eye.

(iv) In the triad (prune belly) hypodysplastic kidney, the ureter is often dysmorphic and dilated and its orifice wide and laterally ectopic (Chapter 37).

Multicystic kidney

Multicystic dysplastic kidney with complete obstruction to the flow of urine along the ureter as with ureteral atresia or its variant, the long impermeable stenosis, has been described in Chapter 14. The renal and ureteric morphologies may result from the combined effects of ischaemia and obstruction.

Pathogenesis of renal dysplasia

Defects of the bud or its branches, or qualitative and quantitative deficiencies of the nephrogenic mesenchyme may lead to dysplasia, which may be total, partial, or focal and intermixed with normal structures.

In occasional families two or more members, usually siblings, have renal dysplasia. It is not known whether this occasional familial distribution is coincidental, is due to an environmental teratogen, or represents a genetically determined variant of the lesion. However, vesicoureteral reflux resulting from congenital defects of the ureterovesical valve is associated with renal dysplasia, and about 10 per cent of vesicoureteral reflux is familial, which may be the reason for the occasional reports of familial dysplasia.

The embryogenesis may be related to defective bud formation, as indicated by abnormal positions of the ureteric orifices; in some instances, the bud may be normal but the metanephric tissue may be absent, defective, or placed out of the territory of induction by the bud; or in others, as with some triad (prune belly) kidneys, both the bud and the metanephros may be at fault qualitatively, creating extremely dysmorphic and dysplastic ureters and kidneys.

Not all kidneys with ureteric orifices abnormally placed, however, are hypoplastic or dysplastic. In such instances, both the bud and the corresponding metanephric parenchyma may be mutually dystopic retaining good inductive capability (see Fig. 30.7).

Multicystic kidneys (Fig. 35.3), which have either a characteristic grape-like appearance or a small, solid-looking dysplastic kidney with microcysts and some minicysts have, in most instances atresia of the ureter (Bernstein, 1968) or long impermeable stenoses (Chapter 14). The ureteric orifice, when present, may be normal in location or ectopic, in which case the ureter caudal to the abnormal segment may be larger than normal. Dysplasia of the nephrons and stroma is present in all multicystic kidneys and often patches of normal-looking nephrons can be found deep in the kidney substance. Complete obstruction of the ureter together with ischaemia of ureter and kidney caused by faulty vascularization during rapid elongation of the ureter and migration and differentiation of the kidney, may account for the cystic dysplasia (see Fig. 26.5). The ischaemic process may continue after birth accounting for diminution in size or disappearance of the affected kidney and ureter. The ureteric atresia may be similar in its aetiology to that of atresia of the bowel (Louw and Barnard, 1955).

Reflux nephropathy

The term 'reflux nephropathy' is used to describe any dysmorphic kidney associated with vesicoureteral reflux. It is a useful, non-committal, radiological and clinical term that embraces, but does not specify, the aetiologies or morphologies of the dysmorphic kidneys; it can be conveniently used by clinicians and radiologists when viewing and describing radiographs of reflux kidneys. It behoves the pathologist, however, to identify the morphology of the defective kidney, including not only the presence of infection but also congenital hypoplasia and dysplasia of the nephrons. The pathologist should take into account the dimensions and morphology of the accompanying ureter and the location of its orifice in the urinary or genital tracts. From the total data obtained from clinician, radiologist, ultrasonologist, cystoscopist and pathologist, it may be possible to specify the aetiology of the reflux nephropathy. In clinical practice, however, the pathological input is unavailable and the specific aetiology or aetiologies remain conceptual and, under these circumstances, the term 'reflux nephropathy' is appropriate.

When the reflux nephropathy is discovered in the neonate or infant, the dysmorphism is more likely to result from congenital hypoplasia with or without dysplasia, whereas, in the older child the nephropathy may be congenital or may be acquired from the effects of reflux urodynamics with or without superimposed infection. The radiographical criterion of reflux infection of the kidney is the Hodson 'scar' characterized radiographically by an indentation of the renal outline overlying a medullary excavation and calyceal elongation—in essence, a parenchymal thinning between capsule and papilla (Hodson, 1979). When these 'scars' affect a greater part of the parenchyma of the kidney following overwhelming infections, the thinning becomes generalized and the calyces bulbous. This kidney, with its acquired lesions, may then resemble radiographically the congenital thin hypoplastic or dysplastic kidney, which

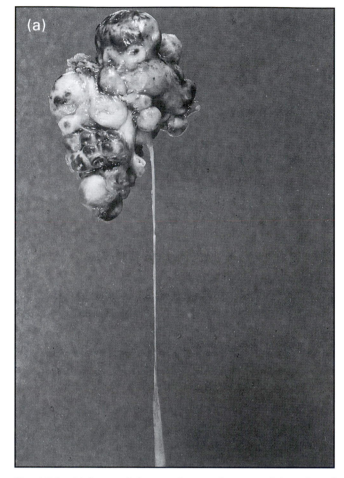

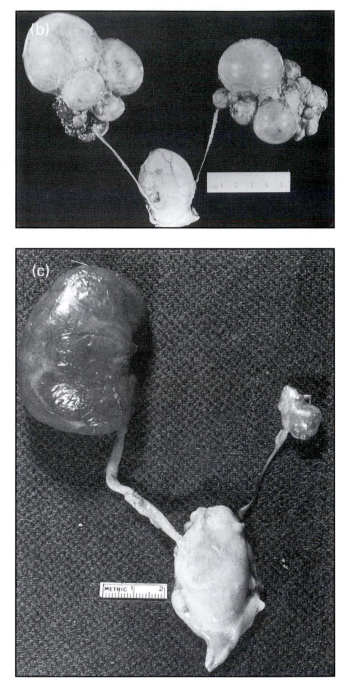

Fig. 35.3 *Multicystic kidneys with ureteral atresias. (a) Unilateral with long upper ureteral atresia. (b) Bilateral with large cysts and areas of compact dysplasia, right atresia of pelvis and calyces, and left lower ureteral atresia. (c) Left-sided mini-kidney with small cysts and dysplasia and atresia of ureter. (Reprinted, with permission, from Stephens, F.D. and Cussen L.J. (1983), In Congenital Malformations of the Urinary Tract, F.D. Stephens (ed.), Fig. 31.3, pp. 477–478. New York: Praeger.)*

also may be further modified radiographically by effects of infection. Hence, in older children especially, the term 'reflux nephropathy', if the meaning as described is understood, is appropriate and useful. The resemblance of the congenital and acquired reflux lesions and the admixture of both has caused a continuing controversy among radiologists, urologists and pathologists as to the effects of primary reflux without infection on the kidney and ureter of the fetus and child. In Stephens' view

(Stephens, 1979d), the effects of vesicoureteral reflux, if any, on the kidney take decades to appear radiographically; the presence of ectasia of the pelvis and ureter, and the ectopic location of the ureteric orifice, which he considers to be part of the pan-bud-metanephros anomaly, provides the clue to the presence of an underlying congenital hypoplasia or dysplasia. Pyelonephritic scarring, which occurs much more rapidly, in months or years, may be superadded, eroding the papillae, clubbing calyces, and still further modifying and complicating the morphogenesis. Scars superimposed upon a hypoplastic thin kidney exhibit no trace of dysplasia, but when superimposed upon a hypodysplastic kidney, traces of primitive ducts and mesenchyme may remain with 'insight' of the ultrasonologist, an earlier and more accurate differentiation between oligonephonia and scarred kidney is now possible.

Renal cystic dysgenesis

Genetic

Autosomal dominant (adult type) polycystic kidneys

Progressive hereditary polycystic disease of the kidneys is usually diagnosed in adult life. It is characterized at the time of clinical presentation by markedly enlarged irregular kidneys with innumerable cysts interspersed among small zones of normal or compressed renal parenchyma. The ureters issue in normal locations on the trigone and are normal in dimensions. As the cysts enlarge, the contiguous parenchyma undergoes progressive ischaemic strangulation and atrophy and hypertension develops in about 50 per cent of the patients. Cystic change in the liver and pancreas is present in a minority of cases.

This is the commonest type of hereditary cystic kidneys, the prevalence in the general population being roughly 1 in 1000 individuals. It is usually diagnosed when symptoms appear, most commonly after the age of 40, but cystic changes have been found in some patients in infancy or even in fetal life. Both sexes are equally affected and there is no known racial, geographical or social factor affecting the incidence.

The disease is usually transmitted in an autosomal dominant pattern, although a few cases are apparently sporadic and may represent new mutations. Type 1, due to an abnormal gene on the short arm of chromosome 16, affects about 90 per cent of patients and is clinically more severe than Type 2, which is due to an abnormal gene on the long arm of chromosome 4. It is not known if there are more than two types.

Factors possibly involved in the pathogenesis of autosomal dominant polycystic kidneys include environmental factors in the host, abnormality of extracellular matrix or of tubular basement membranes, expression of *c-myc* proto-oncogene, production of cAMP and the location and function of the sodium–potassium ion pump.

Cysts of various sizes are present in both kidneys, although one may be more severely affected than the other. The kidneys in adults are usually four or five times their normal size and are distorted by the cysts, which may be up to 4 cm in diameter and involve both cortex and medulla (Fig. 35.4a). The cysts are round and translucent with smooth inner linings of flattened or cuboidal epithelium, and most contain clear fluid, although a few are filled with gelatinous semisolid material, and others contain blood-stained fluid. The cysts may arise in any part of the nephron, some being cystic diverticula of nephrons. In the later stages of the disease, the cysts usually occupy most of the kidney, but strands and islands of functional renal parenchyma and fibrous tissue may be found among the cysts (Fig. 35.4b). The renal pelvis and calyces are usually distorted by the cysts, which radiographically present the appearance of bubbles in the renal shadows, and create the 'spider-like' calyces.

The hepatic cysts are derived from bile ducts (Fig. 35.4c) and those in the pancreas from the branches of the pancreatic duct. Risk factors for development of hepatic cysts in this condition include age (prevalence increases from the second to the fifth decade), sex (more frequent in women), pregnancy and the severity of renal cystic change. About 10 per cent of patients have cysts of the pancreas, and occasional patients have cysts of the spleen and lung.

Renal parenchymal compression and atrophy of nephrons are associated with renal failure and hypertension with its attendant problems of cardiac failure, encephalopathy and visual disturbances. Cerebral aneurysms and aortic and mitral valvular lesions are other associated conditions. Carcinoma of the kidney may supervene in adult polycystic disease, but is a rare complication.

Autosomal recessive (infantile type) polycystic kidney

Infantile polycystic disease is characterized pathologically by markedly enlarged reniform kidneys with very numerous, fine, elongated, ectatic collecting ducts radiating from pelvis to the cortex, as seen on the cut surface of the kidney. The ureters open normally on the trigone and their lumina are usually decreased in comparison with normal ureters.

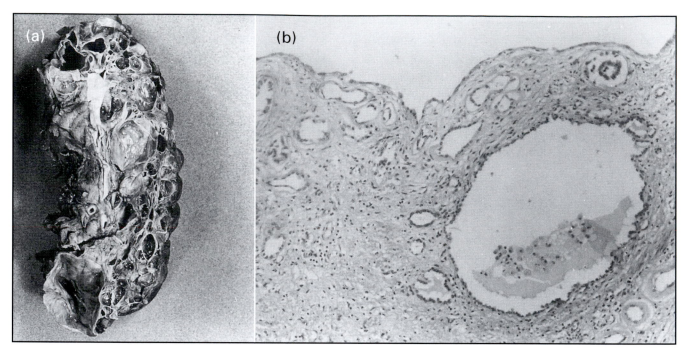

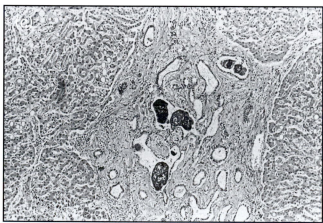

Fig. 35.4 *Polycystic kidney, adult type. (**a**) Polycystic kidney, both cortex and medulla are almost completely replaced by cysts of varying size (×⅓). (**b**) Renal tubules in the septum between cysts (×2). (**c**) Cystic change in the intrahepatic bile ducts of a patient with adult polycystic kidneys (×⅔). (Reprinted, with permission, from Stephens, F.D. and Cussen, L.J. (1983), In Congenital Malformations of the Urinary Tract, F.D. Stephens (ed.), Fig. 31.4, p. 479. New York: Praeger.)*

Proliferation and mild cystic dilation of the intrahepatic bile ducts with variable degrees of fibrosis of the portal tracts is a constant feature.

This comparatively uncommon type of bilateral cystic kidney occurs in between 1 in 10 000 and 1 in 40 000 live births. Most patients die in the first few hours of life but a few survive for months or even years. There is usually a reciprocal degree of severity between the renal and hepatic lesions, such that patients dying in the perinatal period have severe renal involvement and much less severe hepatic involvement, while patients surviving into the second or even the third decade have only minor renal lesions with severe hepatic involvement, a condition often referred to as 'congenital hepatic fibrosis'. Both sexes are affected in equal numbers, and there is no known racial, geographical, or social factor affecting the incidence.

The disease is transmitted in an autosomal recessive pattern. It has been stated that the age at death tends to be similar in affected members of the one family, i.e. there are genetic variants of the disease that breed true (Blyth and Ockender, 1971).

Apart from the fact that it is genetically determined, nothing is known about the pathogenesis of the disease, and there is no indication as to the reason for the variable involvement of liver and kidneys in patients of different ages.

Both kidneys are involved, usually to a similar extent. In newborn infants, the kidneys retain their reniform shape but are enlarged to up to 10 times their normal size (Fig. 35.5a). The fine renal cysts just visible on the cortical surfaces are formed by the projecting ends of the ectatic collecting ducts. On the cut surface, these ducts are readily seen to be linear cystic structures radiating from the pelvis to the cortex (Fig. 35.5b). The cylindrical cysts are translucent, filled with clear fluid, and involve predominantly the collecting ducts in both cortex and medulla (Fig. 35.5c); they are lined by flattened or cuboidal epithelium (Fig. 35.5d). They are joined by normal numbers of normal or mildly ectatic nephrons in the cortex. In older surviving patients, the renal cysts usually take the form of diverticula arising from the collecting ducts chiefly in the medulla. There is no obstructive lesion in the urinary tract.

The hepatic lesion in the newborn infant comprises proliferation and mild dilation of intrahepatic bile ducts with a mild increase in portal fibrous tissue (Fig. 35.5e), while in the older patient, the increase in portal fibrous tissue is more marked.

The commonest complications are respiratory distress in the neonatal period, hypertension and renal failure in infants, and portal hypertension with haematemesis in children in their second decade.

Medullary cystic kidneys including nephronophthisis

Medullary cystic kidneys comprise a group of hereditary diseases characterized by progressive renal failure. They are associated with the development of cystic changes mainly in, but not confined to, the renal medulla. The ureters appear to be normal in all respects.

This group of diseases is uncommon, although the juvenile form is said to be responsible for about 20 per cent of childhood deaths from chronic renal failure (Betts and Forrest-Hay, 1973).

There are two distinct genetic variants of medullary cystic kidney, an autosomal recessive disease affecting children and adolescents, and an autosomal dominant disease affecting young adults. Both of these variants have similar clinical and pathological features. In addition, in a few families with the autosomal recessive variety of the disease, some, but not all, patients have tapetoretinal degeneration or hepatic fibrosis or both. It seems probable that retinal degeneration and hepatic fibrosis are variable features of the autosomal recessive variety of medullary cystic disease. Medullary cystic disease also apparently occurs sporadically in some patients with no family history of the disease, possibly as the result of a new mutation.

The kidneys are characteristically smaller than usual, although they may be of normal size and the lesion is bilateral. There is poor demarcation between the medulla and the attenuated cortex, with cystic change chiefly in the medulla. Microscopically, many tubules are atrophic, while others are dilated, with characteristic marked thickening of the basement membranes. Interstitial fibrosis and mild infiltrates of lymphocytes are present.

Patients with the autosomal recessive disease present usually with polyuria and polydipsia in the first decade, and the disease usually progresses to renal failure over the next 10 years; anaemia and the excessive loss of salt in the urine are common features, but hypertension is uncommon. Patients with the autosomal dominant disease have similar features but develop symptoms in the second to fourth decades. The duration of disease is similar in both groups.

Microcystic disease (congenital nephrosis)

Microcystic disease is a form of nephrotic syndrome, usually leading to death in the first year of life, and characterized by cystic dilation of the proximal convoluted tubules. The disease is rare except in Finland, and is transmitted as an autosomal recessive condition.

The kidneys and ureters are usually of normal size and shape, but on microscopic examination, characteristic cysts are present in the proximal convoluted tubules of both kidneys (Fig. 35.6). The placenta is notably very large. The patients are often oedematous at birth or in the first two months of life, resulting from proteinuria and hypoalbuminaemia.

Cysts associated with malformation syndromes

Chromosomal abnormalities. Patients with monosomy X (Turner's syndrome) and trisomies C, G (Down's syndrome), E (Edwards' syndrome) and D (Patau's syndrome) have, in increasing order, a propensity to develop microscopic cysts, usually involving glomerular spaces of the renal cortex. These are found on pathological examination and are usually of no clinical significance. The ureters appear normal in most instances. However, an occasional patient with a chromosomal abnormality, particularly trisomy D or E, may

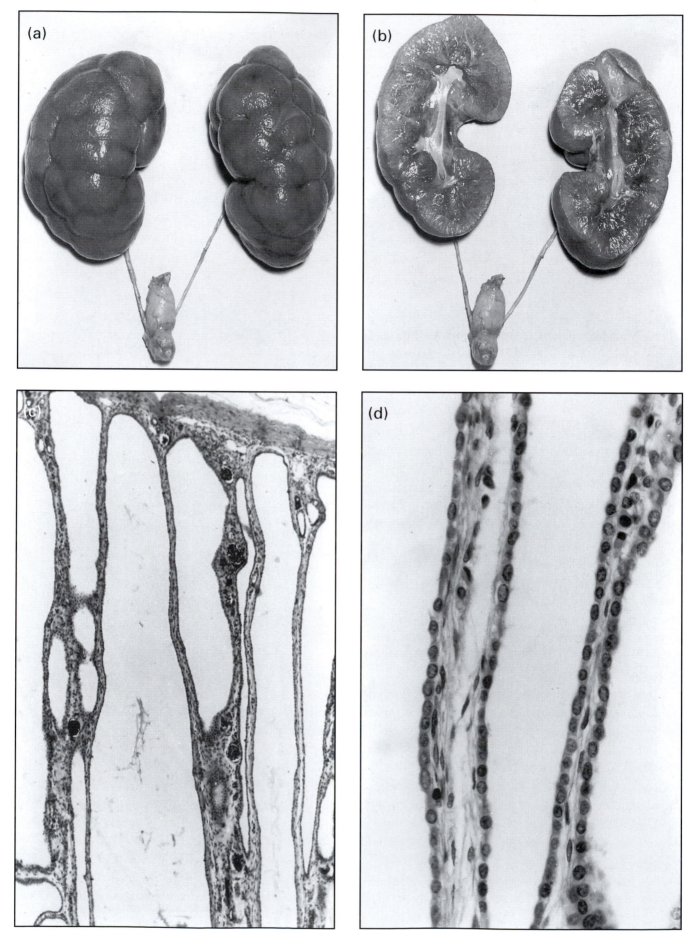

Fig. 35.5 (*continued*)

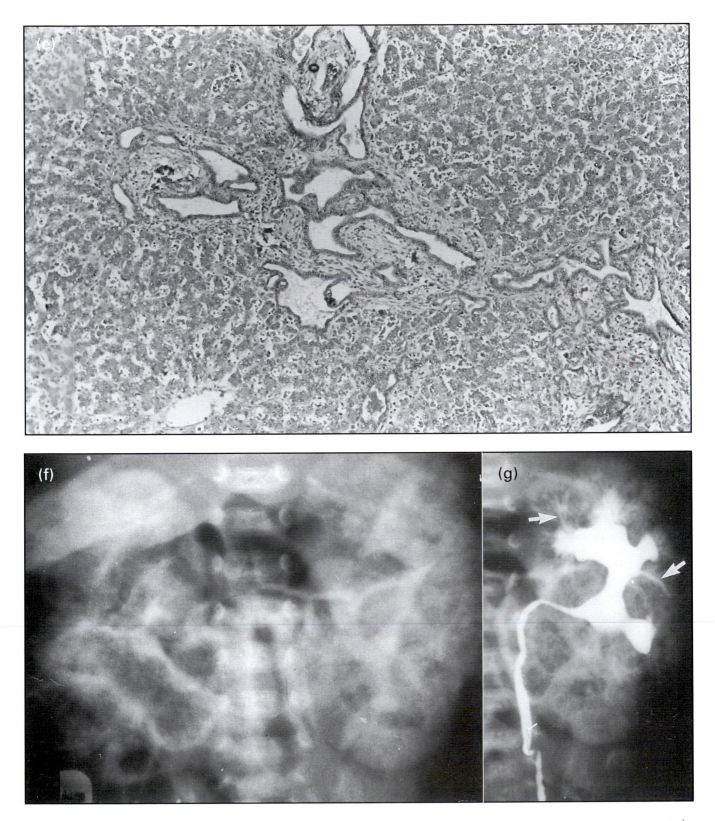

Fig. 35.5 *Infantile polycystic kidney.* (**a**) *Markedly enlarged granular kidneys with small cystic protrusions on the cortical surfaces* ($\times\frac{1}{2}$). (**b**) *Cystic dilatation of the collecting ducts disposed in a linear radiating pattern on the cut surface of the kidneys* ($\times\frac{1}{2}$). (**c**) *Cystic dilatations of the collecting ducts in the cortex, the outer ends of which create the granular appearance on the surface of the kidneys* ($\times\frac{2}{3}$). (**d**) *The ducts are lined by flattened or cuboidal epithelium* ($\times\frac{2}{3}$). (**e**) *Proliferation of bile ducts in the liver of a patient with infantile polycystic kidneys* ($\times\frac{2}{3}$). (**f**) *Intravenous pyelogram of another patient showing pooling of opaque medium.* (**g**) *Retrograde pyelogram showing reflux into the wide collecting ducts (arrows).* (*Reprinted, with permission, from Stephens, F.D. and Cussen, L.J. (1983), In* Congenital Malformations of the Urinary Tract, *New York: Praeger, Fig. 31.5, pp. 480–481.*)

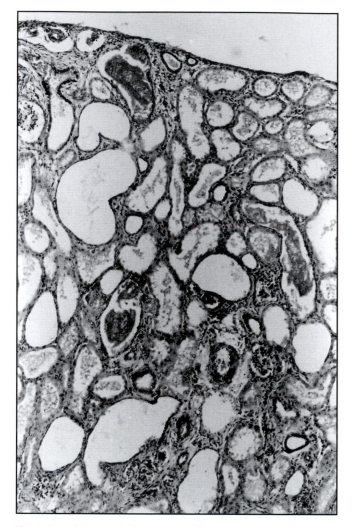

Fig. 35.6 *Microcystic disease; cystic dilatation of proximal collecting tubules in the renal cortex ($\times\frac{2}{3}$). (Reprinted, with permission, from Stephens, F.D. and Cussen L.J. (1983), In Congenital Malformations of the Urinary Tract, New York: Praeger, Fig. 31.6, p. 482.)*

have severe glomerulocystic change or even renal dysplasia, which may have clinical consequences.

Mutant gene anomalies. Cystic disease of the kidneys is a common finding in the following genetically determined malformation syndromes.

Autosomal recessive. Meckel syndrome (encephalocele, polydactyly), Jeune syndrome (asphyxiating thoracic dystrophy), Zellweger syndrome (cerebrohepatorenal syndrome), Majewski and Saldino–Noonan syndromes (short rib polydactyly syndromes), glutaric aciduria Type 2 and carbohydrate-deficient glycoprotein syndrome.

Autosomal dominant. Bourneville syndrome (tuberous sclerosis), von Hippel–Lindau syndrome (retinal angio-

mata and cerebellar haemangioblastoma). Renal carcinoma is a recognized complication of both these conditions.

X-Linked dominant. Oral–facial–digital syndrome Type 1. *Cystic changes in the kidneys in association with other malformation syndromes.* These have also been reported in the following syndromes: Ehlers–Danlos; Dandy–Walker; Ivemark, Goldston, Goldenhar, and Dekaban, Robinow, Laurence–Moon–Bardet–Biedl; Kaufman–McCusick, Roberts, Fryns, Apert; DiGeorge; Marden–Walker; Cornelia de Lange; Smith–Lemli–Opitz; lissencephaly. *Glomerulocystic kidney.* This term, coined by Taxy and Filmer (1976), describes a group of uncommon diseases characterized by the presence of cysts involving the Bowman capsules and adjacent dilated abnormal tubules of both kidneys. In some patients, the disease has a genetic basis, while in others it appears to be sporadic. The sporadic cases are often, but not always, associated with obstruction of the urinary tract. There is rarely any significant effect on renal function. The topic is covered fully by Bernstein (1993).

Non-genetic

Simple cysts

Simple cysts are thin-walled and unilocular, often single, and usually situated in the cortex of the kidney.

The cause of simple cysts is unknown, but the fact that they are frequent in adults and very rare in children suggests that they may be acquired.

There is no familial incidence of simple cysts. The pathogenesis is uncertain. They may be retention cysts caused by persistence of the earliest rudimentary glomeruli, which normally undergo absorption, or by tubular obstruction due to local ischaemia or inflammation (Siegel and McAlister, 1980). Rapidly elongating tubules of the nephron in the embryonic and early fetal stages may sustain an impairment of blood supply with glomerular or tubular cyst formation.

Simple cysts are unilocular, often single, but sometimes multiple, usually filled with clear, serous fluid and lined by a single layer of flattened cells resting on a narrow strip of fibrous tissue. They are usually situated in the renal cortex, may be small or large, often asymptomatic, and occasionally cause hypertension. Simple cysts in children are benign lesions.

Medullary sponge kidney

Medullary sponge kidney is a non-hereditary disease characterized by the development of cysts localized to the collecting tubules in the pyramids of both kidneys.

The incidence has been calculated to be about 1 in 20 000 (Mayall, 1970). Males and females are equally affected, and the disease is very rare in infants and children.

There is no familial tendency, and the few reports of multiple cases in one family may be coincidental, or attributable perhaps to misdiagnosis of conditions such as medullary cystic disease or congenital hepatic fibrosis, both of which are genetically determined and have cystic change in the medullary pyramids.

The condition is bilateral, although one kidney may be more severely affected than the other, and may affect only one or a few pyramids in a kidney. The cysts affect the terminal part of the collecting tubule in the medullary pyramids, and the remainder of the nephron is normally formed. The kidneys are of normal, or slightly increased size and weight, and the cortices and medullae are well demarcated. There are no associated malformations in the urinary tract or elsewhere.

Symptoms related to renal or ureteric calculi or to the presence of infection occur in the fourth or fifth decade. The cysts are usually small and can be detected by excretory pyelography and a few patients progress to renal failure, brought on by damage to the kidneys from nephrocalcinosis and repeated urinary tract infections.

Acquired cystic kidney disease

This condition occurs in patients with chronic renal failure and is characterized by bilateral cysts occurring in both cortex and medulla in any part of the nephron. Acquired cystic kidney disease occurs in both children and adults with an equal incidence in males and females, and its occurrence is not dependent on either previous drug therapy or dialysis. However, the frequency of the condition and the number of cysts are proportional to the duration of chronic renal failure. Three years after the onset of chronic renal failure, up to 40 per cent of patients have acquired cystic kidney disease and this figure may rise to 90 per cent five years after the onset of chronic renal failure. However, acquired cystic kidney is apparently somewhat less common in the native kidneys of patients who have received a renal transplant than in patients who are on dialysis, and it has been claimed that acquired cystic kidney disease may regress, to some extent at least, following a renal transplant.

Neoplasms of the kidney, both adenoma and carcinoma, are a recognized complication of acquired cystic kidney disease. The frequency of neoplasia does not seem to be related to whether or not the patient is on dialysis, but, in one study, the incidence of renal carcinoma was less in patients on peritoneal dialysis than in those on haemodialysis (Katz et al., 1987). Carcinoma of the kidney in patients with acquired cystic kidney disease is five to seven times commoner in males than females.

Neoplasms with cystic changes

Mutilocular cystic kidney (cystic adenoma). Multilocular cystic kidney is characterized by cysts that are solitary, multilocular with loculi that do not communicate with each other or with the renal pelvis, contain no nephrons in their septa, occupy only part of the kidney, and are usually unilateral (Fig. 35.7) (Boggs and Kimmelstiel, 1956). However, bilateral multilocular cystic kidneys have been reported (Chatten and Bishop, 1977).

Multilocular cyst of the kidneys is rare. The condition is about as frequent in children as in adults.

The cause of multilocular cyst of the kidney is unknown. It has been described in a patient who had had a normal intravenous pyelogram four years previously (Uson et al., 1960), suggesting that it may be an acquired lesion. Some authors consider that it is a neoplasm (Datnow and Daniel, 1976), while others regard it as a hamartoma (Fobi et al., 1979). There is no familial tendency.

The cysts form a multilocular, circumscribed mass, occupying part of the kidney and compressing the adjacent renal tissue. The pelvis and calyces are distorted by the mass but are otherwise normal. There is no lesion of the ureter or bladder, and the contralateral kidney is rarely involved.

Multilocular cystic kidneys clinically resemble renal neoplasms, and in several patients were associated with Wilms' tumour or carcinoma of the kidney.

Cysts in other neoplasms. Cysts may be present in intrarenal teratoma (Dehner, 1973), mesoblastic

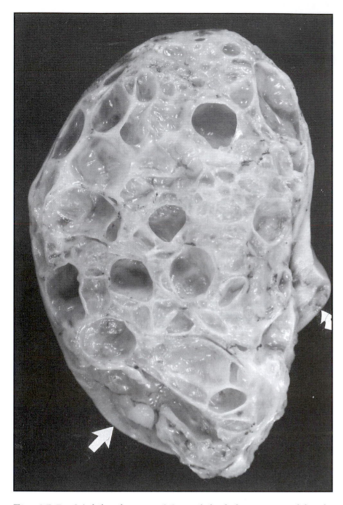

Fig. 35.7 *Multilocular cyst. Most of the kidney occupied by the encapsulated cysts, which compress the remaining renal parenchyma (arrows) ($\times\frac{3}{4}$). (Reprinted, with permission, from Stephens, F.D. and Cussen J.L. (1983), In* Congenital Malformations of the Urinary Tract, *New York: Praeger, Fig. 31.7, p. 482.)*

nephroma, Wilms' tumour and carcinoma of the kidney. They may resemble clinically multilocular cystic kidney, necessitating exploration and biopsy of part or whole of the kidney for histological confirmation of the diagnosis.

Pyelogenic cysts (calyceal diverticula)

A cystic diverticulum situated in the kidney substance arises from a calyx and communicates with it by a narrow channel (Wulfsohn, 1980). These are rare, sporadic, and usually unilateral, and are found in children and adults. They are usually small and situated at one or other pole of the kidney. The cysts are lined by transitional epithelium and contain urine.

In most cases, no associated malformation is present, but in one report (Amar, 1975), about 70 per cent of patients also had vesicoureteric reflux.

Parapelvic cysts

Parapelvic cysts are rare, sporadic, and situated at the hilum of the kidney adjacent to the renal pelvis (Spence *et al.*, 1957). Some parapelvic cysts may arise from obstructed lymphatic vessels, and it has been suggested (Spence *et al.*, 1957) that some may represent cysts derived from mesonephric remnants.

Perinephric cysts

Perinephric cysts are also rare and caused by a collection of fluid outside the renal cortex but bounded by the renal capsule. The fluid, which may be blood, urine or lymph, accumulates following trauma, urinary tract obstruction, or in association with renal lymphangiectasia.

Deformations as opposed to malformations

VI

Moulding and pressure pits on the bodies of 'normal' and abnormal children are generally presumed to be evidence of late fetal compression. Many of these moulded and dimpled children have internal and external anomalies of the genitourinary tracts and often spinal defects that suggest a dysgenesis in the early embryonic period of development. One of the authors (F.D.S.) examined 50 'normal' newborn babies and 102 babies and children under four years of age with multiple anomalies and documented the occurrence of these compression features. Abnormal moulding of head, body or limbs and pressure dimples were not uncommon in the normal babies and were found in 50 of 102 patients with multiple anomalies. These abnormal babies or young children were investigated to detect suspected anomalies of other systems. The diagnoses and clinical features were analysed to explore for a possible cause-and-effect relationship between compression and the multiple anomalies, especially those of the internal and external genitourinary organs.

It is postulated that very early minor rupture of the delicate amniotic membrane or leakage of amniotic fluid cause collapse of the membrane and growth constriction of the embryo or fetus in whole or part. With subsequent early sealing of the perforation, fluid re-accumulates, the membrane expands but the deformations incurred by the temporary compression remain.

The criteria of moulding and focal pressure on the fetus were: asymmetry of head, face or earlobe; scoliosis; rolled feet or talipes; overlap of toe or toes; and pressure dimples on the sacrococcyx, knees and ankles or deep dimples on the elbow. Compression of the elongating embryo or focal pressure on the developing limbs, perineum and genitalia offer plausible explanations of the deformities.

Major rupture of the amnion or chorion usually leads to death of embryo or fetus, respectively, but the few survivors may be mutilated by compression and amniotic bands that disrupt the tissues and constrict or amputate limbs.

A deformation as opposed to a malformation is not hereditary and therein lies the importance of recognition of this ubiquitous entity.

In this chapter, a congenital anomaly is designated a 'malformation' when the dysmorphosis is genetic, chromosomal or teratogenic. A 'deformation' is when a developing external or internal organ is altered by external forces. A 'disruption' is when previously normal tissue breaks down (Smith, 1981).

Occurrence of compression in 50 'normal' newborn babies on clinical examination only

Asymmetry of the head or face was apparent in 24 per cent; the earlobe was tilted up and forward by the shoulder in 54 per cent; the spine had a lateral C-shaped convexity in 20 per cent and seemed to be abnormally hyperextended in two and hyperflexed in two; the foot of one third of the babies exhibited partial folding of the forefoot with abnormal alignment of the toes and 8 per cent had valgus foot deviation; sacrococcygeal pressure dimples either as a discrete pit or deep linear groove occurred in 66 per cent of babies; elbow dimples over the ulna and lateral humeral epicondyle were shallow, occurring in 70 per cent of babies, and knee dimples were found in 26 per cent; overlap of toe or toes was apparent in 70 per cent of babies; and the plantar aspect of the foot was longitudinally folded, with the fourth and fifth toes and metatarsals opposing the first metatarsal. The feet were in valgus or varus positions in 40 per cent of the babies.

The 'position of comfort' or that posture into which the baby may be folded and remain in peaceful relaxation was regarded as normal when the head, spine, hips and knees were comfortably flexed. The position of comfort in the newborn baby or neonate reflects the *in utero* fetal posture. Forty-six babies had the flexed bodily

*Reproduced, with modifications, by permission of W.B. Saunders, from Cook, W.A. and Stephens, F.D. (1988), *Pathoembryology of the urinary tract*. In *Urological Surgery in Neonates and Young Infants*, Lowell R. King (ed.), pp. 1–22.

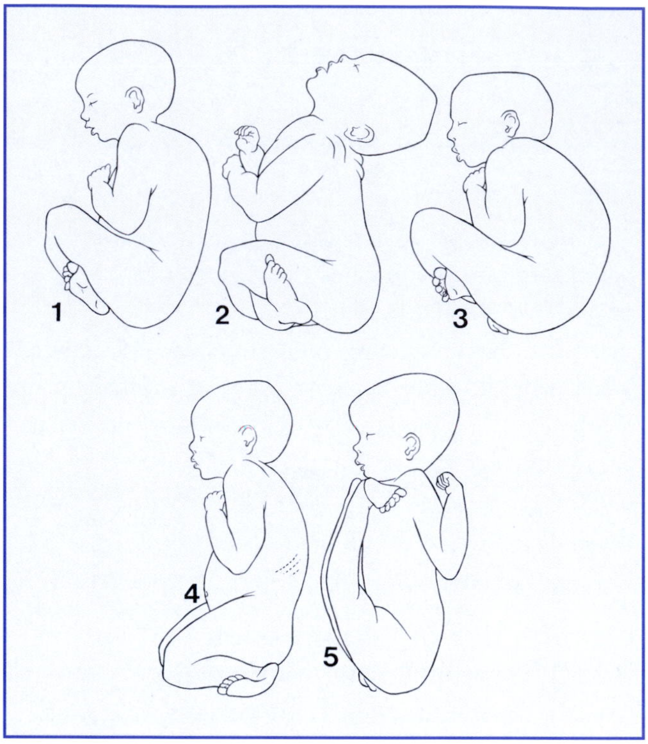

Fig. 36.1 *Positions of comfort of newborn babies. 1. Moderate body flexion, the common normal position. 2. Hyperextension. 3. Hyperflexion. Both (2) and (3) are uncommon normal positions. 4. Body elongation because of extra vertebrae and ribs or by extension of the hips and knees tucked under the buttocks. 5. Extension of the knees folded over the ventral body wall. (Reprinted, with permission, from Cook, W.A. and Stephens, F.D. (1988), Pathoembryology of the urinary tract. In Urological Surgery in Neonates and Young Infants, L.R. King (ed.), Fig. 1.7, p. 11. Philadelphia: W.B. Saunders Co.)*

posture, two babies exhibited hyperflexion, and two had hyperextension of the head and spine (Fig. 36.1). A postural C-shaped curve of the back was noted in some of these babies.

The position of comfort of the legs was that of flexed hips and knees and dorsiflexed ankles in 46 per cent; flexed hips and knees with crossed legs in 24 per cent; and the posture of praying feet in which the hips were abducted, knees flexed, and the plantar surfaces of the feet co-apted over the symphysis pubis or lower abdomen in 30 per cent. Hip flexion with knees hyperextended or partially flexed and rotated to lie over the abdomen and thorax was observed in some otherwise normal babies, but none such was seen in this series of 50 (Figs 36.1 and 36.2).

The asymmetric head and C-shaped curve of the spine suggest longitudinal growth constraint, whereas

foot and toe anomalies and the deep dimples all indicate a measure of focal compression. In combination, asymmetry and crossed or praying feet positions with foot and toe anomalies are suggestive of general compression of the fetus. Moderately late fetal compression features are common but temporary and generally correct spontaneously or by simple forms of treatment.

Occurrence of compression in babies and children under age four with multiple internal and external anomalies

One-hundred-and-two babies with multiple anomalies were examined to detect external signs of intrauterine compression. Fifty per cent of these babies exhibited two or more signs of compression and the clinical features of the multiple defects were analysed. Babies with known inherited or chromosomal defects were not included, even though some had evidence of compression.

The 50 subjects with major multiple defects meeting clinical criteria of more severe grades of compression were diagnosed as spina bifida (20 patients), imperforate anus (23 patients), tracheoesophageal fistula (two patients), triad (prune belly) syndrome (two patients), anterior horn cell deficiency (two patients) and renal hypoplasia (one patient).

Spina bifida

The spina bifida defect was located in the thoracic (two patients), thoracolumbar (four patients), lumbar (one patient), lumbosacral (five patients), sacral (five patients) regions and not known in three patients. Five of the six thoracic or lumbar patients had kyphoses and one also had a deviated sacrum (Fig. 36.3). The sacrum was deviated to one side in five of the seven patients with lower lumbar or sacral spina bifida defects. The temporary lack of amniotic fluid leads to hyperflexion or extension of the embryo that impairs closure of the neural tube.

The accompanying anomalies included myelodysplasia, upper urinary tract agenesis, renal dysgenesis, ectopic kidney, hydronephrosis, incompetent ureterovesical junction and double ureter. The urinary-tract anomalies, apart from neuropathies, occurred in seven of eight patients with sacral deviations, compared with four of 11 patients with normal non-deviated sacra.

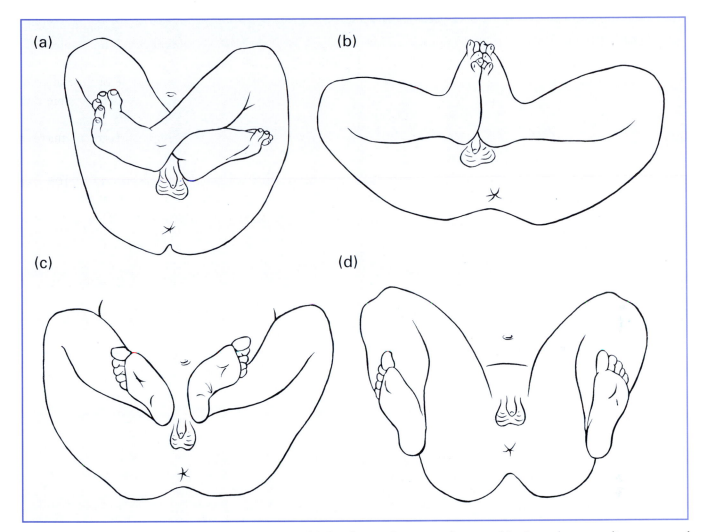

Fig. 36.2 *Positions of comfort of the legs and feet in 'normal' babies showing alteration in alignment of forefoot and toes according to posture of legs and 'normal' late fetal compression. (**a**) Legs crossed and toes tilted or overlap. (**b**) Praying feet and overlapping fifth toes. (**c**) Uncrossed legs, feet flat or valgus. (**d**) Legs uncrossed, feet flat or rolled out. (Reprinted, with permission, from Cook, W.A. and Stephens, F.D. (1988), Pathoembryology of the urinary tract. In Urological Surgery in Neonates and Young Infants, L.R. King. (ed.), Fig. 1.8, p. 12. Philadelphia: W.B. Saunders Co.)*

Spina bifida with posterior gibbus formation was not associated with upper-tract anomalies except in one baby whose sacrum was also laterally deviated. These babies and children exhibited moulding anomalies of the foot or toes in 17 of 19, and cramped positions of comfort with hyperextension or hyperflexion of the neck and spine in 13 of 14 in which these features were noted (see Fig. 36.1).

Imperforate anus

Of these 23 patients, seven were classified as high, nine as intermediate, and seven as low types, and in 17 the sacrum was abnormally developed or deviated. Of these

17 patients, the upper urinary tract was abnormal in 14. In three of these, a hemi-vertebra was also present higher in the spinal column. The sacrum was fully formed and non-deviated in six patients, and of these the upper tracts were abnormal in two and not noted in two.

The position of comfort was regarded as abnormal in 16 of 19 patients. The posture was hyperflexion in 10, hyperextension in four, elongation in two and normal in three. The legs were crossed in 18, in the praying position in one, flexed in one, and hyperextended with genu recurvatum in one, and the position was not noted in two.

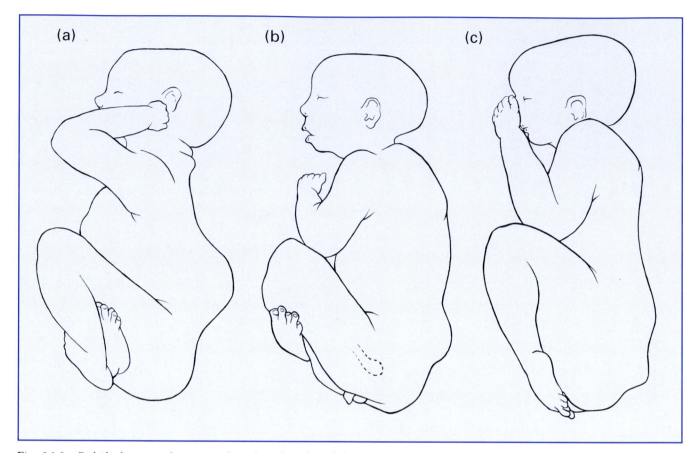

Fig. 36.3 *Bedside drawings of positions of comfort of newborn babies with spina bifida and gibbus formation (**a**), lumbar (**b**) and sacral myelomeningocele (**c**). Note flat heels and end-to-end compression. (Reprinted, with permission, from Cook, W.A. and Stephens, F.D. (1988), Pathoembryology of the urinary tract. In Urological Surgery in Neonates and Young Infants, L.R. King (ed.), Fig. 1.9, p. 13. Philadelphia: W.B. Saunders Co.)*

A skin dimple was noted in the sacrococcygeal region in 19 and foot–toe anomaly was present in 18 (Fig. 36.4). These features, together with the deviation of the sacrum, were compatible with early constraint and moulding of the hind end of the embryo by the shape of the limited space afforded by the amniotic membrane and oligohydramnios at the time of segmentation, elongation and limb bud formation.

Miscellaneous group

Compression signs were very apparent in seven patients whose diagnoses included the triad syndrome (two patients) tracheoesophageal fistula (one patient), VATER (vertebral defects, imperforate anus, tracheoesophageal fistula, and radial and renal dysplasia) syndrome (one patient), two mentally retarded babies with anterior-horn cell deficiency and one baby with whistling face syndrome. The vertebral column was normal in four; the sacrum was deviated to one side in two, and the tip of the sacrum and coccyx was recurved posteriorly in one. The position of comfort was hyperextension in five and not known in two. The legs were crossed in four, knees hyperextended on the trunk in two and flexed in one. Abnormalities of the foot or toes were observed in all seven patients (Fig. 36.5). As expected, the upper urinary tracts were abnormal in the two patients with the triad syndrome, one of whom had a deviated sacrum. The baby with the VATER complex was a twin who had a deviated sacrum, normal kidneys and a rectovaginal fistula. The two babies with anterior horn cell deficiency had muscular weakness; one had deviated fifth sacral vertebra and a rectovaginal fistula, the other had a normal sacrum and pelvic organs and both had normal urinary tracts. Another baby was mentally backward and had a normal spine and dysmorphic urinary tract. All such anomalies may derive from compression of the embryo during the first month of gestation.

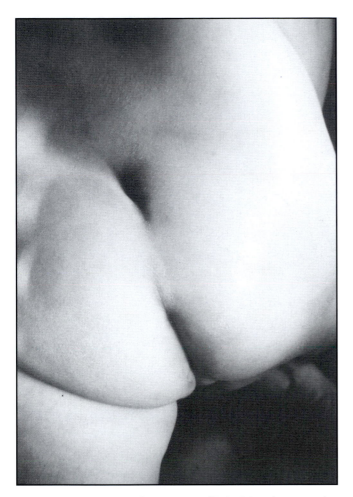

Fig. 36.4 *Sacrococcygeal pressure pit of Baby M. with rectovestibular fistula, indicating counter compression point. (Reprinted, with permission, from Cook, W.A. and Stephens, F.D. (1988), Pathoembryology of the urinary tract. In Urological Surgery in Neonates and Young Infants, L.R. King (ed.), Fig. 1.10, p. 14. Philadelphia: W.B. Saunders Co.)*

Accompanying features of 50 patients with stigmata of compression

Of the 50 babies exhibiting compression features, 40 had major or minor spinal anomalies; of the 40, the spinal anomaly was sacral in 27 (67 per cent). The upper urinary-tract was abnormal in 31 (77 per cent) of these 40 patients.

Of 24 patients with sacral anomalies (excluding those patients with spina bifida plus other sacral defects), upper urinary tract anomalies were present in 17 (70 per cent). When the sacrum was straight with a full complement of vertebral bodies (again excluding spina bifida defects), the upper tract was abnormal in seven of 19 (36 per cent).

Alignment defects of the spinal column in compression patients

When the spine was buckled, forming a thoracolumbar gibbus in the sagittal plane, the kidneys were normally ascended but misplaced medially or laterally. When the spine was deviated by hemi-vertebral anomalies, however, the upper tracts were abnormal in 14 of 22 (64 per cent) patients. These findings, together with the stigmata of compression, suggest that the spine may have been compressed and deformed in the segmentation phase of somite development during the fourth week (Fig. 36.6). The upper tract anomalies associated with these spinal defects may derive from similar disturbances of the wolffian body and its duct which lie alongside the deformed column and the ureteric bud which arises from the duct at the level of the future second sacral vertebra.

Associated external genitourinary anomalies

Thirteen babies and children, nine of whom are included in the previous groupings, had a divided or asymmetric scrotum or labium with or without other perineal anomalies, the cause of which may have been focal compression by the heel of the overlying foot. The labium or scrotum exhibited one-sided defects such as displaced or divided ipsilateral labium major or scrotum (Figs 36.7 and 36.8). In eight, the anorectum was malformed (covered anus in two, high or intermediate anorectal anomaly in four, low anal anomaly in four) and in five the anus was normal. The spine was abnormal in 10 children, normal in one and not known in two. The sacrum exhibited deviation or hemi- or absent segments in these 10, and in three the lumbar or thoracic spine had hemi-vertebral defects as well. Three of the babies had sacral lipomeningoceles. Diastasis of the pubic bones was present in eight of these children (not abnormal in three and not known in two).

In addition to these external genitourinary anomalies, upper genitourinary tracts were abnormal in 10, normal in one and not known in two.

Deep sacral dimples were seen in five of eight (five not known) and foot–toe anomalies were present in nine, not abnormal in one and not known in three.

The features that suggested that focal pressure by the heel of the foot caused the labioscrotal defect were: (1) the heel could be rested in the smooth skin and pit separating the two parts of the divided ipsilateral scrotum

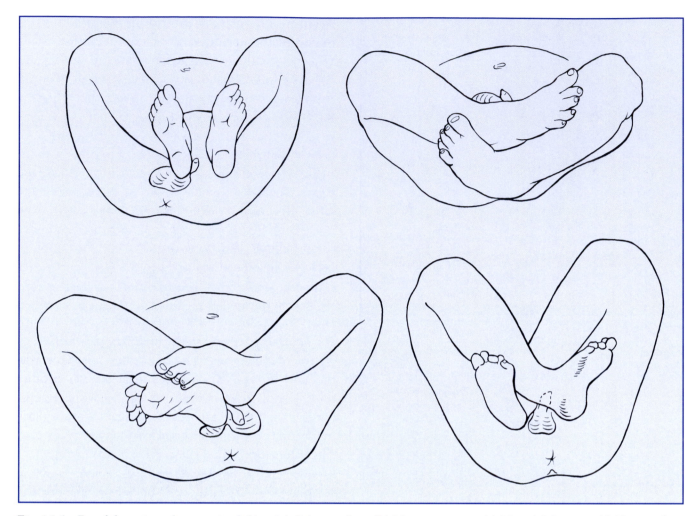

Fig. 36.5   *Foot deformations of compression babies. (**a**) Calcaneovalgus. (**b**) Metatarsus varus. (**c**) Mutual deformities. (**d**) Flat or valgus. Note vulnerability of genitalia to compression by the heels of the feet. (Reprinted, with permission, from Cook, W.A. and Stephens, F.D. (1988), Pathoembryology of the urinary tract. In Urological Surgery in Neonates and Young Infants, L.R. King (ed.), Fig. 1.11, p. 15. Philadelphia: W.B. Saunders Co.)*

or labium major (Figs 36.7 and 36.8); (2) the feet in the position of comfort overlying the labioscrotal defects also exhibited interlocking, or, as Denis Browne termed them, mutual deformities; (3) deep discrete pressure pits persisted over the ankles or knees; and (4) combinations of anomalous sacrum, pubic diastasis, and sacrococcygeal counter pressure pits occurred.

Special examples of deformations

Three patients in addition to the series reported herein and chosen from supplementary series are special examples of deformations presumably caused by external pressure. Baby boy T.H. was born with a deep scarred impression on the undersurface of the penis and adjoining penoscrotal junction. The heel of the foot could be

rested squarely in the pit even when the infant was six months of age (Fig. 36.9; see also Fig. 3.3a).

A deep scar and pressure point through which prolapsed the testis on its spermatic cord pedicle was reported by Heyns (1990). See below and also Fig. 36.9.

Baby D. was an abnormal twin boy with a normal twin sister. His right leg was amputated *in utero* below the knee. The limb below the site of amputation with malformed right foot was autografted *in utero* into the right genital area and perineum. The penis was rudimentary, one testis was intra-abdominal, and the other had descended. The right side of the pelvis was distracted laterally as indicated in Fig. 36.10. Only one kidney was present and this lay in the false pelvis. Extreme mechanical pressure on the somites may have

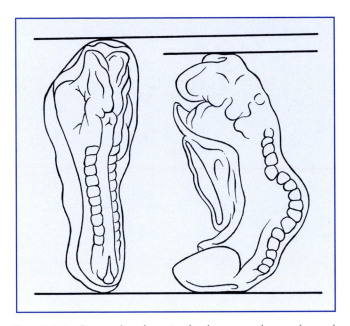

Fig. 36.6 *Stage of embryonic development when end-to-end compression may cause the elongating columns of somites to buckle or deviate. (Left) Normal and (right) embryo of same age (fourth week) restricted by tight amnion. (After Hamilton, W.J., Boyd, J.D. and Mossman, H.W. (1978), In Human Embryology, 4th edn. London: Macmillan.)*

caused scoliosis, the spreading of the pubes, subsequent crossed-leg the amputation and autograft of the partially formed foot into the right genital area (Fig. 36.10).

The following are further examples of the great variety of deformations that may result from temporary early oligohydramnios and compression (Stephens, 1993).

Cloacal exstrophy

Supporting evidence of compression is accompanying talipes, scoliosis or spina bifida, and deformed leg and foot. Failure of or delayed reversal of the hind end of the embryo caused by temporary compression by the amniotic membrane may cause this lesion by distraction of the lower abdominal wall and pelvis.

Vesical exstrophy

The classical examples are usually isolated malformations with a possible genetic tendency (Shapiro et al., 1984). When vesical exstrophy is complicated by talipes, ring constriction of a limb or anoperineal defects, or other clinical evidence of compression, early temporary oligohydramnios may impair the reversal process at a slightly later period than that of cloacal exstrophy.

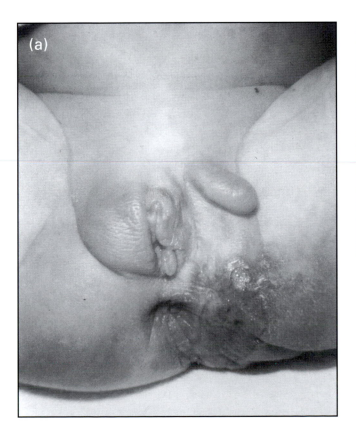

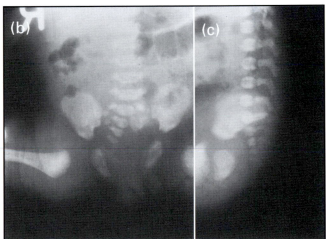

Fig. 36.7 *Effects of compression by heel on left side of perineum. (a) Pressure sore, cutaneous telangiectasia, and partition of the left labium major and gaping anus. (b) Radiographs showing sacral deviation, tilting of left ilium and pubic diastasis. (c) Lack of curve of sacrum. (Reprinted, with permission, from Cook, W.A. and Stephens, F.D. (1988), Pathoembryology of the urinary tract. In Urological Surgery in Neonates and Young Infants, L.R. King (ed.), Fig. 1.13, p. 17. Philadelphia: W.B. Saunders Co.)*

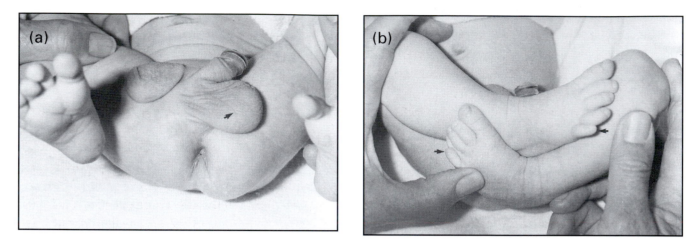

Fig. 36.8 *Compression of genitalia and toes.* (**a**) *Divided right scrotum with testis in upper part. Scrotal raphe indicated by arrow, anocutaneous fistula postanoplasty, and sacrococcygeal pit, (fifth sacral vertebra deviated to left and slight pubic diastasis) not shown.* (**b**) *Crossed ankles with right heel poised near the smooth skin depression between the two parts of the scrotum and compressed overlapping toes (arrows). (Reprinted, with permission, from Cook, W.A. and Stephens, F.D. (1988), Pathoembryology of the urinary tract. In Urological Surgery in Neonates and Young Infants, L.R. King (ed.), Fig. 1.14, p. 18. Philadelphia: W.B. Saunders Co.)*

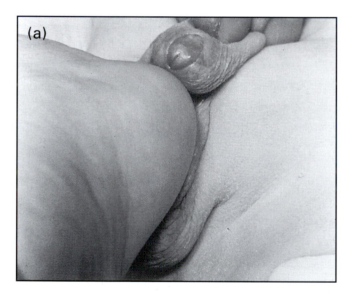

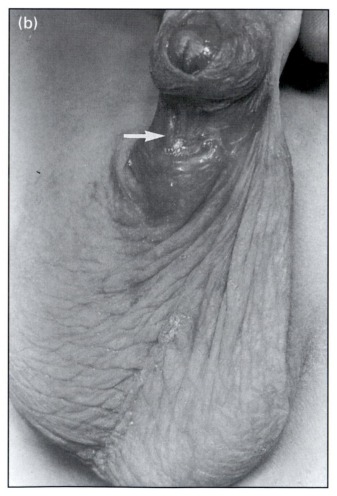

Fig. 36.9 *Effects of foot pressure on penis and upper scrotum.* (**a**) *Position of comfort with heel tucked into a scarred area and* (**b**) *Scar on undersurface of penis and prepuce partially developed (arrow).* (**c**) *Newborn baby with exstrophic testis hanging like a polyp on the spermatic cord from an unhealed ulcer on the upper scrotum. Note the deviation of the penis toward the opposite side; the possible explanation is a pressure sore caused by the heel against the pubis, permitting the testis to deviate externally. ((**a**) courtesy of Casimir Firlit. (**b**) reprinted, with permission, from Cook, W.A. and Stephens, F.D. (1988), Pathoembryology of the urinary tract. In Urological Surgery in Neonates and Young Infants, L.R. King (ed.), Fig. 1.15, p. 18. Philadelphia: W.B. Saunders Co. (**c**) reprinted with permission from Heyns, C.F. (1990), Exstrophy of the testis. J. Urol. 144: 724–725.)*

Hypospadias

Known causes of hypospadias malformations are genetic, chromosomal and endocrine (Bauer *et al.*, 1981). When hypospadias is accompanied by unusual penile configurations, scars, scrotal or perineal defects, or penile torsion, the penile lesion may be a deformation. The most obvious of the deformations in a baby may be the irregular hypospadias but other foot or toe deformations may also be present to support the diagnosis of temporary compression due to early amniotic leakage.

Ipsilateral transverse bifurcation of the scrotum or labium majus

One side of the scrotum or one labium majus is divided transversely by an umbilicated segment of smooth or scarred skin (see Fig. 36.12a–c). Associated lesions may be covered anus, sacropelvic scoliosis, pubic diastasis, myelocystocele, talipes and overlapping toes, and ureter anomalies. Here again, this combination of lesions may share the same aetiology. A sore, scarred skin at birth of the labium majus and gaping anus may also be due to foot pressure (Fig. 36.7).

Testicular defects

Compression by the heel of the foot may impair or delay the maturation of the gubernaculum, causing delay in descent of the testis or cryptorchidism (Luthra *et al.*, 1989) (Fig. 36.11). A pressure sore indicates severe and prolonged compression by the heel of the foot on the pubis (Fig. 36.9). In this case reported by Heyns (1990), ulceration of the skin of the upper scrotum may have been caused by pressure of the heel against the pubis. The testis in its descent toward the scrotum reached the site of the pressure sore and fell through the skin defect (Fig. 36.9c). However, no supporting evidence in the form of foot or toe deformities was noted at the time of operation and the patient could not be traced for verification (C.F. Heyns, pers. comm.).

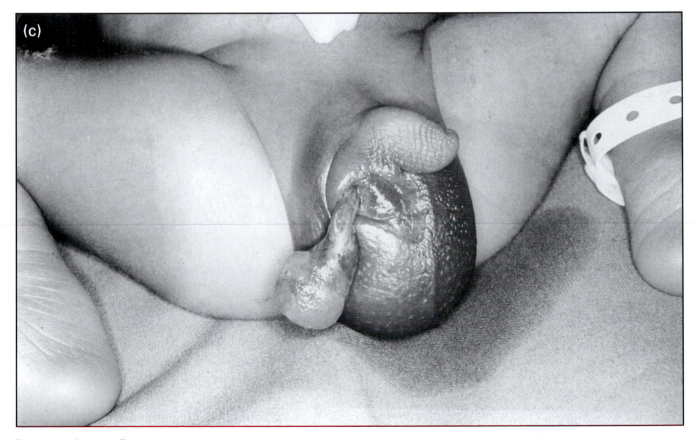

Fig. 36.9 *(continued)*

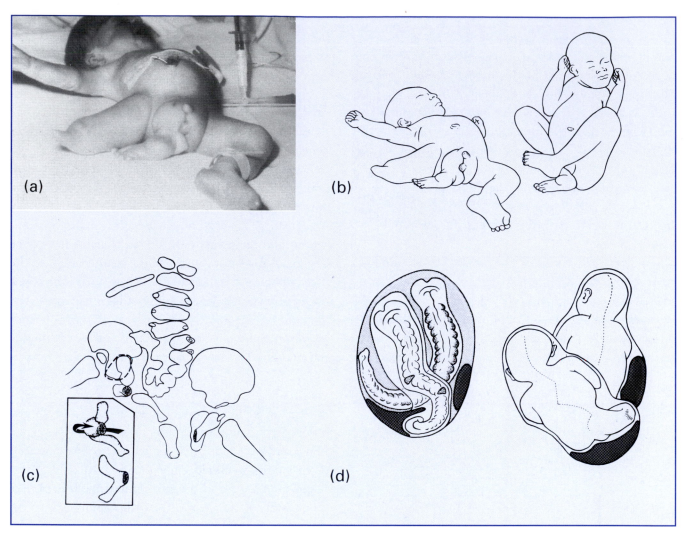

Fig. 36.10 (*a*) *Baby twin D., born with in utero auto-amputation of right leg and dysgenetic right foot grafted into the right perineum and gross deformation of genitalia. Note hypoplastic stump of right tibia and twisted hypoplastic foot emerging from right genital region.* (**b**) *Presumed mechanism of amputation and pressure grafting of right leg by left heel onto right scrotum and the 'sprung' position of tibia after severance of foot.* (**c**) *Tracing of X-ray of pelvis indicating extreme deformation of right pubic bone, distraction of the right ilium, and separation of the ossific centres of the bodies of the sacral vertebrae. Inset diagrams show distorted components of pubic bone and rotational direction (arrow) that would be required if normal orientation could be restored (lower inset diagram).* (**d**) *Possible embryonic relationships of dizygotic diamniotic twins with fused or contiguous placentas and with amniotic spatial constraint of one twin. Also shown is a possible position of discomfort of the eight-week fetuses prior to severance of the leg of the affected twin. (Case report and photo of Baby D. courtesy of Dr Charles Devine.) (Reprinted, with permission, from Cook, W.A. and Stephens, F.D. (1988), Pathoembryology of the urinary tract. In Urological Surgery in Neonates and Young Infants, L.R. King (ed.), Fig. 1.16, p. 19. Philadelphia: W.B. Saunders Co.)*

Preputial defects

The development of the prepuce may be impaired if the developing phallus is squeezed between the heels of the feet during the formative period of the foot and external genitalia. Partial coverage of the glans (natural circumcision) may be caused by such temporary compression. Focal pressure of the heel on the glans and temporary lapping of the developing prepuce around the heel may account for that rare anomaly of coronal hypospadias

with redundant ventral prepuce. Though the focus of attention is on the phallic anomaly, less obvious deformations especially of foot or toes may be present and may be identified if positively sought.

Cloacal septal defects

Hemi-vertebrae in lumbar and sacral regions in some instances result from very early angulation of the embryo by compression. Deformations of the spine in

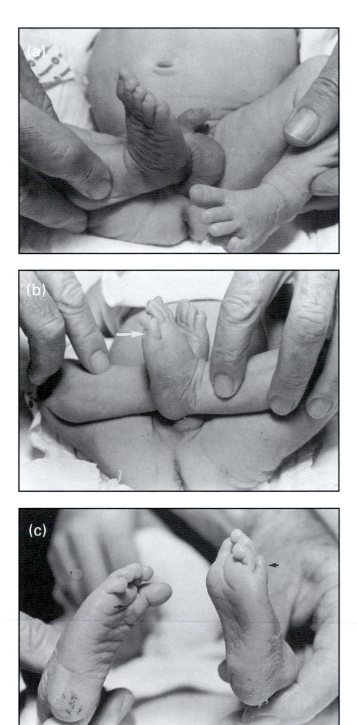

Fig. 36.11 *Oligohydramnios and foot compression on empty right scrotum. (**a**) Heel of right foot overlies empty scrotum. (**b**) Feet placed in position of comfort showing overlapping left fifth toe (arrow). (**c**) Right forefoot rolled from side to side along deep longitudinal groove (arrow); toes of left foot malaligned and fifth overlapping toe (arrow). (Reprinted, with permission, from Luthra, M., Hutson, J.M. and Stephens, F.D. (1987), Effects of external inguinoscrotal compression on descent of the testis in rats. Pediatr. Surg. Int., 4: 403–407.)*

these regions are likely to be accompanied by impaired development of the urorectal septum and cloacal systems as well as other external deformations.

Embryogenesis

The occurrence of multiple anomalies with or without genetic, chromosomal, or environmental aetiology may exhibit evidence of severe compression. In some patients, deforming forces may be the real cause of all the abnormal features. Whereas late fetal compression has been recognized as a natural explanation for those less serious and temporary deformations, doubts have been cast on deformation as the cause of the more serious clubfoot anomalies, congenital scoliosis and others such as dislocated hips, pectus defects and Poland's syndrome, perhaps mainly because they are not usually associated with oligohydramnios at the time of birth. Growth constraint, however, due to leakage of amniotic fluid, may be operating upon the four-week embryo either in a general or focal manner prior to the time that urine begins to swell the volume of amniotic fluid around 10 weeks' gestational age. Any event or defect that impairs the formation or creates temporary leakage of amniotic fluid in the three- to six-week-old embryo may lead to transient oligohydramnios and growth constraint, deviation or suppression of the segments of the rapidly elongating embryo and abnormal moulding of the developing limbs. Scoliosis, kyphosis, clubfoot and asymmetric bodily features accompanying abnormal positions of comfort may result from lack of space within the amnion (see Fig. 36.12). Then the close-fitting amniotic membrane constrains and moulds and deforms the embryo. When eventually the leakage point heals or is plugged and when the normal volume of amniotic fluid is restored by transudation or by urine in normal amounts voided into the amnion, the oligohydramnios is corrected but the deformations remain. These deformations of the embryo are structural and permanent as opposed to those that occur from moulding in late fetal life.

Segmentation of the embryo begins at the age of 21 days at the same time that the lips of the neural plate meet in mid-embryo to form the neural tube. By 28–30 days, 44 segments have formed, the neural tube is closed at each end and the discoid embryo has become cylindrical in shape.

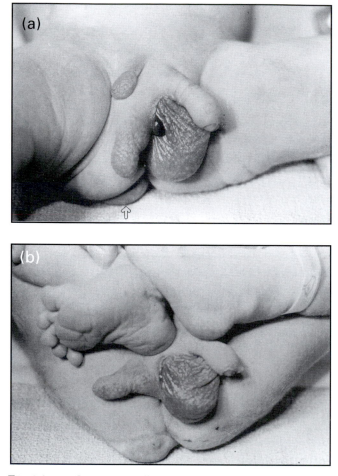

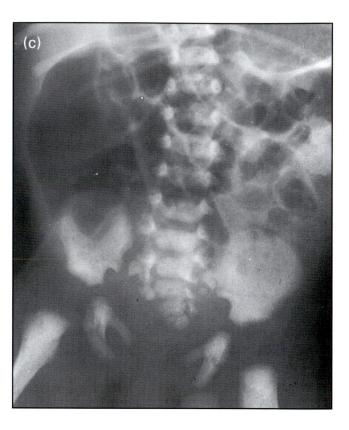

Fig. 36.12 *Compression effects transmitted through feet, genitalia, perineum, pelvis and sacrum in the male (**a**)–(**c**) and the female (see Fig. 36.7). (**a**) Divided scrotum, constricted base of penis, incomplete prepuce, covered anus with anocutaneous fistula; meconium signifies tract of fistula in raphe and myelocystocele (arrow). (**b**) Deformed feet in position of comfort (see also Fig. 36.5c). (**c**) X-ray to show pelvis tilted, pubic diastasis, scoliosis and sacral deviation. (Reprinted, with permission, from Cook, W.A. and Stephens, F.D. (1988) Pathoembryology of the urinary tract. In Urological Surgery in Neonates and Yang Infants, L.R. King (ed.), Fig. 8.4, p. 100. Philadelphia: W.B. Saunders Co.)*

In the fourth week the embryo undergoes 'reversal', which is probably a dangerous phenomenon. Reversal means a change in posture of the embryo from hyperextension of the developing head, tail and spine to one of flexion (Fig. 36.13). Spatial constraint upon the rapidly elongating embryo may cause delay or arrest of reversal (Fig. 36.14). The elongating and folding 'vertebral' column and head and tail may buckle (Fig. 36.6), deviate (Fig. 36.15), or twist in any part and upset the development of structures derived from corresponding segments of the body. The axial tracheoesophageal, urorectal and uroanal septa may be deviated or arrested with ensuing intersystem anomalies. The paraxial wolffian body and duct, the ureteric bud, and the müllerian duct may also be suppressed or impaired in their devel-

opment. All these structures are at critical stages of development in the fourth to sixth weeks.

The external genitalia and perineum undergo morphogenesis at 6–12 weeks, beginning with the partitioning of the external cloaca by the central perineal mound, followed by the inward surge of the genital folds over it. The external genitalia of males and females are similar until the tenth week. By the twelfth week, male and female perineal and external genital organs are completely differentiated. Gubernacular swellings in the scrotum precede the descent of the testes, which appear in the scrotum between 28 and 36 weeks.

The laterally directed lower-limb buds appear during the fourth week, and by the eighth week they have

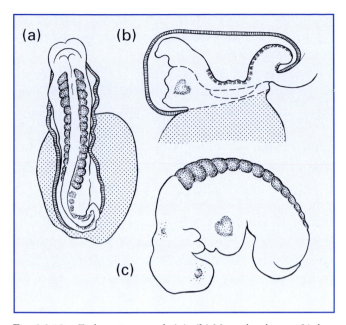

Fig. 36.13 *Embryonic reversal.* (**a**), (**b**) *Normal embryo at 21 days in position of hyperextension of developing head and tail (b traced from photograph of embryo of 21 days' gestation).* (**c**) *Reversal to position of flexion of the head and hind ends of the body at 28 days. (Reprinted, with permission, from Cook, W.A. and Stephens, F.D. (1988), Pathoembryology of the urinary tract. In Urological Surgery in Neonates and Young Infants, L.R. King (ed.), Fig. 1.17, p. 20. Philadelphia: W.B. Saunders Co.)*

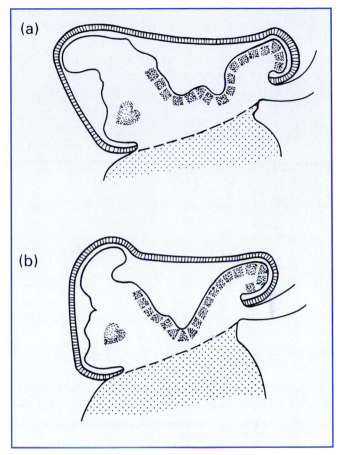

Fig. 36.14 *Effects of oligohydramnios and constraint by the amniotic membrane.* (**a**) *Buckling of the future thoracolumbar region.* (**b**) *Lumbar lordosis and sacral torsion and suppression of cranium. (Reprinted, with permission, from Cook, W.A. and Stephens, F.D. (1988), Pathoembryology of the urinary tract. In Urological Surgery in Neonates and Young Infants, L.R. King. (ed.), Fig. 1.18, p. 21. Philadelphia: W.B. Saunders Co.)*

developed the three basic segments and joints. The knee bends to an angle of 90° and the plantar surfaces of the feet appose beneath the body stalk. Torsion then brings the bent knee to project ventrally. As the legs elongate, they may gain flexed or various crossover positions.

It is during the formation of the perineum and the genitalia, and the descent of the testis from the external ring to the scrotum that compression by the heel of the crossover foot may impair these developmental processes. At 6–12 weeks, heel compression may suppress the perineal mound and inner and outer genital folds, causing anterior location of the anus or covered anus, or hypospadias, torsion of the genital tubercle, split and cleft scrotum, or defective development of the labium major. At a later stage, compression may suppress the temporary swelling of the gubernaculum that normally expands the pathway to the scrotum, thus causing testicular arrest or deviation, or degrees of testicular retraction due to lack of anchorage in the scrotum or initiate torsion of the spermatic cord. The upper scrotum may be pressed hard against the pubis causing ulceration and prolapse of the testes (Heyns, 1990).

Signs of compression

Chapple and Davidson (1941) coined the term 'position of comfort' of the neonate in their study of the causal relationship between fetal position and dislocations of the hip or knee. They found that babies were quietened and consoled when folded up after birth into their abnormal positions of comfort, whatever the deformations, and they claimed that this was the posture preferentially adopted both in and out of the uterus.

When examining the neonate or infant, the clinician notes the position of comfort, the characteristics of the major deformity or deformities, and the minor lesions and other signs of compression. It is the presence of pos-

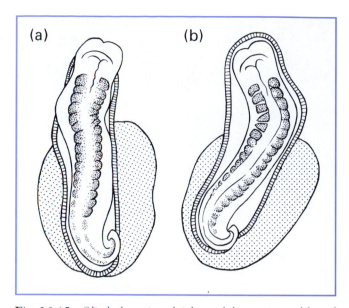

Fig. 36.15 *Oligohydramnios, shrinkage of the amnion and lateral deviation of the developing vertebral column. (a) Convexity to left area. (b) Convexity to the right with wedging of the vertebrae.*

itive external features which support the diagnosis of early amniotic rupture. For example, scoliosis capitis, spinalis and sacralis; pelvic asymmetry; deep dimples, scars on elbows, knees, lateral aspect of ankle, or over other bony prominences of the foot; sacrococcygeal dimpling, talipes and crushed feet and toes of various kinds; overlapping second and fifth toes; deep longitudinal crease on sole of forefoot and free folding of the foot along the axis of the crease (Fig. 36.11c); ring constriction of fingers or limbs; cocked-up lobe of ear; various forms of chest and abdominal wall deformities; and hip subluxations or dislocations. Hemi-vertebra in the lumbar and sacral regions, sacropelvic scoliosis and coccygeal and sacral vertebral agenesis may result from early somite deformations and are pointers to accompanying internal genital, urinary and rectal deformations.

With the likely diagnosis of early amniotic rupture and absence of genetic, chromosomal or known teratogens, the clinician can indicate to the family that this is a sporadic event and such deformations are unlikely to recur in siblings. Beside the most obvious anomaly, other tell-tale signs give the clues to the diagnosis of early lack of amniotic volume. Furthermore, anomalies that are not readily explained according to known embryology are likely to be deformations. Finally, babies

who are malformed from known causes may also be deformed if oligohydramnios occurred during embryonic or fetal development.

Denis Browne (1955), Dunn (1976) and Smith (1981) have been protagonists of the deformation theory of many bodily and orthopaedic anomalies. Emphasis was placed on constraint by the uterine walls as the external deforming force on the developing fetus. An earlier constraint of growth, however, on the embryo in the first month of embryonic life by the amniotic membrane after leakage of amniotic fluid is likely to cause multiple and major deformations. The combination of vertebral defects of babies born with multiple signs of compression may pinpoint the constraint to the fourth week of development. At this time, the fore- and hind-gut midline septa and the wolffian structures may be affected by suppression, buckling or bending of the somites creating the deformations of the VATER syndrome (Pierkarski and Stephens, 1976).

Experiments were conducted on chick embryos to examine the effects of lateral deviation of the developing spine on the internal genitourinary organs. The migrating wolffian and müllerian ducts were arrested in some, and in others the metanephric kidney remained only partially ascended to its normal location (Maizels and Stephens, 1979). These experiments add some support to the aetiological link between internal genitourinary and spinal dysgenesis.

At a later date and consequential to the deformation of the sacral skeleton and with continuing compression, the crossed legs and feet come to exert external compression on the external genitourinary and perineal structures and pubic symphysis, creating yet another set of anomalies. Hence, deformation may explain the combination of multiple external and internal anomalies for which no known cause has hitherto been found. Smith (1982) stated, 'Our knowledge of the impact of early *in-utero* constraint in the human is just beginning to grow.' This dictum of the late David Smith, premier dysmorphologist of his time, together with his recorded observations, may set the stage for a much greater inquiry into the causes of temporary oligohydramnios and its lasting effects on external and internal genitourinary organs and other parts of the body.

Triad (prune belly) syndrome, intersex states and undescended testes

VII

Up-to-date descriptions of the prune belly syndrome (PBS) or triad syndrome by Duckett (1976), Williams (1979) and Welch (1979) summarize the clinical and some of the pathological features of the triad of abnormalities essential to the diagnosis of the syndrome, together with the additional anomalies that sometimes accompany it. This triad, namely abdominal muscle deficiency, urinary tract abnormalities and undescended testes, poses the question as to whether urethral obstruction, a mesodermal defect or a combination of both accounts for this strange association of anomalies. In this chapter, emphasis is laid upon the morphology and embryology of the organs affected in order to provide a plausible explanation for this syndrome.

Osler described the triple anomaly in 1901. This triad of anomalies is graphically etched into the medical literature as the prune belly syndrome. The term, however, is rather harsh when used in conversation with parents or patients and more so when the victim of the syndrome is called a 'prune'. Welch (1979) has avoided the term and adopted 'AMD (abdominal musculature deficiency) syndrome' as an alternative.

Another term perhaps less hurtful should be used in conversation with patients' families; the present author prefers the term 'triad', because the syndrome has three essential components, the abdominal wall defect, the urinary anomalies and the undescended testes in greater or lesser degree; these patients may also have other anomalies.

The lax, wrinkled, redundant abdominal wall, together with the empty scrotum, are outward visible and diagnostic criteria of the syndrome (Figs 37.1 and 37.2). These abdominal muscles may be replaced by aponeurosis without the proper trilamination, especially those derived from the lower thoracic to the first lumbar segments. The muscle components of the abdominal wall may be absent or exhibit grades of development up to near normal amounts.

The urinary tract between the prostatic urethra and the umbilicus and the ureters and renal pelves may be totally or focally ectatic. The testes are intraabdominal. Rarely, the symphysis pubis may be minimally diastatic, in which event, extraordinary phallic and urethral and rectourethral malformations may be present.

The abdominal urinary and genital tracts usually show correspondingly severe or mild spectra of anomalies (Nunn and Stephens, 1961). The severity of the defects of the three systems generally correspond so that

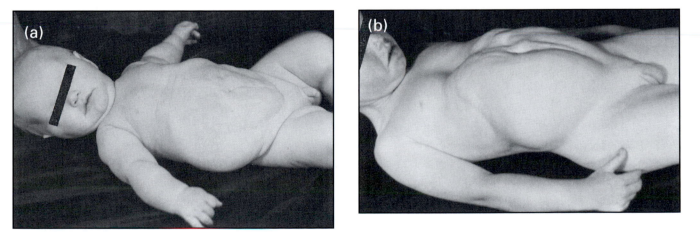

Fig. 37.1 *Abdominal wall in prune belly syndrome.* (**a**) *Aged six months. Note relaxed coarsely wrinkled wall.* (**b**) *Aged six years. Note effect of head raising. Upper rectus muscles draw umbilicus cranially and weaker lower abdomen bulges. Note also pectus excavatum. (Reprinted, by permission, from Nunn, I.N. and Stephens, F.D. (1961), The triad syndrome: a composite anomaly of the abdominal wall, urinary system and testes. J. Urol. 86: 782, Fig. 3.)*

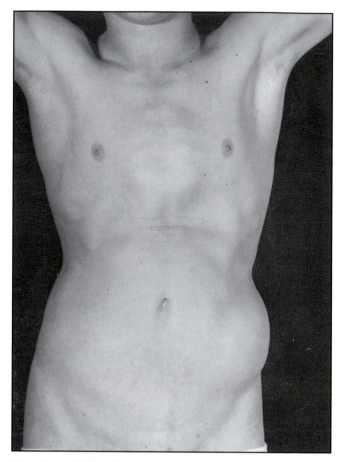

Fig. 37.2 *Abdominal wall and thoracic cage in prune belly syndrome. W.P., aged 15 years. (Reproduced, with permission, from Stephens, F.D. (1983), In Congenital Malformations of the Urinary Tract, Fig. 32.2, p. 502. New York: Praeger.)*

Table 37.1 *Genitourinary abnormalities in 45 patients*

Bladder		52
Megalocystis	39	
Patent urachus	10	
Diverticulum	3	
Ureters		80
Megaureters	76	
Atresia	3	
Double ureters	1	
Kidneys		81
Cystic hypoplasia	67	
Hydronephrosis	12	
Agenesis	2	
Testes		41
Bilateral cryptorchidism	37	
Unilateral anorchia	4	
Urethra		22
Phimosis, meatal stenosis	18	
Atresia	2	
Enlarged prostatic utricle	1	
Coronal hypospadias	1	
Total		276

Source: Welch, K.J. (1979), Abdominal musculature deficiency syndrome (prune-belly). In *Pediatric Surgery*, 3rd edn., M.M. Ravitch, K.J. Welch, C.D. Benson, E. Aberdeen and J.G. Randolph (eds), Chicago: Year Book Medical, p. 1222, Table III–2.

the mildest abdominal wall defects usually occur in children with mildly affected urogenital tracts and vice versa. Occasionally, the redundancy of the abdominal wall is very apparent, yet the urinary tract may be almost normal. Those children that die in infancy, usually from renal malformations, exhibit extreme malformations of the urogenital tracts, abdominal wall, and lesions in other systems, chiefly gastrointestinal, cardiac and the Potter syndrome (Wigger and Blanc, 1977). Welch (1979) listed the genitourinary and associated anomalies found in a series of 45 patients exhibiting the prune belly syndrome (Tables 37.1 and 37.2).

Morphology of necropsy specimens

Twenty-one babies with the prune belly triad of abnormalities died and were subjected to necropsy examinations. Some were stillborn infants and others neonates who survived up to 35 days. Four were fetuses of gesta-

tional ages between 16 and 20 weeks, three between 32 and 38 weeks and 13 were term babies. The data obtained from these specimens, including five originally described by Nunn and Stephens (1961) and 16 others (Stephens and Gupta, 1994), together with reports of necropsy material published by others (Ives, 1974; Wigger and Blanc, 1977) form the basis of the pathological findings. The 21 specimens all exhibited the characteristic features of the triad of anomalies, but with severe renal impairment and some additional bizarre urinary-tract abnormalities. Twenty-three specimens exhibiting posterior urethral-valve obstructive lesions were studied for comparison of the genital tracts with those of PBS specimens. These include 14 of Type 1 and nine of Type 3 valves.

Urogenital tracts in PBS

The important investigations in this system concern the vexed problems of urethral obstruction, the megacystis, the dimensions and musculature of the whole urinary tract, the state of the kidneys, the vas, vesicles and the prostate, and the autonomic nerve supply of the bladder and urethra.

Table 37.2 *Associated anomalies in 45 patients*

Genitourinary		276
Musculoskeletal		37
Metatarsus varus	15	
Congenital dislocation of hips	10	
Polydactylism	5	
Webbing	2	
Arthrogryposis	1	
Scoliosis	2	
Lumbar lordosis	2	
Gastrointestinal		15
Volvulus	7	
Malrotation obstruction	4	
Imperforate anus	3	
Gastric duplication	1	
Chest wall deformity		12
Pectus excavatum	8	
Pectus carinatum	4	
Cardiac		10
Patent ductus arteriosus	4	
Intraventricular septal defect	4	
Patent foramen secundum	1	
Tetralogy of Fallot	1	
Miscellaneous facial		9
Central nervous system		6
Microcephaly	2	
Cerebral hypoplasia	2	
Craniosynostosis	2	
Nose and throat		3
Total		368

Source: Welch, K.J. (1979), Abdominal musculature deficiency syndrome (prune-belly). In *Pediatric Surgery*, 3rd edn., M.M. Ravitch, K.J. Welch, C.D. Benson, E. Aberdeen and J.G. Randolph (eds) Chicago: Year Book Medical, p. 1222, Table III–1.

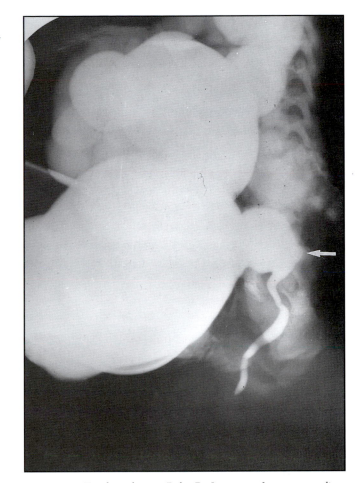

Fig. 37.3 *Triad syndrome, Baby R. Injection of contrast medium into bladder of postmortem specimen showing gross dilatation of bladder and ureters with free vesicoureteral reflux, dilated prostatic urethra with infolded anterior walls, and normal-calibre membranous urethra with no evidence of mechanical obstruction at this point. Note also umbilication instead of eminence where verumontanum should be located (arrow). (Reprinted, by permission, from Nunn, I.N. and Stephens, F.D. (1961), The triad syndrome: a composite anomaly of the abdominal wall, urinary system and testes. J. Urol. 86: 782, Fig. 4.)*

Many of the specimens studied by Nunn and Stephens (1961) and Stephens and Gupta (1994) were subjected to radiographical study of the urinary tract prior to dissection and, subsequently, light microscopic investigation of the three systems involved in the syndrome.

The radiographical features conformed in many respects to those of living patients. In all the specimens fixed in formalin in a state of distension, the bladder neck and prostatic urethra showed the characteristic expansion, the bladder and urachus were enlarged, and the ureters were irregularly dilated; some exhibited vesicoureteral reflux (Fig. 37.3). The kidneys displayed varied and grotesque forms, and many significant anomalies were found in the dissected specimens.

Urethra, prostate gland and seminal ducts

The specimens were preserved in formalin in the fully distended state. After fixation, the formalin was replaced with radiopaque medium, which on radiography displayed the bladder, urethra, and sometimes the ureters and pelves in forms similar to those obtained by micturition cystourethrography in living patients. The internal meatus in the fixed state was widely open, but was demarcated by a shallow collar. The prostatic urethra was about three to four times more expanded than the membranous urethra, which was of normal or smaller than normal calibre. The anterior wall of the posterior urethra was shorter than the posterior wall, and, in some, was infolded. The posterior wall pouched posteriorly, especially at the site of entry of the wolffian ducts (Fig. 37.3).

The internal urinary meatus was widely open so that the lumen of the distended bladder and ectatic prostatic urethra was continuous. The verumontanum was small, flat, absent or replaced by a small, rounded pocket into which the utriculus and seminal ducts issued independently. In nearly all specimens the inferior crest was barely visible on the caudal wall of the expanded urethra.

The utriculus, identified in 14 specimens, varied in size from a short intraprostatic saccule to a blind tubule extending beyond the prostate gland between the seminal ducts.

The trigone in six specimens formed a V-shape with the apex fading in the internal meatus and the ureteric orifices at the ends of very long cornua. In others, the trigone was triangular with the orifices situated on the lateral bladder wall. In 16 specimens, a urachal diverticulum was present and in five of these the urachus was patent but partially obstructive.

The posterior, caudal and side walls of the prostatic segment were extremely dilated in all specimens. We describe three different profiles of the membranous urethra (Fig. 37.4).

1. Membranous urethra exiting from the prostatic urethra along the anterior wall with (a) normal calibre (five examples); (b) narrow calibre (four examples); (c) high 'take-off' (two examples) partly resembling Type 4 valves (Stephens, 1983a).
2. Modified Young's Type 1 valve. One full-term baby and two fetuses (identical twins aborted at 18 weeks gestational age) exhibited a short anterior nipple-like diverticulum of the dilated prostatic urethra directed distally overlying and compressing the narrow calibre eccentrically exiting membranous urethra.
3. Modified Young's Type 3 lesion (five specimens). The prostatic and membranous urethral segments were widely dilated. In the region of the perineal membrane, four exhibited an abrupt narrowing of the exiting urethra, and in the fifth specimen, the lumen was totally occluded.

In all specimens, sections showed a normal transitional cell epithelium and normal striated muscle cells of the

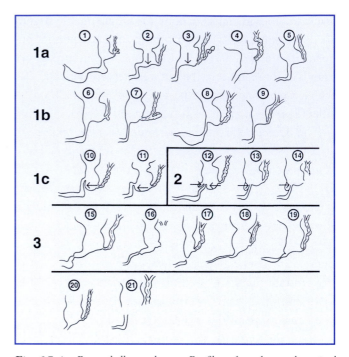

Fig. 37.4 *Prune belly syndrome. Profiles of urethra and seminal ducts and vesicles.* **1a**, **b**, **c**. *Membranous urethra normal and narrow calibre and 'high take off'.* **2** *Modified Young's valve, Type 1.* **3** *Modified Young's valve Type 3; unclassified (20 and 21). Arrows indicate valve or potential activation of valve. Banding of seminal ducts (19 cases) and not known (6 and 16); urachal fistula (5, 19, 21, 42 and 45); scaphoid megalourethra (1 and 8); identical twin fetuses (13 and 14); seminal vesicle present (7), rudimentary (1, 3 and 6), not known (14, 16 and 21), absent in remainder. (Reprinted with permission, after Stephens, F.D. and Gupta, D. Pathogenesis of the prime belly syndrome. J. Urol. 152: 2328–31, Fig. 1.)*

external sphincter surrounding the urethra. In two specimens, the urethra had been transected and the distal part was not examined.

Urethras with profiles (2) and (3) were undoubtedly severely obstructive and with profiles (1b,c) were likely to be mechanically obstructive. Profile (1a) specimens may not be obstructive and may resemble the urethral profile of surviving PBS patients (Stephens, 1983a).

Wigger and Blanc (1977) also concluded from autopsy material and previously published reports that urethral obstruction occurred in one-third of patients with PBS. The lesions were stenosis, atresia, valve, diaphragm, diverticulum and phimosis.

The prostate gland was indistinguishable macroscopically from the surrounding urethral wall in 19 of 21 specimens. Only in one specimen was the prostate gland clearly recognizable. In transverse sections at the level of the verumontanum the prostate gland was found to be mainly fibrous in eight but contained some muscle strands in 12. Prostatic ducts were absent in nine and present but sparse in 11. By comparison, the more bulky prostate glands of three full-term babies were replete with tubules, which were concentrated posteriorly in the region of the sulci (Lowsley, 1912; DeKlerk and Scott, 1978).

The ductus deferens on each side was abnormal in 19 specimens (not known in two) in respect to its course from the level of the bladder base to the urethra (Fig. 37.5). After passing behind the distal ends of the dilated ureters, the seminal ducts veered to the midline meeting one another above the level of the bladder neck. They then turned caudally and coursed side-by-side banded in a delicate fascial investment to the hilum of the prostate gland and urethra. The course was straight in eight and sinuous and ectatic in nine. In four specimens, the course was only partly documented. This abnormal course contrasts with the normal course in which both ducts converge in V-fashion from the interureteric level to coapt at the hilum of the prostate gland.

In 16 specimens, the ductus terminated at the urethra without forming a seminal vesicle. In three, the vesicles were rudimentary—a long non-folded blind tube, a cluster of nipple-like short buds and a globular sac and in one specimen the vesicles were normal macroscopically.

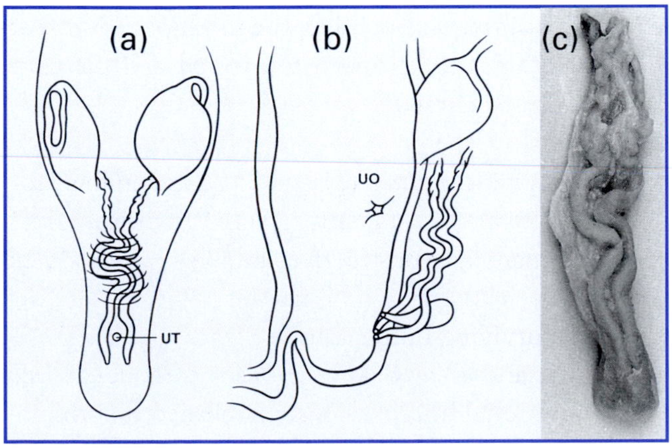

In five specimens, the whole length of the vas deferens on each side was extremely narrow and convoluted from prostate gland to the lower pole of the testis, and in two of these the convolutions of the epididymis were loose and spread out in mini-tortuosities along the body of the ductus. The vas deferens was thick-walled with muscle in two and mainly collagenous in two. An atretic segment was present in the middle of three of these tortuous seminal ducts. The attachment of the epididymis to the upper pole of the testis was extremely tenuous in three of the five specimens (Stephens, 1983b), indicating a marked lack of ductules derived from the wolffian duct (Fig. 37.6).

It was not possible on serial histological examinations to determine whether there was continuity of lumen on these specimens between the ductules and the contiguous rete network of tubules. The head and body of the epididymis were slender in these specimens, and the body was not attached to the testis except for a delicate focal adhesion at the lower pole (Fig. 37.6).

Urogenital tracts in posterior urethral valves (PUV) Types 1 and 3: comparative study

The urogenital tracts of 23 PUV specimens obtained from infants, neonates and fetuses exhibited Type 1 in 14 and Type 3 in nine.

Types 1 and 3 PUV lesions of the urinary tract are well described entities that cause serious back pressure effects (Young and Davis, 1926; Moerman et al., 1984).

Fig. 37.5 *Diagrams and photograph of banded seminal ducts and urethra of profile (Fig. 37.4 specimen 10). (**a**) Posterior view showing tortuous seminal ducts separating around utriculus (UT), absent seminal vesicles, and focal gigantism of ureters and orifices (UO). (**b**) Lateral view showing valve obstruction of membranous urethra, absence of verumontanum and dilated utriculus masculinus. (**c**) Photograph of tortuous seminal ducts, unbanded by dissection. (Reprinted with permission from Stephens, F.D. and Gupta, D. Pathogenesis of the prune belly syndrome, J. Urol. 152: 2328–31, Fig. 2.)*

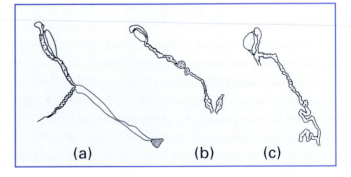

Fig. 37.6 *'Strung-out epididymides'. (**a**) Small testis, pinpoint attachment of epididymis to testis, attachment of gubernaculum to vas, and discontinuity of vas caused by atresia. (**b**) Vas composed of unravelled epididymis with globular mini epididymides along its course. (**c**) Tortuous vas and rudimentary development of the seminal vesicle. (Reproduced, with permission, from Stephens, F.D. (1983). In Congenital Malformations of the Urinary Tract, Fig. 32.8, p. 505. New York: Praeger.)*

In PUV Type 1 the dimensions of the verumontanum and inferior crest of the urethra were large compared with those in normal urethras. In Type 3 valve, the verumontanum and crest were diminutive resembling those features of some of the PBS specimens.

The prostate gland in PUV Type 1 could be readily recognized macroscopically by its bulk and shape and histologically in 10 available specimens by the presence of slightly dilated and compressed peri-urethral ducts and acini embedded in fibromuscular tissue. In PUV Type 3 anomalies the prostate gland was similar to Type 1 in five specimens but in three the ducts were sparse and the stroma fibrous or in the fetal specimens mesenchymal.

The ejaculatory duct, seminal vesicle, ductus deferens and epididymis were present and near normal macroscopically in both types. The seminal ducts from either side curved around the ureterovesical junction in normal manner to meet in V-fashion close to the hilus of the prostate gland (compare Fig. 37.7). The vas deferens and seminal vesicles identified histologically in nine specimens contained well-developed muscular coats. The utriculus was identified in seven and not recorded in 16 specimens.

The location of the testes in PUV specimens was scrotal in two, inguinal in one and intraabdominal in four (including two fetuses < 20 weeks) and not recorded in 11. A 12 per cent incidence of maldescent of the testes in PUV patients was recorded by Barker *et al.* (1993). In the 21 specimens of PBS, the location of the testis was intraabdominal in 16, unilateral scrotal in one and not known in four.

Bladder

The bladder was large and merged cranially into a wide urachal diverticulum in all specimens. In four, this diverticulum was patent at the umbilicus. The walls of the bladder were tough and ≤ 1 cm in thickness in some parts, while in other parts, large segments were of paper thickness only. Some of these thin zones, when small, presented as pocket-like diverticula, but when large in area, showed no tendency to diverticulum formation (Fig. 37.8).

The interior of the bladder was smooth and pale, but laterally some longitudinal folds were visible. The trigone was large and often asymmetrical. The cornua were narrow, elongated and tenuous.

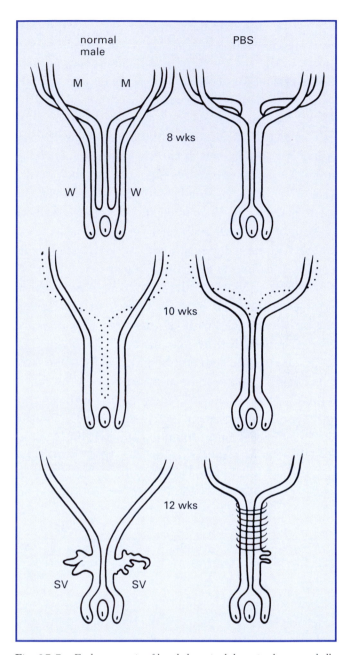

Fig. 37.7 *Embryogenesis of banded seminal ducts in the prune belly syndrome. Normal male, müllerian ducts (M) separate the mesonephric (wolffian) ducts (W) at eight weeks and undergo disintegration at 10 weeks leaving seminal ducts converging in V-fashion at hilus of prostate gland at 12 weeks. Prune belly syndrome müllerian ducts fail to migrate to the midline (or fail to form), disintegrate (dots) leaving the mesonephric ducts to be banded at 12 weeks; note absent (left) or rudimentary (or normal) (right) seminal vesicle. SV = seminal vesicle. (Reprinted with permission from Stephens, F.D. and Gupta, D. Pathogenesis of the prune belly syndrome, J. Urol. 152: 2328–31, Fig. 2.)*

The ureteric orifices were lateral in position, sometimes asymmetrically disposed. In one, the trigone was

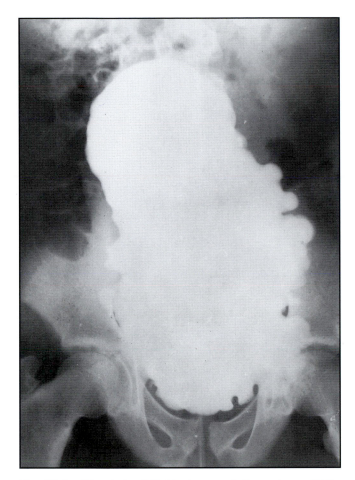

Fig. 37.8 *Diverticula of bladder in prune belly syndrome. W.P., aged 15 years. Multiple small diverticula and a rounded dome with hourglass constriction suggestive of a wide urachal extension of the bladder. (Reproduced, with permission, from Stephens, F.D. (1983), In Congenital Malformations of the Urinary Tract, Fig. 32.5, p. 503. New York: Praeger.)*

only slightly larger than normal and the submucosal segments of the ureter were > 1 cm in length. In others, the orifice lay contiguous with the ureterovesical hiatus ≤ 5 cm from the internal urethral meatus or in the floor of a paraureteral diverticulum. In the majority, the orifices were large and gaping, admitting free reflux in the postmortem state, and only one exhibited stenosis. In none was the ureteric orifice close to or in the urethra.

Ureter

The ureter displayed a remarkable variation in size and tortuosity. The calibre in the megaureters was rarely uniform and varied from end to end. Sometimes, a semblance of symmetry was apparent, but usually,

asymmetry of size and shape predominated. General enlargement of gross proportions was the rule, maximal in the lower third but commonly haphazard focal gigantism or focal narrowing, or atresias occurred in the upper two-thirds of the ureter (Fig. 37.9). Single and multiple pleat valves of the ureter were present in the caudal parts of two ureters respectively (Maizels and Stephens, 1980). In some specimens, both ureters were tremendously dilated, tortuous and 'concertinered', being 9 cm in diameter and > 36-cm long when unravelled. The size and shape of the pelvis and calyces were unpredictable, sometimes conforming with the general state of dilatation of the ureter, but frequently exhibiting marked contrast in dimensions and conformation.

The major and minor calyces varied from large and intrarenal to small or even minuscule, and in some, the infundibula were long and narrow, connecting globular minor calyces of various sizes with a spidery pelvis. Duplication and agenesis of the ureter did not occur in this series.

Histological features of the ureters and bladder. The tissues were prepared and stained with haematoxylin–eosin, Masson and van Gieson's stains. The muscle in the walls varied from absence throughout the ureters, bladder and prostatic urethra in one specimen, to varying degrees of deficit in others.

The walls of the ureters were thick and composed of fibrocytes, collagen and smooth muscle in mixed proportions. In some of the most severe examples of the triad syndrome, the walls exhibited total absence of muscle fibres and were composed of fibrous tissue, which was sparsely cellular compared with the surrounding acellular collagenous ground substance (Fig. 37.10). The total thickness of the ureters in some parts was accounted for by this thick hyaline ground substance. The ureters were all affected to a greater or lesser extent. The giant and narrow areas were similarly affected.

The walls of the bladder were thick in some, thin in others, and a mixture in yet others. Muscle when present was intermixed with fibrocytes and collagen which contributed largely to the thickness of the bladder. In some areas, the wall was devoid of muscle and composed of large or small plaques of collagen, which, under pressure, formed into a bulge or diverticulum (Fig. 37.8).

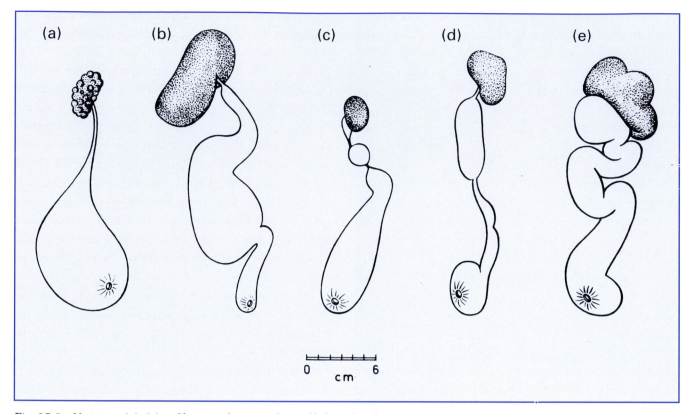

Fig. 37.9 *Variations (**a**)–(**e**) in dilatation of ureter and size of kidneys found in postmortem series of five specimens. (Reprinted, by permission, from Nunn, I.N. and Stephens, F.D. (1961), The triad syndrome: a composite anomaly of the abdominal wall, urinary system and testes. J. Urol. 86: 782, Fig. 6.)*

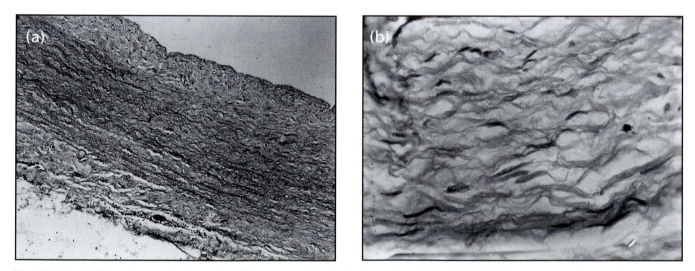

Fig. 37.10   (**a**) *Photomicrograph of ureteral wall showing complete lack of smooth muscle (×100).* (**b**) *High-power magnification of another area showing preponderance of collagen matrix over fibrocytes and occasional smooth muscle cell. ((**a**) reprinted, by permission, from Nunn, I.N. and Stephens, F.D. (1961), The triad syndrome: a composite anomaly of the abdominal wall, urinary system and testes. J. Urol. 86: 782, Fig. 7.)* (**b**) *(reprinted, with permission, from Stephens, F.D. (1983). In Congenital Malformations of the Urinary Tract, Fig. 32.7B, p. 504. New York: Praeger.)*

The thick parts of the bladder wall consisted of muscle, or a mixture, but the very thin areas were composed of fibrous and hyaline tissue. Cussen (quoted by Stephens, 1974) measured the muscle cell size in two of the ureters. The cells were normal in dimension indicating absence of hypertrophy.

Autonomic nerves of the bladder. Henley and Hyman (1953) claimed that two specimens from infants who displayed the triad syndrome lacked ganglion cells in the bladder and ureter and have inferred a close similarity between this condition and aganglionic megacolon (Hirschsprung's disease). On the other hand, McGovern and Marshall (1959) found normal nerves and ganglion cells in four of the specimens examined.

One specimen exhibiting the triad of anomalies (Baby C.) was investigated to trace and plot the ganglion-cell distribution in the pelvic ganglion, the bladder base, urethra, the presacral nerves and nervi erigentes and the rectum. For this purpose, the whole of the true pelvis, including the sacral vertebrae, the symphysis pubis, and the periosteal fibrocartilage of the ischium and ilium, including the soft-tissue content, was removed *en bloc* from the body. This specimen was blocked in paraffin and cut in serial section from side to side in the sagittal plane. The sections were cut at 15-μm thickness and every tenth section was stained with haematoxylin–eosin and every twentieth section with Masson stain; the intervening slides were retained, and, in some important areas, these were also stained and examined. The neuroanatomy was studied and compared with that of six similar blocks taken from normal pelves of stillborn babies.

Ganglion cells do not inhabit the walls of the ureter (Swenson *et al.*, 1951) but congregate around the bladder base and ureterovesical junction. The distribution of ganglion cells in this specimen closely resembled the pattern of the six normal specimens.

The pelvic ganglion on each side consisted of a plexus of large ganglia containing multitudes of ganglion cells, nerves, dendrites and Schwann cells. The plexus was roughly triangular and lay between the vesicourethral structures and the side wall of the pelvis.

The presacral nerves and the nervi erigentes entered the superior and posterior aspects of the plexus, respectively. The pelvic nerves were heavily ganglionated and only an occasional ganglion cell was present in the nervi erigentes, which were traced back to meet the third and fourth spinal nerves.

The sympathetic chains and ganglia were normally located on either side and exhibited numerous ganglion cells.

Ganglion cells were found in the nerves, which were distributed to the bladder base, and some ganglion cells were found in fine nerve terminals amidst the muscle of the wall of the bladder. Large ganglia were situated along the lateral and posterior walls of the prostatic and membranous urethrae. Ganglion cells were identified around the lower end of both ureters adjacent to the bladder wall and in the intramural plexuses of the rectum.

In summary, no abnormality in distribution of ganglion cells of the pelvis could be detected when the findings were compared with those in the normal specimens.

From this study and from the findings of McGovern and Marshall (1959), it appears that dysfunction of the lower urinary tract is not associated with aberrant distribution of the ganglion cells.

Testes

The testes and associated gubernacula were, in some specimens, studied with regard to location and microscopic structure.

Testes were intraabdominal in 16, unilateral scrotal in one and not known in four. The enlarged ureters lifted the testes off the posterior abdominal wall, and 11 testes lay near the ureterovesical junction or at the level of the iliac crest.

Histologically, the germinal epithelium consisted of solid cords of cells that were indistinguishable from the features of normal testes for the age group.

The gubernacula were elongated, attached to the body of the testis or to the tail of the epididymis proximally, and to the pubic tubercle distally. The tail of the gubernacula in all instances passed along the inguinal canal to reach the tubercle. The histological structure included fibrous tissue, collagen, voluntary-muscle cells, nerves and blood vessels. In summary, the structure of the gubernacula revealed no unusual features (Tayakkanonta, 1963).

Kidneys

In these specimens, the kidneys ranged from extreme degrees of hydronephrosis to near normal or to small and dysplastic. When hydronephrotic, the renal parenchyma spread thinly over the clubbed calyces or formed isolated rounded renal nubbins perched on the dilated calyces. In one, the kidneys were composed of a mosaic of thin, flat, isolated plaques of nephrons distributed over the surface of the dilated calyces. When solid, the kidneys exhibited hypoplasia of renal units and dysplastic structures such as embryonic tubules, cartilage, cysts and mesenchymal connective tissue (Fig. 37.11). The structure was composed of near-normal cortex and medulla with minimal dysplasia in one kidney, but, in the others, the cortex and medulla were in part or wholly dysplastic and hypoplastic. Kidneys associated with ureteral atresia were small, solid, and dysplastic.

The abdominal wall

In six specimens, a description of the appearances of the abdominal wall was recorded at the time of autopsy, and the intact specimen was available for special dissection; strips only of the full thickness of the lower abdomen were examined in five. The belly walls were thin and redundant and the skin was wrinkled.

The abdominal wall was dissected in two specimens to display the segmental nerves and the muscle layers,

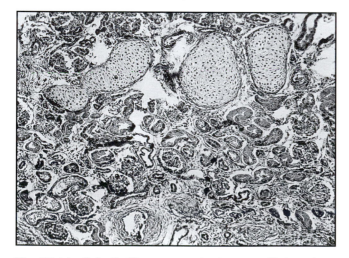

Fig. 37.11 *Baby R. Photomicrograph of section of kidney shows gross renal dysplasia. Islands of cartilage, abnormal tubules, and increase in amount of interstitial connective tissue can be seen (×100). (Reprinted, by permission, from Nunn, I.N. and Stephens, F.D. (1961), The triad syndrome: a composite anomaly of the abdominal wall, urinary system and testes. J. Urol. 86: 782, Fig. 8.)*

and microscopic examinations were made to trace the muscle layers and to study the muscle cells.

Segmental nerves

The full complement of spinal nerves was found. These nerves coursed anteriorly in the normal muscle planes giving twigs at intervals to the muscle layers and terminating in the rectus muscle. Microscopically, these nerves were composed of axon cylinders within the Schwann cell sheaths and appeared normal in formation (Nunn and Stephens, 1961).

Muscle layers

In three specimens in which the abdominal wall was dissected in the fresh state, the muscle layers were thin but arranged correctly. In two, one layer only was found and this observation was confirmed microscopically (Fig. 37.12). Moreover, the muscle cells were deficient in areas of patchy distribution, in which the layers were represented by fibrous laminae or by a single sheet of fibrous tissue.

Muscle cells of abdominal wall

The voluntary-muscle cells, when present, were clear and normal in appearance, especially those of the rectus muscle. Some were larger than usual and appeared to merge with the ground substance, lacking a defined border (Fig. 37.13). Other muscle cells were collected into bundles of fibres to form in some a thin muscle readily identifiable anatomically. In others, the bundles were unevenly distributed, or isolated, and areas within the rectus sheath or in line of the muscle layer were devoid of muscle altogether.

In view of the normal nerve distribution, the patchy distribution of normal striated muscle cells and the irregularity of layers in the abdominal wall, the condition was regarded as, in essence, a developmental malformation of muscle.

Embryology of the bladder and belly wall

In order to explain the occurrence of the abnormalities that comprise the classic triad, it is necessary to trace briefly the embryological events occurring in the cloaca, the urogenital tracts and muscle precursor of the 5-mm

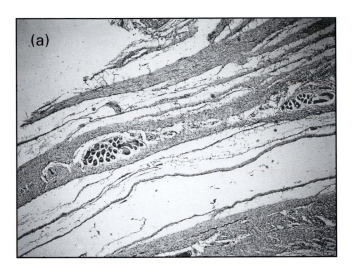

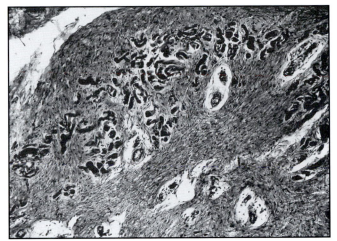

Fig. 37.13 *Triad syndrome, Baby A. Photomicrograph of section of rectus muscle shows disorganized groups of striated muscle fibres merging with dense connective tissue (×110). (Reprinted, by permission, from Nunn, I.N. and Stephens, F.D. (1961), The triad syndrome: a composite anomaly of the abdominal wall, urinary system and testes. J. Urol. 86: 782, Fig. 10.)*

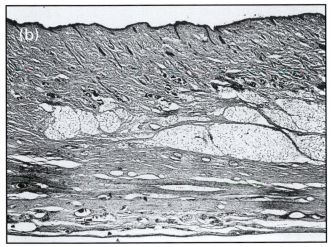

Fig. 37.12 *Photomicrographs of sections of lower anterolateral abdominal wall. Baby A. Only a single incomplete muscle layer is present and there is a great reduction in number of muscle fibres. These are represented as small islands in a single aponeurotic layer (×50). (Reprinted, by permission, from Nunn, I.N. and Stephens, F.D. (1961), The triad syndrome: a composite anomaly of the abdominal wall, urinary system and testes. J. Urol. 86: 782, Fig. 9.)*

(crown–rump length) embryo (late fourth and early fifth week; Carnegie stages 12–13).

The trilaminar discoid embryo during the third week rests upon the yolk sac inside the restricting capsules of amnion and chorion (Fig. 37.14a). It elongates rapidly and folds first at the head end, followed by tail end into a C-shaped organism. The wings of the embryo grow laterally and ventrally to form the thoracic cage and upper abdominal wall. The flexion of the tail end is accompanied by a change in orientation of the body stalk to the embryo (Fig. 37.14b). Its attachment is rotated from the hind end of the disk to the ventrum of the embryo. It comes to lie in contact with the yolk sac stalk cranially and retains contact with the cloacal membrane caudally.

As the embryo grows and folds, its walls tighten around the yolk sac, creating a constriction around the yolk sac and body stalks. The intraembryonic part of the yolk sac undergoes differentiation into the foregut, midgut and hindgut, while the extraembryonic yolk sac resorbs. The midgut elongates and protrudes through the constriction into the yolk sac stalk, where further rapid elongation takes place, and finally, by 11 weeks, the gut returns to the abdomen. With further growth of the hind end, the tail unfolds and the mesoderm of the belly wall grows in between the cloacal membrane and the body stalk.

Cloaca and allantois

Prior to ventral rotation of the tail end, a finger-like diverticulum of the yolk sac grows along the body stalk into the chorion where it ends blindly amongst the umbilical vessels (Fig. 37.14a). With rotation of the body stalk, the open end of the allantoic diverticulum is turned into the cloacal end of the hindgut. The co-apting cranial wall of the allantois and apposing wall of the yolk sac stalk form a wedge of tissue, from which the urorectal septum develops. This septum advances toward the cloacal membrane and partitions the cloaca into the urogenital tract and hindgut in the period of

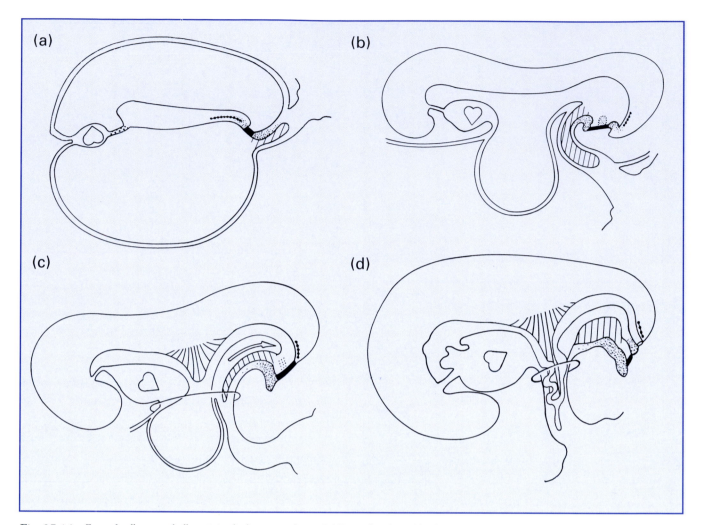

Fig. 37.14 *Fate of yolk sac and allantois in the human embryo. (a) Discoid embryo (third week) showing amniotic and yolk sacs and the allantoic diverticulum in the body stalk. (b) Head and tail rotation, constriction of the abdominal wall around the yolk sac, and inturning of the allantois into cloaca. (c) Body stalk and yolk sac stalk merge, and septum between them, as Tourneux's fold, advances towards the cloacal septum forming from Rathke's plicae (columns of dots). (d) Midgut umbilical herniations; Tourneux's fold meets Rathke's plicae to complete the urorectal septum (arrow). The allantois forms into urachus, bladder and prostatic urethra; genital tubercle and infra-abdominal wall widens in the area between tubercle and body stalk. Hind end is exaggerated in size compared with head end in order to show details of the cloacal development. Heavy black line indicates cloacal membrane; black dots joined together represent the primitive streak; open hatching = allantois; arrow = Tourneux's fold. (Reproduced, with permission, from Stephens, F.D. (1983). In Congenital Malformations of the Urinary Tract, New York: Praeger, Fig. 32.12, pp. 507–508.)*

development between four and six weeks (4–6-mm crown–rump length) (Fig. 37.14c,d).

The mesoderm of the trilaminar disk embryo

In the third week, the mesoderm derived from the primitive streak builds up cranially to form the heart, and laterally to form the somites and the intermediate cell mass and lateral plate. The most caudal migration of mesoderm borders the cloacal membrane and builds up the structures between the membrane and body stalk (Fig. 37.15a–d).

The somites derived from the mesoderm of the primitive streak lying to either side of the midline become segmented and form the extensors and flexors of the spine and, more caudally, the pelvic diaphragm and the voluntary sphincters of the anus and urethra.

The intermediate mesoderm situated more laterally in the trunk remains unsegmented and gives rise to the wolffian bodies, which form kidneys, gonads and their ducts and intrinsic musculature.

The formation of the wolffian duct, ureters and metanephros, and the process by which the ureters are

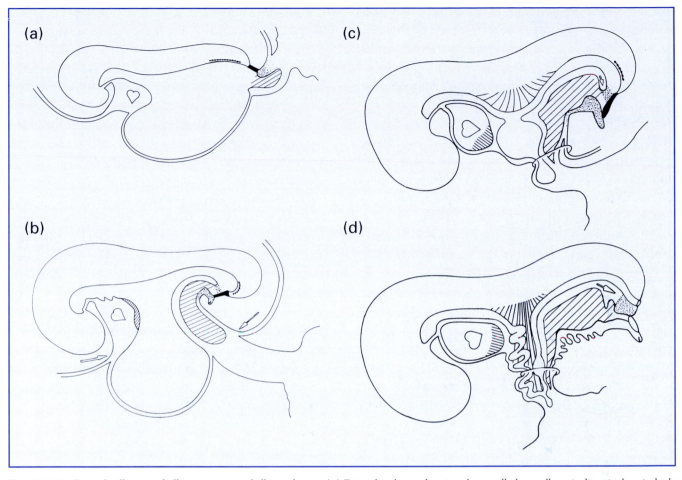

Fig. 37.15   *Fate of yolk sac and allantois in prune belly syndrome. (**a**) Discoid embryo, showing abnormally large allantoic diverticulum in body stalk. (**b**) Abdominal wall forming around the dome of the yolk sac (arrows), and the large allantois turning into the cloaca. (**c**) Yolk sac is contained mainly inside the abdomen, and allantois forms bladder. (**d**) Yolk sac absorbed, abdominal wall redundant; urorectal septum complete and urachus constricted, but patent, bladder and prostatic urethra large. Cloacal urethra near normal in dimensions. (Reproduced, with permission, from Stephens, F.D. (1983). In* Congenital Malformations of the Urinary Tract, *New York: Praeger, Fig. 32.13, pp. 509–510.)*

incorporated into the bladder, are shown in Figs 1.10 and 13.2.

The lateral plate in the wings of the disk give rise to three sets of muscles, the smooth muscle of the urogenital organs, the smooth muscle of the gut and the striped muscle of the thoracoabdominal wall. By eight weeks, that is, two weeks after the internal cloaca has been completely partitioned and the ureteric orifices are located on the trigone, smooth-muscle cells derived from the lateral plate mesoderm have formed around the bowel, bladder and ureters. The lateral plate mesoderm in the lower thoracolumbar region splits around the coelomic cavity and forms into a parietal layer, which becomes the muscle of the anterior wall of the trunk and a visceral layer, which gives rise to the smooth muscle of the bowel and bladder.

The allantois and contribution by it to the bladder and urethra

The bladder is said to be formed from the anterior compartment of the cloaca, which develops as a dilatation of the hindgut in continuity with the allantois. The allantois and the anterior compartment form a tubular structure known as the 'vesicourethral canal'. Together with the trigonal gusset formed by the expanded terminal segments of the wolffian ducts and the globular expansion of the vesical canal, the bladder, bladder neck and urethra take shape. At first, the bladder dilatation extends to the umbilicus, but gradually, the cephalic part of the organ retrogresses, forming the urachus and, finally, the fibrous remnant, which is the middle umbilical ligament (Fig. 37.14c,d). Opinions of embryologists, however, differ as to the extent of the allantoic contribution to the formation of the bladder.

Felix (1912c) and Arey (1947c), who quotes Chwalla (1927), considered that the allantois contributes nothing to either the bladder or urachus. Frazer (1931d) and Patten (1947c) considered that part of the bladder is derived from allantois. Hamilton, Boyd and Mossman (1978c) attribute to the allantois the urachus and middle umbilical ligament. Some evidence may be forthcoming from the study of the prune belly syndrome to support the views of Patten (1947d) who stated that the advance of the urorectal septum toward the cloacal membrane 'makes it difficult to keep track of the original limits of the allantois'. He regarded the bladder, from the region of the ureteric orifices and the urachus to the umbilicus, as being formed from allantois. Some of the malformations of the bladder and urethra noted in the prune belly syndrome, together with the embryopathy of the rectourinary cloacal anomalies, support the contention that the bladder derives from the allantois and wolffian ducts, and that the prostatic urethra derives also in part from these same structures.

Embryogenesis

Stumme (1903) and many others since then have considered that the laxity is caused by pressure atrophy or deformity of the muscle by obstructed, enlarged urinary organs. Most patients exhibit urethral obstruction with extremely large vesicourachal reservoirs that fill and distend the whole of the abdomen. Because not all patients with hypoplastic, redundant belly walls exhibit enlarged urinary organs, it is claimed that the obstruction or dysfunction may have been transient events *in utero* in triad patients. As previously described, urethral obstructions due to Young's valves do not affect the abdominal wall and urogenital organs in the manner of the urethral obstruction of the PBS. Hence, other explanations have been sought and evolved.

Another reason proposed for the laxity and redundancy of the belly wall is that of a primary malformation of muscle and fascial components. Light- and

electron-microscopy studies (Nunn and Stephens, 1961; Wigger and Blanc, 1977) reveal hypoplasia with excess collagenous tissue between islands of muscle cells, absence of muscle over wide areas, and plaques of fibrocartilage. Electron-microscopy studies have indicated abnormalities in the ultrastructure of the muscle cell— namely, disarray of the Z-lines, and arrangement of the glycogen granules (Mininberg *et al.*, 1973). The belly wall may lack lamination and appear as a thin, fibrous, or fibromuscular, single, sheet-like structure.

The redundancy in some babies is extreme, involving all the muscles of the abdomen, while in others, it predominates in the flanks or lower recti muscles or is somewhat unilateral (Fig. 37.2). Occasionally, the belly wall is so mildly affected as to escape notice until the boy seeks medical advice concerning undescended testes.

A yolk sac theory of abdominal wall and vesicourethral ectasia

This theory based on an error of embryogenesis of the yolk sac and allantois could account for the spectra of redundancy and of vesicourachal enlargements. The theory incriminates the yolk sac and its relationship to the lateral folds of the discoid embryo. As the embryo enlarges and folds inside the chorionic cavity, the yolk sac normally shrinks and constricts at the 'umbilicus'. The greater part of the sac lies outside the embryo and undergoes progressive absorption and atrophy. The lesser part is retained inside the embryo as the primitive midgut, which then undergoes progressive elongation on the dorsal mesentery to form the midgut components. The coils of the elongating gut protrude into the umbilical stalk until the abdominal cavity is sufficiently enlarged to receive them back inside. Under abnormal circumstances, it can be envisaged that a much greater part of the yolk sac may be retained inside the embryo. The side wings of the folding discoid embryo may overgrow and constrict the yolk sac into an hourglass shape, with the greater part inside instead of outside the embryo. Almost immediately afterward, the inner and outer component of the hourglass resorb, leaving the abdominal walls redundant. The spectrum of redundancy may depend on the volume of yolk sac retained temporarily inside the abdomen (Stephens, 1983).

Linked to the fate of the yolk sac is the allantoic diverticulum. This structure grows out from the yolk sac into the contiguous body stalk and ends blindly amidst the blood lakes of the chorion (Fig. 37.15a). This yolk sac diverticulum inverts into the cloaca in the hind end and elongates as the body stalk rotates ventrally. In the event that the intraabdominal part of the hourglass yolk sac is larger than normal, the allantoic diverticulum, being part of it, is also large (Fig. 37.15b).

This augmented allantois becomes incorporated into the urinary tract as the typical oversized urachus, bladder and prostatic urethra of PBS. Resorption of the large urachus may be lacking in part or wholly, resulting in a urachal extension of the bladder, which may remain widely open or closed at the umbilicus depending on the extent of regression and the site of constriction by the body wall (Fig. 37.15c,d).

Under these abnormal circumstances, the bladder and urethra remain ectatic to the caudal limit of the prostatic urethra in midpelvis. Beyond this point, the membranous urethra may be small, normal or large in size. The embryological contribution of the allantois to the urinary tract may include urachus, bladder and prostatic urethra, and the cloacal contribution may be only the membranous urethra.

This theory *per se* does not account for the dilatations and errors of development of the ureters and genital tracts. The terminal ends of the wolffian ducts (common excretory ducts) issue into the cloaca prior to partition and become absorbed *pari passu* with the development of the urorectal septum into the vesicourethral canal (see Figs 1.10 and 13.2). After divesting the ureters to the bladder, the wolffian ducts then become the ejaculatory ducts, which open into the prostatic urethra. The trigonal gussets, the ureteric buds, and sometimes the ejaculatory ducts in the PBS all are large, all share the excessive capaciousness of the bladder and prostatic urethra with the overgrown allantois. The ureters, especially the lower ends and the pelves, and calyces may exhibit general, local or irregular dilatation and narrowing and erratic lengthening, shortening, or atresia.

Streak theory of myopathies and urogenital anomalies

Myopathy

The yolk sac theory does not account for the defective development of muscle in the abdominal wall and urinary tracts or for the dysplasia of the kidneys. Ives

(1974) traced the origin of the dysgenesis of the PBS back to the trilaminar disk stage of embryogenesis in the third week. She attributes the anomaly to defective formation and distribution of the mesoderm to each side of the embryonic disk from the primitive streak. At that time, mesoderm is being distributed to the somites, the intermediate cell mass and the lateral plate on both sides of the embryo (Fig. 37.16a–d). Defects of distribution or quality of the mesoderm from the primitive streak to these starting points on each side would undermine the subsequent morphogenesis of the thoracoabdominal muscles, the muscle of the ureters, bladder and prostatic urethra, and the quality of the metanephric blastema.

The distribution of mesoderm to the parietal layer and intermediate cell masses may be asymmetrical and may vary in the amount from mild-to-severe deficiencies of muscle. The lower abdominal musculature is most commonly and severely affected. Visceral mesodermal hypoplasia affects the musculature of the bladder and prostatic urethra. The sacrococcygeal outflow to the perineum, when also deficient, may cause defects in the urorectal septum (Rathke's plicae) incurring cloacal anomalies and defects of the spongy tissue of the anterior urethra, resulting in megalourethra and penile anomalies.

Renal dysgenesis

At least three factors may determine the abnormal hypoplastic and dysplastic development of the kidney:

1. The intermediate cell mass and metanephros may be devoid of its full share of mesoderm from the primitive streak.
2. The ureteric bud may arise from an ectopic location on the wolffian duct and lack induction capability.
3. The stepwise substitution of ladder-like mesonephric vessels by the ascending kidney and hyperelongating ureter may fail, leading to ischaemia of the ureter and kidney, resulting in ureteric atresia or stenosis and renal hypodysplasia.

Undescended testes, gubernaculum and vas deferens

The intraabdominal gonads in the most severe examples of the syndrome are small and may lack some of the germ cells, which stray from the path in their long trek

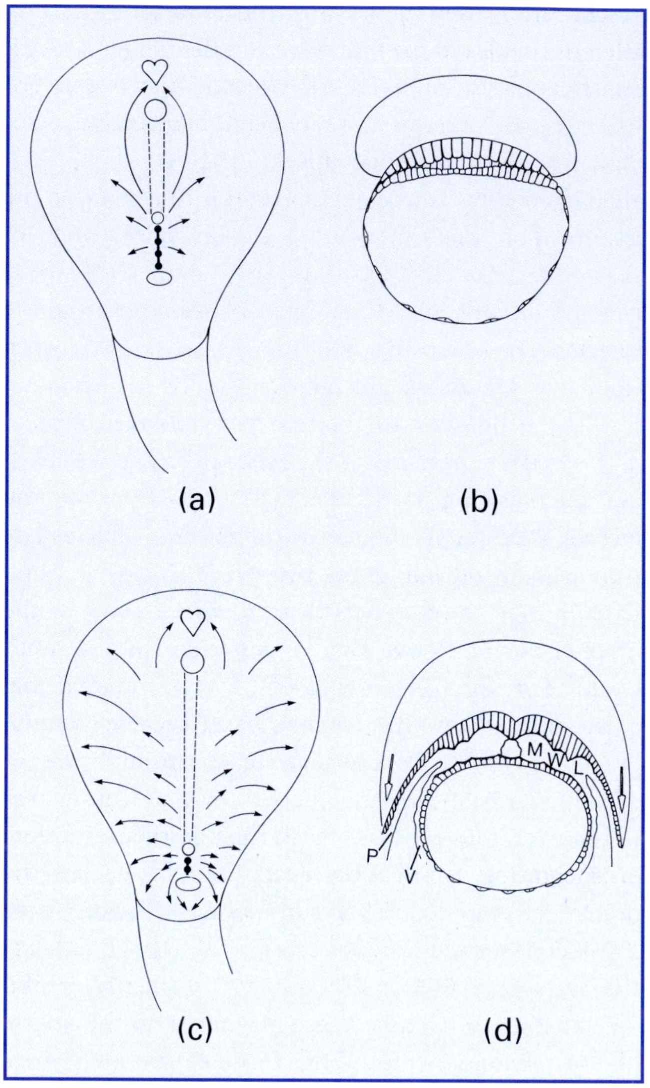

Fig. 37.16 *Trilaminar discoid embryo.* (**a**) *View of disk (amnion removed), showing direction of distribution of mesoderm from primitive streak to notochord (dotted) around the buccopharyngeal membrane (large circle) laterally and to heart (black dots joined = primitive streak; oval = cloacal membrane).* (**b**) *Transverse section through primitive streak showing trilamination: epiblast, mesoderm and endoderm. Also amnion and yolk sac.* (**c**) *Discoid embryo showing wider and now posterior distribution of mesoderm around cloacal membrane.* (**d**) *Transverse section through primitive streak showing mesoderm (unshaded) divided into myotome (M) intermediate cell mass, or wolffian body (W) and lateral plate (L), which is separating into parietal (P) and visceral (V) layers, which in turn, form muscle of abdominal wall and viscera, respectively. Note the encroachment of amniotic cavity over the yolk sac domain. (Reproduced, with permission, from Stephens, F.D. (1983). In* Congenital Malformations of the Urinary Tract, *New York: Praeger, Fig. 32.14, p. 511.)*

from the extra wide allantoic diverticulum and yolk sac to the wolffian ridge. Tayakkanonta (1963) compared the light-microscopic features of the gubernaculum in the triad syndrome with those of normal subjects and found no abnormality or intraabdominal gubernacular cause for the lack of descent of the testes.

The muscularization of the vas (and epididymis) was deficient in two specimens, the muscle being replaced by thick collagenous tissue concentrically arranged around the lumen. In others, the collagen was interspersed between the muscle cells and, in yet others, the muscle cells were normally packed around the lumen. Muscle deficiency in the vas may also be traced to mesodermal deficiencies in the wolffian ridge.

Defective mesoderm of the genital ridge and mesonephric duct

A recent study of the urethral and genital tracts by Stephens and Gupta (1994) throws some light on the pathogenesis of PBS. In that study, many PBS specimens and all of those with PUV valves exhibited obstructive lesions in the posterior urethra. The explanation of the differences in the urogenital tracts of PBS subjects may lie in the common origin of the organs in defective mesoderm of the genital ridge.

The mesonephric (wolffian) duct normally forms in the intermediate mesoderm at the cranial end of the genital ridge and elongates distally to finally penetrate the cloaca in its anterolateral wall contiguous with the anterior end of the cloacal membrane (Felix, 1912), early in the fourth gestational week. It courses obliquely and distally around the side wall of the cloaca from back to front. The orifice recedes rostrally to the level of the future verumontanum by expansion and incorporation of the terminus of the duct into the wall of the vesicourethral canal. This occurs at the same time that the urorectal septum divides the cloaca. The right- and left-duct components in the membranous urethra are demarcated medially by the inferior crest and laterally by the side ridges that converge onto the crest (Stephens, 1983a) (Fig. 37.17). Incorporation of both ducts at a higher level forms a medial strip of prostatic urethra and the trigone. In this manner, a mesodermal gusset is formed in the vesicourethral canal that augments the breadth of parts of the membranous and prostatic urethra and the base of the bladder. The orifices of the ureter and seminal ducts are also incorporated in this gusset. The ducts of the prostate gland appear in the vicinity of the verumontanum in the twelfth gestational week. The seminal vesicle arises from a lateral outpouch of the juxtaprostatic mesonephric duct in the thirteenth

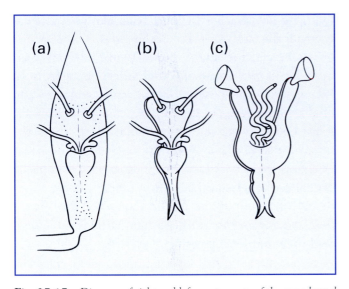

Fig. 37.17 *Diagram of right and left components of the mesodermal gusset in posterior urethra and trigone. (**a**), (**b**) Normal male. (**c**) Prune belly specimens. Note in (**c**) the possible irregular expansions in membranous urethra that may develop into the various profiles; dots outline gusset in vesicourethral tract and broken line divides the halves of the gusset. (Reprinted with permission from Stephens, F.D. and Gupta, D. Pathogenesis of the prune belly syndrome, J. Urol. 152: 2328–31, Fig. 4.)*

gestational week and the ampulla of the duct is yet another focal but tubular dilatation of the subterminal part of the duct (Fig. 37.7).

Abnormal development of the urogenital tracts in PBS

It is proposed that in the PBS subject a faulty hyperectatic process occurs in the terminal mesonephric duct during the fourth to sixth gestational weeks, extending rostrally in the duct from its orifice near the cloacal membrane to much beyond the normal limits causing posterior saccular and often valvular lesions in the posterior urethra (Fig. 37.17).

Hyperectasia of the terminal segment of the mesonephric ducts extended so far rostrally beyond the normal limits that the zones of origin of the ureteric buds and seminal vesicles were affected. This overexpansion process also continued into the ureters causing focal gigantism as well as extreme lateral ectopy and widening of ureteric orifices. The developing buds of the seminal vesicles were absorbed or lost in the ductal ectasia and in nine specimens the 'ampulla' was unusually wide and tortuous. At least part of the prostate gland arises in the mesodermal gusset in which the interaction of epithelial and mesenchymal elements was impaired.

The unravelled epididymis, the tenuous linkage of efferent tubules to the rete testis and the highly tortuous and hypoplastic or segmentally atretic ductus deferens in some specimens may also derive from defective mesoderm from which the duct arises.

The banding of the juxtaprostatic segments of the mesonephric ducts may be a direct consequence of abnormal development of the müllerian ducts (Fig. 37.7). The müllerian duct normally forms in the intermediate mesoderm in the sixth gestational week embryo and its caudal end migrates distally on the lateral side of, but in intimate contact with, the mesonephric duct. At the caudal end of the mesonephros, the müllerian ducts swing medially crossing in front of the mesonephric ducts to meet in the midline. There they turn caudally separating the two mesonephric ducts and then migrate side-by-side to Müller's tubercle in the urethra by the eighth week of gestation. By the tenth week these ducts have united and the uterovaginal anlage degenerates. Banding may occur because the müllerian ducts fail to form or fail to reach the midline, thus allowing the mesonephric ducts to become contiguous. If, however, Müller's ducts reach their destination before disintegrating, the seminal ducts then should run the normal V-course to the prostate. Reports (Manivel *et al.*, 1989; Popek *et al.*, 1989; Reinberg *et al.*, 1991), indicate that analogous female PBS subjects frequently exhibit genital-tract anomalies. These may relate to the origins of the paramesonephric and mesonephric ducts in a defective intermediate cell mass.

Other PBS structures that may reflect their origins from the abnormal intermediate mesoderm (genital ridge) are the undescended testis and its gubernaculum and the dysmorphic kidney. The dysmorphic abdominal and urinary-tract musculature may result from defective lateral plate mesoderm that connects with the intermediate cell mass and that hinders myoblast development and migration in the somatopleure and splanchnopleure (Wigger and Blanc, 1977).

PUV Type 1 valves develop during the period of septation of the cloaca. PUV Type 3 may result from incomplete or delayed rupture of the urogenital membrane. Therefore both types of PUV could cause obstruction of urine formed by the mesonephros which is at its height of morphological development at seven weeks of gestation and by metanephric urine which begins to form at about 10 gestational weeks or later.

The development of the prostate gland was only mildly affected by back pressure of obstruction (DeKlerk and Scott, 1978; Moerman *et al.*, 1984; Popek *et al.*, 1989) and the seminal ducts and vesicles progressed normally.

The lesions of the urethra described in PBS profiles 1–3 (see Fig. 37.4) also develop concurrently with septation of the cloaca or disintegration of the urogenital membrane and should cause back pressure effects on the urinary and genital tracts similar to those described in the PUV specimens. However, in the PBS non-survivors, the genital tracts developed abnormally.

For this reason Stephens and Gupta (1994) consider that a basic mesodermal defect as described by Ives (1974) operates in PBS causing not only the genital defects but also the bizarre obstructive and non-obstructive lesions of the urethra and upper tract and the prune belly. PBS urethral valves when present add back pressure damage to already malformed organs.

Popek *et al.* (1989), who concentrated their microscopy studies on prostate glands in PBS and PUV specimens, found impairment of growth in PBS but, in conflict with observations of Stephens and Gupta's stated that the verumontanum and seminal vesicles were relatively normal in all specimens. Further studies will be needed to resolve this issue.

Beasley *et al.* (1988) found that the anterior urethra of PBS patients was several times larger in calibre than normal and postulated that transient obstruction in the developing glandular urethra caused the megalourethra and the triad of anomalies. The onset of obstruction, however, would occur between 13 and 17 weeks of gestation, after the banding of the seminal ducts had been already established (Fig. 37.7).

Banding of the seminal ducts together with agenesis or rudimentary seminal vesicles may be diagnostic features of PBS in the fetal non-survivors whose abdominal wall signs are ill-defined and whose testes are naturally intraabdominal.

Genetics, chromosomes and twinning

Ives (1974) also enquired into the genetics, chromosomes and twinning in PBS. She found no evidence of single-gene or autosomal recessive genetic inheritance. Chromosomes were normal using the available techniques of examination. Harley *et al.* (1972), however, reported two siblings with PBS and chromosomal mosaicism. Their patients, together with other reported cases, revealed an incidence of twinning of 1 in 23 among pregnancies resulting in PBS as opposed to 1 in 80 in all pregnancies. Six pairs of monozygotic twins (one from previous case reports, two from personal communications, and three from their own series) were discordant for PBS. Ives reasoned that the monozygotic diamniotic twinning takes place at the critical time when the primitive streak is forming in the third week and that one of the twins receives an unequal share of the mesodermal cells, accounting for discordancy and PBS.

Anomalies additional to the triad

Compression features and the Potter syndrome

Many patients exhibit signs of intrauterine compression, particularly in the limbs and thorax, resulting from oligohydramnios. The degree of compression varies in proportion to the amount of urine that is secreted and voided into the amniotic cavity. In those with good renal secretion and no leakage of urine from the amniotic cavity, the compression signs are absent; others exhibit only faint dimples and minimal moulding of feet and thoracic cage; yet others have the full-blown Potter syndrome, including facial features, low-set ears, bowed limbs, dislocated hips, deformed digits, talipes and indented thorax. If the urethra is partially or totally obstructed and urine is secreted in moderate quantity, the urachus may remain open; then urine may leak or dialyze into the amniotic cavity either by rupture of the allantois or by dialysis, and the baby may be free of compression stigmata. Leakage at the umbilicus may persist after birth.

Malformations of the midgut

Welch (1979) found in all 45 patients studied that the mesentery of the midgut lacked the normal broad fixation to the posterior abdominal wall, and the midgut was abnormally rotated. Seven of the 45 developed volvulus, and four had duodenal obstruction relieved by Ladd's operation.

The defective fixation and rotation of the midgut may derive from elongation inside the preformed overspacious abdominal cavity. The orderly rotation and fixation that occur normally with the return of the herniated midgut into a restricted space, are not needed. Consequently, the dorsal mesentery is fan-shaped, pivots on narrow pedicle widening to attach to the loops of bowel, and floats with unpredictable twists and twirls in the voluminous abdominal cavity.

Miscellaneous anomalies

Some triad patients exhibit anomalies of other organs such as the heart, brain and intestines (Table 37.2).

Conclusions concerning "mesoderm" versus "obstructive" theories as the cause of PBS

The abnormal distribution of mesoderm to the intermediate cell mass may affect not only the development of all parts of the upper urinary tract and trigone to a variable degree, but also the pelvic urethra distal to the verumontanum. This would account for many of the nonobstructive and obstructive configurations of the pelvic urethra and ureters and also the abnormalities and irregular distribution of smooth muscle in the urinary and genital tracts. The distribution of lateral mesoderm may also be affected accounting for the abnormal muscularization of the abdominal wall. By contrast, severe PUV obstructions of the urethra cause hypertrophy and dilatation of the upper tracts, rarely distort the genital organs and are not associated with muscle defects of the abdominal wall. According to the concepts of pathoembryology as described herein, the syndrome occurs as the results of a primary mesodermal defect with or without obstruction of the urethra.

Abnormalities of genital development

Normal sexual development

Sexual development is a complex process commencing at fertilization of the ovum and continuing during gestation and after birth and culminating with maturation at puberty. Abnormalities at many levels can cause genital anomaly, with defects identified in the genes, gonadal differentiation and in hormone action on the internal and external genitalia. Morphological anomalies also can occur independently of the hormonal control.

All embryos are formed with the capacity to differentiate into either sex, as the internal genitals and the external genitalia initially develop identically. In the early embryo the mesonephros develops in the urogenital ridge. It develops a duct system which drains into the mesonephric duct, also called the wolffian duct, which grows caudally to reach and fuse with the cloaca. Meanwhile, the ambisexual gonad develops on the anteromedial surface of the urogenital ridge. The internal structure of the gonad contains a primitive cortex and medulla; the germ cells form separately from the embryo on the yolk sac and migrate in the caudal wall of the yolk sac at about seven weeks of gestation into the wall of the abdominal cavity and reach the gonads via the posterolateral mesenchyme. The paramesonephric duct, also called the müllerian duct, forms as a longitudinal invagination of the coelomic epithelium at the cranial edge of the urogenital ridge near the commencement of the wolffian duct and then elongates caudally adjacent to the wolffian duct, with which it shares a common basement membrane. By seven to eight weeks, the two müllerian ducts reach the urogenital sinus and induce an elevation on its dorsal wall called the sinus or müllerian tubercle. During the tenth week, the dorsal urogenital epithelium near the müllerian tubercle begins to proliferate in the absence of androgens. The hymen develops later at the same site. The proliferating epithelium grows cranially to form a solid, flat plate, which later becomes canalized to form the lower two-thirds of the vagina. Canalization of the müllerian tubercle cranially forms the fornix of the vagina.

Sexual differentiation begins to diverge between the sexes at seven to eight weeks of gestation, when a particular gene on the short arm of the Y chromosome, the sex-determining region or SRY, triggers, by as yet unknown mechanisms, the formation of a testis in male embryos (Sinclair, 1994). The primitive cords in the medulla develop while the cortex regresses. The migrating germ cells colonize the cords to form the seminiferous cords. The Sertoli cells developing within the cords begin to produce the hormone müllerian inhibiting substance (MIS), also called antimüllerian hormone (AMH), that is thought to have a role in inducing further testicular differentiation (Josso et al., 1993a). Around the testicular cords the stromal cells develop into Leydig cells which produce testosterone (Wilson et al., 1981).

The testicular hormones induce immediate changes in the adjacent genital ducts and later changes in the external genitalia (Fig. 38.1). Testosterone stimulates the

Fig. 38.1 (a) *Schema of sexual differentiation of internal genitalia. Under the control of the SRY gene on the Y chromosome the undifferentiated gonad develops into a testis. In the absence of this gene, the gonad develops into an ovary. Further female development is characterized by passive regression of the wolffian duct in the absence of testosterone, and continued differentiation of the müllerian duct, in the absence of MIS, into fallopian tubes, uterus and upper vagina. Further male development of the wolffian duct occurs, under the action of testosterone, with differentiation into epididymis, vas deferens and terminal vesicles. (b) The external genitalia differentiate into a male or female depending on the presence of an androgen dihydrotestosterone (DHT). In the male, the inner genital folds fuse to form the urethra on the enlarging genital tubercle to form the penis. The outer genital folds fuse superficially to the urethra to form the scrotum. In females the inner and outer genital folds remain separate and form the labia minora and majora, respectively. (Reproduced, with permission, from Hutson, J.M. and Beasley, S.W. (1988), The Surgical Examination of Children: An Illustrated Guide, p. 258. Oxford: Heinemann Medical.)*

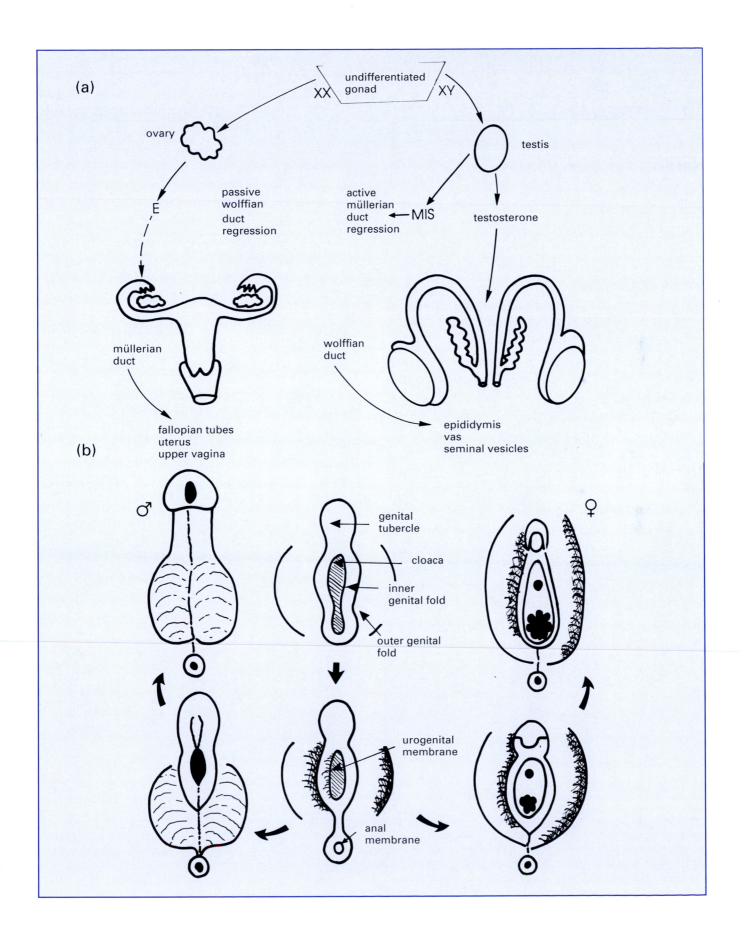

wolffian duct to persist, despite regression of the meso-nephros, and to form the epididymis, vas deferens and seminal vesicle (Wilson *et al.*, 1981; Cunha *et al.*, 1992). The developing testicular cords form a plexus or rete near the cranial part of the testis by fusing with the mesonephric ducts so that the testicular cords are connected directly to the cranial epididymis. The müllerian ducts respond to MIS by regression, so that fallopian tubes, uterus and upper vagina do not persist in the male embryo (Lee and Donahoe, 1993; Josso *et al.*, 1993b). Regression of the müllerian duct is a complex process, and is not simple cell death: receptors for MIS on the

mesenchymal cells around the simple columnar epithelial duct respond initially to the hormone by a combined process of programmed cell death or apoptosis of some epithelial cells and de-differentiation of others into mesenchymal cells (Trelstad *et al.*, 1982). One of the first changes visible microscopically in the müllerian duct is breakdown of the basement membrane and loss of extracellular matrix components around the duct such that on histological fixation shrinkage of the tissue creates a space around the duct (Trelstad *et al.*, 1982). Regression of the cranial regions of the müllerian ducts usually begins before they have reached the urogenital sinus caudally.

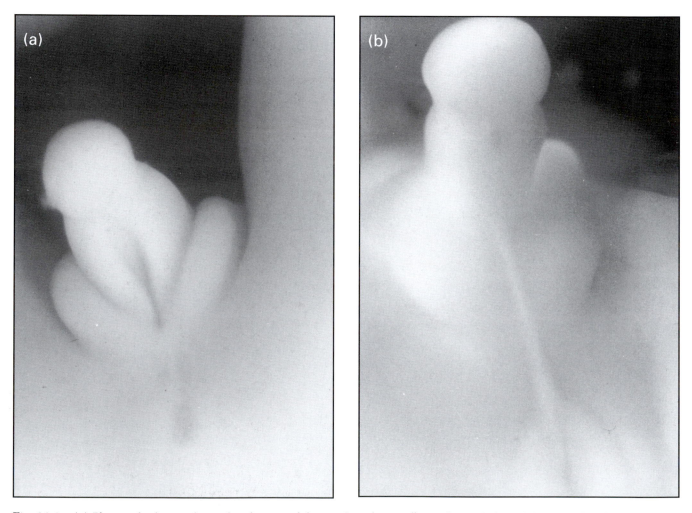

Fig. 38.2   (*a*) *Photograph of external genitalia of nine-week human fetus that is still at ambisexual phase.* (**b**) *Ten-week male fetus showing enlargement of phallus with urethral fusion up to near the coronal groove of the glans penis. The median raphe of the fused scrotum is conspicuous forming a ridge in the perineum extending forward from the anus.* (**c**) *Twelve-week male fetus showing recognizable male genitalia except for development of the prepuce and descent of the testes.* (**d**) *Twelve-week female fetus showing little change from nine weeks except for relative decrease in size of phallus as the adjacent structures have enlarged. (Reproduced, with permission, from England, M.A. (1983), A Colour Atlas of Life Before Birth. Normal Fetal Development, pp. 157–162. London: Wolfe Medical.)*

In the normal female embryo absence of the *SRY* gene allows the ambisexual gonad to continue developing towards an ovary, with enlargement of the cortex and regression of the primitive medulla. The germ cells colonize the cortical region rather than the medullary cords as in the male. The primitive ovary does not manufacture hormones during the first phase of sexual differentiation; oestrogens are produced much later in development (Renfree *et al.*, 1992). Absence of testicular or 'male' hormones in the female genital ridge allows the wolffian duct to degenerate along with the mesonephros, while the müllerian ducts continue their programmed development into fallopian tubes, uterus and fornix of the vagina. The lower two-thirds of the vagina develops from the urogenital sinus (see below).

Up to nine weeks of gestation the external genitalia are still similar in males and females, but testosterone from the testis causes the development in the male to diverge from the basic plan (Fig. 38.2a). The genital tissues contain receptors for androgen as well as an enzyme, 5α-reductase, for converting testosterone to dihydrotestosterone (DHT), which binds 5–10 times more tightly to the androgen receptor than does testosterone itself (Wilson *et al.*, 1981). The conversion to DHT allows the external genitalia to respond to very low levels of androgen in the serum: the developing testis at this time is probably too small to produce sufficient androgen to maintain normal endocrine function as seen postnatally. The wolffian ducts do not contain 5α-reductase, but are exposed to much higher androgen concentrations because of their proximity to

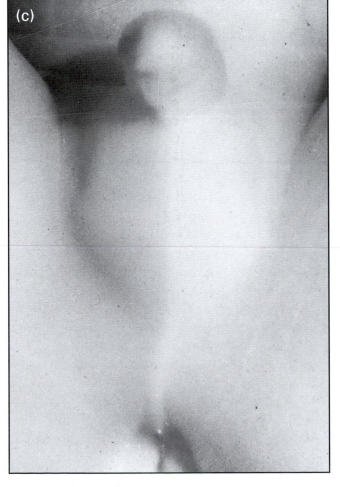

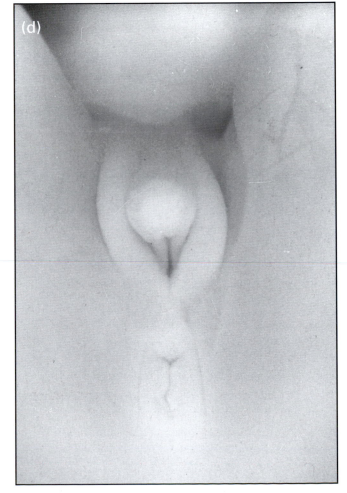

Fig. 38.2 (*continued*)

the testes, which allows local diffusion or may even allow exocrine secretion of testosterone along the ducts (Tong *et al.* 1996).

The genital tubercle in the male responds to DHT by growing faster than the embryo itself such that it enlarges to produce the primitive phallus (Fig. 38.2b). The inner genital folds begin to fuse together posteriorly, covering the urogenital sinus: the fusion continues anteriorly onto the developing phallus, moving the urogenital opening onto the phallic shaft progressively up to the coronal groove at the junction of the glans penis and phallus. Epithelial growth inwards on the ventral glans penis and cavitation forms the glanular urethra which then fuses with the urogenital urethra in midtrimester to form the complete male urethra. The outer genital folds enlarge and fuse with each other superficial to the fusing inner folds, thereby covering over the anterior urethra in the perineum by the developing scrotum. Male genitalia are formed by 10–11 weeks, although further enlargement of the penis and the scrotum continues throughout gestation in response to ongoing androgen production (Fig. 38.2c). The urogenital sinus stops growing in response to androgens, so that with relative enlargement of surrounding tissues, it becomes progressively smaller. The caudal end of the müllerian ducts induces development of the sinovaginal bulbs, which persist as the utriculus masculinus in the verumontanum, adjacent to the openings of the ejaculatory and prostatic ducts. The prostate gland grows from buds from the urogenital sinus into the adjacent androgen-responsive mesenchyme around the ejaculatory ducts.

The external genitalia in the female enlarge with fetal growth although slower growth of the phallus causes it to become relatively smaller as the clitoris (Fig. 38.2d). Absence of androgens allows the urogenital sinus to form the vestibule caudal to the urogenital membrane, which breaks down at about six weeks. Epithelial proliferation of the sinus tubercle where the müllerian ducts had fused previously creates a vaginal plate, which by caudocranial canalization produces the lower two-thirds of the vagina. The exact origin of the hymen is controversial, but may be a persisting remnant of the urogenital diaphragm with secondary mesenchymal ingrowth. Alternatively, it may be derived from the epithelial proliferation of the vaginal

bulb. Maternal oestrogens stimulate vaginal development throughout the latter half of pregnancy, creating a thick, hypertrophied hymen and a significant amount of mucus by the time of delivery; postnatally the hypertrophy regresses and mucus production ceases until puberty.

The position of the gonads is also under complex hormonal control. The human ovaries enlarge on the urogenital ridge, which with growth of the caudal müllerian ducts into a uterus, is held in the enlarging pelvis. The ovaries assume a different position in rodents and ungulates, where the uterus is normally bifid: in these animals the uterus elongates more than in the human such that the ovaries remain high in the lumbar region near the lower pole of the kidneys (Hutson *et al.*, 1992). The female gubernaculum persists as two elongated fibromuscular cords: the ligament of the ovary and the round ligament, linking the lower pole of the gonad to the inguinal region via the body of the uterus just below the attachment of the fallopian tube. The caudal end of the round ligament was believed to be in the labium majus, but recently dissection has demonstrated that it ends just outside the external inguinal ring in the subcutaneous tissues of the groin (Attah and Hutson, 1991) (Fig. 38.3).

The testis begins to move relative to the ovary by 10 weeks of gestation, secondary to hormonally stimulated enlargement of the gubernaculum testis (Hutson and Beasley, 1992). The hormone responsible for this phase is controversial, but is likely to be MIS (Hutson *et al.*, in press). While the ovary moves away from the future internal inguinal ring at 8–10 weeks of gestation, the testis remains very close, held by the shortened and thicker male gubernaculum. This phase has been called the transabdominal phase of testicular descent, but equally could be called the phase of ovarian ascent. By convention, it is the testis which is regarded as moving, as the ovarian position is considered as the starting point because its position is not determined by gonadal hormones.

During the inguinoscrotal phase of descent the testis actually moves through the canal and across the groin to the scrotum in association with the migrating gubernaculum (Fig. 38.4). The testis controls its own movement via testosterone, which acts at least in part indirectly to guide migration via the genitofemoral nerve and

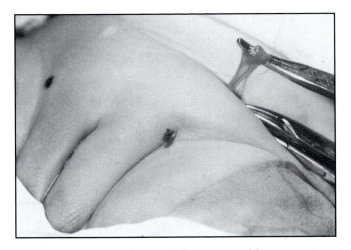

Fig. 38.3 *Operative photograph during inguinal herniotomy in an infant female. Traction on the caudal gubernaculum (round ligament) causes puckering of the skin just outside the external inguinal ring. The palpable ends of the gubernaculum are marked by black dots. Note that the round ligament does not end in the labium majus, as described in current anatomy texts. (Reproduced, with permission, from Attah, A. A. and Hutson, J. M. (1991) The anatomy of the female gubernaculum is different from the male. Aust N.Z. J. Surg. 61: 380–384.)*

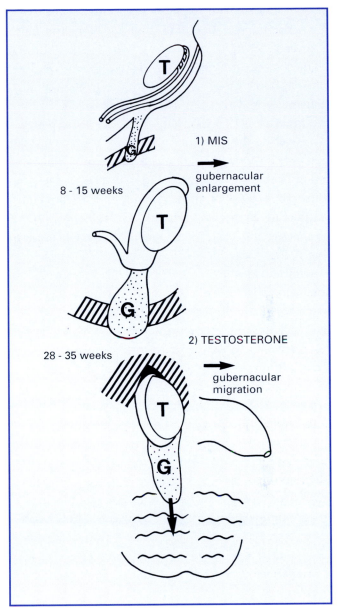

Fig. 38.4 *Testicular (T) descent occurs in two sequential steps at 8–15 weeks and 28–35 weeks, respectively. In the first phase, the gubernaculum (G) enlarges under hormonal control (probably MIS), which anchors the testis near the groin during rapid growth of the embryo. During the second phase, the gubernaculum migrates out from the abdominal wall, across the pubis and into the scrotum. (Reproduced, with permission, from Hutson, J.M. and Beasley, S.W. (1992). Descent of the Testis, p. 14. London: Edward Arnold.)*

release of calcitonin gene-related peptide (CGRP). The reader should consult Chapter 39 for a more detailed description.

Abnormal sexual development

Some sexual anomalies are caused by abnormalities of chromosomal segregation during meiosis in spermatogonia. The ovum may be fertilized by a spermatogonium containing both X and Y (producing a trisomy, 47 XXY; Klinefelter syndrome) or neither sex chromosome (producing 45 XO; Turner syndrome) (Fig. 38.5). Abnormal alignment and separation of chromosomal pairs during meiosis or mitosis may lead to mosaicism, where the embryo contains populations of cells with different numbers of chromosomes. Mosaicism such as 45 XO/46 XY or 46 XX/XY may cause mixed gonadal dysgenesis or true hermaphroditism. Mutations in SRY and other genes may produce pure gonadal dysgenesis.

Even if an ovary or testis develops, intersex can occur if gonadal function is blocked. In the male such conditions are called male pseudohermaphroditism, and may be caused by defects of enzymes in androgen synthesis, anomalies of the androgen receptor causing androgen resistance or insensitivity, or a mutation in 5α-reductase. Mutations in the genes for MIS or its presumed receptor also cause rare forms of male pseudohermaphroditism.

Female pseudohermaphroditism occurs in fetuses where ovarian development is normal but the genitalia are abnormally masculinized by non-gonadal androgens: the commonest anomaly is an enzyme defect in adrenal

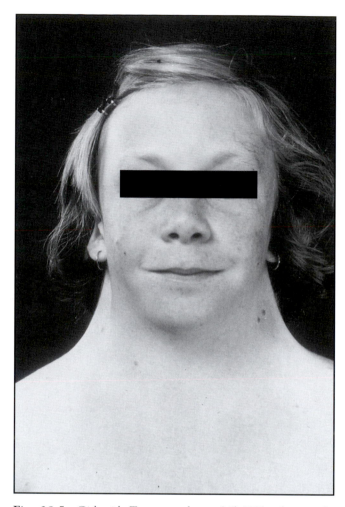

Fig. 38.5 *Girl with Turner syndrome (45 XO), showing the webbed neck caused by spontaneous regression of cervical lymphangiomata in the fetus. The ovaries undergo premature senescence in infancy to form streak gonads. The internal genitalia are normally formed but remain hypoplastic in the absence of ovarian oestrogens.*

Table 38.1 *Eight-year personal experience of patients with genital anomaly*

Female pseudohermaphroditism	
Congenital adrenal hyperplasia	20
Exogenous androgens	2
Male pseudohermaphroditism	
Complete androgen insensitivity	5
Partial androgen insensitivity	5
5α-reductase deficiency	1
Ketosteroid reductase deficiency	2
Drash syndrome	2
Pure gonadal dysgenesis	24
Mixed gonadal dysgenesis	
Persistent müllerian duct syndrome	4
True hermaphroditism	4
Miscellaneous	
Hypopituitarism	1
XO/XY Turner's syndrome	1
Urogenital sinus	2
Secondary androgen failure	1
Buried penis	3
Severe hypospadias/bifid scrotum	3

steroid synthesis such that androgens are produced; alternative sources of androgens include maternal tumours or ingested androgens in the maternal diet.

A review of the patients seen with intersex over recent years shows that congenital adrenal hyperplasia (CAH) is the most common condition (Table 38.1).

Congenital adrenal hyperplasia (CAH)

CAH is a group of autosomal recessive disorders affecting both sexes, but usually only causing intersex in genetic females. In the synthetic pathway from cholesterol via progesterone to cortisol, enzymatic defects at several different levels can cause a build up of intermediary metabolites which are then converted into androgens (Fig. 38.6). The commonest defect is in 21-hydroxylase, which causes

low levels of cortisol and aldosterone in the fetus (and postnatally). Loss of the normal feedback inhibition of the hypothalamus by cortisol causes increased secretion of corticotrophin-releasing factor, which in turn leads to excess production of adrenocorticotrophic hormone (ACTH) and melanin-stimulating hormone (MSH). Excess ACTH causes hypertrophy of the fetal adrenal glands, which convert the cortisol precursors into androgens. Virilization of the fetus is proportional to the severity of the original enzyme defect. Aldosterone deficiency, when present, causes loss of sodium chloride from the kidney and secondary dehydration. Cortisol deficiency reduces resistance to stress, and even trivial infections may induce collapse with vomiting, diarrhoea and dehydration (Addisonian crisis). Less common enzyme defects lead to excess production of deoxycorticosterone which induces hypertension.

The virilization of the external genitalia is quite variable between patients, as the underlying mutations produce different levels of dysfunction in the steroidogenic enzymes. The degree of masculinization is graded according to the Prader scale (Fig. 38.7) (Prader, 1954). Within each patient the degree of virilization of the external genitalia is proportional to that of the internal genitalia. The length and site of opening of the vagina is

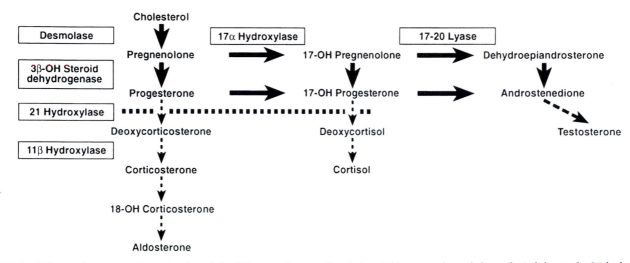

Fig. 38.6 *Schema of enzyme pathway in adrenal gland for manufacture of cortisol and aldosterone from cholesterol. A defect in the 21-hydroxylase, which is the most common anomaly, leads to a build up of intermediary metabolites (e.g. 17-hydroxy progesterone) and abnormal synthesis of the androgen androstenedione.*

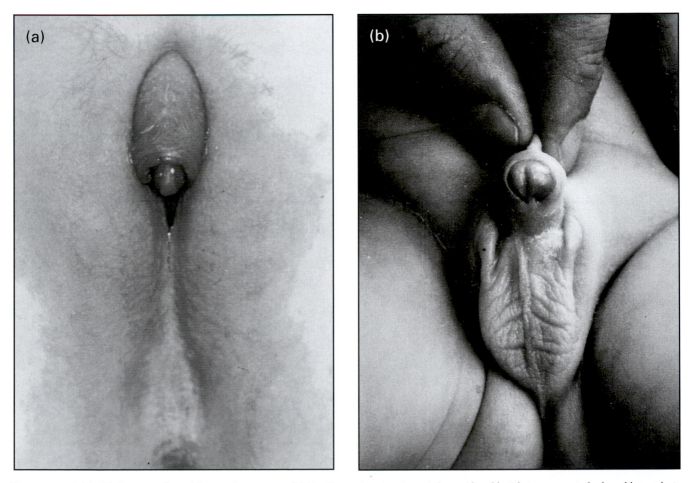

Fig. 38.7 *(a) Mild clitoromegaly and fusion of inner genital folds of cover introitus in an infant with mild virilizing congenital adrenal hyperplasia (CAH). (b) Female infant with severe virilizing CAH showing almost normal penis with chordee. The well-formed scrotum contains no gonads. ((a) Reproduced, with permission, from Hutson, JM. (1995), In Clinical Paediatric Endocrinology, 3rd edn., C.G.D. Brook (ed.). Oxford: Blackwell Science (1995). (b) Reproduced, with permission, from Scheffer, I.E., Hutson, J.M., Warne, G.L. and Ennis, G. (1988) Extreme virilization in patients with congenital adrenal hyperplasia fails to induce descent of the ovary. Pediatr. Surg. Int. 3: 165–168.)*

related to the amount of androgen that the embryo is exposed to: this can be predicted from the size of the phallus and the degree of scrotal development. The more severe the external virilization, the shorter is the vaginal remnant and the higher is its opening into the posterior urethra to form a urogenital sinus (Fig. 38.8). In less severe variants, the opening of the vagina may be visible because the oestrogenized hymen can be seen at the apex of the funnel-shaped urogenital sinus. There is no tendency for the ovaries to descend despite high levels of endogenous androgens (Scheffer *et al.*, 1988).

Mixed gonadal dysgenesis (MGD)

Asymmetrical gonadal dysplasia (MGD) is often caused by mosaicism (XO/XY, XX/XY, etc.). Although both gonads are dysplastic, one has variable testicular develop-

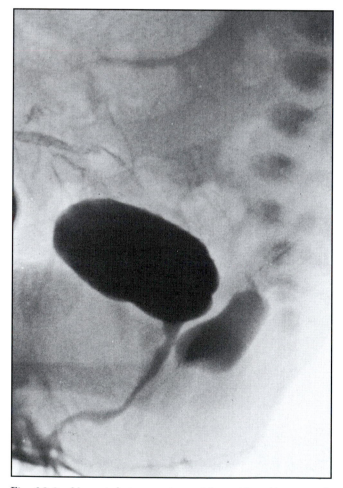

Fig. 38.8 *Urogenital sinugram in an infant with ambiguous genitalia caused by gonadal dysgenesis. Note the large vagina behind the bladder and posterior urethra. (Reproduced, with permission, from Hutson, J.M. (1995), In Clinical Paediatric Endocrinology, 3rd edn. C.G.D. Brook (ed.). Oxford: Blackwell Science (1995).*

ment while the other is an undifferentiated 'streak' gonad. The dysplastic testis induces a variable degree of masculinization and may induce its own descent; the streak gonad remains completely undescended (Fig. 38.9). The genital ducts also are asymmetrical, with some preservation of the müllerian duct ipsilateral to the streak gonad. The degree of müllerian duct development is variable on the side of the dysplastic testis. The amount of retained müllerian duct ipsilateral to the testicular gonad is inversely related to its descent (Scott, 1987; Abe and Hutson, 1994a).

Androgen-insensitivity syndrome (AIS)

Complete or partial AIS is a common form of intersex in genetic males. Mutations in the androgen receptor causing complete AIS (or testicular feminization syndrome) lead to female external genitalia, but with the testes often partly descended in inguinal herniae (Hutson, 1986) (Fig. 38.10). The müllerian duct derivatives are deficient or absent. The lower two-thirds of the vagina is normal but blind-ending because of normal regression of the müllerian ducts. Incomplete AIS leads to variable feminization depending on the severity of the androgen receptor mutation (Fig. 38.11).

Deficiency of 5α-reductase causes partial feminization of the external genitalia in genetic males (Griffin, 1992). The internal genitalia are masculinized relatively normally. This rare mutation is usually seen in very iso-

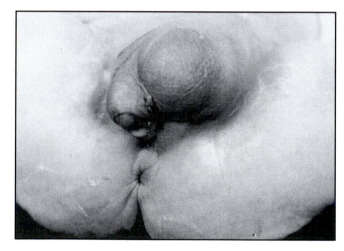

Fig. 38.9 *Infant with ambiguous genitalia caused by mixed gonadal dysgenesis. Note the hypospadiac phallus and one descended gonad in the hemi-scrotum. Just below the phallus is some mucus which was produced in the concealed vagina in response to maternal hormones. (Reproduced, with permission, from Hutson, J.M.; and Beasley, S.W. 1992. Descent of the Testis. p. 29. London: Edward Arnold.)*

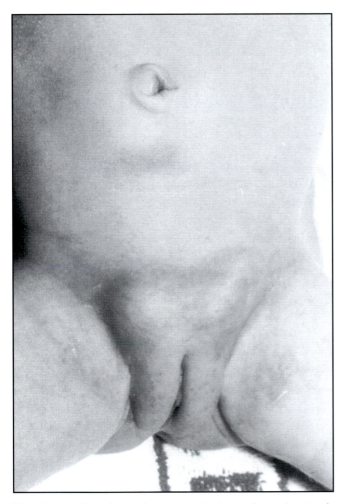

Fig. 38.10 *Complete androgen insensitivity syndrome (previously called testicular feminization). Note the normal female external genitalia but partially descended testes in the inguinal region. (Reproduced, with permission, from Hutson, J.M. and Beasley, S.W. (1992), Descent of the Testis, p. 22. London: Edward Arnold.)*

lated communities with significant inbreeding, hence its first description in Caribbean islands and subsequent recognition in some Pacific islands. The enzyme is no longer necessary at puberty because testosterone secretion is so much greater than during fetal development. Secondary masculinization is, therefore, common at puberty and may lead to gender reversal in an untreated child brought up as a girl.

In patients with both vasa deferentia and a vagina, the vas usually opens into the apex of a bifid vaginal fornix. The seminal vesicles are often absent or open separately into the vaginal remnant, while prostatic development is poor. Such children who are raised as boys would be expected to lack ejaculatory function after sexual maturity.

True hermaphroditism

In ancient times, people who had both breasts and a penis were called hermaphrodites, after the god Hermes and the goddess Aphrodite. The modern definition of a true hermaphrodite is someone with both ovarian and testicular tissue with potentially viable ova and spermatogonia, respectively (Fig. 38.12). Such patients may have mixed gonads, or ovotestes, or have a different gonad on each side (Fig. 38.13). The genetic cause of true hermaphroditism is sometimes obvious mosaicism (e.g. XX/XY) although many have 46 XX chromosomes and are presumed to have occult mosaicism within the gonads.

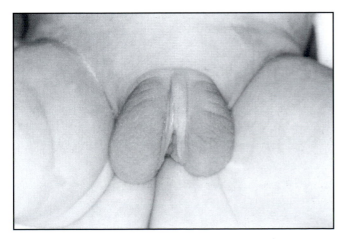

Fig. 38.11 *Partial androgen insensitivity syndrome with descended gonads in hemi-scrota but hypoplastic (concealed) phallus.*

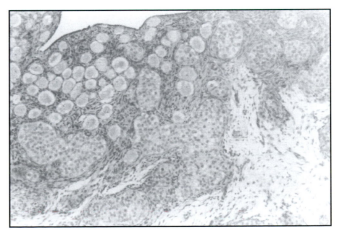

Fig. 38.12 *Photomicrograph of the ovotestis in an infant with true hermaphroditism. Note the presence of ovarian follicles adjacent to seminiferous tubules.*

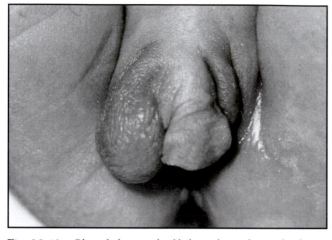

Fig. 38.13 *Clinical photograph of baby with true hermaphroditism. The left gonad, which was an ovotestis, is incompletely descended.*

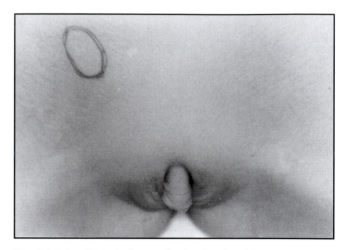

Fig. 38.15 *Clinical photograph of a female adolescent presenting with primary amenorrhoea. Note the clitoromegaly and palpable gonad (testis) marked on the inguinal region. There was a defect in androgen synthesis caused by a mutation in the gene for 17-ketosteroid reductase.*

Other anomalies

Partial virilization of the external genitalia, usually manifested as an enlarged phallus, can occur where the female fetus is exposed to exogenous androgens, such as maternal tumours or dietary ingestion (Fig. 38.14).

Genetic defects in the gonadal steroidogenic enzymes can lead to feminine phenotype in a genetic male. Like complete androgen resistance, the normally-formed testis may be palpable in the groin. These children may

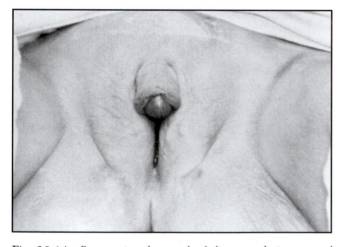

Fig. 38.14 *Preoperative photograph of clitoromegaly in a normal female infant exposed to androgens* in utero *from the maternal diet.*

present in adolescence with primary amenorrhoea and/or partial virilization (Fig. 38.15).

Vaginal atresia is a rare genital anomaly and does not present with ambiguity or intersex at birth. Maternally-stimulated vaginal mucus (mucocolpos) may accumulate behind an imperforate hymen producing bulging at birth. If not diagnosed the mucus is gradually resorbed and the girl develops pain at the onset of puberty with haematometrocolpos. Labial adhesions commonly are confused with vaginal atresia but are merely secondary adherence of ulcerated labia minora in an infant with ammoniacal dermatitis (Leung *et al.*, 1993). Abnormal masculinization is readily excluded by the fact that there is neither clitoral enlargement nor wrinkling and pigmentation of the labia.

Vaginal atresia may be secondary to deficient/arrested caudal migration of the müllerian ducts: no ureteric bud forms leading to ipsilateral absence of the kidney and the ipsilateral müllerian duct ends blindly. One half of the bifid genital tract is atretic, causing haematometrocolpos in adolescence; because the contralateral side is patent, the menstral cycle seems normal but the child has cyclic abdominal pains and an enlarging pelvic mass (see Chapter 4).

Normal testicular descent

Testicular descent is not a simple one-stage mechanism, but a complex multistaged process occurring only in mammals. The result of this complex developmental process is location of the postnatal testis in the subcutaneous scrotum, which functions as a specialized, low-temperature environment for the testis (Zorgniotti, 1991).

After sexual differentiation begins, between seven and eight weeks in the human, the fetal testis starts to move to a different position from that of the ovary. The testis remains close to the site of the future inguinal canal, while the ovary moves away from the inguinal canal as the embryo enlarges. The gonads are held by the cranial suspensory ligament superiorly, and the gubernaculum inferiorly (Fig. 39.1). The cranial suspensory ligament persists in the female, holding the ovary near the pelvic brim in humans, or near the lower pole of the kidney in rodents (van der Schoot, 1993). Caudally, the female gubernaculum elongates in simple proportion to the enlargement of the abdominal cavity to form the ligament of the ovary and the round ligament. In the male, the cranial suspensory ligament regresses while the caudal gubernaculum enlarges, especially at its distal end, where it is embedded in the inguinal abdominal wall.

The inguinal canal is formed by condensation of the mesenchyme around the gubernaculum to form the inguinal musculature. The gubernacular mesenchyme persists to form a solid cord which will later become hollowed out by a diverticulum of the peritoneal membrane, the processus vaginalis. The enlargement of the gubernaculum is caused by deposition of extracellular matrix and uptake of water to form a gelatinous structure (Backhouse, 1982). The proximal end of the gubernaculum, which is initially attached to the gonad, becomes expanded by growth of the developing caudal epididymis. By 15 weeks of gestation, the ovary has moved cranially to the brim of the developing pelvis, while the testis remains in close proximity to the inside of the future inguinal canal. The processus vaginalis grows caudally into the gubernacular mesenchyme, partly hollowing out the gubernaculum. At the caudal end, the gubernaculum remains solid but the proximal part within the developing inguinal canal is divided into a central column attached to the epididymis and an annular parietal layer, in which the cremaster muscle develops.

At about 25 weeks in the human fetus, the caudal end of the gubernaculum begins to bulge out beyond the inguinal and abdominal wall, and migrates across the pubic region to the scrotum (Heyns, 1987). This is accompanied by elongation of the processus vaginalis within the gubernaculum, so that the testis can exit from the abdominal cavity within it. The migration phase of the gubernaculum and testis is completed at approximately 35 weeks, at which time the testis takes up a permanent position within the scrotum. The residual gelatinous bulk of the distal gubernaculum is then resorbed (Backhouse, 1982). During the migration phase, the gubernaculum appears to burrow its way through the inguinoscrotal mesenchyme. Macroscopically, the end of the gubernaculum is completely loose within the tissues (Fig. 39.2), consistent with enzymatic digestion of the adjacent mesenchyme. Eventually the gubernaculum anchors itself to the tissues at the bottom of the scrotum once migration is complete. Surprisingly, little is known about the enzymes produced during this process, or their hormonal control.

The entire mechanism of testicular descent is believed to be hormonally regulated, as are other aspects of sexual differentiation in mammals (Wilson *et al.*, 1981). There is considerable controversy over which hormones are involved in the process, and the reader

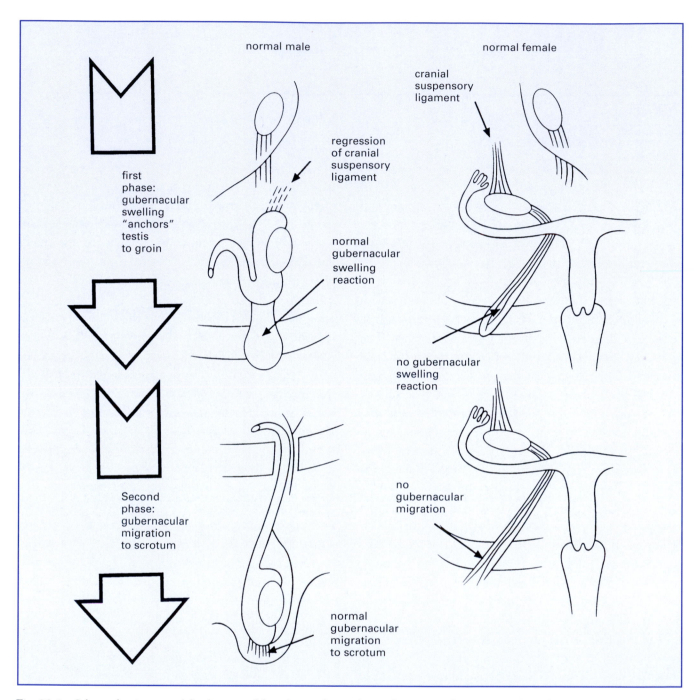

Fig. 39.1 *Schema showing normal development of the gubernaculum and cranial suspensory ligament in males and females. In the first phase of testicular descent (8–15 weeks) the gubernaculum swells while the suspensory ligament regresses. The gubernaculum migrates to the scrotum during the second phase (28–35 weeks).*

should consult several recent reviews discussing these issues (Hutson *et al.*, 1996; Heyns and Hutson, 1995).

Two hormones appear to be important for testicular descent, with the early phase of relative descent within the abdomen being under separate regulation from the subsequent inguinoscrotal phase, where the gubernacu-

lum migrates to the scrotum (Hutson, 1985; Hutson and Donahoe, 1986). Evidence from animal experiments and human mutants shows that the relative positions of the testis and ovary can be accounted for by hormonal control of the gonadal attachments. Androgens are responsible for regression of the cranial suspensory liga-

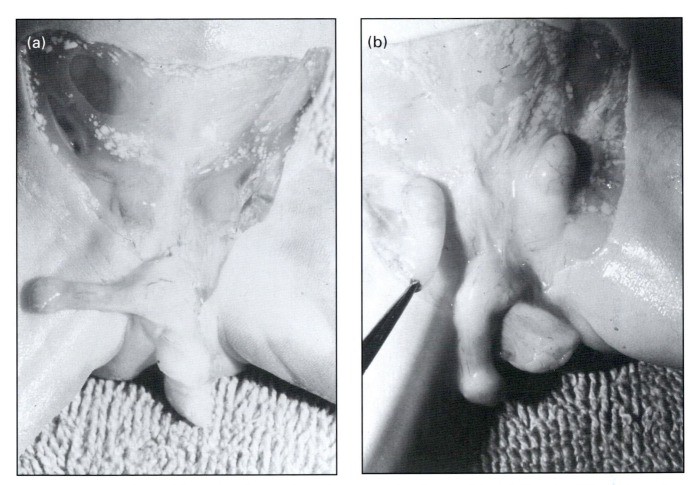

Fig. 39.2 *Dissection of 23-week human fetus showing gubernaculum emerging from the external ring (**a**). Dissection of 25-week human fetus showing the gubernaculum and testis migrating across the pubic region towards the scrotum. A pair of forceps holds up the free caudal end of the right gubernaculum (**b**). (Reprinted, by permission, from Heyns, C. F. (1987), The gubernaculum during testicular descent in the human fetus. J. Anat. 153: 93–112.)*

ment of the testis (van der Schoot and Elgar, 1992), which facilitates, but is not essential for, testicular descent. The enlargement of the gubernaculum testis is controlled by a non-androgenic hormone, the likeliest agent being müllerian inhibiting substance (MIS), also called anti-müllerian hormone (AMH). MIS is a glycoprotein hormone produced by the Sertoli cells in the testis, which induces regression of the embryonic paramesonephric or müllerian duct (Lee and Donahoe, 1993; Josso et al., 1993a). The evidence for and against a role for MIS is summarized in Table 39.1.

Migration of the gubernaculum and testis from the inguinal canal to the scrotum is controlled by androgens, as it is completely absent in syndromes of androgen resistance or gonadotrophin deficiency (Hutson, 1986; Grocock et al., 1988).

The mechanism of androgenic control of gubernacular migration remains uncertain, but there is now a large body of evidence to suggest that the genitofemoral nerve is an important factor (Table 39.2). The gubernaculum is innervated by the genitofemoral nerve (Tayakkanonta, 1963) and recent studies in rodents suggest that the genitofemoral nerve is modified by androgen exposure to become sexually dimorphic. The larger nerve in the male produces an increased amount of a specific neurotransmitter, known as calcitonin gene-related peptide (CGRP) which, at least in rodents, appears to have a major role in gubernacular migration. The gubernaculum contains receptors for CGRP (Table 39.3) and the rodent gubernaculum has rhythmic contractility in organ culture in response to CGRP (Table 39.4). Furthermore, *in vivo* studies in rodents

Table 39.1 *Evidence for and against a role for MIS* in the first phase of testicular descent*

For:
- First phase independent of androgens (Wensing, 1973).
- Low MIS activity in undescended testes (Donahoe *et al.*, 1977).
- Maldescent proportional to müllerian duct retention in intersex patients (Scott, 1987).
- Maldescent proportional to müllerian duct retention in oestrogen-treated mice (Hutson *et al.*, 1990).
- Maldescent and abnormal gubernacular development in persistent müllerian duct syndrome (Hutson *et al.*, 1994).
- Severe maldescent and persisting müllerian ducts in transgenic mice with combined MIS deficiency and androgen resistance (Behringer *et al.*, 1994).

Against:
- Fetal rabbits immunized against MIS still have testicular descent (Tran *et al.*, 1986).
- MIS does not cause cell division of cultured fibroblasts from fetal pig gubernaculum (Fentener van Vlissingen *et al.*, 1988).
- Ovaries not descended (?) in female transgenic mice over-expressing human MIS (Behringer *et al.*, 1990).
- Testes descended in transgenic mice with MIS deficiency but normal androgen levels (Behringer *et al.*, 1994).

*MIS is also called AMH; see page 423.

Table 39.2 *The role of the genitofemoral nerve (GFN) in normal and abnormal testicular descent*

- GFN transection blocks testicular descent (Lewis, 1948; Beasley and Hutson, 1987).
- GFN transection blocks gubernacular migration (Fallat *et al.*, 1992).
- Spinal cord transection blocks testicular descent (Hutson *et al.*, 1988).
- High lumbar myelomeningocele with 35–40 per cent undescended testes (UDT) (Hutson *et al.*, 1988).
- GFN motor nucleus sexually dimorphic (Larkins *et al.*, 1991).
- GFN sexual dimorphism absent after flutamide (Goh *et al.*, 1994).
- GFN sexual dimorphism absent in TS rat (Goh *et al.*, 1994a).
- Capsaicin treatment does not block migration (Shono and Hutson, 1994).

Table 39.3 *CGRP receptor in the rodent gubernaculum*

- CGRP Type-2 binding sites maximal in 1–10-day-old rats (Yamanaka *et al.*, 1992, 1993).
- CGRP binding sites located on developing cremaster muscle.
- Binding increased with flutamide treatment (Terada *et al.*, 1994).
- Binding decreased in TS rat (Terada *et al.*, 1994).
- Binding increased after GFN transection (Yamanaka *et al.*, 1993).
- Binding increased in TS rat after GFN transection (Terada *et al.*, 1995).

Table 39.4 *Contractility of cremaster in organ culture of neonatal rodent gubernaculum*

- Endogenous contractions stimulated by exogenous CGRP (Park and Hutson, 1991; Momose *et al.*, 1992).
- Acetylcholine does not cause rhythmic contractions (Shono *et al.*, 1995).
- CGRP causes increased tone and frequency of contractions (Shono *et al.*, 1995).
- Contractility maximum in 1–10-day-old rats (Terada *et al.*, 1994).
- Cyclic AMP stimulates rhythmic contractions (Momose *et al.*, 1993).
- TFM mouse gubernaculum hypersensitive to CGRP (Momose *et al.*, 1992).
- Flutamide-treated gubernaculum hypersensitive to CGRP (Goh *et al.*, 1993).
- TS rat gubernaculum resistant to CGRP (Goh *et al.*, 1993).
- TS rat gubernaculum sensitive CGRP after GFN transection (Terada *et al.*, 1995).

Table 39.5 *In vivo studies in rodents*

- CGRP(8–37) delays descent in mice (Samarakkody and Hutson, 1992).
- Ectopic CGRP diverts gubernaculum in flutamide rat (Abe and Hutson, 1994).
- CGRP stimulates gubernaculum in TFM mouse (Griffiths *et al.*, 1993).

show that CGRP can modulate gubernacular migration (Table 39.5).

During the migration phase, the force for migration is likely to be provided by intraabdominal pressure within the processus vaginalis as it forms a diverticulum within the gubernaculum. The proximal attachment of the gubernaculum to the developing caudal epididymis and testis provides just enough traction to ensure that the testis and epididymis enter the processus vaginalis and will be pushed down by abdominal pressure. CGRP released from the genitofemoral nerve may direct migration of the gubernaculum and testis towards the scrotum.

Undescended testes

Undescended testes, or cryptorchidism, is a common but poorly understood abnormality, affecting 2–5 per cent of children. Where the testis fails to reach the scrotum, secondary degeneration occurs which is likely to be secondary to the abnormally high temperature of the maldescended testis (Zorgniotti, 1991). The quest for understanding of this complicated anomaly is driven by the desire to prevent the subsequent infertility and risk of testicular tumours which afflict boys with cryptorchidism.

Aetiology

Cryptorchidism is the end result of any anomaly preventing or disrupting normal testicular descent (Hutson and Beasley, 1992). Because of the complexity of the normal process, it is not surprising that the cause of undescended testes is multifactorial. The common causes are not known, but since most undescended testes are located in the groin, it can be seen that the migratory inguinoscrotal phase is more commonly deranged. Intraabdominal testes, by contrast, are relatively uncommon, and only occur in 5–10 per cent of cryptorchid boys. By contrast, most maldescended testes are near the neck of the scrotum, or are just at, or a little lateral to, the external inguinal ring in a space previously called the superficial inguinal pouch. The common forms of maldescent are likely to be abnormalities of gubernacular migration, which may be secondary to defects in the migratory mechanism, or failure of the genitofemoral nerve to release adequate amounts of calcitonin gene-related peptide. Defects of the nerve in turn may be caused by deficiency of androgens during the second and third trimester. Standard endocrine disorders affecting MIS or testosterone do cause failure of descent of testes, but are rare compared with abnormalities of gubernacular migration. Transient deficiency in testosterone during the second and third trimester could be caused by an abnormality of the placental production of chorionic gonadotrophin or an abnormal hypothalamic–pituitary–gonadal axis.

Maldescent of the testes in rare or specific anomalies

Ectopic testes

Maldescended testes lying outside the normal line of descent are quite rare. The testis may be in the perineum, femoral, pubopenile, or may even descend out of the contralateral inguinal canal (transverse ectopia). Ectopic migration beyond the ipsilateral inguinal canal

may be caused by an abnormal location of the genitofemoral nerve. If, as suspected, the genitofemoral nerve attracts the gubernaculum via chemotaxis, then an abnormal site of the nerve will induce abnormal migration. A perineal testis, for example, may therefore be secondary to perineal location of the genitofemoral nerve (Fig. 39.3). Transverse ectopia is likely to be caused by completely different mechanisms. In animal models, transverse ectopia can be readily induced by cutting the gubernacular attachment to the testis, so that the gonad is no longer obliged to exit from the ipsilateral inguinal canal. Gonadal mobility then permits accidental descent through the contralateral inguinal canal. This is a very rare abnormality in otherwise normal males (Beasley and Auldist, 1985), but is common in children with a mutation of the gene for MIS, known as persistent Müllerian duct syndrome (Fig. 39.4) (Hutson et al., 1987, 1994).

Multiple malformation syndromes

Numerous sporadic or inherited syndromes of multiple anomalies cause undescended testes (Table 39.6). In some of these syndromes associated with microcephaly deficiency of pituitary hormones or gonadotrophins may be the underlying cause of the failure of migration of the testes. In recognizable chromosomal disorders, such as a number of trisomies and aneuploidies, prenatal growth deficiency and cryptorchidism suggest either a disorder of the hypothalamus or placental insufficiency. Recognizable disorders of the hypothalamus and pituitary

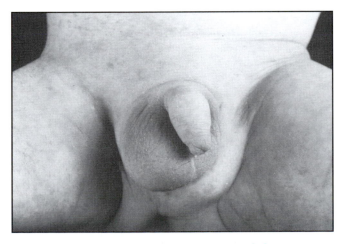

Fig. 39.3 *Perineal ectopic left testis. (Reprinted, by permission, from Hutson, J.M. and Beasley, S.W. (1992), Descent of the Testis, p. 54. London: Edward Arnold.)*

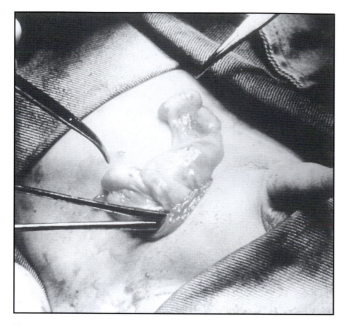

Fig. 39.4 *Persistent müllerian duct syndrome. Operative photograph showing two testes (indicated by forceps) and attached uterus and tubes, all emanating from an inguinal hernial sac (forceps inside sac). Note how far the testes lie not only far from the scrotum but also far from the normal position of ovaries. Abnormal gubernacular development in the absence of MIS allows the testes to be hypermobile intra-abdominal organs. (Courtesy of Dr W-D. Ng, Hong Kong.)*

Table 39.6 *Multiple malformation syndromes with cryptorchidism*

Aaskog syndrome
Beckwith–Wiedemann syndrome
Cockayne syndrome
Cornelia de Lange syndrome
Fraser syndrome
Lowe syndrome
Noonan syndrome
Smith–Lemli–Opitz syndrome

are associated with undescended testes, as expected. This includes a number of syndromes with specific hypothalamic hypogonadism (Table 39.6). Many polymalformation syndromes are also associated with neurogenic and mechanical anomalies. For example, arthrogryposis multiplex congenita causes joint contractures and congenital deficiency of muscle groups, leading to dislocations and deformities. The cause of the abnormality is unknown, but may be related to degeneration of anterior horn cells early in gestation. A review of 57 males with arthrogryposis showed that 18 (32 per cent) had undescended testes (Fallat *et al.*, 1992). Multiple malformation syndromes are also commonly associated with

external compression of the fetus. Inguinal compression during the third trimester may lead to undescended testes at birth, as can be demonstrated experimentally (Luthra *et al.*, 1989).

Prune belly syndrome

High intraabdominal testes is one of the recognized features of the triad syndrome or prune belly syndrome (see Chapter 37). Controversy surrounds the proposed aetiology of prune belly syndrome, which has been proposed as a defect in the mesoderm (Nunn and Stephens, 1961) or a prenatal urinary obstruction (Pagon *et al.*, 1979; Moerman *et al.*, 1984). The site of putative urinary obstruction has not been identified, although it has been proposed that transient obstruction of the developing urethral meatus at the coronal groove may be the cause. Subsequent development of the urethra within the glans, creating a lumen, would overcome the obstruction in mid-trimester (Hutson and Beasley, 1987). Massive enlargement of the bladder has been documented in mid-trimester in prune belly infants (Anderson *et al.*, 1979). During this time, the testes are normally held near the future inguinal canal by the enlarged male gubernaculum. With massive enlargement of the bladder, the gubernaculum might be displaced or torn as the peritoneum is pulled away from the posterior inguinal region (Fig. 39.5). The testes would then come to lie on the posterior surface of the bladder, which is the site normally found in children at operation.

Posterior urethral valves with secondary bladder distension is also related to an increased frequency of cryptorchidism compared with normal males. In most series, this is > 10 per cent (Kreuger *et al.*, 1980). Urethral obstruction in both urethral valves and prune belly syndrome may be responsible. Measurement of the anterior and posterior urethra from micturition cystourethrograms (MCUs) performed postnatally demonstrates abnormal dilatation consistent with prenatal obstruction in both anomalies (Beasley *et al.*, 1988).

Exomphalos and gastroschisis

Cryptorchidism is common in defects of the ventral abdominal wall. In gastroschisis, the incidence of cryptorchidism is > 15 per cent (Kaplan *et al.*, 1986). In exomphalos, cryptorchidism occurs in at least one third (Kaplan *et al.*, 1986). This suggests that there is a correla-

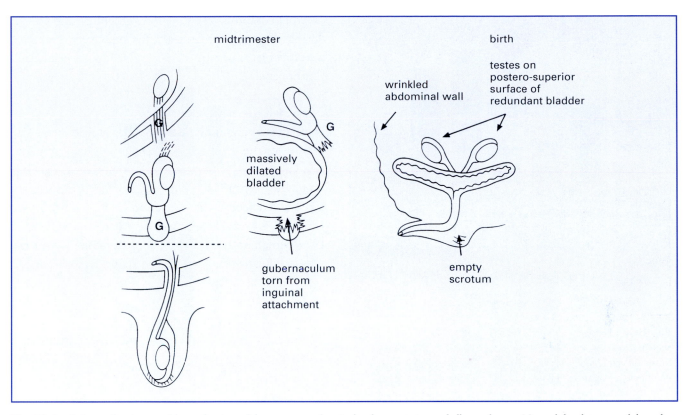

Fig. 39.5 *Schema showing possible mechanism of derangement of testicular descent in prune belly syndrome. Normal development of the gubernaculum (G) is shown down the left side. Massive enlargement of the bladder in midtrimester may disrupt the gubernacular attachment to the inguinal region, leaving the testes located on the superior surface of the bladder at birth.*

tion between cryptorchidism and abnormal abdominal pressure, since in both conditions, the abdominal pressure is lower than normal. Animal experiments confirm that abdominal pressure has a role in normal descent (Attah and Hutson, 1993). Other explanations include the possibility of concomitant brain anomalies causing hypothalamic defects (Hadziselimovic *et al.*, 1987). A further possibility in ventral abdominal-wall defects, particularly gastroschisis, is sudden disruption of the gubernaculum at the time of formation of the defect. There is ultrasound evidence to suggest that gastroschisis may occur secondary to rupture of a physiological hernia or small exomphalos. The gubernaculum may be ruptured by the sudden change of abdominal pressure, and the testis is frequently described as part of the extraabdominal viscera in gastroschisis. This mechanism is analogous to that described previously for transverse ectopia.

Neural-tube defects
Myelomeningocele affecting the upper lumbar spinal cord is associated with undescended testes in more than one-third of boys (Fig. 39.6). This may be caused by dysplasia of the genitofemoral nerve or ganglia at the site of the myelomeningocele (Hutson *et al.*, 1988).

Cloacal exstrophy
Cryptorchidism is relatively common in this rare anomaly, and is likely to be related to severe derangement in the inguinoscrotal anatomy (Hutson and Beasley, 1989).

Cerebral palsy
A high incidence of cryptorchidism, ≤ 50 per cent (Rundle *et al.*, 1982), has been reported in adult males with cerebral palsy. The cause in this multifactorial problem is unknown, but has been postulated to be a secondary abnormality postnatally, related to an upper motor neurone lesion affecting the cremaster muscle. A study of children with cerebral palsy shows a clear trend towards an acquired abnormality with age (Fig. 39.7) (Smith *et al.*, 1989).

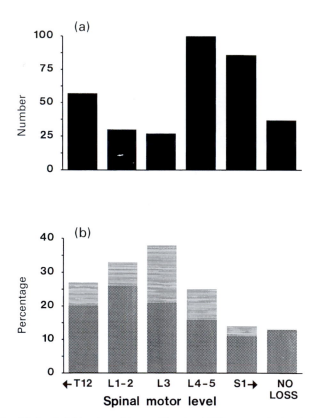

Fig. 39.6 (*a*) *Number of boys with spina bifida versus the level of the spinal motor level.* (**b**) *Percentage of boys with spina bifida who have cryptorchidism versus spinal level of the defect. Cross-hatched bars: unilateral cryptorchidism; horizontal bars: bilateral cryptorchidism.*

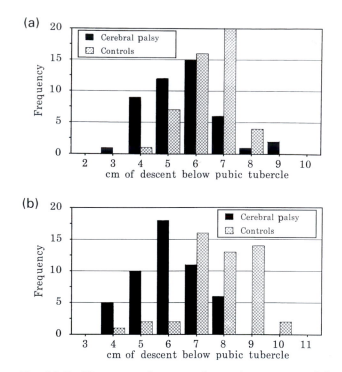

Fig. 39.7 *Histograms of position of testis (in centimetres below pubic tubercle) versus frequency in boys with cerebral palsy (dark bars) and normal males (cross-hatched bars).* (**a**) *Infants < 30 months of age.* (**b**) *Boys between 5 and 10 years of age. (Reproduced, with permission, from Smith, J.A., Hutson, J.M., Beasley, S.W. and Reddihough, D.S. (1989), The relationship between cerebral palsy and cryptorchidism. J. Pediatr. Surg. 23: 275–277.)*

Testicular epididymal fusion anomalies

Separation of the body of the epididymis from the testes occurs frequently in undescended testes (Gill *et al.*, 1989), but its significance is uncertain. Recent experimental evidence in rodents treated with anti-androgens suggests that the epididymal deficiency is secondary to *in utero* androgen deficiency (Cain *et al.*, 1994).

Some cryptorchid testes are associated with anomalies of the vas deferens: impalpable, intracanalicular testes may have a long vas deferens forming a loop that protrudes from the external inguinal ring (Fig. 39.8).

Fowler and Stephens (1959) confirmed by angiography that both the normal and cryptorchid testis with a long-loop vas are supplied by anastomoses from the internal spermatic (testicular), vasal and external spermatic (cremasteric) vessels. The Fowler–Stephens operation, therefore, was developed for the undescended testis with a looped vas deferens: ligation and transection of the internal spermatic vessels would allow the testis to reach the scrotum on a vascular pedicle of the cremasteric and vasal arteries. The results of orchidopexy by the Fowler–Stephens method were encouraging (Gibbons *et al.*, 1979), but recently described two-stage procedures have also been successful (Ransley *et al.*, 1984). This procedure has been of benefit in prune belly syndrome and now the first stage (ligation of testicular vessels on the psoas muscle) is commonly performed laparoscopically (Elder, 1989).

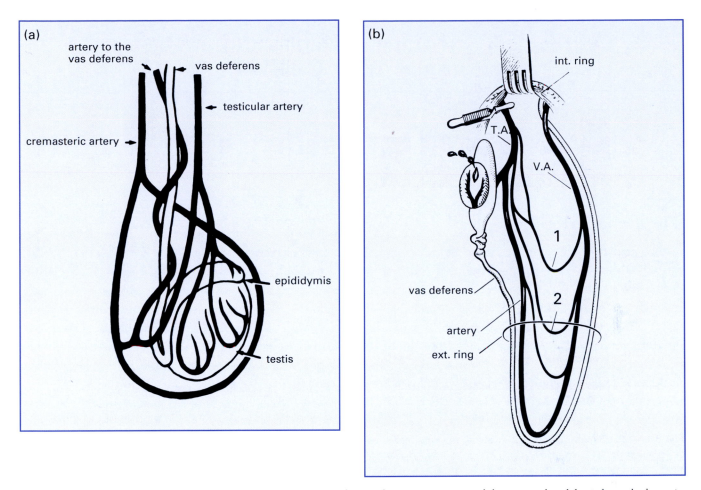

Fig. 39.8 (*a*) *Normal blood supply of the testis. Three arteries contribute to the anastomosis around the testis and epididymis but only the testicular artery supplies the testis directly.* (*b*) *The 'long-loop' vas associated with an undescended testis located at the internal inguinal ring. The artery to the vas (VA) runs along the loop with several anastomotic branches (1 and 2). The adequacy of the anastomoses is tested by whether the testis bleeds when incised while a bulldog clamp is placed on the testicular artery (TA).(a) Reproduced, with permission, from Lee, L.M., Johnson, H.W. and McLoughlin, M.G. (1984) Microdissection and radiographic studies of the arterial vasculature of the human testes. J. Ped. Surg. Vol. 19, No. 3: 287–301, Fig. 5. ((b) Reproduced, with permission, from Fowler, F. and Stephens, F.D. (1959), The role of testicular vascular anatomy in the salvage of high undescended testes. Aust. N.Z. J. Surg. 29: 92–106.)*

40

Ontogeny of congenital anomalies of the kidney and urinary tract, CAKUT

Yoichi Miyazaki, John C. Pope IV, Fumiyo Kuwayama, F. Douglas Stephens and Iekuni Ichikawa

The term, CAKUT

Although congenital anomaly of the kidney is closely related to that of the ureter and the other portions of the urinary tract, there has been little exchange of scientific information between the urology and nephrology scientific communities. For example, while the quarter-century old bud theory (described in detail below) of Mackie and Stephens (1975) is familiar to all urologists today, it remains virtually unknown to nephrologists, even though the theory refers not only to the ureter but also very much to the renal anomalies. Conversely, although many, if not all, nephrologists are familiar with the recent notion that the metanephric mesenchyme induces the ureteral budding from the wolffian duct through regulatory molecules, urologists are aware only of the notion on the reverse relationship, namely that the ureter promotes the differentiation of the metanephric mesenchyme.

Through discussions among the present authors—urologists and nephrologists—we realized that this lack of communication between the two communities is attributable largely to the long-held dogmatic views that each of the communities had been harbouring. Thus, whereas the nephrology community considers the ureter and everything below it as just a conduit, the urology community regards the kidney as a part of the urinary tract. The latter led to implicit inclusion of kidney anomalies when urologists described anomalies of the urinary tract, although they did not explicitly state the term 'kidney' in their title (Stephens *et al.*, 1996). As a result, excellent investigative work by urologists has not been brought to the attention of nephrologists. Obviously, the kidney is not just an excretory tract but also an endocrine organ, producing an active form of vitamin D and erythropoietin, while the ureter (and

below) is not just a conduit but a dynamic organ performing a complex task.

In the hope of increasing the exchange of scientific information between the urology and nephrology communities, therefore, we have recently coined the term 'CAKUT' (congenital anomalies of the kidney and urinary tract), so that not only urologists but also nephrologists will recognize the relevance of these anomalies to the organ of their interest.

The CAKUT's are a family of diseases with a diverse anatomical spectrum. They include kidney anomalies, (e.g. kidney aplasia, multicystic dysplastic kidney, hypoplastic kidney), ureteropelvic anomalies (e.g. ureteropelvic junction obstruction, ureterovesical junction obstruction, vesicoureteral reflux, ectopic ureteral orifice, megaureter, duplex collecting system) and anomalies of the bladder and urethra (Brown *et al.*, 1987).

It is of note that these abnormalities are often concurrent. For instance, hypoplastic kidney and dysplastic kidney are often accompanied by vesicoureteral reflux or ureteropelvic junction obstruction involving the ipsilateral or contralateral kidney (Atiyeh *et al.*, 1992). It is also noteworthy that these anomalies have a familial pattern, showing incomplete and variable penetrance (Squiers *et al.*, 1987).

It has been speculated, therefore, that they share a common pathogenic mechanism and genetic causes. In this regard, *PAX2*, the gene for a paired-box transcription factor, has been identified as the responsible gene, the mutation of which is associated with a special subgroup of CAKUT seen in the renal-coloboma syndrome (Sanyanusin *et al.*, 1995). In addition, it has been shown that haploinsufficiency for *EYA1*, a homologue of *Drosophila melanogaster* gene eyes absent (*eya*), results in the dominantly inherited disorders branchio-oto-renal

(BOR) syndrome, which involves kidney and urinary tract anomalies (Chen *et al.*, 1995; Abdelhak *et al.*, 1997). It has not been well understood, however, how these mutations result in the diverse spectrum of CAKUT.

Ontogeny of CAKUT

To explain how such a wide spectrum of anomalies occur in the kidney and urinary tract system, several theories have been proposed.

1. Physical stress as a result of urinary tract obstruction.
2. Physical stress as a result of dysfunction of bladder or vesicoureteral junction.
3. Ectopic initial budding of the ureter.
4. Primary defect in the metanephric mesenchyme–ureteric bud interaction.

It has been long thought that renal dysgenesis, often seen in combination with other phenotypes of CAKUT, is caused by urinary tract obstruction. Indeed, Peters *et al.* (1992) created complete obstruction at various anatomical levels along the urinary tract of fetal sheep at 55 to 66 days of gestation (comparable to 14 to 16 weeks' gestation in humans) and found a variety of responses by the renal parenchyma. They noted that the most remarkable consequence of fetal obstructive uropathy was its effect on renal parenchymal growth. Specifically, kidneys with unilateral obstruction were always small and cystic/dysplastic in comparison with controls. These observations led some investigators to believe that some degree of urinary tract obstruction and the resultant abnormal physical stress are the intermediary insults for the development of renal hypo/dysplasia. However, other investigators question the role of obstruction in the development of renal parenchymal lesions in CAKUT, on the grounds that many human specimens have shown a lack of correlation between the degree of obstruction and the severity of renal parenchymal abnormality (Stephens *et al.*, 1996).

The development of the kidney and urinary tract depends on reciprocal interactions between the ureteric bud and the surrounding metanephric mesenchyme. Thus, their development begins with the budding of the ureter from the wolffian duct towards the metanephric mesenchyme. Subsequently, the ureteric bud undergoes

dichotomous branching under the influence of metanephric mesenchyme, and finally differentiates into the ureter, the pelvis and the collecting duct. Meanwhile metanephric mesenchyme is induced by factors derived from the ureteric bud to differentiate into epithelial cells that finally give rise to the proximal and distal tubules and the glomeruli (Saxen, 1987). Therefore, interference in the interaction between the ureteric bud and the metanephric mesenchyme in the initial step of kidney and urinary tract development concurrently can bring about both renal parenchymal dysgenesis and urinary tract malformation. Thus, it is plausible that the renal parenchymal anomalies are a result of an abnormal ureteric bud–metanephric mesenchyme interaction, where the obstruction may be merely an epiphenomenon.

Bud theory
Mackie's and Stephens' hypothesis

A unique but now popular theory was derived from a different perspective, via extensive inspection of numerous specimens from human embryos and neonates. This theory stems from observed morphological correlations between the location of the ureteral orifice, the degree of renal hypoplasia and/or dysplasia, and abnormalities of the ureter (Mackie and Stephens, 1975). The hypothesis proposes that these abnormalities are derived from a single common mechanism and are programmed at the time of initial budding of the ureter from the wolffian duct (Fig. 40.1). Note that in the developing embryo, the terminal segment of the wolffian duct is absorbed into the cloaca to form the hemitrigone of the developing bladder. In this process, therefore, the initial budding site of the ureter (normally at Site B) will normally migrate and reach its final destination, i.e. the corner of the bladder trigone (Site B), to form the ureteral orifice in the bladder. Mackie and Stephens postulated that when ureteral budding occurs at an abnormal site (e.g. Site A), the final site of the ureteral orifice will be abnormal (e.g. Site A) as well, thereby often resulting in ureterovesical reflux. In addition, the ectopia has the potential to produce anomalous kidney parenchyma because the bud from the ectopic site makes contact with poorly differentiated portions of the metanephric mesenchyme, which become the precursor for the later hypoplastic and/or dysplastic kidney.

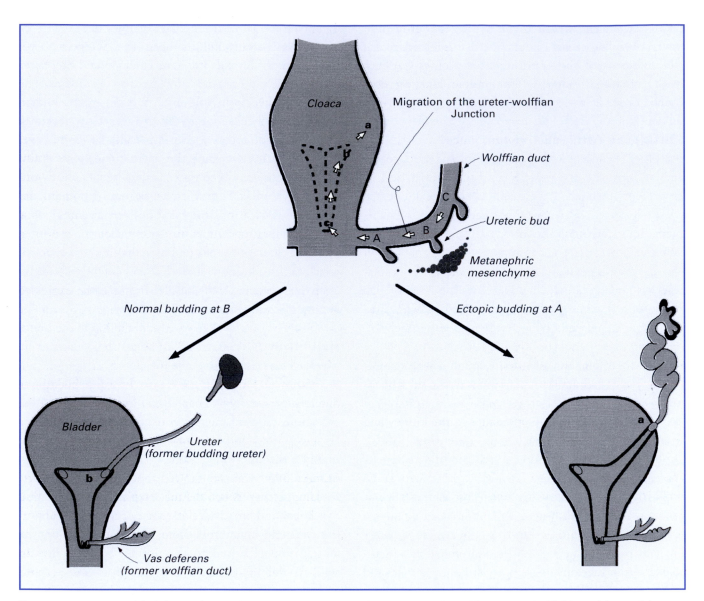

Fig. 40.1 *Dynamics of the kidney and ureteral development and the 'bud theory'. The orifices of the ureter in the bladder and the vas deferens in normal mature animals are located at the corner of the hemitrigone and in the prostatic urethra, respectively. These sites are the result of migration and incorporation of the terminal segment of the wolffian duct into the urogenital sinus, ultimately forming the hemitrigone of the developing bladder. The migration places the normal ureteric bud orifice 'B' on the corner (Site b), and an ectopic bud orifice, 'A', on the lateral and cranial end of the hemitrigone (Site a). The ureterovesical junction from the 'A' ureteral bud results in a vesicoureteral reflux. The metanephric (mesoderm) is well differentiated when interacting with a bud at the normal site 'B' but sparse and poorly differentiated around bud 'A' (and bud 'C'). The interaction between bud and blastema is thus critical for the ontogeny of both ureter and metanephros, and abnormal interactions can result in various forms of CAKUT (reflux, hypodysplasia, obstruction, etc.).*

Therefore, anomalies in three different tissues constituting CAKUT (i.e. abnormal ureterovesical junction, abnormalities of the ureter and dysmorphic kidney) can be derived from a single abnormal embryonic event (i.e. ectopic ureteral budding).

Ectopic initial budding of the ureter in mouse models of CAKUT

Although the Mackie's and Stephens' hypothesis can comprehensively explain the ontogeny of CAKUT, it has been neither proven nor disproven, since it is impossible, ethically or technically, to verify that ectopic budding occurs in humans. In this regard, recent studies of several congenital mouse models of CAKUT have provided evidence that ectopic budding does indeed occur at the early stage of the development of CAKUT.

CAKUT in Agtr2 null mutant mice. Of the two receptors for angiotensin II, angiotensin Type 2 receptor (AT2) is the one more recently identified, and its gene (*Agtr2*) cloned (Kambayashi *et al.*, 1993). Located on the X chromosome, *Agtr2* has been shown to be primarily an embryonic gene in rodents and humans, i.e. it is actively transcribed at the onset of and throughout the embryonic development of the kidney and urinary tract system and largely inactivated by the time of birth (Gasc *et al.*, 1994; Kakuchi *et al.*, 1995). When *Agtr2* was target-inactivated by genetic engineering technology, and its phenotype was screened, no apparent anatomical anomaly was initially found in the mutant (Hein *et al.*, 1995; Ichiki *et al.*, 1995). In the subsequent extensive observations, however, it was noted that 2–3% of mutant mice had anomalies in the kidney and urinary tract system, which were absent in normal, wild-type animals. To increase the penetrance rate of this abnormal phenotype, mutants which had given birth to anomalous offspring were cross mated, and, by repeating this inbreeding, the penetrance rate reached approx. 20%, indicating that this anomaly is also regulated by other gene(s). Detailed anatomical and histological examinations of *Agtr2* mutant embryos and neonates revealed that the abnormal phenotype mimics all the key features that characterize human CAKUT (Nishimura *et al.*, 1999). Thus, in *Agtr2* mutants, a wide anatomical spectrum of anomalies (e.g. ureteropelvic junction stenosis, hypoplastic kidney, vesicoureteral reflux, megaureter, double collecting system) were seen within the same pedigree in a random manner, with each specific anatomical pattern having its own counterpart in humans (Brown *et al.*, 1987). Also, as in humans, CAKUT of *Agtr2* nullizygotes appear predominantly in males, and in a highly asymmetrical manner (Johnston *et al.*, 1977; Najmaldin *et al.*, 1990; Coret *et al.*, 1994). Furthermore, mice and humans also share renal histological characteristics, namely lack of interstitial fibrosis at birth, with some hypoplastic, cystic and/or dysplastic parenchyma.

Finally, some *Agtr2* null mutants have a duplex system, which universally fulfills both the Weigert–Meyer (Weigert, 1877) and Stephens (Mackie and Stephens, 1975) rules established for human CAKUT. The Weigert–Meyer principle predicts that, in the human duplex kidney/ureter system, the upper kidney mass drains into the orifice within the bladder at a site lower than the orifice to which the lower kidney mass drains (Weigert, 1877). According to the Stephens relationship, if a duplex kidney/ureter system in humans has both histologically normal and dysplastic renal masses, the normal tissue drains into the bladder at a normal site, whereas the dysplastic tissue drains at an aberrant site (Mackie and Stephens, 1975).

In the normal, *Agtr2* mRNA begins to be expressed intensely in the mesenchymal cells that surround the wolffian duct at the time of initial budding of the ureter (embryonic day 11.0, E11.0, in mice) (Nishimura *et al.*, 1999). This finding gave rise to the first suggestion that *Agtr2* may play a role in regulating the initial budding of the ureter from the wolffian duct. Most recently, analysis of whole tissues and sections showed that ectopic budding does indeed occur in *Agtr2* null mutant embryos (Oshima *et al.*, 2000). Thus, approximately half of the mutant embryos showed abnormal initial ureteric budding, either as two distinct buds or as one bud that was larger and broader, relative to normal. These abnormal ureteric buds arose from an ectopic site on the wolffian duct cranial to the normal budding site. In wild-type embryos, *Agtr2* is expressed at this 'ectopic' cranial site between the wolffian duct and metanephric mesenchyme, beginning at E11.0, but is not expressed at the normal budding site, i.e. the caudal end of the wolffian duct. Thus, *Agtr2* can play a role in the embryonic development of the urinary tract by preventing aberrant ureteric budding from the wolffian duct. A defect in this regulatory process results in ectopic ureteric budding and subsequently leads to a duplex collecting system and other CAKUTs, as noted in Mackie's and Stephens' hypothesis. Furthermore, the observation that the incidence of ectopic initial budding of the ureter in mutant embryos is higher than the actual phenotypic expression of urinary tract anomalies in mature form suggests that most ectopic ureteral budding can be repaired by some regulatory mechanisms during embryonic development.

CAKUT *in heterozygous Bmp4 null mutant mice.*
Bone morphogenetic protein 4 (BMP4), a member of the transforming growth factor β (TGF-β) superfamily of secretory signalling molecules, has been implicated in many aspects of embryonic development, ranging from establishment of the basic embryonic body plan to morphogenesis of individual organs, by regulating cell proliferation, differentiation, apoptosis and cell fate determination (Hogan, 1996). The essential role of BMP4 in embryonic development is confirmed by the lethality between E6.5 and E10.0, in mouse embryos (E20 is full term in mice), of homozygosity for null mutations in *Bmp4* (*Bmp4* –/–) (Winnier *et al.*, 1995; Lawson *et al.*, 1999). Moreover, even in heterozygous mutants (*Bmp4* +/–), several defects have been described, including skeletal abnormalities, eye defects and cystic kidneys accompanied by urinary tract anomalies (Dunn *et al.*, 1997). Detailed examination of the excretory system revealed that some 50% of *Bmp4* +/– mice have anomalies that closely mimic human CAKUT, including hypoplastic/dysplastic kidneys, hydroureter and double collecting systems (Miyazaki *et al.*, 2000a). Of note, similar to human CAKUT, this mouse CAKUT includes ectopic ureterovesical junction, i.e. the location of the ureteric orifice being abnormally caudal to the normal site. Analyses of the mutant embryos showed that this ectopia of the ureteric orifice is a consequence of the ectopic initial ureteric budding from the wolffian duct. Thus, in *Bmp4* +/– embryos, the initial ureteric bud emerges from the wolffian duct at the site more cranial than in wild-type embryos (Fig. 40.2). This connection between the initial ureteric bud in embryos (cranial) and the final ureteric orifice in mature mutant animals (caudal) is predicted in Mackie's and Stephens' hypothesis. In addition to the ectopic budding of the initial ureter, some *Bmp4* +/– embryos show accessory budding from the main trunk of the initial ureter, which can lead to the formation of the double collecting system, an anomaly commonly found in the mutants at birth.

One essential regulator of ureteric budding is glial cell-derived neurotrophic factor (GDNF), which acts on the wolffian duct and ureter epithelium through its receptor tyrosine kinase, c-ret (Pichel *et al.*, 1996; Sanchez *et al.*, 1996). The GDNF expressed in the metanephric mesenchyme regulates the initial budding and subsequent branching of the ureter by stimulating bud initiation and by determining bud orientation (Sainio *et al.*, 1997; Tang *et al.*, 1998). However, the precise mechanism for determining the correct site of

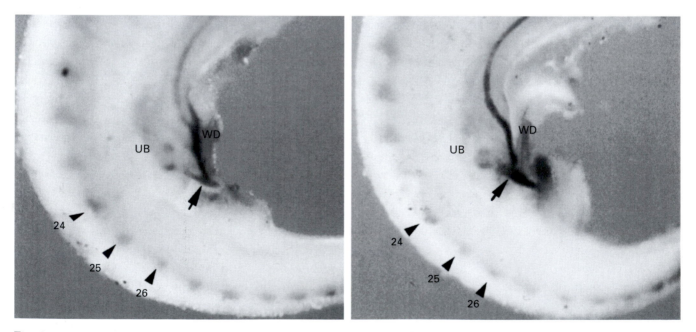

Fig. 40.2   *c-ret and Wnt 11 whole mount in situ hybridization for wild-type +/+; left and Bmp4 +/– mutants at E11.0. The position of the initial ureteric budding (UB) from the wolffian duct (WD) is indicated by arrows, and the 24th, 25th and 26th somite pairs are marked by arrowheads. The position of the initial budding in the wild-type corresponds to the ~26th somite, whereas that in the mutant corresponds to the ~25th somite.*

the ureteric budding has heretofore been largely unknown. Although the tightly regulated expression pattern of c-ret and GDNF could be a part of the mechanism to specify the site of branching (Schuchardt et al., 1996), both c-ret and GDNF are expressed surprisingly broadly throughout the wolffian duct/ureteric epithelium and metanephric mesenchyme, respectively, at an early stage of kidney development (E10.0 to E12.0) (Miyazaki et al., 2000a). In normal wild-type embryos undergoing the initial ureteric budding, Bmp4 is expressed in the loose stromal mesenchymal cells located between the wolffian duct and the cranially extending metanephric mesenchyme, whereas Bmp4 expression is absent in the wolffian duct and metanephric mesenchyme per se. Given this expression pattern of Bmp4 in normal wild-type embryos and the observed ectopic and accessory budding in Bmp4 +/− heterozygous embryos, it is conceivable that BMP4 serves as an inhibitory factor for the bud-inducing GDNF-ret signalling along the wolffian duct and the stalk of the ureter, thereby determining the site of new bud formation. Indeed, in vitro studies on a metanephric explant culture system showed that BMP4 can inhibit the GDNF signalling within the wolffian duct and the ureteric epithelium, without directly modulating the expression pattern of GDNF itself. Therefore, a defect in this function of BMP4 causes ectopic and accessory budding of the ureter, which can lead to a wide spectrum of CAKUT in Bmp4 +/− mice (Mackie and Stephens, 1975).

CAKUT in Foxc1 null mutant mice. The Foxc1 gene (formerly Mf1) encodes a forkhead/winged helix transcription factor, which plays several essential roles in embryonic development, including cell fate determination, proliferation and differentiation (Kaufmann and Knochel, 1996). Mice homozygous for a null mutation of Foxc1 gene die perinatally with multiple abnormalities, including haemorrhagic hydrocephalus and skeletal, ocular and cardiovascular defects (Kume et al., 1998). Moreover, depending on the genetic background, most Foxc1 homozygous mutants have duplex kidneys and double ureters (Kume et al., 2000). In these, the upper kidney and ureter are always enlarged and fluid-filled, and the abnormal ureter, but not the normal ureter, connects aberrantly to the wolffian duct derivatives such as the seminal vesicle or vas deferens in males. Analysis of embryos reveals that Foxc1 homozygotes have an accessory ectopic ureteric bud which emerges from the wolffian duct more cranially than the normal bud. Thus, in this mutant also, an abnormality in the number and the site of the initial ureteric bud leads to a duplex collecting system and an ectopic ureteric orifice, respectively, that accompany anomalous kidney tissues, as described by Mackie and Stephens. In Foxc1 homozygotes, for a reason yet to be determined, expression of GDNF in the intermediate mesoderm is found to be extended much more cranially, when compared to wild types. Taken together, these findings suggest that, in Foxc1 null mutants, abnormally cranial extension and persistence of the normal GDNF expression domain underlies the formation of ectopic and accessory budding of the initial ureter, which then leads to the duplex kidney/ureter system.

Multifunction of regulator genes; a paradigm shift from the early anatomical theories

The above findings demonstrate that ectopic initial budding of the ureter is a universal phenomenon preceding the ontogeny of CAKUT. However, it is worth noting that the expression of the regulatory molecules for organogenesis of the kidney and urinary tract is not limited to the site and time of initial ureteric budding, but instead continues throughout kidney development. It is possible, therefore, that a given molecule which regulates the initial budding of the ureter can regulate the subsequent process of kidney and urinary tract development. For example, while BMP4 has an important function in specifying the site of the initial ureteric budding as documented above, intense Bmp4 expression continues beyond the initial budding stage and throughout the rest of intrauterine life at various sites of the excretory system, including loose stromal mesenchymal cells around the main trunk and the stalk of the branching ureter, and the epithelium of comma- and S-shaped bodies. Indeed, studies on both Bmp4 heterozygous embryos in vivo and cultured explants in vitro showed that BMP4 has multiple biological functions in the morphogenesis of the excretory system (Miyazaki et al., 2000b). First, in addition to its inhibitory effect on the ureteric bud formation, BMP4 promotes the growth and elongation of ureteric buds once buds have formed. Second, BMP4 acts on the metanephric mesenchyme to prevent apoptosis, promotes growth of the stromal cell population and inhibits condensation of the mesenchymal cells around the ureter bud. Furthermore, BMP4 can serve as a chemoattractant for the periureteral mesenchymal cells and, in so doing, induce locally the smooth muscle layer of the ureter.

Likewise, *Agtr2* and *Foxc1* can have diverse regulatory roles as well, as their expression also continues throughout kidney development. Indeed, it has been shown *in vivo* and *in vitro* that activation of the *Agtr2* receptor promotes timely apoptosis of the undifferentiated mesenchymal cells that surround the smooth muscle layer of the ureter, and a defect in this function of *Agtr2* may lead to the atresia of the ureter found in some *Agtr2* null mutant mice, by not permitting normal enlargement of the ureter and/or supplying vessel calibre (Nishimura *et al.*, 1999). In conjunction with the notion that many embryonic genes govern organogenesis at various stages and tissues, the diversity of CAKUT can be attributed to the fact that each gene responsible for the formation of CAKUT functions as a multifunctional regulator for the excretory system. Thus, a wide spectrum of anomalies are the result of a mutation in a gene that can regulate not only the site of the ureterovesical orifice (via determination of the site of the initial ureteric bud), but also the site of the kidney and the ureter at later stages, each through a distinct mechanism (Fig. 40.3).

CAKUT as a multigenic disease

By studying a variety of mutant strains of mice, to date more than 30 genes have been found to be essential for mammalian kidney development (see http://www.golgi.ana.ed.ac.uk/kidhome.html). Moreover, several gene mutations have been identified as a cause of human CAKUT. These include *PAX2* (Sanyanusin *et al.*, 1995), *KAL* (Franco *et al.*, 1991), *EYA1* (Abdelhak *et al.*, 1997) and *AGTR2* (Hohenfellner *et al.*, 1999; Nishimura *et al.*, 1999). In the human *AGTR2* gene (capitalization indicates a human gene), a single nucleotide transition (A to G in intron 1) has been found, which causes an abnormality in the quantity and quality of the *AGTR2* mRNA. Studies on genomic DNA from two groups of patients who have common forms of CAKUT, with general populations as controls, revealed that while this mutation is found in the patients at a significantly higher incidence than the control group, some normal controls

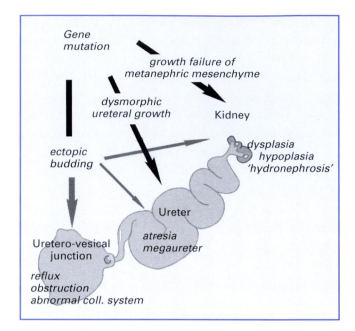

Fig. 40.3 *Pluripotentiality of the single gene mutation underlies the wide spectrum of clinical anomalies involving the ureterovesical junction, the ureter and the kidney. The loss-of-function mutation of the single gene can produce multiple anomalies: first, due in part to its multiple biological actions on the morphogenesis of the three tissues of the excretory system, i.e. the ureterovesical junction, the ureter and the kidney (black arrows); second, due to the multipotentiality of the initial ectopic budding to produce three clinical entities, ectopic ureteral orifice, anomalous ureter and hypoplastic/dysplastic kidney as postulated by Mackie and Stephens (grey arrows).*

do have this transition. This suggests that while the *AGTR2* mutation is involved in the development of human CAKUT, this mutation alone does not result in the disease. In this regard, in *Agtr2* null mutant mice also, the penetrance rate of CAKUT was, at best, imperfect, and the rate increases through cross mating phenotype-positive pairs. Thus, *AGTR2* is one of multiple genes involved in the common forms of CAKUT, and some genetic modifiers are necessary for the development of the anomalies. In this regard, *AGTR2* is distinctively different from *PAX2* (Sanyanusin *et al.*, 1995), *KAL* (Franco *et al.*, 1991) and *EYA1* (Abdelhak *et al.*, 1997), mutation of which produces a rare form of congenital anomalies of the kidney and urinary tract, which is accompanied by malformation of other organs with a high penetrance rate. In most cases of human CAKUT, however, anomalies in other organs are commonly absent, and the mode of inheritance is not typical mendelian, but instead is somewhat sporadic (i.e. incomplete penetrance). Overall, therefore, the development of the common forms of human CAKUT is attributed to an accumulation of minor mutations in multiple genes, each of which has multiple ontogenic functions on the excretory system.

These multiplicities in the genetic mechanism underlie the multiple theories for the mechanism of CAKUT formation that were offered by early scholars based on their excellent anatomical studies.

Summary

In summary, we have discussed the ontogenic mechanism for the diversity of CAKUT (Fig. 40.3). Ectopic initial budding of the ureter is important, as it precedes three clinical entities concurrently, i.e. ectopic ureterovesical orifice, anomalous ureter and hypoplastic/dysplastic kidney as postulated by Mackie and Stephens (1975). Recent gene targeting studies on mice demonstrated that ectopic ureteric budding indeed occurs prior to the formation of CAKUT. The wide spectrum of CAKUT is also related to other functions of the gene responsible, because the gene is expressed at multiple sites at different ontogenic stages and directly regulates the morphogenesis of the several sites of the excretory system.

41

Embryogenesis of deformations

F. Douglas Stephens and John M. Hutson

Disproportion between the size of the developing embryo or fetus and the uterine cavity has been regarded as a cause of compression and moulding defects since the time of Hippocrates (Ballantyne, 1904; Browne, 1936); Oligohydramnios has also been recognized as a cause of deformation, a well-known example being a deformed fetus with absent or hypoplastic kidneys (Potter's syndrome). More recently rupture of the amnion during the embryonic and early stages of fetal development has been shown to be a cause of multiple deformations, either by compression of the conceptus within the chorionic membrane, or by the entanglement of external structures by amniochorionic strings (Torpin, 1968). Some degree of scepticism prevails as to the mechanical explanation of some deformations when at no time in the pregnancy has oligohydramnios been observed.

Deformation resulting from amniotic rupture occurs in about one in 2000 surviving neonates (Smith, 1981; Jones, 1988). In spontaneous abortuses the incidence is much higher. After necropsy and clinical studies of deformed fetuses and infants with suspected compression *in utero* without evidence of frank rupture of the amnion, it is proposed that deformations by amnion constraint on the growing embryo can occur during a period of temporary oligohydramnios. During the brief period, the amniotic membrane shrinks on the fragile embryo/fetus, causing multiple permanent deformations of the head, hind end, body or limbs. An embryological and mechanical explanation is offered, both for the transient oligohydramnios and the deformations resulting from the accompanying compression by the temporarily shrunken fetal membranes. The embryo develops in a craniocaudal sequence so that earliest temporary compression affects the head, and later compression involves the trunk and ventral body wall and spares the head and, later still, the hind end.

Previous studies of ruptured amniotic sequence

Torpin (1965, 1968) clearly demonstrated the association of rupture of the amnion sac in his studies of membranes of fetuses and survivors exhibiting amputations, constriction rings and talipedic moulding. He reviewed 400 case reports of amniogenic compression and examined 14 fetuses or infants suspected of amnion rupture, with their corresponding placentas and membranes, using an underwater suspension technique to display the rupture site of the amnion and chorioamniogenic strings. He concluded (1) that the amniotic membrane was formed from ectoderm on the inside and extraembryonic mesoderm on the outside with variations in total thickness; (2) that rupture of the amnion allows the embryo to pass from the amniotic cavity into the chorionic space and survive for varying periods of time; (3) that the ruptured amnion may shrink to a small globule attached only to the placenta around the insertion of the umbilical cord, or the amnion may shred into dangerous strings or bands; and (4) that the embryo or fetus may continue to develop within the chorion, or may die and be absorbed, or abort, or become entangled in strings that strangulate limbs or other parts of the body. He also considered that in some instances the fetus can develop without deformation in the chorionic cavity even though the space after rupture of the amnion may be temporarily oligohydramniotic until the rates of formation and absorption of amniotic fluid adjust to restore adequate volume. (5) Between 10 and 12 weeks of gestation, the amnion becomes loosely sealed to the chorion thus eliminating the chorionic space. In this state a rupture of the amnion is accompanied by dissection of the loosely attached amnion from chorion, with formation of chorioamniotic strings and collapse of part or all of the amniotic membrane. A more severe rupture may include the chorionic wall with leakage into the vagina or even abortion.

Experimental evidence of effects of amniotic rupture

Poswillow and Roy (1965) demonstrated that following puncture of the amnion at 15.5 days and sacrifice on day 22, rat embryos exhibited cleft palate, micrognathia, glossoptosis and other deformations such as talipes, syndactylism, ring constrictions of limbs, amputations and phocomelia. They found that cleft palate deformity was accurately related to the timing of the puncture and that the amnion contracted on the embryo, creating widespread compression effects. The amniotic membrane pressed the head and mandible against the thorax and inhibited the normal extension of the neck. The tongue was forced between the palatal shelves and the nasal septum thus creating a cleft palate deformity. This, together with micrognathia, resembled the Pierre–Robin syndrome in humans. Their experiments indicate that amniotic membrane compression can also cause widespread deformities of the limbs and body in addition to the analogous Pierre–Robin anomalies.

Kennedy and Persaud (1977) performed amniocentesis on Sprague–Dawley rats at 16 days' gestation. The fetuses were recovered from 15 minutes to 38 hours after the procedure. These authors found intense vascular damage, hypoxia and postural moulding, especially affecting the head and limbs. Cranioschisis, digital reductions, amputations, bowing of the long bones and scoliosis, and ischaemic tissue necrosis were observed as a consequence of amniocentesis. In one rat, amputation of a leg occurred and the limb was recovered in the membranes.

Clinical evidence of amniotic rupture

Higgenbottom *et al.* (1979), Miller *et al.* (1981), Kalousek *et al* (1990) and Smith (1981) have all recognized the entity of amniotic rupture and amniotic band complex and have described the multifarious moulding deformations resulting from early rupture, oligohydramnios and chorioamniotic band disruption of the embryo, and those occurring later from leakage of amniotic fluid. Miller *et al.* (1981) collected autopsy reports of 27 fetuses with limb/body-wall deformities. Forty-one per cent had amniotic bands or adhesion-related defects, but some of these also exhibited other non-band- or adhesion-related anomalies. These include scoliosis or neural tube or postural deformations and short umbilical cord, which Miller *et al.* attribute to oligohydramnios and uterine compression. Furthermore, they believed that temporary loss of amniotic fluid following rupture without band formation can lead to a wide range of lethal or non-lethal compression deformations. Elias and Simpson (1992) reported constant leakage of amniotic fluid after midtrimester amniocentesis until birth of

normal infants in several women. Laurence (1974) reported two examples of amniotic membrane perforation, one with constant leakage into the vagina and one without leakage, and in both instances the mothers had given birth to normally developed babies. Ashkenazy *et al.* (1982) showed that amniocentesis in one patient at 14 weeks' gestation caused amnion membrane rupture resulting in a single band which partially constricted the umbilical cord. The fetus matured in the chorionic cavity and was a normal baby at birth.

In summary, with rupture of the amnion, the embryo or fetus is extruded from the amniotic cavity into the chorionic sac where it may die from compression or umbilical cord strangulation, or may survive with or without moulding from compression and with or without partial or a total strangulation of limbs or torso by amniogenic bands. Even with frank rupture or leakage of amniotic fluid, some survive without abnormality. Some will show evidence of fragmentation of the amniotic membrane, revealed by meticulous examination of the placental membranes and umbilical cord.

Cause of rupture of amnion

The actual cause of the rupture is in general not known, though case reports of typical fetal deformations following maternal trauma are cited by Torpin (1968). Five examples of trauma showed indisputable evidence that typical deformations of these fetuses had resulted from injury of the amnion with band formation. These include trauma early in pregnancy in one case with the amnion shrunken to a globule around the umbilical cord and with amniotic strings (Greeff, 1892, quoted by Torpin, 1968); trauma early in pregnancy in two mothers, followed by fetal deformation and shredding of the amnion (Mayer 1952, quoted by Torpin, 1968); and trauma in one mother in late pregnancy with fetal death due to a ruptured amnion and a string which strangulated the umbilical cord (Hahn, 1938; quoted by Torpin, 1968).

Meyer-Ruegg (1939, quoted by Torpin, 1968) reported a case of trauma to the conceptus in an unwanted pregnancy secondary to attempted abortion with a knitting needle through the cervix into the gestational sac. At 7 months the baby was born accompanied by a large quantity of amniotic fluid. The amnion had peeled away from the wall of the chorion and was attached to the anterior aspect of the head and body, which exhibited cerebral and abdominal herniations and facial fissures.

Ashkenazy *et al.* (1982) reported a case of amnion rupture following amniocentesis performed at 16 weeks' gestation. No complications were noted during pregnancy and mother gave birth to a normal full-term 3530-g male baby, but examination of the placenta and membranes revealed (1) an amniotic band partially constricting the umbilical cord, (2) the chorion and placenta were denuded of amniotic lining, and (3) the baby had survived in the chorionic cavity. This shows that the chorionic cavity is a buffer against harmful uterine muscular contractions. Elias and Simpson (1992) have reported persistent leaking of amniotic fluid into the vagina after amniocentesis, yet with normal pregnancy and baby. Presumably fluid formation exceeded fluid loss through the needle puncture wound, the volumes being adequate, and no compression anomalies followed.

Penso *et al.* (1990) reported 407 amniocenteses at ages ranging from 11 to 14 weeks' gestation. Amnion fluid leakage occurred in 2.2 per cent. There were eight instances of congenital orthopaedic deformities: four babies had clubbed feet and one each had hyperextended knees, scoliosis, congenital dislocation of the knees and congenital dislocation of the hips. In three of the eight deformations (scoliosis, dislocation and club feet), leakage followed the amniocentesis.

There is much clinical evidence to suggest that multiple deformations may occur from moulding at specific times in development in otherwise normally developed infants. In order to explain the occurrence of this group, it is proposed that the following errors in embryogenesis may account for a state of temporary oligohydramnios that induces permanent deformations.

Proposed embryological explanation of temporary oligohydramnios

Normal embryogenesis

In normal circumstances, between 18 and 28 days, the wings of the flat discoid embryo wrap ventrally to form a cylindrical shape. During this time the heart, head and tail ends fold ventrally; the notochord or temporary 'spine' is formed; up to 29 somites are aligned on each side of the notochord; the notochord changes its orientation from dorsiflexion to ventroflexion, a process termed 'reversal' or 'flexion'; and the neural plate is formed into the neural tube and both the anterior and posterior neuropores close (Fig. 41.1). During this

period amniogenic constriction due to temporary fluid loss may cause temporary compression and impair reversal and renders the embryo vulnerable to moulding deformations.

Formation of the notochord and neurenteric canal

In the bilaminar flat discoid embryo of 16 days (fertilization age), mesoderm from the region of the primitive streak begins to separate the ectodermal from endodermal layers of the inner cell mass of the blastocyst embryo. Henson's node or primitive pit is situated at the cranial end of the dorsal groove, called the primitive streak. The node is the site of rapid multiplication of mesodermal cells from each side that push cranially in the midline as a rod-like structure—the so-called notochord—between ectoderm and endoderm as far as the buccopharyngeal membrane. Beginning at the pit in Henson's node, a lumen extends progressively along the notochord. The floor of the notochord then fuses with the contiguous endoderm and then the common wall breaks down bringing the amniotic fluid into communication with the yolk sac. The opened out walls of the notochord form a longitudinal inlay in the endodermal roof of the yolk sac. The longitudinal edges of this inlay then unite in a craniocaudal direction to reconstitute the notochordal canal while at the same time the co-apting edges of the endodermal layer also reunite. On reaching the site of the primitive pit, the uniting edges of the neurenteric canal occlude the lumen at the level of the future mid sacrum on about the 28th day. Very soon afterwards, the overlying neural folds of the neural plate come together under the influence of the notochord to close the caudal neuropore. Caudal to the site of occlusion of the lumen of the neurenteric canal, the notochord overtakes the shrinking primitive streak and continues to pay out mesoderm to the end of the transient human tail. The notochord is the primary organiser of all the somites and vertebrae, septation of the foregut and cloaca and neurulation (Fig. 41.1).

Defects in the timing of the closing of the neurenteric canal and patchy porosity of the amnion may cause temporary amniotic fluid leakage without actual rupture of the membrane. The temporary oligohydramnios leads to shrinkage of the amnion and compression of the embryo and permanent deformations. If the leakage

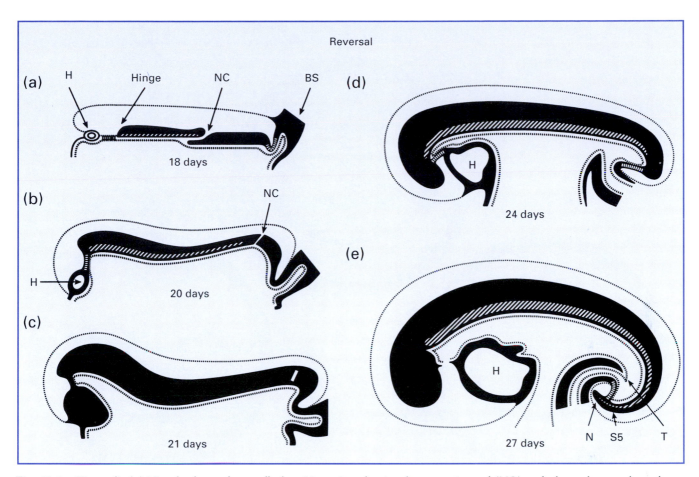

Fig. 41.1 *'Reversal'.* (**a**) *Notochord extends rostrally from Henson's node, site of neurenteric canal (NC) to the buccopharyngeal membrane where the hinge of reversal is sited.* (**b**) *and* (**c**) *Heart rotates ventrally, notochord and neurenteric canal (NC) grow caudally; head process enlarging.* (**d**) *Head and heart (H) rotation complete, tail end beginning rotation, body stalk (BS) and allantois infolding.* (**e**) *Notochord extends into primitive tail, allantois in body stalk rotated into hindgut forming Tourneux's fold (T). S5, Region of future fifth sacral vertebra.*

stops, amniotic fluid reaccumulates and development of the embryo with its deformities continues unabated.

The amnion first appears in the inner cell mass of the blastocyst embryo during its implantation into the uterine wall. The floor of the amnion is formed of a single layer of epiblast cells of the bilaminar disc and the roof is contiguous with the cytotrophoblast cells, to which it remains attached as the future body stalk. The amniotic fluid forms at first by diffusion from maternal blood and the trophoblast cells of the chorion and steadily increases in amount. By the third week, blood lakes and blood vessels arise in the extra-embryonic mesodermal coat of the yolk sac, forming the vitelline vascular system, whilst blood vasculature develops in the body stalk and links with the placental vasculature. The heart tubes form and heart beat begins at about 18 days. With the development of the primitive circulation, the amniotic fluid increases in volume. After about 10 weeks

of age, the metanephric kidney secretes urine which is voided into the amnion and, by 18 weeks, becomes the main contributor to amniotic fluid circulation.

Abnormal embryogenesis of the notochord and amnion

Notochord

The neurenteric canal connecting the lumina of the amnion and yolk sac normally obliterates spontaneously at 28 days. The amniotic fluid increases in amount and the amnion expands, presumably because the intra-amniotic pressure is higher than in the surrounding chorionic sac. If the notochordal canal closure is unduly delayed, amniotic fluid may escape into the yolk sac and be absorbed by the endoderm. The amniotic membrane then may shrink, constraining and dangerously impairing the process of 'reversal' of the embryo which may die or be deformed (Fig. 41.2). When the canal

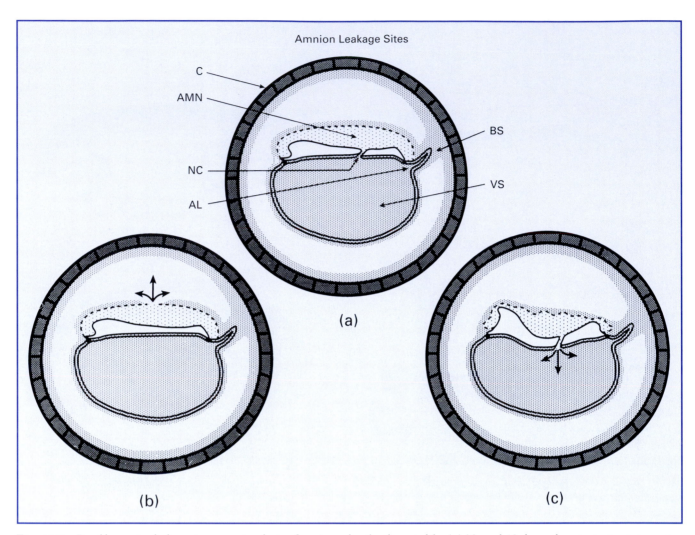

Fig. 41.2 *Possible amnion leakage sites occurring during first six weeks of embryonic life. (**a**) Normal 18-day embryo projecting into amnion (AMN) with normal temporary patency of the neurenteric canal (NC). (**b**) Tension pore (or pores) opens up, permitting leakage into fluid containing chorionic sac and shrinkage of amnion membrane, with compression of elongating embryo similar to that occurring after leakage via abnormally prolonged patency of neurenteric canal, as shown in (**c**). C, Chorion wall; AL, allantois; BS, body stalk; YS, yolk sac.*

occludes, amniotic fluid volume is restored and the development of the deformed embryo continues.

Porosity of the amnion

Between 14 and 28 days the amnion expands to maintain an envelope of fluid around the enlarging and folding embryo. The amniotic membrane, being at this stage extremely thin, may develop a pinpoint pore or pores between the lining cells, permitting leakage of fluid from the amnion into the chorionic sac (Fig. 41.3). Leakage leads to shrinkage of the amniotic membrane which, in the collapsed state, may repair itself. The amnion then re-expands to normal fluid volume. Brief compression of the embryo by the tightly fitting amnion,

however, may cause permanent deformations without any trace of rupture in the form of amniogenic bands.

Normally, the amnion steadily expands within the chorion until the fetus is approximately 10 weeks of age, when the amnion and chorionic walls appose. Spontaneous leakage and frank rupture then are less likely to occur; though, if the amnion wall is breached, it is liable to peal away from the chorion and create amniochorionic bands and compression anomalies if the fetus survives.

Effects of temporary oligohydramnios

Whether the lack of amniotic fluid is due to patency of the neurenteric canal, pores in the amnion or other

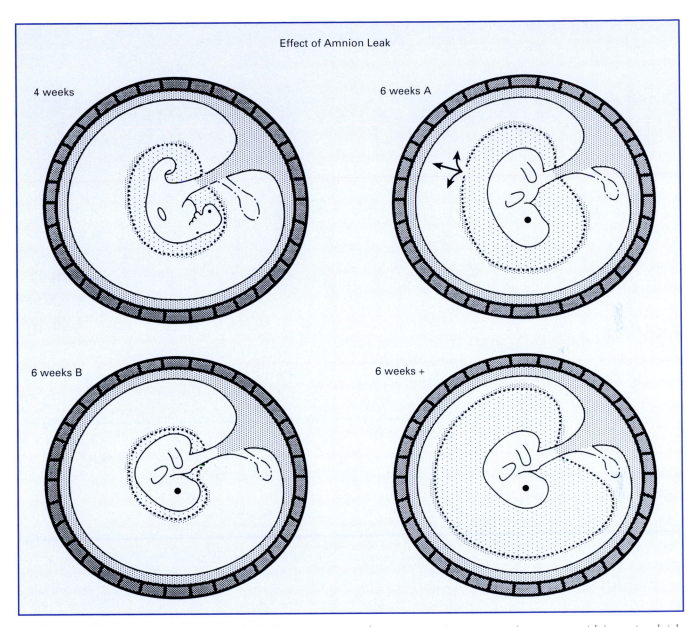

Fig. 41.3 *Effect of amnion leakage. Amnion fluid volume increases as embryo grows, tension pore opens (arrows upper right), amnion shrinks compressing embryo (lower left), and pore closes; amniotic fluid reaccumulates, compression injuries remain and embryonic development continues (lower right).*

causes, compression by the contracted membrane on the fragile embryo is similar, though patency of the neurenteric canal may account for earliest deformations.

The notochord, being the precursor and early substitute for the future spinal column is the axial strut that directs and maintains the appropriate axis of body development. In the discoid embryo the notochord is almost straight, with faint dorsal curvature at the head and hind ends. As the embryo elongates and assumes a cylindrical shape, it undergoes 'reversal' and flexes ventrally. Compression may exaggerate the dorsal curvature or arrest, delay or increase ventral flexion of the notochord. Deformations caused by compression result from distortions of the notochordal zones of the developing organism.

Notochordal zones

For the purpose of description, the notochordal zones are referred to as cranial, cervical, dorsolumbar and lumbosacral. Non-notochordal compression zones include protruding parts such as limbs, genitalia (see Chapter 36), ears, nose and mandible.

Cranial zone

The head, being the early part of the embryo to grow, may be warped or mutilated by end-to-end compression of the embryo. The neural folds flatten or fail to unite creating cranial anomalies such as anencephaly, exencephaly or iniencephaly and forms of ocular hypertelorism and clinocephaly and defects of the lips, nose, palate and jaw (Fig. 41.4).

Cervical zone

Delayed or excessive reversal or torsion in the future neck region of the notochord interferes with midline septation of the foregut, creating forms of tracheoesophageal anomalies and vertebral lesions such as fused or hemivertebra or butterfly vertebra (right and left vertebral bodies unfused; see p. 325). The notochord may continue to elongate against end-to-end compression, causing distortion of the developing column of cervical vertebra (Fig. 41.4).

Dorsolumbar region

Flexion of the dorsolumbar notochord may be delayed when the mesodermal wings are timed to wrap the discoid embryo into a cylindrical shape. The wings may then fail to unite in the ventral midline, though the abdominal musculature is well differentiated. The result is a central divarication or splaying of the rectus muscles in the region of the umbilicus, epigastrium or sternal attachments, resulting in exomphalos and rarely pericardial defects. The degree of retraction of the body of the embryo is proportional to the extent of divarication and extrusion of the viscera.

Rarely the notochord is retracted into the shape of a hairpin, with the pelvis and lower limbs and spinal column and chord bent backwards, with feet positioned behind the head (Fig. 41.5) and occasionally with a loose 'rocker' false joint between the upper and lower halves of the body. Compression may cause the lower body to twist sideways at the dorsolumbar junction, in which case the ribs on one side are crushed together or fused and on opposite side are splayed (Fig. 41.6).

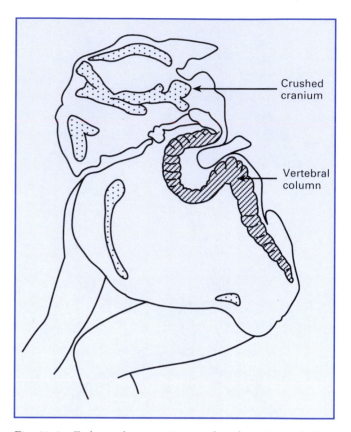

Fig. 41.4 *End-to-end compression in early embryonic period. Fetus at 10 weeks' gestation showing concertinad cervicothoracic spine, compressed calvarium and rachischisis.*

Lumbosacral region

This is the last part of notochordal differentiation, which occurs concomitantly with final segmentation of the coccyx and tail. Five lumbar, five sacral, four coccygeal and seven tail segments are laid down but the seven tail segments undergo apoptosis.

The notochordal canal closes at its caudal end near the second sacral segment at about 28 days, thus cutting off the confluence of amniotic and yolk sac fluids. The notochord, however, continues and governs segmentation to the end of the tail and determines the normal shape and curvature of the hind end of the body. It also is implicated in its own apoptosis in the transient human tail.

Any abnormal amniotic compression on the hind end of the 28 to 35-day embryo may twist, deviate, damage or disrupt the notochord and somites, creating agenesis of vertebrae and nucleus pulposis or hemivertebrae or fusion of vertebrae. A torsion effect may create a 'scimitar' deformation of the sacrococcygeal vertebrae

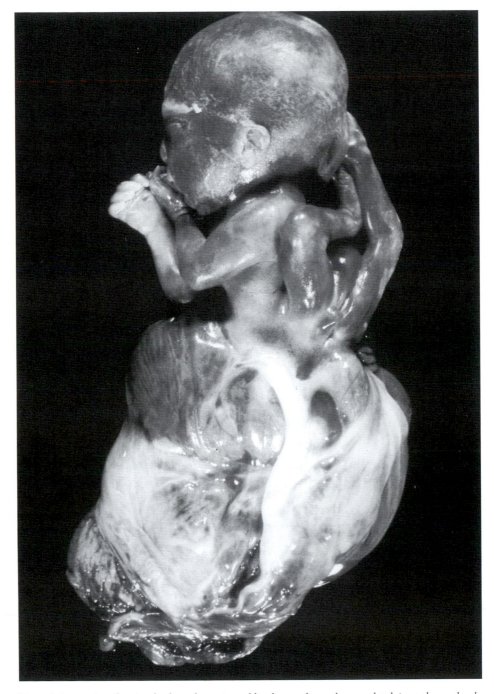

Fig. 41.5 *Fetus at 24 weeks' gestation showing backward rotation of lumbosacral vertebrae and pelvis at thoracolumbar junction. Note feet resting on occiput and total exomphalos; all viscera in embryonic mesodermal sac attached to amnion; skin covered meningomyelocele. (Bilateral distal ureteral atresia and oligohydramnios). See Fig. 36.14.*

(Fig. 36.7). The midline septation of the cloaca and the developing wolffian bodies that follow closely the orientation of the notochord also may be impaired. Such anomalies as absent kidney and reflux nephropathy are commonly associated. Furthermore, the abnormal posture taken up by the limbs because of the vertebral

defects may cause pressure effects on the developing external genitalia and perineum (see Figs 36.5 and 36.12).

External compression of the developing notochord may arrest the process of ventral rotation of the hind end so that the infolding of the allantois is delayed,

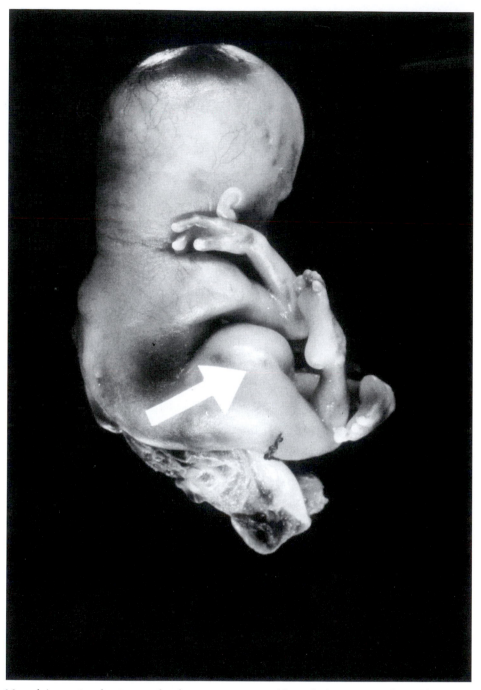

Fig. 41.6 *Fetus at 16 weeks' gestation showing non-band compression; twisted lower body position with moulding of limbs. Exomphalos (and wide divarication of rectus muscles), Viscera exteriorized in a mesodermal sac. Note pressure dimple on right thigh (arrow).*

arrested or skewed, in which event Tourneux's septum fails to progress to its rightful destination and Rathke's plicae fail to eventuate (see Fig. 2.11). The result is union of the rectum with bladder or urethra, forming cloacal defects known clinically as the rectovesical, recto-prostato-bladder-neck and recto-urethro-prostatic fistulae (see Fig. 2.5).

If Tourneux's septum advances to the normal situation, Rathke's plicae are activated and complete the partition. Compression forces acting after completion of this stage affect perineal development of the anus and genitalia (see Fig. 36.12).

Torsion of the caudal notochord by external compression creates tangential malalignment of the two sides of the os coxae, with diastasis of the pubic bones, the degree depending on the timing, degree and duration of the twisting forces (see Fig. 36.12).

During this period also, developing bilateral facial and palatal structures are vulnerable to compression if the head and neck are twisted or pressed unduly sideways or upon the developing sternum. Severe compression of the head upon the sternum has been shown experimentally to occur following amniocentesis in rats, as described by Poswillow and Roy (1965), supporting the concept of moulding as a cause of the Pierre–Robin sequence in humans. Lateral compression of the developing facial components may disrupt their union, deviating the first arch or the nasal prominence, inducing facial clefts or asymmetry of face and cranium and anomalies of the nasal septum. Lateral tilt of the head occurs when compressed by the amnion. The ipsilateral mandible is forced against the chest, sometimes with the clenched hand tucked between jaw and ribs. The head and spine become scoliotic, the mandible indented and the developing toothbuds displaced. The ipsilateral ear may be flattened between head and shoulder.

Tracheo-Oesophageal anomalies and spinal deformation

Because the VATER (vertebral defects, imperforate anus, tracheo-oesophageal atresia and fistula, and radial and renal dysplasia) syndrome may derive from impairment of the 'reversal' process and amniogenic compression, each anomaly deserves special explanation concerning embryogenesis.

Embryogenesis of human foregut and tracheo-oesophageal anomalies

Septation of the foregut into oesophagus and trachea begins at the embryonic age of 3.5 weeks (4 mm in length). When associated with notochordal defects, septation may be impaired. It is proposed that compression of the embryo by the amniotic membrane in a state of oligohydramnios may bend the notochord and future developing spinal column at this early period, causing both vertebral and foregut septal defects. Analysis of records of 285 patients with tracheo-oesphageal anomalies revealed that 53 (19 per cent) had scoliosis with vertebral anomalies (Dickens, 1991).

Stevenson (1972) found that vertebral anomalies, including extra vertebrae and sacral defects, were present in 75 per cent of patients with congenital tracheo-oesophageal defects. Thirteen of fourteen patients with VATER syndrome, investigated by Piekarski and Stephens (1976), exhibited butterfly vertebrae, fusions or extra vertebrae in the thoracic column, extra vertebrae or fusions in lumbar region, and fusions or agenesis of the sacrococcygeal vertebrae. Amniogenic constraint may induce hyperflexion, hyperextension or scoliosis of the cervicothoracic notochord and interfere with septation of the foregut, accounting for some non-VATER tracheo-oesophageal anomalies.

Embryogenesis of foregut septation into trachea and oesophagus

In order to explain the occurrence of tracheo-oesophageal deformations, Piekarski and Stephens (1976) reasoned that the septation of the tracheal bud from the foregut takes place by a two-part septum. The first is a 'catenoidal' (Sutliff and Hutchins, 1994) or saddle-like indentation on the caudal aspect of the bud, separating it from the foregut. This indenting saddle progresses cranially to meet a second septum formed by the meeting of lateral indentations in the foregut. The meeting of these indentations takes place at first distally, progressing cranially to the future hypopharynx, thus separating the respiratory tract from the oesophagus (Fig. 41.7). This two-part septation is coordinated with normal rotation of the notochord or future cervicothoracic spine during the process of 'reversal'.

Distortion of the notochord and foregut anomalies

Experimental: chemical teratogen

The notochord governs septation of the foregut and is the axis around which the vertebrae form. Merei et al. (1998), using the adriamycin fetal rat model, demonstrated tracheo-oesophageal anomalies and abnormal endodermal adherence, kinking, bending and cranial splitting of the notochord. They proposed that disorganized function of the notochord was responsible for the tracheo-oesophageal and vertebral anomalies. Possoegel et al. (1998) found similar anomalies in the

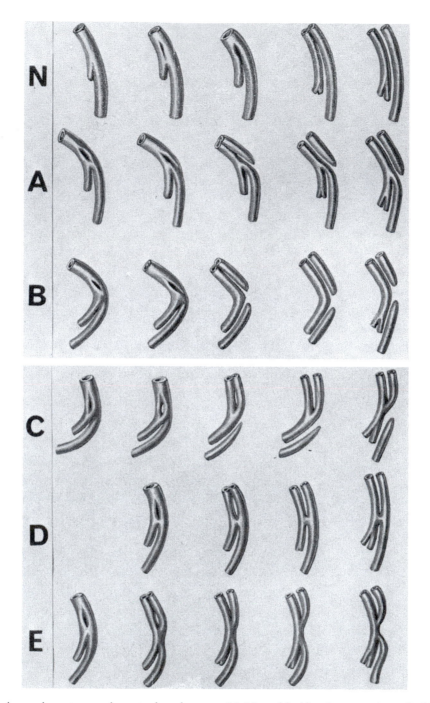

Fig. 41.7 *Normal and abnormal two-part tracheo-oesophageal septum. N, Normal budding from anterior wall of foregut at 2.5-mm stage. Septum formation progresses cranially, starting with a coronal (carinate) saddle indentation which meets in continuity with independently developing lateral folds. These lateral folds meet each other in midline and continue cranially, completing subdivision into trachea and oesophagus. (**a**) Proximal oesophageal atresia with distal tracheo-oesophageal (T-O) fistula. With hyperangulation of the foregut, the cranial septum slews towards the dorsal wall and separates off blind upper oesophageal pouch and fails to connect with caudal septum. (**b**) Oesophageal atresia; with midforegut hyperangulation, both cranial and caudal septa slew into dorsal wall separating the oesophagus into blind pouches above and below. (**c**) Proximal T-O fistula with a distal oesophageal atresia. With low hyperangulation, the caudal septum slews toward the dorsal wall and separates off the blind lower oesophageal pouch. (**d**) H-Type fistula; failure of septa to meet over a short distance, possibly due to hyperextension, results in a narrow fistula between trachea and oesophagus. (**e**) Distal and proximal T-O fistulas, failure of septa to meet over a longer distance leaves patent communications above and below. Reprinted, by permission from Piekarski, D.H. and Stephens, F.D. (1976). The association and embryogenesis of tracheo-esophageal and anorectal anomalies. In Progress in Pediatric Surgery, P.P. Rickham, W.Ch. Hecker and J. Prévot (eds), vol. 9, pp. 63–76. Munich: Urban & Schwarzenberg.)*

notochord and foregut in their adriamycin-treated fetal rat experiments.

Qi and Beasley (1999) noted notochordal abnormalities, especially the abnormal persisting attachment to the foregut and acute flexion, in the adriamycin model and reasoned that the abnormal notochord caused the tracheo-oesophageal dysgenesis.

Xia et al. (1999) considered that the adriamycin-induced anomalies in the rat model were similar to those in the human VATER association.

Mechanical compression

In the fourth week in the 2.5- to 5.5-mm embryo, the head and cervical notochord normally flex ventrally over the developing heart, angulating the undivided foregut. Hyperflexion, or lateral angulation may compress the notochord, thus interfering with the extent, direction and alignment of one or both parts of the two-part septation of the foregut. Furthermore, the focal point of acute angulation may vary in its location, being at the region of the future T3 or higher or lower. With cervical hyperangulation, the rostral part of the septum may skew tangentially from the axis to meet the posterior wall of the foregut, whilst the caudal septal component fails to shut off the future trachea from the oesophagus (Fig. 41.7a). With more caudal thoracic hyperangulation of the embryo, the reverse may happen so that the distal septal component of the foregut skews posteriorly, clipping off the distal oesophagus from the future trachea whilst the rostral component only partially separates trachea from oesophagus (Fig. 41.7c). With pinpoint T3 hyperangulation, both components of the septa may skew posteriorly, dividing the foregut into upper and lower blind segments with a short or long gap between (Fig. 41.7b). Notochordal injury at corresponding pinpoint levels may be expected to deform the developing vertebrae.

H-Type communications between trachea and oesophagus may be due to dorsal angulation, resulting in delayed 'reversal'. In this event the rostral and caudal components fail to meet in continuity (Fig. 41.7d). Depending on the lateness of 'reversal', the communication between the trachea and oesophagus may be pinpoint (Fig. 41.7d) or extensive (Fig. 41.7e). Vertebral defects are uncommon in this type of tracheo-oesophageal fistula (Dickens, 1991).

Anomalies of the VATER association

The non-random association of vertebral, anal, tracheo-oesophageal, radial and renal anomalies constitute the VATER association (Quan and Smith, 1973). Approximately 10% of tracheo-oesophageal septal anomalies are accompanied by anorectal septal defects, and vice versa (Stephens and Smith, 1971).

Similar septation defects may arise in cloacal septation due to impairments of reversal of the hind end of the embryo. The same amniogenic deforming forces caused by temporary oligohydramnios operate at each end of the embryo on the very rare occasion when timing of the impairment of 'reversal' of the rostral and hind-end flexions overlaps. Normally 'reversal' of the head and heart precede that of the hind end.

The vertebral anomalies in 17% of 387 patients with tracheo-oesophageal atresia or fistula are consistent with distortion of the notochord by external forces. Two-thirds of the vertebral anomalies lay in thoracic and one-third in the lumbosacral or sacral vertebrae. In a series of 31 VATER subjects, 11 had sacral vertebral fusions or short sacrum, seven had lumbar and five thoracic anomalies (Piekarski and Stephens, 1976). Compression effects at both ends of the notochord account for these vertebral and septation anomalies in the VATER syndrome.

Radial club hand, radial anomalies and thumb defects sometimes feature in the VATER syndrome. It is possible that compression injures the protruding arm bud or, alternatively, the neural crest at the level of the fifth cervical segment, thus impairing the radial side of the arm at the critical time of development (McCredie, 1974). More extensive neural crest injury may lead to suppression of limb development (amelia) or partial suppression (meromelia). If the condition is bilateral, compression occurs when the two lips of the neural plate, with the underlying neural crest cells, come into apposition at approximately the 25th day (Moore, 1977).

Urogenital anomalies form part of the VATER sequence. Compression that deforms the developing lumbosacral or sacral vertebrae may be accompanied by deformation of the mesoderm of wolffian ridge that runs parallel with the notochord (future developing lumbar and sacral vertebrae), leading to impairment or arrest of development of the wolffian duct, or absence of the ureteric bud or renal anomalies, and to defects in the müllerian ducts in the female.

Abdominal wall deformities

Exomphalos and exstrophic anomalies of the bladder and urethra may be caused in some instances by amniotic membrane constraint of the 'reversal' process during embryonic development.

Exomphalos

Exomphalos has many forms ranging from a central herniation of a peritoneal sac at the umbilicus to a large sac protruding between the widely divaricated rectus muscles. The sac contains coils of midgut and may contain solid organs.

One possible explanation for the persistence of the omphalocele and the divaricated abdominal wall may be delay in the 'reversal' process in the fourth week of embryonic development, affecting chiefly the notochord in the region of the future 10th thoracic vertebrae.

Extreme retroversion instead of flexion of the embryo may occur at a mid-spinal level if oligohydramnios (leakage of amniotic fluid) occurs temporarily before reversal occurs (see Fig. 36.14). Then the future elongating spinal column bends backwards in the thoracolumbar region, with pelvis and lower limbs approximating the thoracic spine and back of the head. In this instance, the lateral body walls divaricate, and all the abdominal contents develop in an extra-abdominal coelomic sac covered only by extraembryonic mesoderm. The umbilical cord is central, extremely short and located on the convexity of the sac (Fig. 41.5).

Another fetus studied by the author exhibited acute retroflexion of the body, occurring between 19 weeks, when ultrasound examination revealed the fetus to be in a flexed position, and 34 weeks, when the baby was born. The retroversion possibly resulted from oligohydramnios and compression of the fetus. The baby was delivered by caesarian section because of hydramnios probably caused by hyperextension of the neck and functional oesophageal obstruction.

If the embryo is acutely twisted to one side during 'reversal', the abdominal wall together with the umbilical cord form on the concave side, but the muscles on the convex side divaricate to produce a huge type of gastroschisis. The abdominal content protrudes in the gap. In three fetuses examined by the author, there was no coelomic sac covering the intestines which were shiny and normal in appearance. Less severe twists during 'reversal' may account for the regular types of gastroschisis.

If the acute 'reversal' was temporarily halted at the time of maximum flexion in the future abdominothoracic region, the central deficit may cleft the epigastrium and sternum and expose the heart and pericardium, as in the so-called Cantrell's pentalogy.

Deformations of the hind end

Delay of 'reversal' at the caudal end may impair the closure of the caudal abdominal and perineal folds and the caudal neuropore. Caudal retroversion could create such anomalies as exstrophy of the bladder and urethra, cloacal exstrophy, anorectal and spinal anomalies and the so-called OEIS syndrome, the omphalocele–exstrophy–imperforate anus–spinal defects complex (Smith et al., 1992).

Forces acting on the tail end during rotation may arrest segmentation (agenesis of terminal vertebrae), impact segments (fused vertebrae) or deviate the somites and the pelvic skeleton to one side as they form (hemivertebrae or hemisacrum), including degrees of pelvic asymmetry and widening of the pubic symphysis (see Figs 36.7 and 36.12).

Transmission of compression forces that disturb the pelvic skeleton may affect developing pelvic organs and perineal structures (see Fig. 36.7). The midline septation of the cloaca during the fourth to sixth weeks may be deviated or disrupted causing an array of anorectourogenital anomalies. The developing external genitalia adapt to the abnormal external orifices of the internal organ anomalies. Later, the external genitalia or anorectum may be impaired by direct pressure of the overlying foot on the perineum (see Figs 36.5 and 36.7 to 36.12).

Coincidentally with these sacral vertebral disruptions occurring during 'reversal', the posterior neuropore and developing spinal cord are hindered in their development. Spina bifida, myelomeningocele, lipomeningocele, myelocystocele, neurenteric cysts, dermoids or tethered cord may result from external deforming forces occurring during the period of 'reversal' of the hind end of the embryo.

Congenital dislocation of the hip

Denis Browne (1959) has attributed the dislocation of the femoral head to abnormal uterine muscle pressure exerted on the flexed knee held in adducted and flexed position of the hip joint, which is consistent with the accompanying valgus moulding. A skin dimple on the knee denotes the point of maximum pressure.

The lower limb buds appear in the embryo of four weeks, project laterally, then elongate as unbending legs without joints until around seven to eight weeks when the hip and knee joints mobilize. The knees then flex to an angle of 90° and the feet appose beneath the body stalk. Moulding and torsion then bring the bent knees to project ventrally and, as the limbs elongate, the feet take up other positions (see Fig. 36.2).

These changes in lower limb posture take place in the embryonic stage of development when the volume of amniotic fluid is adequate. Leakage of amniotic fluid at this period may cause the amnion to shrink and restrain growth and exert pressure on the protruding knee, as indicated by a pressure dimple. Forces generated are conducted along the femur, the head of which over-rides and disrupts the posterior lip of the glenoid cup. The femoral head dislocates posteriorly and remains dislocated even when the normal amniotic fluid volume is restored. The head, developing in the false joint, lags in its ossification.

Browne noted that in the common form of congenital dislocation of the hip, the ipsilateral foot is moulded into the valgus position, which tilts the leg into adduction. Pressure on the knee forces the head of the femur out of the acetabulum posteriorly.

In the uncommon form, where the knee is hyperextended over the abdomen, the foot may be moulded into severe varus deformation and the pressure dimple is then located on the foot. Depending on the timing and duration of the oligohydramnios, the disruption of the posterior lip of the acetabulum may lead to posterior dislocation of the femoral head.

Deformations of the feet

During the early stage of limb development when the joint regions are rigid, temporary compression by the shrunken amnion can create 'club foot' deformations.

The earliest laterally directed limb bud is moulded by the restraining amnion into talipes calcaneovarus, in which the heel is twisted permanently into severe fixed varus position with the forefoot elevated. Talipes equinovarus and talipes varus are moulding deformities arising later when the moulding force impacts on the dorsum of the foot of the elongating rigid limb. After eight weeks when the joints mobilize and the feet cross over the midline beneath the body stalk, milder forms of inversion and eversion of the forefoot occur often with disruption of the alignment of the toe or toes. Moulding and fixation of the bones and joints of the foot are associated with under-development of the calf muscles proportional to the severity of the rigid foot deformity.

Discussion

Torpin (1968) focussed attention on (1) the range of malformation caused by entanglements of amniotic strings; (2) the pathological features of the ruptured amnion, chorion and placenta; and (3) the compression effects caused by uterine contractions. Amnion rupture has been impugned as one of the causes of cranioschisis– limb/body wall dysgenesis and the OEIS syndrome, and the 'amniotic deformity, adhesions mutilations' (ADAM) complex (Keller et al., 1978; Yang, 1990).

Higginbottom et al. (1979) associated the deformities in the amnion rupture sequence with the timing of the rupture and Miller et al. (1981) considered that the amniogenic rupture causes band defects, moulding or a combination of both, and that oligohydramnios may be temporary. Commonly, compression is unrelated to the direct effects of uterine muscle contraction on the embryo or fetus during the period of oligohydramnios.

Based on clinical observations of infants with suspected moulding deformities, and on necropsies of fetuses, it is proposed that non-band compression anomalies may result from temporary leakage of amniotic fluid into the yolk sac via the neurenteric canal, or into the chorionic sac via pores in the amnion membrane, without frank rupture of the amnion; that moulding and restraint on growth of the fast-developing embryo occurs by the sudden collapse and envelopment by the close-fitting amnion; and that moulding occurs by either direct pressure of the amnion on projecting body parts or indirectly by pressure transmitted to the notochord. Direct pressure moulds, whereas the pressure damage to the notochord interrupts its organizing signals that promote the development of the somites, neurulation and endodermal structures, resulting in deformities of the ano-rectum and in VATER syndrome and OEIS complex.

The temporary leakage phenomenon and the moulding is most likely to occur prior to eight weeks, well before the amnionic membrane becomes adherent to the chorion, thus eliminating the chorionic sac and reinforcing the wall of the conceptus.

The lack of evidence of oligohydramnios at the time of birth casts doubts on the role of moulding as a cause of the deformations. However, the concept of very early temporary oligohydramnios resulting from short-lived accidental leaks in early embryogenesis provides a reasonable explanation for the non-band deformations, both moderate and severe. Moulding of the fetus in late pregnancy only augments the early pre-formed deformations.

42

Epispadias and exstrophy of the bladder:
Pathological anatomy and methods of treatment, including radical soft tissue mobilization, an alternative to pelvic osteotomy

Justin Kelly

Abnormal pelvic anatomy in epispadias, exstrophy and variants

The spectrum and subgroups of malformations within the epispadias/exstrophy complex, from continent epispadias to cloacal exstrophy, were well described by Marshall and Meucke (1962). The most common abnormality is classic bladder exstrophy and this will be described in more detail below.

The spectrum of malformations
Continent epispadias

Continent epispadias (Fig. 42.1) is the least serious abnormality in the spectrum. In the male, the epispadiac orifice is on the dorsum of the penis and may be glandular or penile in position. In penile epispadias usually a groove extends from the epispadiac orifice to the glans, which itself is usually deeply grooved in the midline dorsally. As the prepuce may fully cover the penis and may be unretractable, the epispadias may be concealed. More usually, however, the penis is short and almost buried, the prepuce is deficient dorsally and the condition is obvious at birth. In the female the urethral opening extends towards the clitoris, which may be bifid, but in the absence of obvious genital abnormality, a minor degree of epispadias may go undiagnosed.

Incontinent epispadias

When epispadias is more severe it is usually associated with urinary incontinence. With incontinent epispadias the urethral meatal orifice tends to be more proximal, the urethral lumen wider, the pubic symphysis absent, and in either sex, the genital appearance more obviously abnormal.

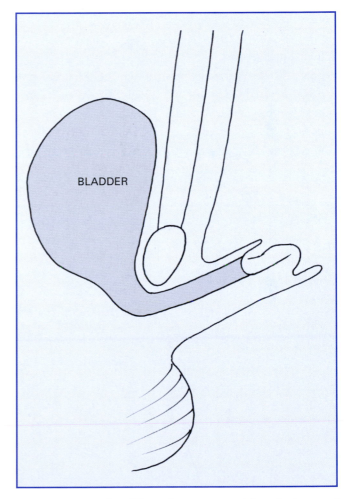

Fig. 42.1 *Epispadias. The urethra opens in a cleft on the dorsum of the penis. The pubic symphysis is present, suggesting that the child may be continent.*

Pubovesical fissure (cleft)

Pubovesical fissure refers to a complete cleft involving the bladder neck, but with the bladder otherwise intact. Continuous urinary leakage occurs from this deep cleft in the pubic region, and the genitalia are malformed.

The urethra is represented by a mucosal strip, in the male this being on the dorsum of the penis.

Classic bladder exstrophy

In classic or typical bladder exstrophy (ectopia vesicae; Fig. 42.2) the mucosal surface of the back wall of the bladder is open on the surface of the lower abdomen and there is a completely open urethral strip. A detailed description follows below. The association of classic bladder exstrophy with imperforate anus usually indicates a more serious anomaly.

Cloacal exstrophy

In cloacal exstrophy the exstrophied bladder, urethral strip and phallus are in two widely separated halves. There is often an exomphalos. Between the two bladder halves lies the exposed ileocaecal mucosa of the bowel, and one or both limbs of the exposed bowel may be prolapsed. There is associated colonic hypoplasia and imperforate anus. Myelomeningocele and other major spinal abnormalities are common and there may be other malformations of the bowel, including a very short small bowel.

Summary

The above definitions are arbitrary, and within the epispadias/exstrophy complex there is considerable variability in almost every detail (Marshall and Meucke, 1962). Also there are rare variants with bladder duplication, genital duplication or skin-covered bladder, and many other variations. The 'typical' anatomy is described below as a basis for surgical management because the surgeon needs to understand the detailed anatomy and its variations.

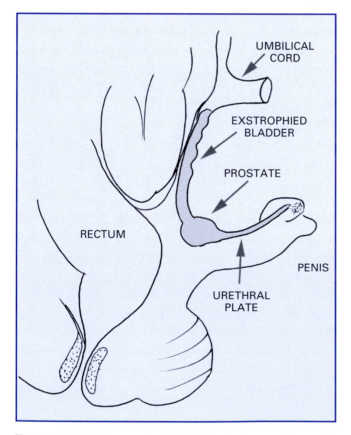

Fig. 42.2 *Classic exstrophy. The bladder is open and lies on the surface of the lower abdomen. The penis is short and curved with the urethral plate on its dorsal surface. The umbilical cord is at the upper margin of the bladder. There is no pubic symphysis.*

The anatomy of 'typical' classic bladder exstrophy

These are operative descriptions as death is rare and autopsy specimens of unoperated classic exstrophy are exceedingly rare. The anatomy will be described under the headings of pelvic girdle and pelvic wall, abdominal wall, bladder, pelvic viscera, both male and female, pudendal vessels and nerves, rectum and anus, and urinary and anal sphincters.

Pelvic girdle and pelvic wall

The pelvic girdle is an open 'C'-shaped structure instead of a complete bony ring, so that the pubic bones are widely separated. The pubic symphysis is replaced by a soft-tissue space of variable width. There is external rotation of the hips, and the thighs are widely separated by a broad perineum. The inside of the pelvic girdle has a normal configuration apart from the laterally displaced pubis and ischium, but the anterior pelvic wall structures are somewhat smaller than normal.

Abdominal wall

The rectus abdominis muscles diverge inferiorly to attach to the superior aspect of the widely separated pubic bones, producing a triangular defect in the lower abdominal wall. In the lower part of this defect lies the exstrophied bladder with no anterior wall and the mucosa of the back wall is on view. Sometimes what appears to be a small bladder is merely a small opening in a capacious bladder which may evert on straining. Usually, however, the exposed surface is flat and represents the entire bladder. The bladder muscle merges with the fascia of the medial aspect of each rectus sheath. The area superior to the bladder varies in size, and the skin almost directly overlies the peritoneum as there is usually little fat. The umbilical cord attaches in this area, although occasionally the umbilicus is situated further superiorly and even in an apparently normal situation. The single umbilical vein passes superiorly and enters the extraperitoneal plane deep to the rectus muscles. The two umbilical arteries arise from branches of the internal iliac arteries and pass on the back wall of the exstrophied bladder in the extraperitoneal plane to reach the umbilicus. The urachus may be an obvious thick cord from the bladder to the umbilicus, or may be absent. A small exomphalos (omphalocele) may be present in the less severe cases, but in the more severe, there may be a large exomphalos. The lateral (oblique) muscles of the abdomen are shortened because of the lateral displacement of the recti and the inguinal canals. The processus vaginalis is frequently patent and an indirect inguinal hernia may result, but otherwise the contents of the inguinal canal are normal.

Bladder

In classic bladder exstrophy, the bladder is a single structure lying on the surface of the lower abdomen and has the appearance of missing its anterior wall. The bladder mucosal area may be normal, but more usually it is so small that, after operation, the volume is only a few millilitres. Nevertheless, a very small bladder closed shortly after birth will often become soft and pliable and increase in volume despite total lack of outlet obstruction (Jeffs, 1983). Apart from a smooth trigone, the bladder mucosa is usually grossly irregular. The mucosa is often congested at birth, but over a few days the degree of congestion and oedema increases rapidly. Frequently there are mucosal polyps above the trigone. Even when the mucosa appears to be macroscopically normal at birth, there is always some microscopic abnormality, with ulceration, metaplasia and cystitis cystica (Culp, 1964). The trigone is less swollen than the rest of the bladder mucosa, and while the ureteric orifices are often widely gaping, sometimes they are small and not

easy to identify. Each ureter after reaching the floor of the pelvis curves superiorly to reach the bladder, so that a catheter passed into the ureteric orifices will tend to pass downwards and laterally. Between the bladder mucosa and the surrounding skin laterally is a layer of smooth epithelium which has been used as 'para-exstrophy flaps' in reconstructive surgery. Deep to the bladder mucosa is a submucosal plane that is usually very congested and adherent in the newborn, and beneath the submucosa lies the bladder muscle. The muscle may be thick or thin, rigid or supple, and extends out to the medial margin of the rectus muscles. The normal prenatal filling and emptying does not occur in exstrophy, and may account for some of the changes in the bladder muscle. The peritoneum covers most of the back of the bladder.

Pelvic viscera

The anatomy of the pelvic viscera and their relationships can be appreciated well in sagittal section. The umbilical cord attachment is usually lower than normal, and below the umbilicus the abdominal wall consists only of the bladder, comprising a layer of altered urothelium on a sheet of bladder muscle. Immediately deep to the bladder is the peritoneal cavity and its contents.

Urethra and genitalia

Male   The penis is curved upwards, so that the glans penis is very close to the mucosal surface of the bladder. Therefore the urethral plate is acutely curved from its commencement at the inferior end of the trigone to its end as a groove in the glans penis.

Urethral plate   The urethral plate is usually much less than half the length of the normal male urethra, and lies on the dorsal surface of the penis. After an indistinct transition from the bladder, the proximal urethra is flat or slightly concave with occasionally some longitudinal grooves. The exposed verumontanum (and the underlying prostate) is small but is usually quite obvious. The urethral plate from this point onwards is smooth, and on the dorsum of the penis consists of an epithelial surface covering the corpus spongiosum. The normally cylindrical corpus spongiosum is splayed out under the mucosal strip, and often extends down between the corpora cavernosa. Distally the corpus spongiosum is continuous with the erectile tissue of the glans penis. There is a midline cleft on the dorsum of the glans penis, and here the surface usually exhibits longitudinal ridges and grooves.

Prostate   The verumontanum is exposed but normal. Beneath the veru is the entire prostate, and this expands at puberty. Between the inferior margin of the prostate and the anal sphincters is the urogenital diaphragm, a thin sheet of skeletal muscle between two flimsy fascial layers described more fully below. After urethral repair, reflux of urine into one or both vasa may occur and may predispose to epididymo-orchitis.

Penis   The penis in exstrophy is short, wide and curved, with small corpora cavernosa. Because the pubic bones are widely separated, the attachments of the corpora cavernosa to the ischiopubic rami are also widely apart, and so the corpora use most of their length reaching the midline before forming the shaft, and as a consequence the shaft is very short. The wide shape of the penis is produced by the corpora being separate. Unlike the normal corpora fused at the base of the penile shaft and sharing a common incomplete fibrous wall, in exstrophy the corpora are entirely separate right to the glans, each having its own dense fascial covering. Proximally the corpora diverge to produce an even wider almost conical appearance to the base of the penis. A short urethral plate and an inbuilt curvature of the corpora cavernosa cause the dorsal curvature of the penis. The glans is cleft dorsally into two lobes, each of which caps the respective corpora cavernosa, and between the lobes is a thin isthmus of glans. The coronal sulcus is absent dorsally but is usually obvious laterally and ventrally. The prepuce is present ventrally as a flap of skin connected by a frenulum to the glans. In cross section, the shaft of the penis in exstrophy consists of the two separate corpora cavernosa, between which is a variable extension of the erectile tissue of the corpus spongiosum as it underlies the mucosa of the urethral plate.

Scrotum and testes   Unlike the normal penoscrotal junction, there is usually a 1 to 2-cm gap of smooth skin between the scrotum and the base of the penis. This skin is said to be hair-bearing after puberty (Kulkarni, personal communication, 2000). The testes may be undescended, but more usually the widely separated testes are in the flat, wide scrotum.

Urogenital diaphragm   The normal urogenital diaphragm is triangular. The transversus perinei muscles form the posterior border, and these connect in the midline with the anterior fibres of the external anal sphincter. Anterolaterally are the crura of the penis covered by the ischiocavernosus muscles and the ischiopubic rami which meet at the pubic symphysis. The urogenital diaphragm is perforated by the urethra. Surrounding the urethra is the sphincter urethrae muscle which is continuous superiorly with the external sphincter of the urethra and inferiorly with the bulbocavernosus muscle.

In exstrophy the ischiopubic rami are widely separated and lie approximately parallel. The urogenital diaphragm is rectangular in shape and contains mainly transversely running skeletal muscle fibres which are continuous laterally with the ischiocavernosus muscles covering the crura of the corpora of the penis. There is no urethra to perforate the urogenital diaphragm. The prostate is situated anterior and superior and somewhat deep to the urogenital diaphragm, and the urethral plate has no urethral bulb or obvious bulbospongiosus muscle. The transversely running skeletal muscle is important for the repair. The posterior fibres of this muscle fuse in the midline with the most anterior fibres of the external anal sphincter.

Female   *Urethral plate*   The urethral plate is short and superiorly merges with the lower portion of the trigone and inferiorly with the hymen which may have several openings. Behind the urethral plate is the anterior wall of the vagina with no plane between the two. The vagina seems short and the uterus is normal. The lower vagina is displaced forwards, so that from the front the vaginal opening passes directly backwards. Behind the lower vagina is the urogenital diaphragm which, as in the male, is a thin sheet of skeletal muscle with a flimsy fascial layer on either surface, and which fuses with the anterior fibres of the external anal sphincter.

Female genitalia   Instead of the mons pubis there is a depressed midline area consisting of the exposed bladder, the urethral strip and the vaginal introitus. The clitoris is in two halves, one on either side of the central strip, and each continuous with a small labium minus. The labia majora are very widely separated and not prominent, and there is a slight elevation at the superior end of each labium majus corresponding to half the mons. The urethral strip is short, flat and blends with the inferior part of the trigone. In classic bladder exstrophy a double vagina is not unusual, particularly in the more severe forms.

Perineum and urogenital diaphragm The urogenital diaphragm in the normal female is triangular and is perforated by the urethra and the vagina. Laterally it is bordered by the ischiopubic rami and the crura of the clitoris as far forward as the pubic symphysis. The transversus perinei muscle forms the posterior border. In the midline the transversus perinei fuses with the most anterior fibres of the anal external sphincter at the perineal body.

In exstrophy, as the ischiopubic rami run parallel with one another, the urogenital diaphragm is rectangular rather than triangular. The anterior border is a variably developed fibrous band connecting the pubic bones and passing deep to the vagina. The crura of the clitoris and the ischiocavernosus muscles appear normal. Neither the urethra nor the vagina perforate the urogenital diaphragm. The muscles of the urogenital diaphragm (sphincter urethrae, sphincter vaginae and transversus perinei) are represented by skeletal muscle running transversely behind the vagina and fusing in the midline posteriorly with the perineal body.

Pudendal vessels and nerves

In exstrophy the pudendal vessels and nerves have normal courses and relationships, apart from being widely separated (Fig. 42.3). In the repair of bladder exstrophy described below, the anatomy of the pudendal vessels and nerves is of great importance. This surgical correction involves the lateral pelvic wall remaining unchanged but the pelvic viscera and particularly the sphincters and the phallus being mobilized medially. It is therefore necessary to mobilize the pudendal vessels and nerves. This means detaching and mobilizing them as far back as the ischial spine, and then drawing them medially and straightening their curve.

Branches of the second, third and fourth sacral nerves join in the posterior part of the pelvis to form the pudendal nerve. The nerve is joined by the pudendal vessels, and, entering the pelvic cavity from behind and below the spine of the ischium and the sacrospinous ligament, it runs on the medial surface of the pelvic wall lying between the obturator internus muscle laterally and the fat of the ischiorectal fossa medially. The pudendal nerve and vessels reach the medial aspect of the ischium where they lie in the fibrous pudendal canal (Alcock's canal, an extension of the sacrotuberous ligament), and at the anterior end of this canal they curve superiorly along the line of the ischiopubic ramus. The pudendal nerve sends branches to the rectum, and then divides before the base of the penis into the perineal branches and the dorsal nerve of the phallus. In the male, the dorsal nerve of the penis runs on the deep aspect of the crura and corpora cavernosa of the penis and emerges from the pelvis on the dorsum of the corpora cavernosa to supply the shaft and glans of the penis and, in the normal male, the distal penile urethra (Yang and Bradley, 1998). It is generally accepted that an intact dorsal nerve of the penis is essential for normal erection and ejaculation (Bors and Comarr, 1954; Seftel et al., 1994). The perineal branches of the pudendal nerve run onto the superficial aspect of the urogenital diaphragm and supply the muscles of the urogenital diaphragm and the skin of the scrotum and, in the normal male, the proximal penile urethra. In the female the pudendal nerves and vessels are as for the male, the relationships of the branches of the pudendal nerve to the clitoris being as of the penis and to the labia as of the scrotum. The nerve supply follows a similar pattern.

Rectum and anus

The rectum and anus appear anterior, although they are normally positioned in relation to the ischium. This is probably because of the relative failure of development of the anterior pelvic structures. In the male the rectum lies just behind the region of the bladder neck.

Sphincter muscles

Urinary sphincters

The urinary sphincters are grossly abnormal. There is smooth muscle deep to the mucosa of the proximal part of the urethral strip, representing the internal urethral sphincter. Use of a muscle stimulator at operation indicates no evidence of skeletal muscle near the urethra. However, there is skeletal muscle in the urogenital diaphragm, which is situated some distance from the urethral plate.

Anal sphincters

The levator ani, and particularly the puborectalis sling are abnormal. In the normal pelvis the puborectalis attaches to the pubic bones close to the midline,

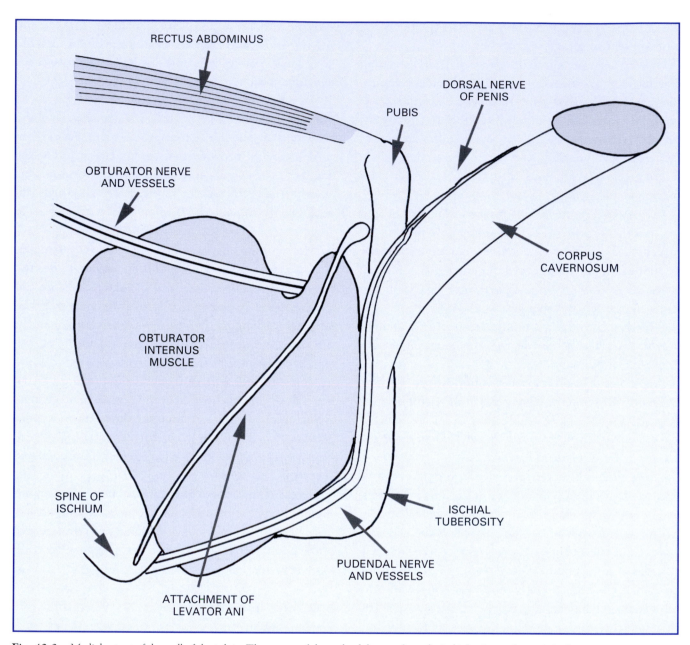

Fig. 42.3 *Medial aspect of the wall of the pelvis. The course of the pudendal nerve from the ischial spine to the penis is shown.*

forming a tight 'U' sling supporting the anorectal junction. In exstrophy, the puborectalis shows an open 'C' shape, resulting in a less efficient support and sphincter. Rectal prolapse is not uncommon. The external and internal anal sphincters appear to be normal.

Sacrum

The sacrum is usually normal, although in the more severe forms of exstrophy, sacral agenesis or some form of spina bifida is often present.

Developments in the management of bladder exstrophy

Exstrophy of the bladder is described on an Assyrian tablet dated from 2000 BC (currently in the British Museum) (Jeffs, 1986). Perhaps the earliest subsequently recorded description of the malformation is that of Schenk von Grafenberg (1644). The first illustration was made by Christian Gockels (Gockels, 1686). The first complete description is attributed to James Mowat

(Mowat, 1747). According to Mazel (1899), the term 'exstrophie' was coined by Chaussier in 1780.

The management of exstrophy was initially non-surgical. In the 18th and early 19th centuries the management concentrated on collecting devices to reduce somewhat the misery of a life of unceasing wetness (Murphy, 1972).

Reconstructive surgery commenced in the latter half of the 19th century and has followed five different paths:

1. covering the exposed bladder with local skin flaps,
2. closing the anterior bladder wall and having urinary drainage by means of an artificial urethra or some other route,
3. providing urinary diversion,
4. reconstructing the exstrophied bladder and urethra with the aim of achieving both anatomical and functional normality, or
5. providing functional reconstruction with deliberate departure from reconstructing normal anatomy.

Covering the exposed bladder with local skin flaps

Covering the bladder with local skin flaps was advocated as early as 1825 (Murphy, 1972), but it was not until 1858 that Daniel Ayres in New York successfully covered over a woman's bladder (Ayres, 1859), and subsequently a number of reports of various modifications appeared in the literature, with Karl Thiersch describing in 1876 the use of raw flaps to cover the bladder to avoid the problems of incorporation of hair-bearing skin (Thiersch, 1876).

Closing the anterior bladder wall, with urinary drainage by artificial urethra or other route

Closing the anterior bladder wall and providing drainage by an artificial urethra or other route has provided an opportunity for a number of ingenious operations with occasional success but significant morbidity and a high mortality. The anal sphincters could be used to provide continence by bringing a neo-urethra through the anus, the neo-urethra being constructed from the rectum (Soubottine, 1901), from the divided lower ureter after transureteroureterostomy (Murphy, 1972), or from pedicle and Thiersch grafts (Murphy, 1972). After a left

colostomy, anastomosis between bladder and rectum could give good urinary control (Murphy, 1972). Alternatively the whole exstrophic bladder could be implanted into the bowel (Moynihan, 1906).

Providing urinary diversion

Urinary diversion was initiated in the 1850s with attempts at creating anastomoses between the ureters and the rectum, but the techniques were crude by modern standards and the mortality was very high. In 1892 Maydl implanted the trigone into the sigmoid colon with success (Maydl, 1894), and Bergenhem included a separate rosette of bladder around each ureter in a ureter-to-sigmoid implantation in an adult presenting with malignancy in an exstrophied bladder (Bergenhem, 1896). Subsequently this technique was used by many others (Murphy, 1972). Eventually, anti-refluxing ureterosigmoidostomy with cystectomy became the treatment of choice in most centres, and it still has its advocates despite overwhelming evidence of the eventual development of aggressive malignant change in the bowel near the anastomosis (Mayo, 1908; Bagchi, 1990). Following the work of Bricker in the 1940s in patients with cystectomy for malignancy, ileal conduits became accepted as a method of urinary diversion (Bricker, 1950). Some were performed for bladder exstrophy, either as an initial treatment or as a salvage procedure in cases where anatomical reconstruction had failed (Rickham, 1956). It was soon apparent that ileal conduits were particularly likely to fail if there was dilatation of the upper urinary tracts (Johnston, 1958). Nevertheless from the 1960s to the late 1970s there was considerable enthusiasm for ileal conduits for many conditions of bladder dysfunction and incontinence. By the early 1980s evidence was mounting that after 10 or more years of relatively trouble-free diversion, ileal conduits gradually failed and stenoses, calculi, infections and renal damage became very common. Colonic conduits, being suitable for antireflux ureteric anastomoses, were considered to be more appropriate and they enjoyed brief popularity, but it soon became apparent that they suffered the same problems as ileal conduits.

Continent diversion has the very considerable appeal of the lack of an external collecting device and is enthusiastically recommended by some workers (Bassiouny, 1992), but as the abnormal physiology of urine in isolated small or large bowel is similar in many ways to that of conduits, it seems not unlikely that continent diversions will eventually fail also.

Closing and reconstructing the bladder and urethra, aiming for anatomical and functional normality

Bladder closure was recommended from 1844 but it was not until 1885 that Wyman achieved the first successful closure in a 5-day-old baby (Murphy, 1972). Poppert in 1896 described a three-stage operation with bladder closure and urethral construction, which he claimed gave the 13-year-old boy a bladder 'physiologically virtually perfect' (Poppert, 1896). It was realized that the wide separation of the pubic bones in exstrophy made bladder closure and abdominal wall closure difficult, and in 1892 Trendelenberg divided the ligaments of the sacroiliac joints and placed the patients in a pelvic sling to maintain apposition of the pubes prior to bladder closure (Trendelenberg, 1892). He argued that in bladder exstrophy the physiological factors necessary for both retention of urine and voluntary micturition were present (Trendelenberg, 1906). However, he noted that the pubes tended to distract again and revert to their original positions, and he commented upon the likelihood of such changes interfering with urinary sphincter function. A number of reports of osteotomies of the ilium or of the superior or inferior rami of the pubic bones appeared in the first few years of the 20th century (Murphy, 1972). So-called 'new' osteotomies reported in recent years can be often traced back to this era. However, various osteotomies, improved surgical techniques and newer methods of external and internal fixation continue to be utilized and reported (Gearhart and Jeffs, 1996).

Anatomical reconstruction has remained an elusive goal. In 1922 Young reported an operation for the production of continence in incontinent epispadias (Young, 1922). Subsequently he reported a successful bladder closure with continence in bladder exstrophy in a female (Young, 1942) and this technique was modified by Dees (1942) to incorporate the prostatic urethra and bladder neck in the plication of the urethra. In 1949 Chisolm was instrumental in setting up a multidisciplinary team (the Minnesota Exstrophy Team) devoted to the anatomical and physiological repair of bladder

exstrophy (Sweetser et al., 1952). They performed staged repair and stressed the importance of accurate co-aption of the pubic bones, which could be achieved at the definitive operation by a posterior iliac osteotomy being performed up to 2 weeks earlier. The pubic apposition was produced by wire sutures and maintained by 4 months of body cast. Epispadias repair was performed as a separate stage. There was low mortality, the rate of kidney damage was very low and the continence results were far superior to those previously reported, with a long-term review of almost 100 patients showing an incontinence rate of only 35%, and 45% showing very acceptable continence, being dry except for stress incontinence (Chisolm, 1979). Jeffs and his team followed a similar plan, concentrating upon improvements in all aspects of the management and particularly operative technique, and their results have been excellent, with up to 86% continence in 22 patients (Lepor and Jeffs, 1983). It was accepted that bladder closure was most easily performed in the first day or two after birth, and while most authors preferred a staged approach, Ansell (1979) recommended neonatal functional repair. He subsequently reported 43% continence in 23 patients (Ansell, 1983).

Anatomical reconstruction without osteotomy has been described by the present author, the soft tissues of the pelvis being mobilized from the lateral pelvic wall, dividing the attachment of the levator ani from the surface of the obturator internus muscle and, using a subperiosteal plane, mobilizing the corpora and the sphincters from their bony attachments on a pedicle of the pudendal vessels and nerves (Kelly, 1995). The principles and details of this operation are given below.

The anatomical reconstruction of the male urethra in epispadias was advocated by Cantwell over 100 years ago (Cantwell, 1895). Ransley and his co-workers extended this operation to the urethra in bladder exstrophy (Ransley et al., 1988). In constructing the urethra, this technique moves it from the dorsum of the penis to its normal ventral position and the associated glans repair leads to a very normal appearance. However, the penis in both epispadias and exstrophy is short, conical and has a dorsal curvature, worse on erection. The Ransley–Cantwell repair incorporates cavernosa-cavernostomy and this reduces chordee and helps with the conical appearance, but does not correct the shortness. Mobilization of the corpora cavernosa from their attachments on the ischiopubic rami has been shown to elongate and straighten the penis (Kelly and Eraklis, 1971), but has the potential to render the penis ischaemic, and if the urogenital diaphragm is used to wrap around the urethra, this latter manoeuvre tends to pull the penis back into the pelvis.

Kulkarni (personal communication, 2000) has observed that the skin between penis and scrotum has the appearance of the skin normally in the pubic region superior to the penis. She has therefore mobilized this skin to its normal position and in the process the penis becomes more pendulous and the urethral length more adequate. The Cantwell principle can be used then to retain the urethra while still wrapping it with the bladder neck and membranous sphincters.

Providing functional reconstruction with deliberate departure from reconstructing normal anatomy

Many authors have departed from the principle of recreating entirely normal anatomy in functional closure. The high incidence of vesicoureteric reflux following sphincter construction in exstrophy, together with infection and raised intravesical pressure, has contributed to a number of children with exstrophy developing renal damage. Anti-reflux surgery is therefore common and transtrigonal reimplantation is used frequently, a deliberate distortion of the normal anatomy.

Guy Leadbetter extended the short urethral plate by incorporating the medial portion of the trigone as the proximal part of a Young–Dees repair, mobilizing and reimplanting the ureters to a higher level on the back wall of the bladder (Leadbetter, 1964). Incorporation of the lower trigone without resiting of the ureters was recommended by Williams, with a layered wrap to tighten the bladder neck (Williams and Savage, 1966). Mollard has reported a variation of the Leadbetter principle by using asymmetric flaps of trigone to reconstruct the bladder neck and increase outlet resistance (Mollard et al., 1994). Duckett described the elongation of the proximal urethra by division of the urethral plate and the interposition of para-exstrophy flaps created from the shiny epithelium found to either side of the lower part of the exposed bladder (Duckett, 1978). Finally the

congenitally short urethra may be elongated by bringing its distal end into a hypospadiac position, and subsequently repairing the hypospadias (Kelly, 1995).

The mucosal area at birth is variable, but is usually much smaller than the normal bladder. Although it is common for the bladder to enlarge and become supple after closure, even when there is no sphincteric or other outlet obstruction, there is considerable variation in bladder wall compliance and bladder growth, so that its volume may be inadequate for continence and there may be high intravesical pressures. Indeed it has been questioned whether many of the children with exstrophy can ever have a normally functioning bladder. Augmentation of the bladder volume using an isolated segment of bowel, enterocystoplasty, was carried out firstly in animal experiments and then in exstrophy patients in 1899 (Rutkowski, 1899). More recently enterocystoplasty has been used, sometimes at the initial operation but particularly in 'failed' repair, usually using small or large bowel (Gearhart, 1988). In exstrophy, the use of stomach to augment the bladder (gastrocystoplasty) has been reported as producing intolerable pain and so is contraindicated. Following enterocystoplasty, clean intermittent catheterization is often necessary, and this may be difficult through the reconstructed urethra. An alternative abdominal catheterizing channel may need to be provided using appendix (Mitrofanoff, 1980), tubed small bowel (Monti and Carvalho, 1997) or disconnected ureter (Duckett and Lofti, 1993). The short- and long-term problems of exposure of enteric mucosa to urine have been recognized and efforts made to use urothelium where possible. In the presence of a megaureter, the ureter itself can be utilized for augmentation, but this is not a common scenario in exstrophy (Bellinger, 1993). There is considerable ongoing research, and eventually it is possible that a generally applicable urothelial-lined bladder augmentation will become a clinical reality.

In every reported series there is a proportion of repaired children who are unable to achieve acceptable urinary continence even with adequate bladder capacity, and alternative measures have been described, particularly the use of submucosally injected inert substances, implanted mechanical sphincter devices (Aliabadi and Gonzalez, 1990) or valve closure of the bladder neck with or without an abdominal stoma.

Staged repair of classic exstrophy using radical mobilization of soft tissues

At the Royal Children's Hospital, Melbourne, we see one or two new patients with bladder exstrophy each year. Prior to 1985 we performed staged repair using posterior iliac osteotomy, but, in our hands, the osteotomy had invariably failed in the long term, with the pubic bones eventually reverting to their original positions. No child with staged repair using osteotomy developed and maintained useful bladder control, and for all patients ultimately we proceeded to some form of urinary diversion. The need to close the bladder and abdominal wall meant we had to perform some form of anatomical repair, even if urinary diversion was eventually performed.

In 1986 the fortuitous intraoperative use of a muscle stimulator during such a repair improved our knowledge of the anatomy of the skeletal muscle in the pelvis in exstrophy. It was recognized that skeletal muscle appropriate for use as a urethral sphincter was nowhere near the bladder neck but lay in two areas: in the urogenital diaphragm behind the vagina in the female and beneath the scrotum in the male, and in that part of the levator ani which could be seen to run from the medial aspect of each pubis to pass behind the vagina in the female and behind the proximal urethra in the male. Both the urogenital diaphragm and the levator ani would need to be detached from the pelvic wall to utilize them as sphincters. Some years ago we had described the concept of detachment of the penis from the pelvic wall in exstrophy, including dissection and mobilization of the pudendal neurovascular bundle (Kelly and Eraklis, 1971). It was therefore logical to use this principle to release the muscle attachments for both the urogenital diaphragm and the levator ani and to use these in sphincter construction. In the male the detachment needed to include the penis, and thus the operation of total radical mobilization was conceived.

It was assumed that in the male the urethra constructed from the urethral plate would be too short to reach the sphincter muscle area and still remain attached to the tip of the penis. Rather than using para-exstrophy flaps, it was decided to detach the urethral plate from the glans and to bring the urethral opening into a proximal penile hypospadiac position, and to later perform hypospadias correction as a further stage (Kelly, 1995). Recently the work of Kulkarni has led to a change in this approach, the penis being moved downwards towards the scrotum and the urethral plate being tubed and mobilized as in the Cantwell procedure, thus avoiding the construction of a hypospadiac urethra (Kulkarni, personal communication, 2000).

It became apparent that in the female the sphincter muscles would need to be wrapped around both the constructed urethra and the vagina, which in turn would need to be mobilized into a more posterior position. The operation using radical mobilization of the soft tissues, which was devised 15 years ago is described below. It has been modified in many ways for easier access, less blood loss, less tissue damage and more accurate repair, but the key principles have remained unchanged.

Key principles

To improve the technique of this surgery, we have studied children in whom the results of previous surgery have been poor. By analysing the previous treatments and operations and particularly the findings at re-operation, we have identified several factors needed for optimum results:

1. The bladder neck must be a sudden and definite junction between the spherical bladder and the tubular urethra. A gradual narrowing leads to urinary incontinence and, in the male, retrograde ejaculation and, with the urine being at bladder pressure in the posterior urethra, epididymo-orchitis. Support of the bladder neck to the back of the pubis is probably important also.

2. When dissecting the penis, it is necessary to preserve intact both the urethral plate and its underlying corpus spongiosum on the one hand and the corpora cavernosa on the other. As there is no clear plane of dissection between them, sharp dissection is necessary. Damage to the urethral plate and corpus spongiosum produces a thin urethra, prone to infarction, diverticulum formation or stricture. Without a pad of soft tissue for the sphincters to squeeze upon, continence will be compromised. Damage to the corpora cavernosa leads to growth failure of the penis, to deformity from growth disturbance or to tethering from fibrous bands of scar, or to failure of erection of one or both sides of the penis. In the most severe

situation, infarction and necrosis could occur to the glans or distal shaft of the penis. Any of these problems may defy later attempts at salvage. It is critical that the dissection between corpora and urethral plate is meticulous, even though it may be very time consuming.

3. The bladder muscle and its nerve and blood supply must be preserved. Denervation may produce a small, fibrotic, high-pressure neuropathic bladder. There are several possible causes, both at initial closure as a newborn and at the later stage during bladder and sphincter reconstruction and reimplantation of the ureters. The bladder muscle extends under the 'para-exstrophy' tissues to the margins of the recti, and the lateral muscle margins are easily lost in freeing the bladder from the recti. The nerve supply to the bladder runs beside the ureters to the trigone and is then distributed on the peritoneal aspect of the bladder wall. Nerves for erection and ejaculation pass close to the prostate. To minimize bladder and nerve damage our current practice is:

a. to close the bladder as soon after birth as possible to prevent mucosal fibrosis,

b. to follow the medial margin of the recti and preserve the bladder muscle margins,

c. to minimize dissection on the peritoneal aspect of the bladder,

d. when reimplanting the ureters, to dissect only transvesically and very close to the ureters,

e. to avoid incising the trigone or using the trigone to augment the urethral length,

f. to keep clear of the prostatic venous plexuses and their attendent nerves and

g. to carefully identify and preserve the pudendal nerves and their branches.

With this as a background, the operation as currently performed is described in detail as follows.

Classic bladder exstrophy: the newborn male patient

A staged repair is performed: stage 1, bladder closure as a newborn; and stage 2, functional repair with radical mobilization at 2–6 months of age. If at the second stage a hypospadias is constructed, it is repaired as a third stage at 3–5 years.

Stage 1: bladder closure at birth

The bladder should be closed soon after birth, as mucosal congestion rapidly increases, and the pelvic girdle becomes less pliable. An incision is made around the base of the umbilicus and is continued around the margin of the bladder as far as the bladder neck region. The bladder portion of this incision should be undermined laterally so that the underlying bladder muscle is preserved. The urachus, if present, is divided. The umbilicus may be excised or, more usually, it is mobilized superiorly by dividing the obliterated umbilical arteries and passing the umbilical stump up behind the linea alba to emerge through a surgically created circular skin defect in the centre of the abdominal wall. The medial margins of the rectus abdominus muscles are identified and followed inferiorly to detach the bladder muscle from the recti without damage to either. Preserving the bladder muscle ensures the largest possible bladder capacity. The bladder is closed in the midline down to the bladder neck. When the recti are closed in the midline the bladder becomes an extraperitoneal structure behind them, a position maintained by a couple of sutures anchoring the front wall of the bladder to the back of the rectus muscles. Thus, at the level of the bladder neck, a suprapubic urinary stoma is produced. This stoma must be small, about 10–12 F gauge, to prevent bladder prolapse and subsequent dehiscence. The ureters are catheterized and the catheters either emerge through the bladder and abdominal wall or emerge through the stoma. Closure of the abdominal wall may be easily accomplished in some children, but sometimes the pubic bones and the lower rectus muscles are too widely separated. If so, the recti are closed in the midline as low as reasonably possible, and then bilateral flaps of anterior rectus sheath, hinged on their medial margins, are created and are used as a double layer to close the midline defect down to the stoma. Only absorbable sutures are used, as non-absorbable sutures migrate into the urinary tract and cause calculi. Inguinal hernial sacs are frequently present, and the extraperitoneal exposure provided by the above dissection affords an opportunity for repair. Alternatively, transinguinal repair can be performed at birth as a preventative measure, or later if a hernia becomes clinically apparent.

Several days of postoperative ureteric drainage are recommended to prevent ureterovesical obstruction and postrenal anuria. No suprapubic catheter is necessary. Vertical skin traction of the legs, just enough to lift the buttocks off the bed, can be used to reduce tension on the repair and to facilitate nursing in the early post-operative phase, or alternatively crêpe bandages can be used to bring the thighs together gently so as to reduce the tension on the abdominal closure with adduction of the thighs.

Stage 2: aged 2–6 months

This stage involves functional repair with radical soft tissue mobilization, construction of the urethra and urethral sphincters, penile mobilization, bilateral anti-reflux ureteric reimplantation and, if desired, production of penoscrotal hypospadias.

The principles of the radical repair are to detach the pelvic soft tissues from the wall of the pelvis so they are freed from tension, and then to construct urogenital structures from the normal tissues which are present but not properly formed.

This repair should not be undertaken unless the first stage has been successful and is fully healed. If there has been any wound breakdown or if the bladder has pro-lapsed even partly through the stoma, it is recommended that the first-stage repair be re-done rather than attempt this major operation. Unless the mucosa of the bladder has been inside an intact bladder for a month or more, the technical aspects of reimplantation will be unnecessarily difficult. On occasion reimplantation has been delayed until after radical repair, but the risk of renal damage occurring in the interim, due to infection plus increased bladder pressure plus reflux, is very real. Any excoriated or inflamed skin is vigorously treated before commencing surgery.

Re-opening the bladder, defining of the bladder neck and reimplanting the ureters   A midline abdominal incision is made through the scar of the old repair, dividing the abdominal wall and anterior bladder wall through the stoma (Fig. 42.4). The level of the bladder neck may be indistinct and if so it is judged to be half-

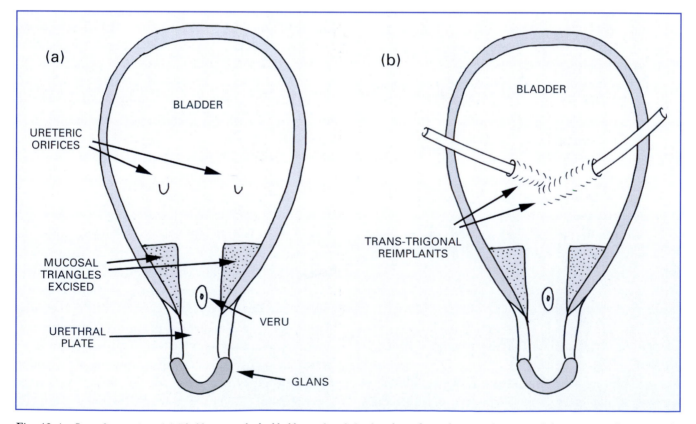

Fig. 42.4 *Stage 2 operation.* **(a)** *Bladder opened: the bladder neck is defined at the midpoint between the veru and the ureteric orifices. Triangles of mucosa are excised to produce a urethra of uniform calibre.* **(b)** *Reimplantation of ureters. Bilateral transverse advancement ureterocystoplasty is performed.*

way between the apex of the verumontanum and the level of the ureteric orifices. The urethral strip below the bladder neck level should be 12 mm in width and above this level it should rapidly widen to the full width of the bladder wall. To achieve this a triangle of mucosa is excised from each side to expose the muscle of the bladder neck. This muscle is not incised, but later it is used to help strengthen the bladder neck closure. Usually the bladder mucosa is normal, but it may still be friable. If mucosal polyps are present they may be excised. After sphincter construction one can expect that vesicoureteric reflux will become apparent, so that anti-reflux reimplantation of the ureters is strongly recommended, and it is convenient to perform re-

implantation early during this repair, before the bladder mucosa becomes swollen. The ureters usually enter the bladder from the inferior aspect, and either transtrigonal or superior advancement of the ureters may be performed. The plane of dissection needs to be close to the adventitial surface of the ureters to minimize damage to the bladder innervation. Sometimes the bladder seems too small to allow reimplantation, but anti-reflux surgery is still recommended, as persisting reflux after sphincter construction is a major concern, particularly in a small tight bladder.

Dissecting the penis   The lateral margins of the urethral plate (about 12 mm wide) on the dorsum of the penis are outlined with a marking pen. Shallow inci-

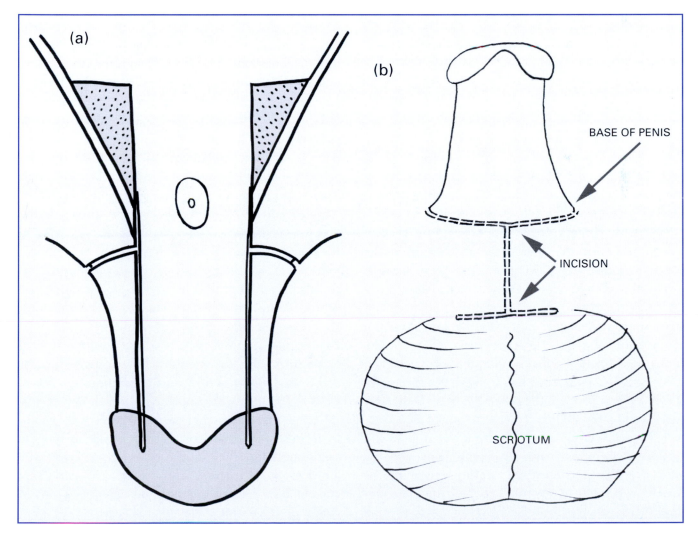

Fig. 42.5 *(a) Urethral plate incised. Parallel incisions are made along the margins of the urethral plate and onto glans. An incision is made around the base of the penis commencing at the margins of the urethral plate. (b) Incisions in penoscrotal region. Note the incision around the base of the penis. A midline incision is made from base of penis to scrotum. Short incisions are made along superior margin of scrotum.*

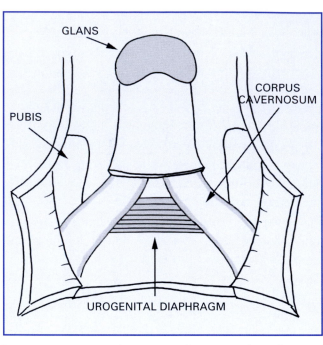

Fig. 42.6 *Exposure after penoscrotal incision. After reflection of flaps the corpora and urogenital diaphragm are on view. Retraction exposes the ischiopubic rami.*

sions are made along these margins and then, as they are deepened, each is shelved outwards so as to reach the covering of the corpora cavernosa at the lateral side of the penis (Figs. 42.5 and 42.6). The urethral plate is then dissected from the corpora cavernosa (Fig. 42.7). Between the corpora lies a midline strip or 'keel' of erectile tissue continuous with the undersurface of the urethral plate. By following a plane close to each corpus, the urethral plate with the attached keel can be dissected free from the corpora and the corpora themselves separated almost down to the intact ventral penile skin. It requires patience to remain in the correct plane between the corpora cavernosa and their covering tunica on the one hand, and the erectile tissue of the urethral plate on the other, but it is essential for a good long-term result and there is minimal blood loss. As discussed above, damage to the urethral plate will produce scarring and later major problems with the urethra and/or incontinence, while damage to the corpora will result in deformity of the penis. The urethral incisions are extended about half-way to the end of the glans, and are deepened to almost reach the skin on the underside of the penis. At no stage is the skin of the penis mobilized.

Pelvic soft tissue mobilization *Exposing the urogenital diaphragm and incising the subcutaneous border of the ischiopubic ramus* An incision is made around the base of the penis. Below the penis a midline incision connects the above incision to the scrotum, and short incisions are made on either side along the scrotal margin (Fig. 42.5b). This produces two skin flaps hinged laterally, and undermining these in the subcutaneous plane and retracting them exposes the corpora cavernosa and, between the bases of the corpora, the urogenital diaphragm (Fig. 42.6). The muscle stimulator is useful in identifying the latter. The base of each corpus cavernosum is freed from the overlying tissues and from its fellow on the opposite side. The urogenital diaphragm is preserved and will later provide a bed into which the urethral plate will be laid. Care must be taken to preserve also the dorsal nerves of the penis (and their accompanying vessels), which are adherent to the corpora cavernosa on their dorsal and lateral aspects. A relatively bloodless plane is dissected laterally under the flaps to expose the pubis and ischiopubic ramus and ischium as far back as the ischial tuberosity. The periosteum/perichondrium of the ischiopubic ramus and pubis is scored with diathermy along the subcutaneous surface, and the dissection deepened to include a thin flake of the underlying cartilage and bone (Fig. 42.9). The dissection stops short of going right through to the deep side of the ischiopubic ramus for fear of damaging the nerves and vessels on the deep aspect. At the superior end, the incision is carried through and over onto the medial aspect of the pubic bone, incorporating part of the pubis down to and including the attachment of the puborectalis part of the levator ani.

Exposing the superior aspect of the levator ani An extraperitoneal plane is dissected between the bladder and rectus muscles and is carried down into the pelvis, exposing the iliac vessels, obturator vessels and nerves, the obturator internus and the medial wall of the pelvis, including the superior surface of the levator ani and the posteromedial aspect of the pubic bone below the attachments of the recti. This dissection is quick, easy and bloodless, but the vas needs to be identified early in dissection to prevent inadvertent damage.

Exposing and mobilizing the pudendal neurovascular bundle The next part of the dissection occurs beside the 'white line' which is the attachment of the levator ani to the

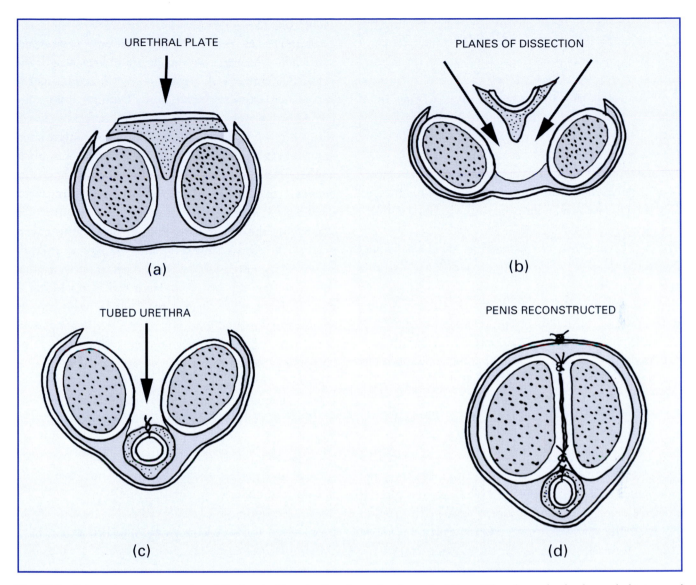

URETHRAL PLATE

(a)

PLANES OF DISSECTION

(b)

TUBED URETHRA

(c)

PENIS RECONSTRUCTED

(d)

Fig. 42.7 *Schematic transverse section of distal penis. Note the dissection to free the urethral plate. When the urethra has been tubed it is moved into a normal relationship with the corpora. When the corpora are sutured in midline, the penis is reconstituted and the dorsal skin margins lie close together and are readily closed.*

fascia overlying the obturator internus muscle. An incision is made through the levator ani about 2 or 3 mm from the white line and parallel to it (Fig. 42.10). A plane is developed between the under surface of the levator ani and the surface of the obturator internus muscle. It may be difficult to develop this plane initially, and it is not uncommon to enter the obturator internus muscle. However, this seems to do no demonstrable damage. Within about 1 cm of deeper blunt dissection the fat of the ischiorectal fossa is encountered. By keeping between the fibrous envelope of the ischiorectal fat, and the obturator internus fascia, a straightforward

dissection can be carried down to the ischial spine, which can be readily palpated as a guide. The pudendal neurovascular bundle (Fig. 42.11) is found anterior to the ischial spine, either on the surface of the fat or on the medial surface of the obturator internus muscle. The pudendal vein usually receives a tributary from the obturator internus and this needs to be divided. It is then possible to follow the pudendal neurovascular bundle anteriorly as far as the ischiopubic ramus.

Separating the flake of the ischiopubic ramus to free the central pelvic structures When the pudendal neurovascular bundle has been identified, it is now safe to continue the dissection of the ischiopubic ramus, dividing the periosteum/perichondrium and incorporating a flake of underlying bone and cartilage through to the medial surface of the pelvis and back to the ischial tuberosity. Any subcutaneous fibrous attachments of the mobilized segment are divided. Some additional mobilization of the pudendal neurovascular bundle from its surrounding fibrous attachments may be required.

Following the above dissections the central structures of the pelvis are freed from all lateral attachments (Fig. 42.11) and can be brought to the midline without tension.

Tubing the urethra, reconstructing the penis, creating the sphincters The urethral plate is infolded with fine absorbable sutures to create a urethral tube (Figs. 42.7 (a, b), 42.8 (a, b)) and the lumen of the urethral tube so created is usually between 8 and 10 F

gauge. Distally the urethra continues to the tip of the penis and the glans is reconstructed on the dorsal aspect of the urethra using several layers of fine absorbable sutures. The meatus so created is surprisingly normal in appearance and no need has been found to perform the IPGAM procedure of Ransley. The shaft of the penis, still wrapped in undisturbed skin on its lateral and ventral aspect, is now reconstructed. A 7/9 urethral sound is introduced into the urethral tube through the meatus and is used to gently draw the urethra down (Figs. 42.7 (c) and 42.8 (c)) between the corpora to lie under the skin on the ventral aspect of the penis. The corpora are then approximated with fine absorbable sutures (Fig. 42.7 (d)) and in the process the urethra comes to lie in its normal position and the skin margins become drawn together on the dorsum. Proximal to the skin-covered segment of the penis is the urogenital

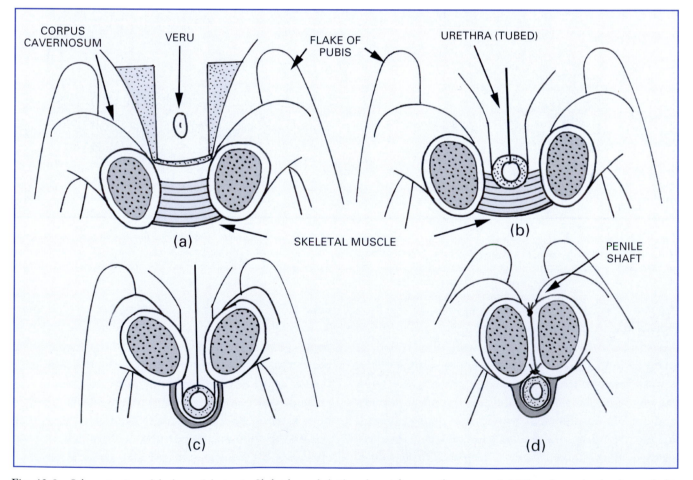

Fig. 42.8 *Schematic view of the base of the penis. Skeletal muscle bridges the gap between the corpora.* (**a**) *When the urethra has been tubed it is placed within this muscle.* (**b**) *By bringing the corpora together at the attachment of the muscle, the urethra becomes encircled with muscle.* (**c, d**) *As corpora are brought together the flakes of pubis come close to the midline and are later sutured together.*

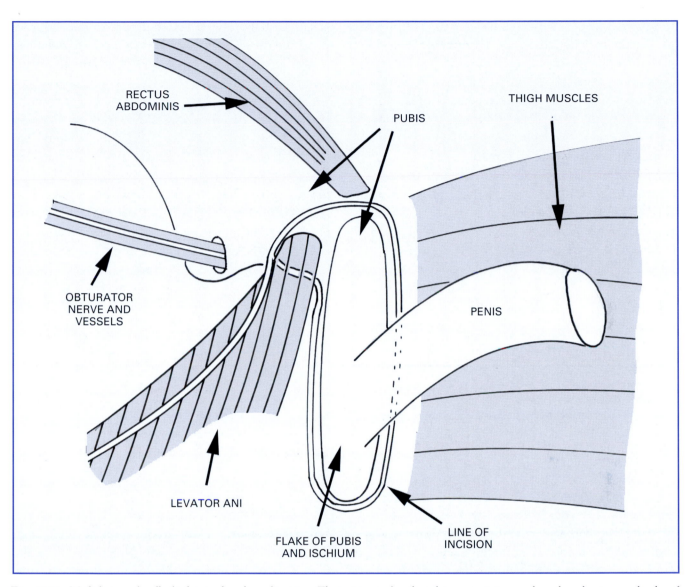

Fig. 42.9 *Medial view of wall of pelvis to show line of incision. The incision to free the pelvic contents passes along the subcutaneous border of the ischiopubic ramus just medial to the attachments of the thigh muscles. The incision then carries over the top of the pubis medial to the rectus abdominis and deviates laterally to include the origin of the puborectalis with the flake of bone/cartilage. Further back, the levator ani is incised close to its origin from the 'white line'. Once the pudendal nerve and vessels are identified and preserved, the flake of pubis and ischium is dissected free by incising the periosteum deep to the attachment of the penis.*

diaphragm bridging the gap between the corpora. A series of sutures are placed between each corpus cavernosum at its attachment to the urogenital diaphragm. When these are tied the urethra is on the ventral aspect and is surrounded by the urogenital diaphragm. Proximal to the urogenital diaphragm is the prostatic urethra and the bladder neck and several layers of fine sutures reconstruct the bladder neck. At this point the flakes of pubis are nearly in the midline and these are sutured together with heavier absorbable sutures. A 5

feeding tube is used temporarily during sphincter construction. If there is any doubt about the urethra, a heavy thread of monofilament nylon is passed through the urethral lumen and out through the bladder and abdominal wall and is tied to itself as a loop. This directs dilators if needed. Without this thread, postoperative dilatation may be difficult and hazardous.

Closing the bladder For ease of access it is important to close the bladder before the bladder neck is finally constructed. A single layer of absorbable sutures may

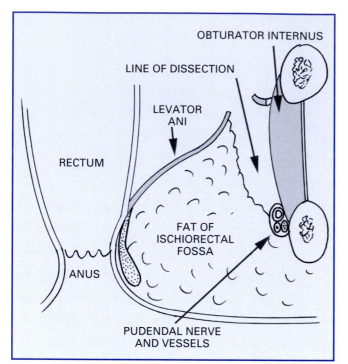

Fig. 42.10 *Coronal section through pelvis at level of the anal canal to show the surgical approach to the pudendal nerve. The levator ani is incised near its attachment to the 'white line', a thickening of the obturator internus fascia. A plane is dissected between the fat of the ischiorectal fossa and the surface of the obturator internus. The pudendal nerve and vessels lie close to the ischium.*

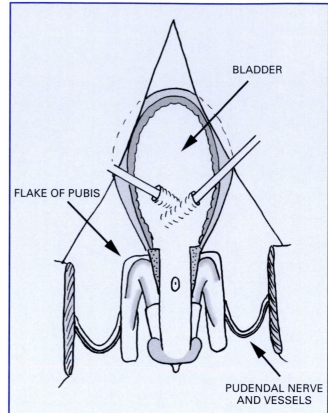

Fig. 42.11 *Release of central pelvic structures. The flakes of pubis and ischium have been mobilized medially on the pudendal nerves and vessels. The central structures are now freely mobile and repair can be completed without tension.*

suffice, but a second layer can be used, although care must be exercised not to reduce the bladder capacity in so doing. A suprapubic catheter and both ureteric catheters pass through the anterior bladder, and also, if used, the heavy monofilament nylon thread from the urethra.

Closing the abdominal wall   The abdominal wall is closed in layers. The rectus abdominus muscles are closed in the midline commencing superiorly, although the margins may not be able to be approximated in the suprapubic region, requiring flaps of rectus sheath, hinged medially. They form two fibrous layers being sutured to one another and to the flakes of pubis. Occasionally the bodies of the pubic bones are particularly prominent, and bilateral osteotomy or excision may be employed to improve the cosmesis. The previous dissection makes these osteotomies quick and easy. If possible, fat should be mobilized to lie under the surface of the lower abdominal skin. Suction drains are placed into the extraperitoneal, extravesical plane and the subcutaneous layer beside the scrotum.

Closing the skin   Skin closure must be meticulous. The shaft of the penis is already skin covered. The skin flaps mobilized from under the penis are brought superior to the penis and this provides adequate skin for closure. A zig-zag suture line is preferred because a straight midline scar on the lower abdomen will contract. The skin covering the penile shaft is sutured to the scrotal margin and the nearby skin.

Postoperative management   If possible continuous epidural anaesthesia is given during the operation and for several days postoperatively, to reduce pain and movement. Blood transfusion may be necessary and antibiotics are given intravenously. The ureteric catheters can be removed on day 4 or 5 but the suprapubic catheter should be left for 2 weeks or more. A trial of clamping should precede its removal. A cystogram might be used if there is difficulty in voiding after about 3 or 4 weeks; if voiding is still not achieved, gentle urethral dilatation under anaesthesia may help (facilitated if there is a thread through the urethra). No catheter is left in the urethra immediately postoperatively as mucosal compression may occur. Although it may indicate stricture formation, early postoperative urinary retention suggests the development of intermittent voiding and later continence.

The timing of urinary continence varies considerably. Occasionally a child is dry day and night by 2 years, but others are wet at 5 or more and still eventually achieve control. This is in keeping with individual variation both of the basic pathology and of the surgery, and the normal individual variation between children.

Classic bladder exstrophy: the newborn female patient

There are three stages in the repair in the female child: 1, bladder closure at birth; 2, urethra and sphincter construction at 3–6 months of age, with bilateral reimplantation and the first genital surgery; and, 3, ultimately further genital surgery to be performed at or after puberty.

Stage 1: bladder closure at birth

The first stage repair in the female is neonatal closure of the bladder and abdominal wall, leaving a small stoma in the bladder neck. The procedure is very similar to that in the male. As it is difficult in the female to identify the junction between bladder and urethra, the stoma is sited about 1 cm inferior to the level of the ureteric orifices and should be 10–12 F gauge in diameter.

Stage 2: aged 3–6 months—urethra and sphincter construction, bilateral reimplantation and genital construction

The old lower midline scar is re-opened through to the bladder. Bilateral transtrigonal anti-reflux reimplantations are performed. Parallel incisions outline a 12-mm urethral strip extending up to the bladder. By shelving these incisions obliquely outwards to a depth of about 2 mm, and then undercutting the margins, a thick-walled urethra can be constructed. The urethra can be constructed now or after the mobilization of the vagina. The vagina may be opened unintentionally, particularly if there is vaginal duplication, and therefore the anterior vaginal wall should be identified. The skin incisions encircle the glans of each half clitoris, continue around the vaginal orifice to the midline and then extend about 1 cm further posteriorly. Each half clitoris is dissected down to its attachment to the ischiopubic ramus. The clitoris is a very slender structure and care must be taken not to divide or damage it or its nerves.

The wall of the pelvis is dissected as in the male, noting the obturator neurovascular bundle, the obturator internus muscle and the superior aspect of the levator ani where it attaches along the white line to the obturator internus fascia. The subcutaneous border of the ischiopubic ramus is exposed by tunnelling beneath the labium majus lateral to the clitoris. The periosteum of the pubis and ischiopubic ramus are incised with diathermy. The pubic end of the periosteal incision is carried on to the medial aspect of the pelvis to encompass the attachment of the puborectalis. The attachment of the levator ani is divided a few millimetres from the obturator internus muscle, and the dissection is carried down between the surface of the obturator internus and the fat of the ischiorectal fossa. The pudendal neurovascular bundle is seen coming from behind the spine of the ischium and is followed forward. Near the ischial tuberosity it curves forwards to supply the bladder and urethra and the structures of the perineum.

The separation of the periosteum and perichondrium together with an underlying flake of bone and cartilage from the pubis and the ischiopubic ramus can be performed once the neurovascular bundle has been identified and dissected. Any fibrous strands attaching the perineal structures to the subcutaneous tissues of the buttock are divided. Dissection behind the vagina exposes the uro-genital diaphragm. Use of the muscle stimulator makes accurate identification of the muscle of the uro-genital diaphragm possible. The dissection is carried around the lateral wall of the vagina, and the urethra and vagina are mobilized posteriorly. Both the urethra and vagina are now able to be surrounded by the muscle of the uro-genital diaphragm. Absorbable sutures are used, being preplaced along the lateral margins of the muscle and subsequently tied as in the male. The flakes of pubis are approximated in the midline with absorbable sutures. This produces a wrap of tissue at the bladder neck, helps to force the urethra and vagina into in a more normal position and brings the two half clitorises together, which are then denuded where the glans touch and are approximated as a single clitoris. The mons is repaired, mobilizing subcutaneous fat to make the mons look more normal.

The abdomen is closed, anterior rectus flaps often being employed. Drainage includes ureteric catheters, a suprapubic bladder catheter, and bilateral extra peritoneal suction drains.

Stage 3: adolescence—introitoplasty

Most girls will need the introitus enlarged at or after puberty. It is important that the girl and her parents are aware of this at an early age.

Revision surgery

When the more standard operations for bladder exstrophy such as pelvic osteotomy and Young–Dees bladder-neck reconstruction have been performed without producing satisfactory results, the radical mobilization operation described above can be undertaken at any age with a good chance of improving the genitalia and a reasonable hope of providing worthwhile continence. Usually the deep tissue planes have not been dissected to any extent, and although there may have been some previous damage to the penile structures, the penis can usually be straightened and elongated, and this may include mobilizing the urethra from the dorsum of the penis to a hypospadiac position. However, any pre-existing urethral strictures do make satisfactory repair very difficult, and it seems almost impossible to obtain continence with a tiny rigid bladder.

When previous pelvic osteotomy has been successful and has resulted in pubic approximation or near approximation, the child may still remain totally incontinent, and there may be a place for limited exposure and reconstruction of the proximal urethra using the skeletal muscle described above. If investigation reveals a compliant bladder but a patulous bladder neck region and urethra, in such cases the present author has had experience in secondary repair which may be undertaken below the pubes. The urethra is superficial on the dorsum of the penis or lying between the separated corpora cavernosa, and it may be very wide at this point. It is possible to mobilize the urethra from the corpora, and, having identified the skeletal muscle, to narrow the urethra as necessary and bring it between the corpora to a more ventral position and wrap the skeletal muscle around the urethra as an external sphincter. The bladder

neck also can be tightened if necessary, including, if appropriate, removing some of the mucosa at the bladder neck to make a tubular proximal urethra and an abrupt transition from bladder to urethra. Where osteotomy has successfully approximated the pubes, the muscle is under little tension and can be wrapped around the urethra without extensive mobilization of the pudendal nerves. If the distal urethra and penis are satisfactory, and the urethral length allows, this surgery can be performed without disrupting the glans or distal penis. However the intact penis does reduce the exposure and makes accurate sphincter construction somewhat more difficult, and no increase in penile length can be achieved although chordee can be corrected. Previous cavernosa-cavernostomy increases the difficulty of dissection.

In female children with adequate bladder capacity but patulous inert urethras, but with the pubes approximated by previous surgery, it may be possible to operate between the clitoris and urethra, and by drawing the urethra and vagina more posteriorly, identify the perineal skeletal muscle and suture it anterior to the urethra and the bladder neck.

Where the bladder is a small fibrous rigid chamber, secondary surgery is not indicated. However, the bladder may enlarge so that later the child may become suitable for revision surgery. The decision whether or not to augment the bladder and/or provide an alternative catheterizing channel may be very difficult in the young child with good upper tracts. However, a small rigid bladder with reflux and upper tract dilatation or damage probably commits one to augmentation or diversion.

Complete dryness may first occur up to 12 years post radical mobilization, and in the meantime the management of the partially continent child can present a significant challenge, particularly from the psychological viewpoint, and considerable pressure may be exerted by the family and others to divert or augment.

Modifying the radical mobilization operation to fit into other surgical protocols
Total reconstruction in the newborn
There is a very considerable theoretical advantage to closing the bladder, constructing the urethra and performing sphincter wrap as a newborn. The disadvantages of staged repair are avoided and the constructed

sphincter is present from the earliest possible time and therefore the child has the maximum chance of adapting to the surgically created repair. The author's experience shows that there are major problems in his hands with full repair in the neonate, mainly due to the oedematous inflamed bladder, which makes anti-reflux surgery all but impossible. Total repair in the newborn is not recommended.

Posterior osteotomy with radical mobilization

The appeal of having an intact pelvic girdle may suggest that it could be incorporated with the dissection as described, but the rotated pelvic girdle distorts the anterior pelvis so the penis is drawn inwards and almost disappears.

Radical mobilization surgery in variants of epispadias and bladder exstrophy

The principles of radical mobilization can be applied to variations of the spectrum of epispadias and exstrophy. Continent epispadias does not require radical mobilization, and the Cantwell–Ransley operation has proven to be most satisfactory. However, radical mobilization can be employed with the full range of anomalies from incontinent epispadias to cloacal exstrophy.

Incontinent epispadias

In children with incontinent epispadias radical mobilization is performed similarly to the second stage of bladder exstrophy. It may be necessary to divide the interpubic band to open the pelvis enough to obtain access. Sphincter construction is as for classic exstrophy, but in the young child it may be possible to approximate the pubic symphysis.

Cloacal exstrophy

In cloacal exstrophy the bladder segments are usually tiny and there are often abnormalities of pelvic innervation. It has not been possible to achieve continence in any of these children, although radical mobilization can help closure of the bladder and abdominal wall. Spinal abnormalities are common and are associated with pelvic nerve deficiencies, and the small and large bowel segments are not infrequently short, with the small bowel deficiencies being sometimes incompatible with exclusively enteral nutrition.

Advantages of soft tissue mobilization

There are several advantages of extensive soft tissue mobilization as against pelvic osteotomy.

Pelvic osteotomy, when performed well, does significantly reduce the tension in the tissues of the anterior pelvis. However, the bones tend to drift apart again, and this may result in deterioration of function of those soft tissues attached to the bones, particularly those of the bladder and urethra. Protracted immobilization with or without internal or external osseous fixation has been employed to minimize this tendency. Osteotomy through the posterior pelvis has on occasion led to later pain in the area, and over recent years osteotomies have been more frequently performed through the pelvic girdle anterior to the acetabula. Whether through the anterior or posterior pelvis, rotating the pubes medially tends to rotate the base of each half of the penis medially but deeper, and this may increase the genital deformity.

Extensive soft tissue mobilization does not require prolonged immobilization or bony fixation. It does not increase the abnormal appearance of the genitalia, and in fact usually significantly improves it. It does allow anatomical reconstruction of the bladder neck and posterior urethra. Most of the children are in hospital for less than 10 days for the operation.

Disadvantages of soft tissue mobilization

Soft tissue mobilization requires extensive dissection in areas which may be unfamiliar to the paediatric urologist. Some of the structures are easily damaged, particularly the pudendal neurovascular bundle, and damage is likely to have permanent unfortunate effects. The mobilization of the penis is extensive and risky. It is a multistaged procedure, which is a significant disadvantage.

Results

The wide variation in the epispadias – exstrophy spectrum makes comparison of results difficult unless the initial pathology is detailed. Even with classic exstrophy, there is very significant individual variation. For example, children with a minute bladder disc are unlikely to do as well as children with a much larger bladder area.

The results of surgery will depend on many factors as well as the pathology at birth. With these provisos, the following results of the radical soft tissue mobilization are presented in 26 children with classic exstrophy operated by the author at the Royal Children's Hospital, Melbourne.

Urinary continence

Few children with bladder exstrophy develop continence under the age of 6 months or less than a year following sphincter surgery, so the time elapsed since surgery must be included.

The 26 patients have been assessed more than 2 years after sphincter surgery and all are over 6 years of age. They are recorded in Table 42.1.

The definitions used for 'physiological continence', 'social continence' and 'incontinence' are as follows.

Physiological continence This is defined as being able to control urine without effort, being able to remain dry without a pad, medications or catheters. These children are able to hold their urine for at least 2 hours, detect the need to void, and then able hold on to their urine until an appropriate time and voluntarily void so as to fully or nearly fully empty their bladder. Most are dry at night, but some wet the bed occasionally. Of the 26 children, 10 are have 'physiological continence'.

Social continence This has been defined as children who have to make some adjustment to their lives because of imperfect bladder control. It may be the occasional accident that means they need to wear a pad, they may need to catheterize, or they may have to void by the clock or void significantly more frequently than their peers. 'Social continence' has been achieved in eight of the 26 children.

Incontinent These children are unable to prevent urine leakage and need a pad or appliance. Some may be able to void on the toilet on occasion, but usually urine leakage is continual. Of the 26 children, eight were incontinent, and subsequently seven of the eight have had further surgery, most usually bladder augmentation with small bowel and a continent abdominal stoma.

Other parameters of outcome

Many important parameters of outcome can be assessed only after many years, and it is too early to assess the status of the children in this study. These parameters include acceptable genital appearance, satisfactory sexual function, normal fertility and satisfactory pregnancy outcome. Also the long-term preservation of renal function, the late appearance of urinary or genital malignancy and the development of psychological disturbances are aspects needing long-term follow-up.

Surgical complications

Almost every patient has had some surgical complications. A few are listed below.

Urinary infection In this series every patient has had urinary infection, the first usually within the first few months of operation. Antibiotics are given with the induction of anaesthesia and continued for 3 or 4 days. This has prevented severe postoperative sepsis, but local infection in relation to catheters and drains has been noted in about half the patients. The frequency of urine infection and the tendency for bladder stasis in the early months after operation underlies the recommendation for anti-reflux surgery.

Wound dehiscence In the first-stage bladder closure (without release of tension by osteotomy), over 25% of patients have had some wound breakdown. This has usually resulted in partial or complete bladder prolapse. The alternatives are to re-attempt a repeat simple bladder closure or to incorporate bladder closure at the same operation as the sphincter repair. This latter option has been followed in five children, and in no child has anti-reflux surgery been possible at that time. Therefore it is not recommended that bladder closure be combined with sphincter repair.

Suprapubic leak After sphincter construction most children have a temporary suprapubic leak, and some have a prolonged leak. This leak acts as a safety valve while the recently operated urethra and sphincter are oedematous and there is a high-pressure obstructed bladder. The leak occurs usually either at the site of the suprapubic catheter or the loop of thread. Spontaneous closure is usual once the thread is removed, but may

Table 42.1 *Urinary continence in 26 patients with bladder exstrophy over 6 years of age and over 2 years after sphincter construction performed at The Royal Children's Hospital Melbourne*

Continence	Males	Females	Total
Physiological	5	5	10 (40%)
Social	4	4	8 (30%)
Incontinent	5	3	8 (30%)
Totals	14	12	26

take several months. If the leak occurs near the base of the penis it may indicate proximal urethral and sphincter disruption.

Penile ischaemia Ischaemia of the penis is a risk after extensive mobilization. In this series two boys required release of tight sutures because of acute penile ischaemia, with return of the circulation and salvage of the penis. Loss of the whole penis has not been noted, but in the later follow-up, in some boys a degree of asymmetry of the penile shaft has been seen, suggesting occasional damage to the corpora cavernosa, and in two cases there has been the loss of a small part of the glans. Penile asymmetry also occurred after reconstruction without radical mobilization, possibly due to direct damage to the corpora. With radical mobilization there is the added risk to the pudendal neurovascular supply with subsequent partial or complete infarction of the corpora. Sometimes the lengthening of the penis by the mobilization is not as great as expected from the immediate postoperative appearance. Whether this is due to ischaemia and fibrosis or to a gradual return to the original state of the penis is not immediately apparent.

Penile urethral fistula Urethral fistulae are common after the hypospadias repair, occurring in four of the 14 boys. The lack of available skin not only increases the likelihood of fistula formation but also the difficulty of repairing a fistula, should one occur.

Urethral stricture or stenosis Urethral stricture or meatal stenosis has occurred in the majority of children, leading to a routine examination under anaesthesia a few weeks after sphincter construction and to the need to gently dilate the urethra. Repeated dilatations have been required in six children and in three of these it is suspected that urethral stricturing has contributed to a poor continence result. Ensuring that the urethra has a thick well-vascularized wall has considerably reduced the stricture rate in more recent operations.

Calculi Bladder and urethral calculi have occurred in four children. Three were in children who had non-absorbable sutures in the bladder and/or abdominal wall closure. However, calculi must be likely to occur in any of the children, as infection, incomplete bladder emptying and abnormal mucosa are frequent and in theory must predispose to calculi. Hair-bearing skin in the urethra is a possible long-term problem.

Renal damage Fortunately in these 26 patients, only four renal units have shown long-term damage, though temporary upper-tract dilatation has been common.

Conclusion

Children born with the epispadias/bladder exstrophy range of anomalies can be surgically corrected, the results of surgery being dependent not only on the original pathology but also on the subsequent surgery and the complications encountered. In children with the most common anomaly, the results of staged surgery using extensive soft tissue mobilization would indicate that over half will achieve normal or socially acceptable urinary continence in childhood. The long-term outcome of this surgical programme will need to be assessed.

Appendix 1: 'Forgetmenots':
Measurements of urogenital organs of infants and children, calendar of embryological events, catheter gauges and classifications of vesicoureteral reflux

The purpose of this Appendix is to assemble for ready reference many urological facts and figures published in books and journals subserving diverse disciplines. The data are of special interest to paediatric urologists who are intrigued by anomalies, who need to refer to standards of normality for comparison with abnormal states and who wish to theorize on the embryogenesis. The information is grouped into the following categories:

1. Renal dimensions in children: intravenous pyelogram measurements of length according to (a) age and (b) intervertebral distance; (c) and (d) nomograms which determine deviations from the mean renal length and area.
2. Renal length of duplex kidneys.
3. Renal weights.
4. Glomerular diameters and nephron lengths.
5. Dimensions of normal ureter.
6. Calibre of ureter as measured radiographically.
7. The structure of the normal ureter.
8. Bladder capacity.
9. Urine output per day according to age.
10. Trigonal measurements.
11. Urethral calibrations, male and female.
12. Penile measurements.
13. Blood pressures.
14. Muscle and skin segments of lower limbs.
15. Developmental homologues of genital systems.
16. Chronological development of urogenital tracts and concurrent key events in other systems.
17. Catheter gauges.
18. Classifications of vesicoureteral reflux.

1. Renal dimensions in children

(a) Normal range of renal lengths according to age (Fig. 1a)

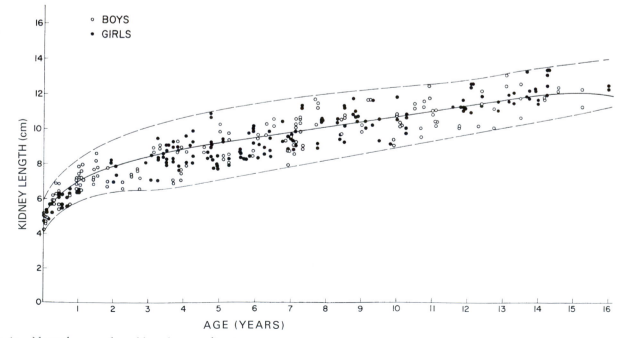

Fig. 1a   Normal range of renal lengths according to age.
Source: Stolpe, Y., King L.R. and White, H. (1967) The normal range of renal size in children. *J. Urol.* 4: 600 (Fig. 2).

Kidneys were measured from outlines shown on three- or eight-minute postinjection films obtained with the subject supine and film-focus distance of 100 cm.

Renal length is plotted against age in children, newborn to 16 years of age. In the newborn, the renal length ranges from 4 to 6 cm. By the age of three years, kidney length may be as great as 10 cm, or as little as 6 cm. This 4-cm variation is 50 per cent of the mean renal length at this age. The 4-cm range in normal length then remains relatively constant, so that by the age of 14 years, the normal variation is 36 per cent of the mean length.

(b) Normal renal length plotted against distance between top of first lumbar and bottom of fourth lumbar vertebrae (Fig. 1b)

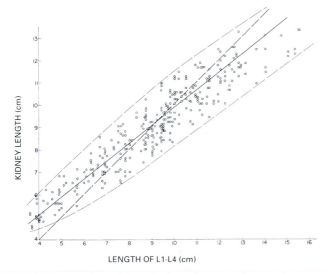

LENGTH OF L1-L4 (cm)

Fig. 1b. Normal renal length plotted against distance between top of first lumbar and bottom of fourth lumbar vertebrae.
Source: Stolpe, Y., King, L.R. and White, H. (1967) The normal range of renal size in children. *J. Urol.* 4: 600 (Fig. 6).

When mean lengths are compared, a linear relationship is present (solid line). This departs from a 1:1 ratio (heavy broken line) so that below 9.25 cm the renal length tends to be greater than the L1 to L4 distance, while in larger patients the L1 to L4 distance tends to be slightly greater.

(c) Nomogram for length of given kidney in standard deviation (Fig. 1c)

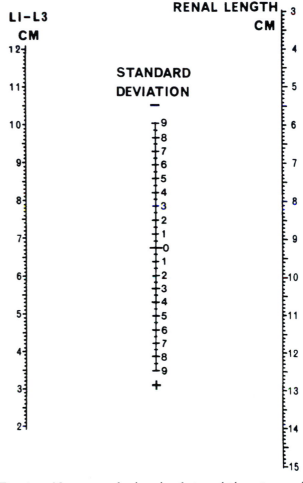

Fig. 1c. Nomogram for length of given kidney in standard deviation.
Source: Eklof, O. and Ringertz, H. (1976) Kidney size in children: a method of assessment. *Acta Radiol. Diagn.* 17: 617 (Fig. 3).

Intervertebral length from top of the first lumbar to the bottom of the third lumbar vertebrae is marked on left vertical scale. Renal length (supine, film in nephrographic phase) is recorded on the right vertical scale. A straight line joining the two points crosses the central scale at a point which indicates precisely the deviation from the mean of the length of the kidney at any length of the lumbar spine. (X-ray beam coned to cover solely the kidney areas.)

(d) Nomogram for the renal parenchymal area (in square centimetres) of any given kidney in standard deviations, using the height L1–L3 as reference Fig. 1d)

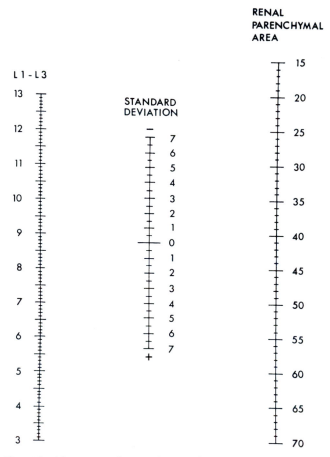

Fig. 1d Nomogram for renal parenchymal area of any given kidney in standard deviations, using the height L1–L3 as reference.
Source: Jorulf, H., Nordmark, J. and Jonsson, A. (1978) Kidney size in infants and children assessed by area measurements. *Acta Radiol. Diagn.* 19: 154 (Fig. 3).

Film focus distance = 100 cm, table top film distance = 12 cm, and measurements made on film exposed 10 minutes after injection of contrast medium, compression having been applied 5 minutes after the injection.

2. Renal length of duplex kidneys (Table 1)

The radiographic lengths of non-diseased unilateral bifid kidneys (including duplication of at least the proximal one-third of the ureters) of 45 patients (38 adult, 7 children) were compared by Amar and Scheer (1965) with renal lengths of contralateral non-duplicated kidneys. The measurements of kidneys of control patients, matched for age and sex, fell within an average of 3 mm of those of the contralateral unduplicated kidneys. The bifid kidneys averaged 13 mm longer than the non-bifid contralateral kidneys.

Table 1. *Differences in length between non-diseased bifid kidneys and contralateral normal non-bifid kidneys*

Difference between bifid and non-bifid kidney (mm)	Cases (n)
<–4	2
–4–0	1
1–5	8
6–10	6
11–15	16
16–20	5
21–25	2
> 25	5
Total	5
Average	13

Source: Amar, A.D. and Scheer, C.W. (1965), Comparative length of unilateral bifid kidney and its single counterpart. *N. Engl. J. Med.* 273: 211, Table 4.

3.   Normal renal weights

Age	Body length (cm)	Kidneys (g)	
		Right	Left
Birth–3 days	49	13	14
3–7 days	49	14	14
1–3 wks	52	15	15
3–5 wks	52	16	16
5–7 wks	53	19	18
7–9 wks	55	19	18
9–3 months	56	20	19
4 months	59	22	21
5 months	61	25	25
6 months	62	26	25
7 months	65	30	30
8 months	65	31	30
9 months	67	31	30
10 months	69	32	31
11 months	70	34	33
12 months	73	36	35
14 months	74	36	35
16 months	77	39	39
18 months	78	40	43
20 months	79	43	44
22 months	82	44	44
24 months	84	47	46
3 years	88	48	49
4 years	99	58	56
5 years	106	65	64
6 years	109	68	67
7 years	113	69	70
8 years	119	74	75
9 years	125	82	83
10 years	130	92	95
11 years	135	94	95
12 years	139	95	96

Source: Coppoletta, J.M. and Wolbach, S.B. (1933), Body length and organ weights of infants and children. *Am. J. Pathol.* 9: 55, Table 1. Reprinted with permission of the American Association of Pathologists.

4. Glomerular diameters and nephron lengths. Mean glomerular diameter and proximal length for three cortical levels of nephrons in 23 patients

Age of patient	Mean glomerular diameter (mm)			Mean proximal length (mm)		
	Outer	Middle	Inner	Outer	Middle	Inner
Newborn (full term)	0.106	0.115	0.129	1.26	1.73	2.46
1 month	0.105	0.109	0.123	2.29	2.94	3.37
$3\frac{1}{2}$ months	0.101	0.125	0.142	2.83	3.19	4.12
5 months	0.155	0.151	0.163	6.54	6.78	7.17
6 months	0.150	0.165	0.184	4.84	6.05	6.74
11 months	0.122	0.122	0.131	4.87	4.70	4.86
12 months	0.124	0.177	0.132	6.38	6.01	6.37
14 months	0.168	0.168	0.173	7.16	7.98	7.86
20 months	0.152	0.157	0.158	5.52	5.74	5.39
22 months	0.173	0.175	0.174	7.53	8.52	8.36
27 months	0.175	0.162	0.186	7.99	8.24	8.51
3 years	0.170	0.164	0.176	8.03	8.24	6.99
3 years	0.169	0.166	0.181	7.37	7.28	7.82
$3\frac{1}{2}$ years	0.178	0.178	0.188	6.29	7.14	7.50
$3\frac{1}{2}$ years	0.201	0.201	0.200	8.61	9.15	8.17
5 years	0.146	0.155	0.154	7.05	6.93	6.91
6 years	0.190	0.204	0.212	8.34	9.92	9.51
$7\frac{1}{2}$ years	0.215	0.221	0.230	10.72	10.94	12.91
$8\frac{1}{2}$ years	0.192	0.196	0.204	12.29	13.73	13.82
12 years	0.241	0.249	0.249	11.74	11.95	12.70
13 years	0.243	0.235	0.237	12.72	13.06	12.84
15 years	0.222	0.212	0.229	15.21	12.99	13.47
18 years	0.196	0.207	0.197	11.68	12.78	11.53
35 years* (average)	0.287	0.280	0.283	21.5	19.4	17.8

* Data are for composite kidney at age 35. Source: G.H. Fetterman *et al.* (1965), *Pediatrics* 35: 601.

Sources: Fetterman, G.H., Shuplock, N.A., Philipp, F.J. and Gregg, H.S. (1965), The growth and maturation of human glomeruli and proximal convolutions from term to adulthood; studies by microdissection. *Pediatrics* 35: 601.
McCrory, W.W. (1978), Embryologic development and prenatal maturation of the kidney. In *Pediatric Kidney Disease*, C.M. Edelmann, Jr. (ed.), Table 1–2, p. 23. Boston: Little, Brown.

5(a). Dimensions of normal ureter in infancy and childhood (ready reckoner of approximate ureteric dimensions)

Parameter	30 weeks gestation	3 months	3 years	6 years	12 years
Height (cm)	40	60	90	120	150
Weight (kg)	2	5	13	20	35
Total length of ureter (cm)	5	10	15	20	25
Histological assessment of length of intravesical ureter (cm)	0.4	0.6	0.8	1.0	1.2
Histological assessment of length of submucosal ureter (cm)	0.2	0.3	0.4	0.5	0.6
Fr-Charrière gauge					
UPJ	Fr2	Fr4	Fr6	Fr8	Fr10
Mid-spindle	F4	F10	F12	F14	F16
Distal end and UVJ	F2	F3	F4	F5	F6

Source: After Cussen, L.J. (1967a), Dimensions of the normal ureter in infancy and childhood. *Invest. Urol.* 5: 164, Table 6.

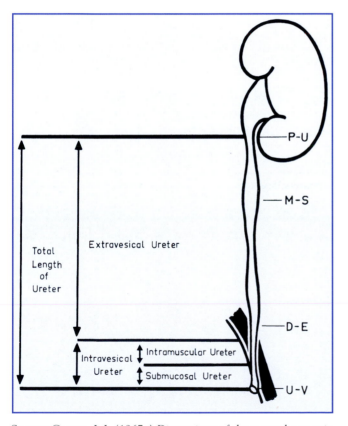

Source: Cussen, L.J. (1967a) Dimensions of the normal ureter in infancy and childhood. *Invest. Urol.*, 5: 164, Table 6.

5(b). Length of submucosal ureter (orifice to hiatus inside bladder (cm) — postmortem assessment)

30 weeks gestation	3 months	3 years	6 years	12 years	15 years
0.2	0.5	0.6	0.8	1.0	1.5

Source: After Hutch, J.A. (1961), Theory of maturation of the intravesical ureter. *J. Urol.* 86: 534.

6. Calibres of ureter and megaureter as measured radiographically in children

With the patient supine and X-ray source 100 cm from the film, the body of the normal ureter in its extravesical course measures up to 0.7 cm in diameter in infants and children up to 12 years.

A megaureter is one which, when fully distended by vesicoureteral reflux, retrograde injection, renal excretion or obstruction measures > 0.7 cm in diameter.

The upper limit of the range of diameter measurements of the middle spindle from birth to 12 years is 0.5–0.65 cm and allowing for 10 per cent magnification, the upper limit of normal may be regarded as closely approximating 0.7 cm.

Source: Cussen, L.J. (1967a) Dimensions of the normal ureter in infancy and childhood. *Invest. Urol.* 5: 164, Table 1.

7. The structure of the normal human ureter in infancy and childhood: a quantitative study of the muscular tissue (ready reckoner of approximate microscopic measurements of ureter)

Parameter	30 weeks gestation	3 months	3 years	6 years	12 years
Height (cm)	40	60	90	120	150
Weight (kg)	2	5	13	20	35
Muscle cell population*					
P-U	1200	1700	2200	2700	3300
M-S	1600	2200	2600	3200	4000
D-E	1400	1500	1900	2500	3100
U-V	900	1000	900	1400	2000
Muscle cell size (μm^3)	1500	1500	1500	1700	1700
Area of muscle in section of ureter (mm^2)*					
P-U	0.2	0.2	0.4	0.5	0.6
M-S	0.3	0.5	0.5	0.8	1.0
D-E	0.2	0.2	0.3	0.5	0.8
U-V	0.1	0.2	0.2	0.3	0.3

*P-U, Pelviureteric junction; M-S, middle spindle; D-E, distal end of extravesical ureter; U-V, ureterovesical junction.
Source: Cussen, L.J. (1967b), The structure of the normal human ureter in infancy and childhood. A quantitative study of the muscular and elastic tissue. *Invest. Urol.* 5: 179, Table 6.

8. Bladder capacity

Normal bladder capacity in conscious children can be calculated from the equation as follows:

Bladder capacity (ounces) = age (years up to 11) +
          2 ounces
          (± 2 ounces standard
          deviation)

Source: Berger, R.M., Maizels, M., Moran, G.G., Conway, J.C. and Firlit, C.F. (1983) Bladder capacity (ounces) = age (years) + 2—predicts normal bladder capacity and aids diagnosis of abnormal voiding patterns. *J. Urol.* 129: 347.

9. Urine output per day according to age

Age	Output (cc)
0–48 hours	15–60
3–10 days	100–300
10–60 days	250–450
2 months–1 year	400–500
1–3 years	500–600
3–5 years	600–700
5–8 years	650–1000
8–14 years	800–1400

Source: Campbell, M. (1951g), *Clinical Pediatric Urology*, p. 29. Philadelphia: W.B. Saunders Co.

10. Trigonal measurements. Normal position of the ureteral orifice in infancy and childhood

Table 1 *Distance (cm) between vesicoureteral orifice and internal urethral orifice according to age*

Age	Measurements (n)	Mean	Standard deviation	Standard error of mean
<37 weeks gestation	186	0.9	0.2	0.01
0–3 months	166	1.2	0.2	0.02
3–12 months	32	1.3	0.4	0.07
1–3 years	26	1.6	0.4	0.08
3–6 years	34	1.8	0.5	0.08
6–12 years	24	1.8	0.3	0.07
12–18 years	8	2.3	1.9–2.7*	—

*Because of the small number of measurements the range is given instead of the standard deviation.

Appendix 10   *continued.*

Table 2   *Distance (cm) between vesicoureteral orifice and internal urethral orifice according to height*

Height (cm)	Measurements (n)	Mean	Standard deviation	Standard error of mean
30–40	114	0.9	0.2	0.02
40–50	130	1.1	0.2	0.02
50–60	120	1.2	0.3	0.02
60–80	34	1.6	0.4	0.07
80–100	26	1.6	0.4	0.09
100–120	26	1.9	0.3	0.06
120–140	8	2.1	1.9–2.4*	–
140–180	6	2.3	2.0–2.7*	–

*Because of the small number of measurements the range is given instead of the standard deviation.

Table 3   *Estimate of approximate distance (cm) between vesicoureteral orifice and internal urethral orifice according to age*

Distance from ureteral orifice to urethral orifice (cm)*	Age	Height (cm)	Weight (kg)
0.9	30 weeks gestation	40	2
1.3	3 months	60	5
1.6	3 years	90	13
1.9	6 years	120	20
2.2	12 years	150	35

*The two vesicoureteral orifices and the internal urethral orifice formed an equilateral triangle, with no more than a 0.2 cm difference in length of the sides in 92 per cent of the 239 subjects.
Source: Cussen, L.J. (1979), Normal position of the ureteral orifice in infancy and childhood: a quantitative study. *J. Urol.* 121: 646, Tables 1, 2 and 6.

11.   Urethral calibrations

(a)   Normal size of urethral meatus in boys

Age	Size	n (%)		Size	n (%)	
Group 1						
6 weeks to 1 year	Below 8F	22/160	(14)	10F	138/160	(86)
1 year	Below 8F	10/63	(14)	10F	53/63	(86)
2 years	Below 8F	17/109	(16)	10F	92/109	(84)
3 years	Below 8F	13/93	(14)	10F	80/93	(86)
Group 2						
4 years	Tight 8F	7/83	(8)	12F	70/83	(84)
5 years	Tight 8F	10/111	(9)	12F	92/111	(83)
6 years	Tight 8F	8/87	(9)	12F	61/87	(82)
7 years	Tight 8F	4/56	(7)	12F	43/56	(77)
8 years	Tight 8F	5/61	(8)	12F	41/61	(67)
9 years	Tight 8F	4/60	(7)	12F	40/60	(67)
10 years	Tight 8F	3/50	(6)	12F	37/50	(74)
Group 3						
11 years	Below 10F	2/45	(4)	14F	36/45	(80)
12 years	Below 10F	2/40	(5)	14F	28/40	(69)

Source: Livak, A.S., Morris, J.A., Jr. and McRoberts, J.W. (1976), Normal size of the urethral meatus in boys. *J. Urol.* 115: 736, Table 1.

Appendix 11   *continued.*

(b) Urethral calibre in normal girls

Table 1   *Urethral meatus*

Age (years)	Patients (n)	Mean	Median
2	14	14	14
4	20	15.6	16
6	27	16.1	16
8	27	16.9	16
10	18	19.6	20
12	6	23.3	22
14	4	24.5	24
16	9	25.8	26
18–20	6	27.3	26

Table 2   *Distal urethra*

Age (years)	Patients (n)	Mean	Median
2	15	14	14
4	18	15.3	14
6	23	15.4	16
8	25	16.8	16
10	16	19.5	16
12	6	21.0	20
14	7	23.4	24
16	9	25.6	26
18–20	6	26	24

Source: Immergut, M., Culp, D. and Flocks, R.H. (1967), The urethral caliber in normal female children. *J. Urol.* 97: 693.

12. Penile measurements. Stretched penile length (cm) in normal males[*]

Age	Mean ± S.D.	Mean – $2^1/_2$ S.D.
30 weeks gestation	2.5 ± 0.4[**]	1.5
34 weeks gestation	3.0 ± 0.4[**]	2.0
Term	3.5 ± 0.4[†]	2.5–2.4
0–5 months[***]	3.9 ± 0.8	1.9
6–12 months	4.3 ± 0.8	2.3
1–2 years	4.7 ± 0.8	2.6
2–3 years	5.1 ± 0.9	2.9
3–4 years	5.5 ± 0.9	3.3
4–5 years	5.7 ± 0.9	3.5
5–6 years	6.0 ± 0.9	3.8
6–7 years	6.1 ± 0.9	3.9
7–8 years	6.2 ± 1.0	3.7
8–9 years	6.3 ± 1.0	3.8
9–10 years	6.3 ± 1.0	3.8
10–11 years	6.4 ± 1.1	3.7
Adult	13.3 ± 1.6	9.3

[*]   Record length to tip of glans on a ruler pressed into pubic arch and resting along dorsum of stretched penis.

[**] Based on Feldman, K.W. and Smith, D.W. (1975), Fetal phallic growth and penile standards for newborn male infants. *J. Pediatr.* 86: 395.

[***] Data for 0–5 months through to adult are based on Schonfeld, W.A. and Beebe, G.W. (1942), Normal growth and variation in the male genitalia from birth to maturity. *J. Urol.* 48: 759.

[†]   Based on Flateau, E., Josefsberg, Z., Reisner, S.H., Bialik, O. and Zaron, Z. (1975), Penile size in the newborn infant. *J. Pediatr.* 87: 663.

Source: Lee, P.A., Mazur, T., Danish, R., Amrhein, J., Blizzard, R.M. Money, J. and Mijeon, C.J. (1980), Micropenis. I. Criteria, etiologies and classification. *Johns Hopkins Med. J.* 146: 156, Table 1.

13. Blood pressures: normal blood pressures in children

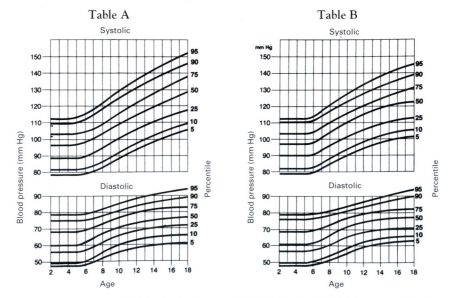

Percentiles of blood pressure measurements. Table A, in boys, and Table B, in girls (right arm with the patient seated). (From Blumenthal, S. *et al.* (1977), Report of the task force on blood pressure control in children. *Pediatrics* 59: 803.

Appendix 13   *continued.*

Table C   *Systolic blood pressures (mmHg) according to age**

Age (years)	Number of patients Boys	Number of patients Girls	Mean Boys	Mean Girls	Standard deviaton Boys	Standard deviaton Girls	90 per cent range Boys	90 per cent range Girls	80 per cent range Boys	80 per cent range Girls
4	79	65	98	98	8.5	9.7	85–114	83–114	88–110	89–113
5	90	80	101	102	9.6	10.1	83–115	84–119	88–113	90–115
6	89	81	105	105	10.5	11.0	91–124	91–125	93–122	93–120
7	77	81	106	107	9.8	10.9	91–122	92–125	93–118	95–122
8	61	70	108	108	10.6	10.3	91–125	94–127	94–123	97–124
9	61	69	111	112	11.3	9.9	94–130	94–129	91–126	88–125
10	53	68	114	114	10.5	11.3	95–133	91–134	102–128	97–129
11	53	61	114	121	11.1	12.2	98–134	103–143	101–130	106–141
12	51	58	116	117	10.3	11.9	100–133	101–136	103–128	104–134
13	47	50	120	121	11.6	12.1	97–144	101–141	103–140	105–135
14	41	33	120	119	10.3	12.0	105–135	93–138	108–133	102–136
15	33	22	125	115	9.8	11.0	112–142	112–142	113–138	106–134
Total	735	738								

*Blood pressures recorded on right arm with patient supine. Data based on blood pressures recorded on right arm with 9- or 14-cm cuffs appropriate to cover two-thirds of arm with the patients supine.
Source: Londe, S. (1966), Blood pressure in children as determined under office conditions. *Clin. Pediatr.* 5: 71–78, Tables 13.3 and 13.3.

Table D   *Diastolic blood pressures (mmHg) according to age**

Age (years)	Number of patients Boys	Number of patients Girls	Mean Boys	Mean Girls	Standard deviaton Boys	Standard deviaton Girls	90 per cent range Boys	90 per cent range Girls	80 per cent range Boys	80 per cent range Girls
4	79	65	57	60	9.6	10.2	40–71	41–76	42–69	45–73
5	90	80	60	60	10.2	9.2	43–75	43–75	48–74	50–73
6	89	81	60	64	10.1	9.2	42–79	44–78	47–74	45–74
7	77	81	63	63	9.4	9.5	45–77	46–79	46–74	51–76
8	61	70	61	65	11.5	8.0	43–76	53–79	51–74	56–77
9	61	69	65	67	9.7	9.5	51–79	52–85	53–77	58–78
10	53	68	66	64	8.6	8.9	51–84	51–79	56–79	53–75
11	53	61	65	69	9.3	8.2	51–81	59–90	53–75	61–80
12	51	58	67	65	7.1	8.0	54–81	52–80	58–78	54–75
13	47	50	65	69	8.4	9.8	57–77	53–88	55–74	58–83
14	41	33	68	67	8.1	9.8	53–80	51–86	60–78	53–84
15	33	22	67	67	8.0	8.3	54–82	53–82	60–78	60–79
Total	735	738								

*Blood pressures recorded on right arm with patient supine. Data based on blood pressures recorded on right arm with 9- or 14-cm cuffs appropriate to cover two-thirds of arm with the patients supine.
Source: Londe, S. (1966), Blood pressure in children as determined under office conditions. *Clin. Pediatr.* 5: 71–78.

14.   Muscle and skin segments of lower limbs

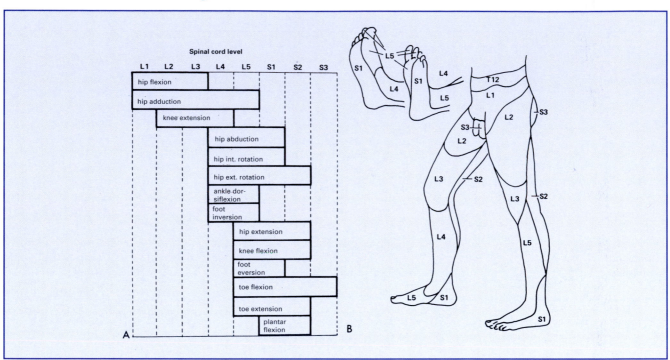

Source: Kaplan, G.W. (1979) Myelomeningocele. In Campbell's Urology, 4th edn., J.H. Harrison, R.F. Gittes, A.D. Perlmutter, T.A. Stamey and P.C. Walsh (eds), Vol. 2, p. 1787, Fig. 53.4. Chicago: Year Book Medical.

15.   Catheter gauges

French gauge—Charriére[*]	French gauge—Béniqué[**]	English gauge	Diameter (mm)
1	2	–	0.3
2	4	–	0.6
3	6	0	1.0
4	8	–	1.3
5	10	–	1.6
6	12	2	1.9
7	14	–	2.2
8	16	–	2.5
9	18	4	2.9
10	20	–	3.2
11	22	–	3.5
12	24	6	3.8
13	26	–	4.2
14	28	–	4.5
15	30	8	4.8
16	32	–	5.1
17	34	–	5.4
18	36	10	5.7
19	38	–	6.0
20	40	–	6.4

15.   Catheter gauges (contd.)

French gauge—Charriére[*]	French gauge—Béniqué[**]	English gauge	Diameter (mm)
21	42	12	6.7
22	44	–	7.0
23	46	–	7.3
24	48	14	7.6
25	50	–	8.0
26	52	–	8.3
27	54	16	8.6
28	56	–	8.9
29	58	–	9.2
30	60	18	9.5
31	62	–	9.9
32	64	–	10.2
33	66	20	10.5
34	68	–	10.8
35	70	–	11.1
36	72	22	11.5
37	74	–	11.8

[*]Joseph Frederic Benoit Charriére. French instrument maker, 1803–1876.
[**]Pierre Jules Béniqué, French physician, 1806–1851.

16. Developmental homologues of male and female genital systems

Male	Indifferent stage	Female
Probably disappears	Pronephros	Probably disappears
Testis	Gonad	Ovary
Seminiferous tubules	Germinal cords	Pfluger's tubes

Collecting tubules of mesonephros — upper/middle/lower:

Male	Indifferent stage	Female
Disappear	upper	Disappear
	middle	
Ductuli aberrantes superiores — cephalic	lower (cephalic)	Ductuli aberrantes superiores
Efferent ducts of epididymis — intermediate	lower (intermediate)	Tubules of epoophoron
Ductulus aberrans inferior, and paradidymis — caudal	(caudal)	Ductulus aberrans inferior and tubules of paroophoron

Male	Indifferent stage	Female
Duct of epididymis; ductus deferens; appendix of epididymis; common ejaculatory duct; seminal vesicle; trigone of bladder	Mesonephric duct (wolffian duct) initially pronephric duct	Straight tube of epoophoron, and Gartner's duct; trigone of bladder
Appendix testis ? Part of utriculus prostaticus (uterus masculinus or vagina musculina)	Paramesonephric duct (müllerian duct)	Uterine tubes; uterus; part of vagina
Part of utriculus prostaticus	Sinovaginal bulb from urogenital sinus	Part of vagina
Bladder and prostatic urethra above the orifices of the ejaculatory ducts (except trigonal region); definitive urogenital sinus	Primitive urogenital sinus	Bladder and greater part of urethra (except trigonal region); definitive urogenital sinus
Prostatic part of urethra below the orifice of the ejaculatory ducts; membranous urethra; penile urethra (except urethra of glans)	Definitive urogenital sinus (lower part of primitive urogenital sinus after the vesicourethral canal has separated from it)	Vestibule and ? distal part of urethra
Prostate gland	Urethral glands and glands of pars pelvina of urogenital sinus	Urethral glands and paraurethral glands (Skene's tubules)
Penile urethral glands (glands of Littré); bulbourethral (Cowper's) glands	Glands of pars phallica of urogenital sinus	Lesser vestibular glands; greater vestibular (Bartholin's) glands
Glans penis	Glans of phallus	Glans clitoridis
Floor of penile urethra	Urethral folds	Labia minora
Scrotum	Genital swelling	Labia majora
Gubernaculum testis	Gubernaculum	Ligament of ovary; round ligament of uterus
No established homologue	Junction of sinovaginal bulbs and urogenital sinus	? Hymen

Source: Hamilton, W. J. and Mossman, H. W. (1978d), in Hamilton, Boyd and Mossman's *Human Embryology*, 4th edn, p. 433. London: Macmillan Press. Baltimore: Williams and Wilkins Co.

17A.   Chronological development of urogenital tracts and concurrent key events in other systems

Age (weeks)	Size (crown–rump) (mm)	Urogenital system	Some key events in other systems
2.5	1.5	Allantois present.	Embryonic disc flat. Primitive streak prominent. Neural groove indicated. Gut not distinct from yolk sac.
3.5	2.5	All pronephric tubules formed. Pronephric duct growing caudad as a blind tube. Cloaca and cloacal membrane present.	Neural groove deepens and closes (except ends). Somites 1–16 present. Cylindrical body constricting from yolk sac. Fore- and hindgut present. Yolk sac broadly attached at mid-gut. Cloaca and cloacal membrane present. Heart tubes fuse, bend S-shape and beat begins.
4	5.0	Pronephros degenerated. Pronephric (mesonephric) duct reaches cloaca. Mesonephric tubules differentiating rapidly. Metanephric bud pushes into secretory primordium.	Yolk Stalk slender. All somites present (40). Limb buds indicated. Body flexed, C-shaped. Intestine a simple tube. Cloaca at height. Trachea and paired lung buds become prominent. Dorsal mesentery a complete median curtain. Neural tube closed.
5	8.0	Mesonephros reaches its caudal limit. Ureteric and pelvic primordia distinct. Genital ridge bulges.	Tail-gut atrophies. Yolk stalk detaches. Intestine elongates into a loop. Bronchial buds pressage future lung lobes. Suprarenal cortex accumulating.
6	12.0	Cloaca subdividing. Pelvic anlage sprouts pole tubules. Sexless gonad and genital tubercle prominent. Müllerian duct appearing.	Limbs recognizable as such. Mesentery expands as intestine forms loops. Heart acquires its general definitive form. Myotomes, fused into a continuous column, spread ventrad.
7	17.0	Mesonephros at height of its differentiation. Metanephric collecting tubules begin branching. Earliest metanephric secretory tubules differentiating. Bladder–urethra separates from rectum. Urethral membrane rupturing.	Digits indicated. Tail regressing. Anal membrane ruptures. Muscles differentiating rapidly throughout body and assuming final shapes and relations. Suprarenal medulla begins invading cortex.
8	23.0	Testis and ovary distinguishable as such. Müllerian ducts, nearing urogenital sinus, are ready to unite as uterovaginal primordium. Genital ligaments indicated.	Small intestine coiling within cord. Definitive muscles of trunk, limbs and head well represented and fetus capable of some movement.
10	40.0	Kidney able to secrete. Bladder expands as sac. Genital duct of opposite sex degenerating. Bulbourethral and vestibular glands appearing. Vaginal sacs forming.	Umbilical hernia reduced. Intestines withdraw from cord and assume characteristic positions. Anal canal formed. Processus (saccus) vaginales forming. Perineal muscles developing tardily.
12	56.0	Uterine horns absorbed. External genitalia attain distinctive features. Mesonephros and rete tubules complete male duct. Prostate and seminal vesicle appearing. Hollow viscera gaining muscular walls.	Sex readily determined by external inspection. Cauda equina and filum terminale appearing.
16	112.0	Kidney attains typical shape and plan. Testis in position for later descent into scrotum. Uterus and vagina recognizable as such. Mesonephros involuted.	
20–40 (5–10 months)	160.0–350.0	Female urogenital sinus becoming a shallow vestibule (5). Vagina regains lumen (5). Uterine glands appear (7). Scrotum solid until sacs and testes descend (7–9). Kidney tubules cease forming at birth.	Testes invading scrotum. Vaginal sacs passing into scrotum (7–9). Perineal muscles finish development. Myelinization of cord begins (5). Myelinization of brain begins (10).

Source: Selected references from Arey, L.B. (1974c), A reference table of correlated human development. In *Developmental Anatomy*, facing p. 106. Philadelphia: W.B. Saunders Co.

17B. Approximate timing of occurrence of deformation caused by amniotic constraint on growth of embryo and fetus

Age wks	CR length mm	Normal embryo-fetal developmental events	Amnion v chorion volumes (normal)	Deformations caused by amniotic membrane constraints
2.5	1.5	Blastocyst embedding in uterine wall-embryonic disc flat; notochordal plate and neurenteric canal patent		Rupture of cyst wall & abortion
3.5	2.5	Dorsiflexed discoid embryo 2–16 somites ± neurenteric canal closes; brain & neural tube forming; cylindrical body constricting from yolk sac heart beat begins; neural crests developing	+ v +++	Dorsiflexion or torsion of notochord; heart mesoderm compressed. Brain defects; meningomyelocele, cranial asymmetry; heart anomalies.
4	5	heart and head followed by hind end rotate ventrally (reversion 23–28 days); wings of ventral body wall uniting in midline; septation of foregut begins; cranial neuropore closes; neural crests continuous bands		Impaired rotation plus compression; anencephaly, exencephaly, axial twists, sacral defects, exomphalos, ADAM Tracheoesophageal and neural crest defects affecting upper limbs.
5	8	40 somites; notochord in tail somites septation of cloaca proceeding; rudimentary tail resorbs; caudal neuropore closes; budding of upper followed by lower limbs; budding of ureters	+ v +++	Distortion of notochord leads to arrest or deviation of tail end rotation; cloacal exstrophy; recto-urinary defects; OEIS sacral anomalies & ureterorenal defects.
6	16	Fore- and hind-gut septation complete Limbs recognizable as such		Tracheoesophageal and anorecto-urinary defects established.
7	18	Tail end straightens Hip & knee joints mobilize Genital tubercle elongates	++ v ++	Compression delays straightening of hind end leading to malplacement of genitals &/or anus; congenital dislocation of hip; penile defects.
8	30	Head lifts off chest perineum differentiates; feet apposed on perineum; gubernaculum at internal ring glans differentiates.	+++ v ++	Compression by fetal feet leads to covered anus, scrotal & labial defects; testicular descent arrested at inguinal canal; penile torsion and hypospadias.
9	50	Gubernaculum outside external ring Feet cross over perineum Legs elongate and overlap	+++ v 0	Testis descent arrested at external inguinal pouch; mutual anomalies of genitalia and feet; talipes and toe alignment defects.
10	60	Male and female external genitalia distinguishable and enlarging	+++ v 0 Amniotic fluid vol 30 cc Amnion fuses with chorion	Pressure sores caused by heel on soft tissues; scrotal and labial anomalies and pelvic girdle torsion and scrotoschisis.
	28–35	Gubernaculum migrates to scrotum	350–1000cc	Foot pressure on gubernacular impairs testicular descent, or prevents gubernaculum from attaching to scrotum causing so-called retractile testes.

After Arey, L.B. *Developmental Anatomy. Revised 7th Edition*, 1974. Philadelphia, W.B. Saunders, Facing page 106.

18. Classifications of vesicoureteral reflux

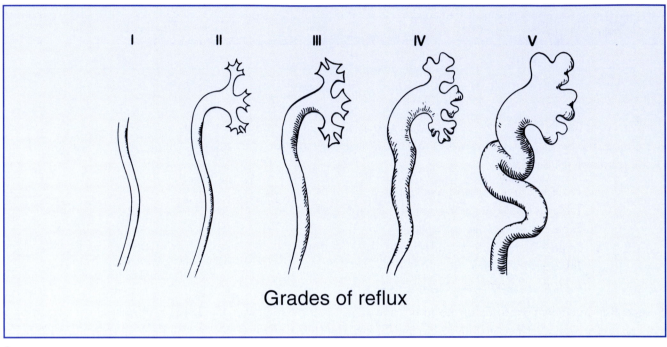

Grades of reflux

Sources:

Dwoskin, J.Y. and Perlmutter, A.D. (1973) Vesicoureteral reflux in children: a computerized review. *J. Urol.* 109: 888.

Heikel, P.E. and Parkkulainan, K.V. (1966) Vesicoureteral reflux in children: a classification and results of conservative treatment. *Ann. Radiol.* 9: 37.

*Levitt, S.B. (1981) Medical versus surgical treatment of primary vesicoureteral reflux: a prospective international reflux study in children. Report of the International Study Committee. *J. Urol.* 125: 277 Fig. 2.

Rolleston, G.L. (1970) The significance and management of vesico-ureteric reflux in infancy. Part 2. Radiologist aspects. In *Renal Infection and Renal Scarring*, P. Kincaid-Smith and K.F. Fairley (eds), p. 246. Melbourne: Mercedes Press.

Smellie, J.M. (1967) Medical aspects of urinary infection in children. *J. Roy. Coll. Phys. (Lond.)* 1: 189.

1. Heikel–Parkkulainan (with minor modifications) and 'International'* classification of grades of reflux— Grade I, reflux into ureter only; Grade II, filling of normal calibre system; Grade III, reflux into mildly dilated upper tract with minimal, if any, tortuosity or blunting of fornices; Grade IV, reflux into moderately dilated and tortuous upper tract, obliterating sharp angle of fornices but papillary impressions maintained in the majority of calyces; Grade V, gross dilatation and tortuosity of upper tract and absence of papillary impressions in the majority of calyces.

2. Smellie Grading—Grade I, reflux not extending above the pelvic brim; Grade II, reflux up to the kidney on micturition; and Grade III, reflux in a normal-sized ureter up to the kidney, both at rest and on micturition as in (II); and Grade IV, reflux extending up to the kidney with dilatation of the renal pelvis and ureter as in (IV) and (V) in diagram.

3. Dwoskin–Perlmutter Grading— Grade I as in (I) in diagram; Grade IIA as in (II) in diagram; Grade IIB as in (III) in diagram; Grade III as in (IV) in diagram; Grade IV as in (V) in diagram.

4. Rolleston Grading—Slight, incomplete filling of the upper urinary tract without dilatation; moderate, complete filling of the upper urinary tract with slight dilatation but without ballooning of the minor calyces; gross, marked dilatation of the upper urinary tract during micturition with marked ballooning of the minor calyces.

Appendix 2:
Syndromes with a renal component[†]

By Cyril Chantler, MD, MRCP
Consultant Paediatrician, Guy's Hospital, London

This appendix is reproduced in order to provide the paediatric urologist with a reference guide to the ever-increasing numbers of syndromes which have a urological component in the perplexing realms of teratology and dysmorphology. It includes:

Table 1   Ears, eyes and renal disease
Table 2   Skeletal malformations
Table 3   Visceral abnormalities
Table 4   Metabolic disturbances
Table 5   Infections
Table 6   Chromosomal abnormalities

Source: Reprinted, by permission of the author and publisher, from Chantler, C. (1975) Syndromes with a renal component. In *Paediatric Nephrology*, M.I. Rubin and T.M. Barratt (eds), pp. 891–902. Baltimore: Williams and Wilkins Co.

Table 1   *Ears, eyes and renal disease*

Syndrome	Principal components	Renal abnormality	Inheritance	Reference
Oculorenal	Tapetoretinal degeneration; retinitis pigmentosa	Juvenile nephrono-phthisis	Autosomal recessive	Senior et al. (1961)
Oculorenal	Retinal aplasia	Renal dysplasia	Autosomal recessive	Loken et al. (1961)
Oculorenal	Retinal dysplasia; cataracts	Polycystic kidneys; medullary cysts	?Autosomal recessive	Fairley et al. (1963)
Oculocerebro-renal; Lowe	Cataracts; mental retardation; rickets	Proximal tubular defects	X-linked recessive	
Hereditary nephritis with deafness; Alport	Nerve deafness; eye abnormalities	Nephritis; nephrosis	Autosomal dominant	
Cockayne	Renal dysplasia; deafness; small stature; photosensitivity	Albuminuria	Autosomal recessive	Ohno and Hirooka (1966)
Fraser	Cryptophthalmos; ear anomalies; genital anomalies	Various	?Autosomal recessive	Ehlers (1966)
Laurence–Moon–Biedl	Mental retardation; polydactyly; obesity; retinitis pigmentosa	Hypoplastic kidneys; obstructive uropathy	Autosomal recessive	Nadjini et al. (1969)
Unnamed	Nerve deafness	Renal tubular acidosis	Autosomal recessive	Nance et al. (1970)
Unnamed	External ear malformations	Various urinary tract malformations	?	Longneck et al. (1965)
Unnamed	Middle ear anomalies; vaginal atresia	Renal dysgenesis	?Autosomal recessive	Winter et al. (1968)

[†]*A more extensive series of tables in which syndromes involving the renal system are clustered according to the primary renal condition is included in* Pediatric Nephrology, *3rd edn, 1993, Chapter 27, p. 491. M.A. Holliday, T.M. Barratt, D.E. Ellis and B.A. Kogan (eds), Baltimore: Williams and Wilkins Co.*

Table 1   *continued*

Syndrome	Principal components	Renal abnormality	Inheritance	Reference
Unnamed	Cataracts	Chronic glomerulo-nephritis	Autosomal recessive	Campbell *et al.* (1972)
Hypopara-thyroidism	Hypoparathyroidism; deafness	Nephrotic syndrome; renal failure	Autosomal recessive	Barahat *et al.* (1979)
Unnamed	Developmental retardation; optic atrophy	Polycystic kidneys	Autosomal recessive	Dekaborn (1967)
Unnamed	Anopthalmia microcephaly	Renal agenesis	X-linked	Hoefnagel *et al.* (1963)
Unnamed	Aniridia hamartoma	Wilms' tumor	?	Haicken and Miller (1971)

Table 2   *Skeletal malformations*

Syndrome	Principal components	Renal abnormality	Inheritance	Reference
Zellweger	Chrondrodystrophy; glaucoma; hepatomegaly; brain anomalies	Polycystic kidneys	Autosomal recessive	Bowen *et al.* (1964)
Unnamed	Polydactyly; internal hydrocephalus	Infantile polycystic kidneys	Autosomal recessive	Simopoulos *et al.* (1967)
Meckel	Encephalocele; polydactyly; sloping forehead	Polycystic kidneys	Autosomal recessive	Tucker *et al.* (1966); Opitz and Howe (1969)
Oral–facial–digital	Cleft tongue; jaw, palate; digital malformations	Polycystic kidneys	Sex-linked lethal	Doege *et al.* (1964)
Onycho-osteo-dysplasia; Nail–patella	Dysplasia of nails and patella; iliac horns	Nephritis nephrosis (including congenital)	Autosomal dominant	Hawkins and Smith (1950); Simila *et al.* (1970)
Potter	Abnormal facies; genital, cardiac skeletal and lung anomalies	Renal agenesis		Potter (1961)
Spina bifida	Meningomyelocele	Double ureter; horseshoe kidney; congenital hydronephrosis; neonatal ascites		Norman(1963); Howat (1971)
Hemihypertrophy	Hemihypertrophy	Wilms' tumour; hypospadias		Ward and Lerner (1947); Miller *et al.* (1964)
Arachnodactyly; Marfan's	Arachnodactyly; cardiac and ocular malformations	Various anomalies including ectopia and duplex systems; pyelonephritis	Autosomal dominant	Loughridge (1959)
Beckwith	Hypoglycaemia; macroglossia	Dysplasia; nephroblastoma	Autosomal recessive	Beckwith (1969)
Fanconi's anaemia	Hypoplastic anaemia; skeletal defects	Various renal anomalies	Autosomal recessive	McDonald and Goldschmidt (1960)
Smith–Lemli–Opitz	Abnormal facies; skeletal abnormalities; small stature; cryptorchidism	Hypospadias	?Autosomal recessive	Smith *et al.* (1964)

Table 2 *continued*

Syndrome	Principal components	Renal abnormality	Inheritance	Reference
Rubinstein–Taybi	Broad thumbs; abnormal facies with hypoplastic maxilla	Dilated ureter		Johnson (1966)
Acrocephalo-syndactyly; Apert	Craniosynostosis; syndactyly	Polycystic kidney; hydronephrosis	Autosomal dominant	Smith (1970)
Unnamed	Osteolysis of carpal and tarsal bones	Renal insufficiency hypertension	?Autosomal dominant	Shurtleff *et al.* (1964)
Acrocephalopolysyndactyly; Carpenter	Acrocephaly; hypoplastic maxilla; exophthalmos	Aminoaciduria	?	Temtamy (1966)
Cutis hyper-elastica; Ehlers–Danlos	Hyperextensibility of joints and skin	Pelviureteric obstruction	Autosomal dominant	McKusick (1966)
Jeune	Thoracic asphyxiant dystrophy	Proteinuria; medullary necrosis		Herdman and Langer (1968)
Unnamed	Agenesis of sacrum	Neurogenic bladder		Koontz and Prout (1968)
Russell-Silver	Hemihypertrophy: short stature; craniofacial dysostosis	Pelviureteric obstruction; vesicoureteric reflux; pyelonephritis		Haslam *et al.* (1973)
Unnamed	Congenital asymmetry	Hypospadias; medullary sponge kidney; non-functioning kidney; adrenal tumours		Parker and Skalko (1969)
Multiple lentigenes	Hypogonadotrophism; hyposmia	Unilateral renal agenesis; hydronephrosis	Autosomal dominant	Swanson *et al.* (1971)
Chondroectodermal dysplasia; Ellis–Van Creveld	Dwarfism; polydactyly; dystrophy of finger nails; cardiac malformations	Nephrocalcinosis glomerulosclerosis	Autosomal recessive	Blackburn and Belliveau (1971)
Acral–renal	Abnormalities of hands, feet and ears	Hypospadias; renal agenesis; duplex system		Curran and Curran (1972)
Unnamed	Lateral displacement of nipples	Renal hypoplasia		Fleisher (1966)
Bloom	Congenital telangiectatic erythema of face; small stature; photosensitivity	Hypospadias	Autosomal recessive	Bloom (1966)
Unnamed	Red and blonde hair	Medullary cystic disease		Rayfield and McDonald (1972)
EEC	Ectrodactyly; cleft lip and palate; ectodermal dysplasia	Renal agenesis		Roselli and Gulienetti (1961)
Oculo-auriculo-vertebral dysplasia; Goldenhar	Epibulbar dermoids; auricular appendages; vertebral anomalies	Various renal anomalies		Holmes *et al.* (1972)
Oral–cranial–digital	Cleft lip and palate; syndactyly; flexion deformities of digits; microcephaly	Horseshoe kidney	Autosomal recessive	Juberg *et al.* (1969)
Ectromelia and ichthyosis	Unilateral ichthyosis; limb anomalies	Polycystic kidney; hydronephrosis	Autosomal recessive	Cullen *et al.* (1969)
Roberts	Tetraphocomelia; cleft lip and palate; genital hypertrophy	Polycystic kidneys and other renal anomalies	Autosomal recessive	Appelt *et al.* (1966)

Table 3 *Visceral abnormalities*

Syndrome	Principal components	Renal abnormality	Inheritance	Reference
Prune belly	Dysplasia of abdominal musculature; cryptorchidism	Urinary tract dysplasia		Eagle and Barrett (1950)
Unnamed	Bladder exstrophia; rectal and other anomalies	Various renal anomalies		Uson *et al.* (1959)
Unnamed	Imperforate anus	Rectourethral fistula		Schaffer and Avery (1971)
Unnamed	Pneumothorax; pneumo-mediastinum	Renal dysplasia; polycystic kidneys		Lieberman *et al.* (1969) Renert *et al.* (1972)
Tuberous sclerosis	Tuberous sclerosis; adenoma sebaceum; white macules	Mixed tumour of kidney; angiolipoma; cystic kidneys	Autosomal dominant	Potter (1961); Kaplan *et al.* (1961)
Ivemark's familial dysplasia	Hepatomegaly; pancreatic dysplasia	Renal dysplasia	Autosomal recessive	Ivemark *et al.* (1959)
Unnamed*	Vaginal atresia	Various urinary tract anomalies		Phelan *et al.* (1953)
Von Hippel–Lindau	Angiomatous lesions of retina, brain etc.; cystic pancreas	Cystic kidneys; renal carcinoma; phaeo-chromocytoma	Autosomal dominant	Simon and Thompson (1955); Christoferson *et al.* (1961); Kaplan *et al.* (1961)
Unnamed	Cystic liver	Infantile polycystic disease	Autosomal recessive	Blyth and Ockenden (1971)
Unnamed	Occluded liver or pancreatic cysts	Adult polycystic disease	Autosomal dominant	Blyth and Ockenden (1971)
Von Reckling-hausen	Multiple neurofibromatosis; coarctation of aorta	Renal artery stenosis; phaeochromocytoma	Autosomal dominant	Fienman and Yakovac (1970)
Unnamed	Giant umbilical cord	Patent urachus		Chantler *et al.* (1969)
Hirschsprung's disease	Congenital megacolon	Obstructive uropathy		Swenson and Fisher (1955)
Unnamed	Lipodystrophy	Chronic nephritis		Senior and Gellis (1964)
Sickle-cell disease	Haemoglobin S	Medullary damage; haematuria		Schlitt and Keitel (1960)
Denis–Drash	Pseudohermaphroditism	Wilms' tumour; degenerative renal disease		Drash *et al.* (1970)
Unnamed	Fetal gigantism	Renal hamartomas; nephroblastoma	Autosomal recessive	Perlman *et al.* (1973)
Lissencephaly	Microcephaly; sloping forehead; polydactyly	Renal agenesis	Autosomal recessive	Miller (1963)
Cerebro-hepatorenal	Hypotonia; hepato-megaly; abnormal ears	Cortical cysts; hypospadias	?Autosomal recessive	Passarge and McAdams (1967)
Leprechaunism	Emaciation; hirsutism; endocrine disorders; failure to thrive	Aminoaciduria	?Autosomal recessive	Dekaborn (1965)
Unnamed	Single umbilical artery	Renal anomalies		Feingold *et al.* (1964)
Unnamed	Leukaemia	Renal involvement		Tucker *et al.* (1962)
Unnamed	Co-arctation of abdominal aorta	Renal artery stenosis		Riemenschneider *et al.* (1969)
Unnamed	Cyanotic congenital heart disease	Glomerulomegaly; proteinuria		Ingelfinger *et al.* (1970)

Table 3 *continued*

Syndrome	Principal components	Renal abnormality	Inheritance	Reference
Cardiofacial	Asymmetric facies when crying; multiple anomalies including congenital heart disease	Various renal anomalies		Pope and Pickering (1972)
Intestinal lymph-angiectasia	Protein-losing enteropathy	Nephrotic syndrome		de Sousa *et al.* (1968)
Baber	Congenital cirrhosis of liver	Aminoaciduria		Baber (1956)
Partial lipo-dystrophy	Facial lipodystrophy hypocomplementaemia	Glomerulonephritis		Peters *et al.* (1973)
The VATER association	Vertebral defects; anal atresia; oesophageal atresia with tracheo-oesophageal fistula; radial dysplasia; cardiac; (single umbilical artery, large fontanel, minor defects of external ear)	Renal anomaly 449	?	Barry and Auldist (1974)

*Sometimes referred to as the Rokitansky sequence. Smith, D.W. and Jones, K.L. (1982), *Recognizable Patterns of Human Malformations*, 3rd edn., p. 483. Philadelphia: W.B. Saunders Co.

Table 4 *Metabolic disturbances*

Syndrome	Principal components	Renal abnormality	Inheritance	Reference
Angiokeratoma; corpora diffusum (Fabry)	Skin angioma; abdominal and limb pains	Nephritis and renal failure	X-linked	Wise *et al.* (1962)
Hepatolenticular degeneration (Wilson)	Extrapyramidal signs; liver damage	Renal tubular dysfunction	Autosomal recessive	Bearin (1972)
Fructosaemia	Hypoglycaemia; hepatic damage; failure to thrive	Proteinuria; aminoaciduria	Autosomal recessive	Froesch (1972)
Galactosaemia	Cataracts; brain damage; hepatic damage; failure to thrive	Renal tubular dysfunction	Autosomal recessive	Segal (1972)
Glycogen-storage disease (Von Gierkel)	Hypoglycaemia hepatomegaly	Renal tubular dysfunction	Autosomal recessive	Howell (1972)
Tyrosinosis	Failure to thrive; fever; hepatomegaly	Renal tubular dysfunction	Autosomal recessive	La Du and Gjessing (1972)
Hydroxyprolinaemia	Mental retardation	Haematuria	?Autosomal recessive	Scriver and Efron (1972)
Hyperprolinaemia	Deafness; epilepsy; mental retardation	Renal insufficiency	Autosomal recessive	Scriven and Efron (1972)
Familial lecithin-cholesterol acetyl transferase deficiency	Corneal opacities; anaemia	Proteinuria; renal failure	Autosomal recessive	Norum *et al.* (1972)
Lesch–Nyhan	Mental retardation; self-mutilation; hyperuricaemia	Renal calculi	X-linked	Kelley and Wyngaarden (1972)
Familial Mediterranean fever	Abdominal pain; fever	Amyloid; proteinuria; renal failure	Autosomal recessive	Cohen (1972)

Table 4 *continued*

Syndrome	Principal components	Renal abnormality	Inheritance	Reference
Unnamed	Urticaria; deafness	Amyloid renal disease	Autosomal dominant	Cohen (1972)
Hypophosphatasia	Low alkaline phosphatase; rickets; hypercalcaemia	Nephrocalcinosis	Autosomal recessive	Bartter (1972)
Unnamed	Hypergammaglobulinaemia; macroglobulinaemia; cryo-globulinaemia	Renal tubular acidosis		Seldin and Wilson (1972)
Infantile hyper-calcaemia	Hypercalcaemia in infancy; mental retardation; abnormal facies; supravalvular aortic stenosis	Renal artery stenosis		Chantler *et al.* (1966)
Vitamin C deficiency (scurvy)	Skin and bone haemorrhage	Aminoaciduria		Jonxis and Huisman (1954)
Hypermethionaemia	Hepatic cirrhosis; pancreatic islet hyperplasia	Enlarged kidneys; aminoaciduria	Autosomal recessive	Perry *et al.* (1965)
Hyperparathyroidism	Hypercalcaemia	Renal calculi; proximal renal tubular acidosis		Sideligui and Wilson (1972)
Unnamed	Hyperuricaemia	Hereditary nephropathy	Autosomal dominant	Neumann and Wegmann (1972)

Table 5 *Infections*

Syndrome	Principal components	Renal abnormality	Inheritance	Reference
Congenital rubella	Cataracts; cardiac anomalies; deafness; microcephaly, etc.	Various renal anomalies		Menser *et al.* (1967)
ECHO; mumps; Varicella infections		Acute nephritic syndrome		Yuceoglu *et al.* (1966, 1967); Masson and Nickerson (1967)
Sarcoid	Pulmonary lesions; skin nodules; lymphadenopathy	Nephrocalcinosis		Kogut and Neumann (1961)
Infectious mononucleosis	Malaise; lymphadenopathy; periorbital oedema; spleno-megaly	Rapidly progressive interstitial nephritis		Lowery and Rutsky (1972)
Schistosomiasis	Haematuria	Nephrotic syndrome; ureteric obstruction		El Said *et al.* (1972)

Table 6 *Chromosomal abnormalities*

Syndrome	Principal components	Renal abnormality	Inheritance	Reference
Trisomy C	Abnormal facies; joint abnormalities, cleft palate	Ureteral atresia; cystic dysplasia		Juberg *et al.* (1970)
Trisomy D (13-15); Patau	Cleft lip and palate; congenital heart disease; abnormal facies	Cystic and other renal anomalies in 60 per cent of cases		Snodgrass *et al.* (1966); Egli and Stalder (1973)

Table 6 *continued*

Syndrome	Principal components	Renal abnormality	Inheritance	Reference
Trisomy E (18); Edwards	Abnormal facies and ears; small for dates; overlapping digits; congenital heart disease	Cystic horseshoe or duplication in 70 per cent of cases		Egli and Stalder (1973)
Trisomy 21: Down	Abnormal facies; brachycephaly; congenital heart disease, etc.	Cystic and other anomalies in 70 per cent of cases		Egli and Stalder (1973)
Cat-eye	Coloboma; rectal anomalies; abnormal facies; congenital heart disease	Agenesis and other anomalies in 60–100 per cent of cases		Egli and Stalder (1973)
5 Short arm deletion; Cri du chat	Abnormal facies; typical cry; mental retardation	Various		Egli and Stalder (1973)
Other autosomal aberrations		Various, but not common		Egli and Stalder (1973)
XO; Turner	Small stature; congenital heart disease; amenorrhoea	Horseshoe, duplication and abnormalities of rotation, etc. in 60 per cent of cases		Egli and Stalder (1973)
XXY; Klinefelter	Gynaecomastia; azoospermia; hypogonadism	Rare		Egli and Stalder (1973)

References

Anderson, D. and Tanner, R.L. (1969) Tuberous sclerosis and chronic renal failure. Potential confusion with polycystic kidney disease. *Am. J. Med.* 47: 163.

Appelt, H., Gerken, H. and Lenz, W. (1966) Tetraphokomelie mit Lippen–Kiefer–Gaumenspalte und Clitoris Hypertrophie—ein Syndrom. *Paediatrie Pathologie* 2. 119: 24.

Baber, M.D. (1956) A case of congenital cirrhosis of the liver with renal tubular defects akin to those in the Franconi syndrome. *Arch. Dis. Childh.* 31: 335.

Barahat, A.Y., D'Albora, J., Hollerman, C.E., Jose, P. and Calcagno, P.L. (1979) Hereditary renal disease associated with hypoparathyroidism. *Abstracts of the Fifth International Congress of Nephrology, Mexico,* p. 99.

Barry, J.E. and Auldist, A.W. (1974) The VATER association. *Am. J. Dis. Childr.* 128: 769.

Bartter, F.C. (1972) Hypophosphatasia. In *The Metabolic Basis of Inherited Disease,* 3rd edn., J.B. Stanbury, J.B. Wyngaarden and D.S. Fredrickson (eds), p. 1295. New York: McGraw-Hill.

Bearn, A.G. (1972) Wilson's disease. In *The Metabolic Basis of Inherited Disease,* 3rd edn., J.B. Stanbury, J.B. Wyngaarden and D.S. Fredrickson (eds), p. 1033. New York: McGraw-Hill.

Beckwith, J.B. (1969) Macroglossia, omphalocele, adrenal cytomegaly, gigantism, hyperplastic visceromegaly: the clinical delineation of birth defects. II. *Malformation Syndromes,* p. 188. New York National Foundation.

Blackburn, M. and Belliveau, R.E. (1971) Ellis–Van Creveld syndrome. *Am. J. Dis. Childr.* 122: 267.

Bloom, D. (1966) The syndrome of congenital telangiectatic erythema and stunted growth. *J. Pediatr.* 68: 103.

Blyth, H. and Ockenden, B.G. (1971) Polycystic disease of kidneys and liver presenting in childhood. *J. Med. Genet.* 8: 257.

Bowen, P., Lee, C.S.N. and Zellweger, H. (1964) A familial syndrome of multiple congenital defects. *Johns Hopkins Med. J.* 114: 402.

Campbell, R.A., Musgrave, J.E., Lourien, E.W., Jacinto, E.Y. and Chan, J.C. (1972) Fatal familial nephropathy cataracts and immunofluorescent glomeruli. *Abstracts of the Fifth International Congress of Nephrology, Mexico,* p. 40.

Chantler, C., Davies, D.H. and Joseph, M.C. (1966) Cardiovascular and other associations of infantile hypercalcaemia. *Guy's Hospital Reports* 115: 221.

Chantler, C., Baum, J.D., Wigglesworth, J.S. and Scopes, J.W.J. (1969) *Gynecol. Obstet.* 70: 273.

Christoferson, L.A., Gustafson, M.B. and Peterson, G. (1961) Von Hippel–Lindau's disease. *J. Am. Med. Ass.* 178: 280.

Cohen, A. (1972) Inherited systemic amyloidosis. In *The Metabolic Basis of Inherited Disease,* 3rd edn., J.B. Stanbury, J.B. Wyngaarden and D.S. Fredrickson, p. 1273. New York: McGraw-Hill.

Cullen, S.I., Harris, D.E., Carter, C.H. and Reed, W.B. (1969) Congenital unilateral ichthyosiform erythroderma. *Arch. Dermatol.* 99: 724.

Curran, A.S. and Curran, J.P. (1972) Associated acral and renal malformations: a new syndrome. *Pediatrics* 49: 716.

Dekaborn, A. (1965) Metabolic and chromosomal studies in leprechaunism. *Arch. Dis. Childh.* 40: 632.

Dekaborn, A.S. (1967) Hereditary syndrome of congenital retinal blindness (Leber). Polycystic kidneys and maldevelopment of the brain. *Am. J. Ophthalmol.* 68: 1029.

de Sousa, J.S., Guerrerro, O., Cunha, A. and Araujo, J. (1968) Association of nephrotic syndrome with intestinal lymphangiectasia. *Arch. Dis. Childh.* 43: 245.

Doege, T.C., Thuline, H.C., Priest, J.H., Norby, D.E. and Bryant, J.S. (1964) Studies of a family with the oral facial syndrome. *N. Engl. J. Med.* 271: 1073.

Drash, A., Sherman, F., Hartmann, W.H. and Blizzard, R.M. (1970) A syndrome of pseudohermaphroditism, Wilms' tumor, hypertension and degenerative renal disease. *J. Pediatr.* 76: 585.

Eagle, J.F. and Barrett, J.S. (1950) Congenital deficiency of abdominal musculature with associated genito-urinary abnormalities. *Pediatrics* 6: 721.

Egli, F. and Stalder, G. (1973) Malformations of kidney and urinary tract in common chromosomal aberrations. *Hum. Genet.* 18: 1.

Ehlers, N. (1966) Cryptophthalmos with orbitopalpebral cyst and micro-ophthalmos. *Acta Ophthalmol.* 44: 84.

El Said, W., Gabal, I.A. and Sabom, M. (1972) Urinary bilharziasis as a cause of nephrotic syndrome? *Abstracts of the Fifth International Congress of Nephrology, Mexico*, p. 93.

Fairley, K.F., Leighton, P.W. and Kincaid-Smith, P. (1963) Familial visual defects associated with polycystic kidneys and medullary sponge kidney. *Br. Med. J.* 1: 1060.

Feingold, M., Fine, R.N. and Inzall, D. (1964) Intravenous pyelography in infants with single umbilical artery. Preliminary report. *N. Engl. J. Med.* 270: 1178.

Fienman, N.L. and Yakovac, W.C. (1970) Hemofibromatosis. *J. Pediatr.* 76: 339.

Fleisher, D.S. (1966) Lateral displacement of nipples, a sign of bilateral renal hypoplasia. *J. Pediatr.* 69: 806.

Froesch, E.R. (1972) Essential fructosemia and hereditary fructose intolerance. In *The Metabolic Basis of Inherited Disease*, 3rd edn., J.B. Stanbury, J.B. Wyngaarden and D.S. Fredrickson, p. 131. New York: McGraw-Hill.

Haicken, B.N. and Miller, D.R. (1971) Simultaneous occurrence of congenital aniridia, hamartoma and Wilms' tumor. *J. Pediatr.* 78: 497.

Haslam, R.H.A., Berman, W. and Heller, R.M. (1973) Renal abnormalities in the Russell–Silver syndrome. *Pediatrics* 51: 216.

Hawkins, C.F. and Smith, O.E. (1950) Renal dysplasia in a family with multiple hereditary abnormalities including iliac horns. *Lancet* 1: 803.

Herdman, R.C. and Langer, L.O. (1968) Thoracic asphyxiant dystrophy and renal disease. *Am. J. Dis. Childr.* 116: 192.

Hoefnagel, D., Keenan, M.E. and Allen, F.H.Jr. (1963) Heredofamilial bilateral anophthalmia. *Acta Ophthalmol.* 69: 760.

Holmes, L.B., Moser, H.W., Halldorsson, S., Mack, C., Pant, S.S. and Matzilevich, B. (1972) In *Mental Retardation: an Atlas of Diseases with Associated Physical Abnormalities*, p. 284. New York: Macmillan.

Howat, J.M. (1971) Urinary ascites complicating spina bifida. *Arch. Dis. Childh.* 46: 103.

Howell, R.R. (1972) Glycogen storage diseases. In *The Metabolic Basis of Inherited Disease*, 3rd edn., J.B. Stanbury, J.B. Wyngaarden and D.S. Fredrickson, p. 1049. New York: McGraw-Hill.

Ingelfinger, J.R., Kissane, J.M. and Robson, A.M. (1970) Glomerulomegaly in a patient with cyanotic congenital heart disease. *Am. J. Dis. Childr.* 120: 69.

Ivemark, B., Oldfelt, V. and Zetterstrom, R. (1959) Familial dysplasia of kidneys, liver and pancreas: a probably genetically determined syndrome. *Acta Paediatr.* 48: 1.

Johnson, C.F. (1966) Broad thumbs and broad great toes with facial abnormalities and mental retardation. *J. Pediatr.* 68: 942.

Jonxis, J.H.P. and Huisman, T.H.J. (1954) Aminoaciduria and ascorbic acid deficiency. *Pediatrics* 14: 238.

Juberg, R.C. and Hayward, J.R. (1969) A new familial syndrome of oral, cranial and digital anomalies. *J. Pediatr.* 74: 755.

Juberg, R.C., Gilbert, E.F. and Slisbury, R.S. (1970) Trisomy C in an infant with polycystic kidneys and other malformations. *J. Pediatr.* 76: 598.

Kaplan, C., Sayre, G.P. and Greene, L.F. (1961) Bilateral nephrogenic carcinoma in Lindau–Von Hippel disease. *J. Urol.* 86: 36.

Kelley, W.N. and Wyngaarden, J.B. (1972) The Lesch–Nyhan syndrome. In *The Metabolic Basis of Inherited Disease*, 3rd edn., J.B. Stanbury, J.B. Wyngaarden and D.S. Fredrickson, p. 969. New York: McGraw-Hill.

Kogut, M.D. and Neumann, L.L. (1961) Renal involvement in Boeck's sarcoidosis. *Pediatrics* 28: 410.

Koontz, W.W. and Prout, G.R. (1968) Agenesis of sacrum and neurogenic bladder. *J. Am. Med. Ass.* 203: 481.

La Du, B.N. and Gjessing, L.R. (1972) Tyrosinosis and tyrosinaemia. In *The Metabolic Basis of Inherited Disease*, 3rd edn., J.B. Stanbury, J.B. Wyngaarden and D.S. Fredrickson, p. 296. New York: McGraw-Hill.

Lieberman, M.M., Abraham, J.M. and France, N.E. (1969) Association between pneumomediastinum and renal anomalies. *Arch. Dis. Child.* 44: 471.

Lieberman, E., Salinas Madrigal, L., Gwinn, J.L., Brennan, L.P. and Landring, B.H. (1971) Infantile polycystic disease of the kidneys and liver. *Medicine* 50: 277.

Loken, A.C., Hansson, O., Halvorsen, S. and Jolstor, N.J. (1961) Hereditary renal dysplasia and blindness. *Acta Paediatr.* 50: 177.

Longnecker, C.G., Ryan, R.F. and Vincent, R.W. (1965) Malformations of the ear as a clue to urogenital anomalies: Report of 6 additional cases. *Plast. Reconstr. Surg.* 35: 303.

Loughridge, L.W. (1959) Renal abnormalities in Marfan's syndrome. *Q. J. Med.* 28: 531.

Lowery, T.A. and Rutsky, E.A. (1972) Infectious mononucleosis and progressive interstitial renal failure. *Abstracts of the Fifth International Congress of Nephrology, Mexico*, p. 39.

Masson, A.M. and Nickerson, G.H. (1967) Mumps with nephritis. *Can. Med. Assoc. J.* 97: 866.

McDonald, R. and Goldschmidt, B. (1960) Pancytopenia with congenital defects (Fanconi's uraemia). *Arch. Dis. Childh.* 35: 367.

McKusick, V.A. (1966) *Heritable Disorders of Connective Tissue*, 3rd edn., p. 179. St. Louis: C.V. Mosby.

Menser, M.A., Robertson, S.E.J., Dorman, D.C., Gillespie, A.M. and Murphy, A.M. (1967) Renal lesions in congenital rubella. *Pediatrics* 40: 901.

Miller, J.Q. (1963) Lissencephaly in two siblings. *Neurology* 13: 841.

Miller, R.W., Fraumeni, J.F. and Manning, M.D. (1964) Association of Wilms' tumour with aniridia, hemihypertrophy and other congenital malformations. *N. Engl. J. Med.* 270: 922.

Nadjini, B., Flanagan, M.J. and Christian, J.R. (1969) Laurence–Moon–Biedl syndrome. *Am. J. Dis. Childr.* 117: 352.

Nance, W.E., Unger, E.J. and Sweeney, A. (1970) Evidence for autosomal recessive inheritance of the syndrome of renal tubular acidosis, with deafness. IX. *The Clinical Delineation of Birth Defects*. Baltimore: Williams and Williams.

Neumann, E.P. and Wegmann, W. (1972) Hereditary nephropathy with hyperuricemia. *Abstracts of the European Society for Pediatric Nephrology, Dublin*.

Norman, A.P. (1963) *Congenital Abnormalities in Infancy*, p. 34. Oxford: Blackwell Scientific Publications.

Norum, K.R., Glomset, J.A. and Gjore, E. (1972) Familial lecithin-cholesterol acetyl transferase deficiency. In *The Metabolic Basis of Inherited Disease*, 3rd edn., J.B. Stanbury, J.B. Wyngaarden and D.S. Fredrickson (eds), p. 531. New York: McGraw-Hill.

Ohno, T. and Hirooka, M. (1966) Renal lesions in Cockayne's syndrome. *Tohuku J. Exp. Med.* 89: 151.

Opitz, J.M. and Howe, J.J. (1969) The Meckel syndrome (dysencephalia, splanchnocystica, the ocular syndrome). II: the clinical delineation of birth defects. In *Malformation Syndromes*, p. 167. New York National Foundation.

Parker, D.A. and Skalko, R.G. (1969) Congenital asymmetry: report of ten cases with associated developmental abnormalities. *Pediatrics* 44: 584.

Passarge, E. and McAdams, J. (1967) Cerebrohepatorenal syndrome. *J. Pediatr.* 71: 6091.

Perlman, M., Goldberg, G.M., Bar-Ziv, J. and Danovitch, G. (1973) Renal hamartomas and nephroblastomatosis with fetal gigantism: a familial syndrome. *J. Pediatr.* 83: 414.

Perry, T.L., Hardwick, D.F., Dixon, G.H., Dolman, C.L. and Hansen, S. (1965) Hypermethioninemia, a metabolic disorder associated with cirrhosis, islet cell hyperplasia and renal tubular degeneration. *Pediatrics* 36: 236.

Peters, D.K., Williams, D.G., Charlesworth, J.A., Boulton-Jones, J.M., Sissons, J.G.P. and Evans, D.J. (1973) Mesangiocapillary nephritis, partial lipodystrophy and hypocomplementaemia. *Lancet* 2: 535.

Phelan, J.T., Counsellor, V.S. and Greene, L.F. (1953) Deformities of the urinary tract with congenital absence of the vagina. *Surg. Gynecol. Obstet.* 97: 1.

Pope, K.E. and Pickering, D. (1972) Asymmetric crying facies: an index of other congenital anomalies. *J. Pediatr.* 81: 21.

Potter, E.L. (1961) *Pathology of the Fetus and Infant*, 2nd edn., p. 432. Chicago: Year Book Medical.

Potter, E.L. (1961) *Pathology of the Fetus and Infant*, 2nd edn., p. 441. Chicago: Year Book Medical.

Rayfield, E.J. and McDonald, F.D. (1972) Red and blonde hair in renal medullary cystic disease. *Arch. Intern. Med.* 130: 72.

Renert, W.A., Berden, W.E., Baher, D.H. and Rose, J.S. (1972) Obstructive urologic malformations of the fetus and infant—relation to neonatal pneumomediastinum and pneumothorax (air block). *Radiology* 105: 97.

Riemenschneider, T.A., Emmanouilides, G.C., Hirose, F. and Linde, L.M. (1969) Coarctation of the abdominal aorta in children: report of three cases and review of literature. *Pediatrics* 44: 716.

Roselli, D. and Gulienetti, R. (1961) Ectodermal dysplasia. *Br. J. Plast. Surg.* 14: 190.

Schaffer, A.J. and Avery, M.E. (1971) *Diseases of the Newborn*, 3rd edn., p. 391. Philadelphia: W.B. Saunders.

Schlitt, L.E. and Keitel, H.G. (1960) Renal manifestations of sickle cell disease: a review. *Am. J. Med. Sci.* 239: 773.

Scriver, C.R. and Efron, M.L. (1972) Disorders of proline and hydroxy-proline metabolism. In *The Metabolic Basis of Inherited Disease*, 3rd edn., J.B. Stanbury, J.B. Wyngaarden and D.S. Fredrickson, p. 351. New York: McGraw-Hill.

Segal, S. (1972) Disorders of galactose metabolism. In *The Metabolic Basis of Inherited Disease*, 3rd edn., J.B. Stanbury, J.B. Wyngaarden and D.S. Fredrickson, p. 174. New York: McGraw-Hill.

Seldin, D.W. and Wilson, J.D. (1972) Renal tubular acidosis. In *The Metabolic Basis of Inherited Disease*, 3rd edn., J.B. Stanbury, J.B. Wyngaarden, and D.S. Fredrickson, p. 1548. New York: McGraw-Hill.

Senior, B. and Gellis, S. (1964) Lipodystrophy. *Pediatrics* 33: 593.

Senior, B., Friedmann, A.I. and Braudo, J.L. (1961) Juvenile familial nephropathy with tapetoretinal degeneration. A new oculorenal dystrophy. *Am. J. Ophthalmol.* 52: 625.

Shurtleff, D.B., Sparkes, R.S., Clawson, D.K., Guntheroth, W.G. and Mottet, N.K. (1964) Hereditary osteolysis with hypertension and nephropathy. *J. Am. Med. Ass.* 188: 363.

Sideligui, A.A. and Wilson, D.R. (1972) Primary hyperparathyroidism and proximal renal tubular acidosis. *Can. Med. Assoc. J.* 106: 644.

Simila, S., Vesa, L. and Wazz-Hockert, O. (1970) Hereditary onycho-osteodysplasia (the nail–patella syndrome) with nephrosis-like renal disease in a newborn boy. *Pediatrics* 46: 61.

Simon, H.B. and Thompson, G.J. (1955) Congenital renal polycystic disease. A clinical and therapeutic study of three hundred and sixty six cases. *J. Am. Med. Ass.* 159: 657.

Simopoulos, A., Brennan, G.C., Alivan, A. and Fidis, N. (1967) Polycystic kidneys, internal hydrocephalus, polydactylism in newborn siblings. *Pediatrics* 39: 931.

Smith, D.W. (1970) Apert's syndrome. In *Recognizable Patterns of Human Malformation*, p. 226. Philadelphia: W.B. Saunders.

Smith, D.W., Lemli, L. and Opitz, J.M. (1964) A newly revised syndrome of multiple congenital anomalies. *J. Pediatr.* 64: 210.

Snodgrass, G.J.A.L., Butler, L.J., France, N.E., Crome, L. and Russell, A. (1966) The D (13–15) trisomy syndrome: an analysis of 7 examples. *Arch. Dis. Childh.* 41: 250.

Swanson, S.L., Santen, R.J. and Smith, D.W. (1971) Multiple lentigines syndrome: new findings of hypogonadotrophism hyposmia and unilateral renal agenesis. *J. Pediatr.* 78: 1037.

Swenson, O. and Fisher, J.H. (1955) Relation of megacolon and megaureter. *N. Engl. J. Med.* 253: 1147.

Temtamy, S.A. (1966) Carpenter's syndrome. Acrocephalo-polysyndactyly: an autosomal recessive syndrome. *J. Pediatr.* 69: 111.

Tucker, A.S., Newman, A.J. and Persky, L. (1962) The kidney in childhood leukaemia. *Radiology* 78: 407.

Tucker, C.C., Finley, S.C., Tucker, E.S. and Finley, W.H. (1966) Oral–facial–digital syndrome with polycystic kidneys and liver. Pathological and cytogenetic studies. *J. Med. Genet.* 3: 145.

Uson, A.C., Lattimer, J.K. and Melicow, M.M. (1959) Types of exstrophy of urinary bladder and concomitant malformations. *Pediatrics* 23: 927.

Ward, J. and Lerner, H.H. (1947) A review of the subject of congenital hemi-hypertrophy and a complete case report. *J. Pediatr.* 31: 403.

Winter, J.S.D., Kohn, G., Mellman, W.J. and Wagner, S.A. (1968) Familial syndrome of renal genital and middle ear anomalies. *J. Pediatr.* 72: 88.

Wise, D., Wallace, H.J. and Jellinek, E.H. (1962) Angiokeratoma corporis diffusum. A clinical study of eight affected families. *Q. J. Med.* 31: 177.

Yuceoglu, A.M., Berkovich, S. and Minkowitz, S. (1966) Acute glomerulonephritis associated with ECHO virus type 9 infection. *J. Pediatr.* 69: 603.

Yuceoglu, A.M., Berkovich, S. and Minkowitz, S. (1967) Acute glomerulonephritis as a complication of varicella. *J. Am. Med. Ass.* 202: 879.

References

Abdelhak, S., Kalatzis, V., Heilig, R., Compain, S., Samson, D., Vincent C., Weil, D., Cruaud, C., Sahly, I., Leibovici, M., Bitner-Glindzicz, M., Francis, M., Lacombe, D., Vigneron., J., Charachon, R., Boven, K., Bedbeder, P., Van Regemorter, N., Weissenbach, J. and Petis, C. (1997) A human homologue of the *Drosophila* eye's absent gene underlies branchio-oto-renal (BOR) syndrome and identifies a novel gene family. *Nat. Genet.*.15: 157–164.

Abe, T. and Hutson, J.M. (1994a) Gonadal migration in ambiguous genitalia. *Pediatr. Surg. Int.* 9: 547–550.

Abe, T. and Huston, J.M. (1994b) Calcitonin gene-related peptide injected ectopically alters gubernacular migration in flutamide-treated rat with cryptorchidism. *Pediatr. Surg. Int.* 9: 551–554.

Abeshouse, B.S. (1943) Ureteral ectopic–report of rare case of ectopic ureter opening in uterus and review of literature. *Urol. Cutan, Rev.* 47: 447.

Abeshouse, B.S. (1947) Crossed ectopia with fusion. *Am. J. Surg.* 73: 658.

Abrahamson, J. (1961) Double bladder and related anomalies: clinical and embryological aspects and a case report. *Br. J. Urol.* 33: 195.

Adamson, A.S. and Burge, D.M. (1990) Megalourethra. *Pediatr. Surg. Int.* 5: 449–450.

Aleem, A.A., El Sheikh, S., Mokhtar, A., Ghafouri, H. and Saleem, M. (1985) The perineal groove and canal in males and females–a third look. *Z. Kinderchir.* 40: 303.

Alfert, H.J. and Gillenwater, J.Y. (1972) Ectopic vas deferens communicating with lower ureter: embryo logical considerations. *J. Urol.* 108: 172.

Aliabadi, H. and Gonzalez, R. (1990) 'Success of the artificial urinary sphincter after failed surgery for incontinence.' *J. Urol.* **143**(5): 987–990.

Altemus, A.R. and Hutchins, G.M. (1991) Development of the human anterior urethra. *J. Urol.* 146: 1085–1093.

Amar, A.D. (1975) The clinical significance of renal caliceal diverticulum in children: Relation to vesico-ureteral reflux. *J. Urol.* 113: 255.

Ambrose, S.S. and Nicholson, W.P. (1962) The causes of vesicoureteral reflux in children. *J. Urol.* 87: 688.

Amsler, E. (1961) Rétrécissements congénitaux de l'uréthre caverneux chez l'homme. *Helv. Chir. Acta.* 28: 99.

Anderson, J.C., Faulder, K.G. and Mpor, J.E. (1979) 'Prune belly' syndrome. *Med. J. Aust.* 314–315.

Ansell, J.S. (1979) Surgical treatment of exstrophy of the bladder with emphasis on neonatal primary closure: personal experience with 28 consecutive cases treated at the University of Washington Hospitals from 1962 to 1977: technique and results. *J. Urol.* **121**: 650.

Ansell, J.S. (1983) Exstrophy and epispadias. *Urologic Surgery*, J.F. Glenn (ed.), p. 647. Philadelphia; J.B. Lippincott.

Anson, B.J. and McVay, C.B. (1936) The topographical positions and the mutual relations of the visceral branches of the abdominal aorta. A study of 100 consecutive cadavers. *Anat. Rec.* 67: 7.

Anson, B.J. and Riba, L.W. (1939) The anatomical and surgical features of ectopic kidney. *Surg. Gynecol. Obstet.* 48: 37–44.

Antony, J. (1977). Complete duplication of female urethra with vaginal atresia and supernumerary kidney. *J. Urol.* 118: 877.

Arant, B.S., Sotelo-Avila, C. and Bernstein, J. (1979) Segmental 'hypoplasia' of the kidney (Ask-Upmark). *J. Pediatr.* 95: 931.

Arey, L.B. (1974) *Developmental Anatomy*, 7th edn., rev. (a) p. 309; (b) p. 317; (c) p. 106; (d) p. 98; (e) p. 311. Philadelphia: Saunders.

Ashkenazy, M., Borenstein, R., Katz, Z. and Segal, M. (1982) Constriction of the umbilical cord by an amniotic band after midtrimester amniocentesis. *Acta Obstet. Gynecol. Scand.* 61: 89–91.

Ask-Upmark, E. (1929) Über juvenile maligne Nephrosclerose und ihr Verhältnis zur Störungen in der Nierenentwicklung. *Acta Pathol. Mircrobiol. Scand.* 6: 383.

Assayer, (1870) Cited by Campbell (1930).

Atiyeh, B., Husmann, D. and Baun, M. (1992) Contralateral renal anomalies in multicystic dysplastic kidney disease. *J. Pediatr.* 121: 65–67.

Attah, A.A. and Hutson, J.M. (1991) The antatomy of the female gubernaculum is different from the male. *Aust. N.Z. J. Surg.* 61: 380–384.

Attah, A.A. and Hutson, J.M. (1993) The role of intraabdominal pressure in cryptorchidism. *J. Urol.* 150: 994–996.

Attalla, M.F. (1991) Subcoronal hypospadias with complete prepuce: a distinct entity and new procedure for repair. *Br. J. Plast. Surg.* 44: 122–125.

Atwell, J.D., Cook, P.L., Howell, C.J., Hyde, I. and Parker, B.C. (1974) Familial incidence of bifid and double ureters. *Arch. Dis. Childh.* 49: 390.

Aulie, R.P. (1966) Caspar Friederich Wolff and his 'theoria generationis'. *J. Hist. Med. Allied Sci.* 16: 124.

Avellan, L. and Knutson, F. (1980) Microscopic studies of curvature-causing structures in hypospadias. *Scand. J. Plast. Reconstruct. Surg.* 14: 249–258.

Avery, M.E. (1964) *The Lung and its Disorders in the Newborn Infant*, p. 56, Philadelphia: W.B. Saunders.

Axelrod, H.D. (1954) Triplicate ureter and renal pelvis. *J. Urol.* 72: 799.

Ayres, D. (1859) Congenital exstrophy of the urinary bladder and its complications, successfully treated by a plastic operation. *Am. Med. Chir. Rev.* 3: 709.

Backhouse, K.M. (1982) Embryology of testicular descent and maldescent. *Urol. Clin. N. Am.* 9: 315–325.

Bacon, S.K. (1947) Large hydronephrosis of a true supernumerary kidney. *J. Urol.* 57: 459.

Badenoch, A.W. (1949) Congenital obstruction at bladder neck. Hunterian Lecture. *Ann. R. Coll. Surg. (Engl)* 4: 285.

Bagchi, A.G. (1990) Seven years' experience of ureterosigmoidostomy in surgically failed exstrophy of the bladder. *J. Indian. Med. Assoc.* **88**: 255–7.

Baggenstoss, A.H. (1951) Symposium on diseases of the kidney: Congenital anomalies of the kidney. *Med. Clin. N. Am.* 35: 987.

Bailey, R.R. (1979) An overview of reflux nephropathy. In *Reflux Nephrology*, J. Hodson and P. Kincaid-Smith (eds), p. 9. New York: Masson.

Ballantyne, J.W. (1904) The embryo. In *Manual of Antenatal Pathology and Hygiene*, Ch. 10, pp. 129–136. Edinburgh: William Green & Sons.

Barker, A.P., McMullin, N.D. and King, P.A. (1993) Posterior urethral valves and testicular maldescent: an underreported association. *Pediatr. Surg. Int.* 8: 51.

Barloon, J.W., Goodwin, W.E. and Vermooten, V. (1957) Thoracic kidney; case reports. *J. Urol.* 78: 356.

Barnett, J.A. and Stephens, F.D. (1962) The role of the lower segmental vessel in the aetiology of hydronephrosis. *Aust. N.Z. J. Surg.* 31: 201.

Barnhouse, D.H. (1972) Prune belly syndrome. *Br. J. Urol.* 44: 356.

Bassiouny, I.E. (1992) Continent urinary reservoir in exstrophy/epispadias complex. *Br. J. Urol.* **70**: 558.

Bauer, S.B., Retik, A.B. and Colodny, H.H. (1981) Genetic aspects of hypospadias, *Urol. Clin. N. Am.* 8: 559–564.

Baurys, W. and Servosa, S. (1949) Eventration of the diaphragm: report of a case involving a kidney. *Urol. Cutan. Rev.* 53: 535.

Bazy, P. (1903) A propos du diagnostic des lésions rénales unilatérales. *Bull. Soc. Chirurgie* 29: 32.

Beasley, S.W. and Auldist, A.W. (1985) Crossed testicular ectopia in association with double incomplete testicular descent. *Aust. N.Z. J. Surg.* 55: 301–303.

Beasley, S.W. and Hutson, J.M. (1987) Effect of division of genitofemoral nerve on testicular descent in the rat. *Aust. N.Z. J. Surg.* 57: 49–51.

Beasley, S.W., Bettenay, F. and Hutson, J.M. (1988) The anterior urethra provides clues to the aetiology of prune belly syndrome. *Pediatr. Surg. Int.* 3: 169–172.

Beck, A.D. (1971) The effect of intra-uterine urinary obstruction upon the development of the fetal kidney. *J. Urol.* 105: 784.

Begg, R.C. (1953) Sextuplicates renum: a case of six functioning kidneys and ureters in an adult female. *J. Urol.* 70: 686.

Behringer, R.R., Cate, R.L., Froelick, G.J., Palmiter, R.D. and Brinster, R.L. (1990) Abnormal sexual development in transgenic mice chronically expressing müllerian-inhibiting substance. *Nature* 345: 167–170.

Behringer, R.R., Finegold, M.J. and Cate, R.L. (1994) Müllerian-inhibiting substance function during mammalian sexual development. *Cell* 79: 415–425.

Bellinger, M.F. (1993) Ureterocystoplasty: a unique method for vesical augmentation in children. *J. Urol.* **149(4)**: 811–813.

Bergenhem, B. (1896) Ectopia vesicae et Adenoma destruens Vesicae. Extirpation af Blasen. Implantation af ureterna i rectum [abstract]. *Zentralbl. Chir.* **34**: 1262.

Belman, A.B. and King, L.R. (1972) Urinary tract abnormalities associated with imperforate anus. *J. Urol.* 108: 823.

Belman, A.B., Filmer, R.B. and King, L.R. (1974) Surgical management of duplication of the collecting system. *J. Urol.* 112: 316.

Ben-Ari, J., Merlob, P., Mimouni, F. and Reisner, S.H. (1985) Characteristics of the male genitalia in the newborn: penis, *J. Urol.* 134: 521–522.

Berger, R.M., Maizels, M., Moran, G.G., Conway, J.C. and Firlit, C.F. (1983) Bladder capacity (ounces) = age (years) *b: 2–predicts normal bladder capacity and aids diagnosis of abnormal voiding patterns. *J. Urol.* 129: 347.

Berkeley, C.H.A. and Bonney, V. (1935) A *Textbook of Gynaecological Surgery*, 3rd edn., p. 511. London: Cassell.

Berlin, H.S., Stern, J. and Poppel, M.E. (1957) Congenital superior ectopia of the kidney. *Am J. Radiol.* 78: 508.

Bernard, R., Reboud, E. and Maestraggi, P. (1959) A propos d'une image en coucher de soleil de l'hemi-coupole diaphragmatique droite (ectopie rénale intra-thoracique). *Pediatrie* 14: 293.

Bernstein, J. (1968) Developmental abnormalities of the renal parenchyma–renal hypoplasia and dysplasia. In *Pathology Annual*, S.C. Sommers (ed.), p. 213. New York: Appleton-Century-Crofts.

Bernstein, J. (1971) The morphogenesis of renal parenchymal maldevelopment (renal dysplasia). *Pediatr. Clin. N. Am.* 18: 395.

Bernstein, J. (1973) The classification of renal cysts. *Nephron* 11: 91.

Bernstein, J. (1993) Glomerulocystic kidney disease–nosological considertions. *Pediatr. Nephrol.* 7: 464–470.

Betts, P. R. and Forrest-Hay, I. (1973) Juvenile nephronophrisis. *Lancet* 2: 475.

Bialestock, D. (1960a) Microdissection of specimen of hydronephrosis with comparative nephron measurements. *Aust. N.Z. J. Surg.* 29: 211.

Bialestock, D. (1960b) Morphogenesis of unilateral multicystic kidney in childhood. *Aust. Ann. Med.* 9: 53.

Bialestock, D. (1963) Renal malformations and pyelonephritis–the role of vesicoureteral reflux. *Aust. N.Z. J. Surg.* 33: 114.

Bialestock, D. (1965) Studies of renal malformations and pyelonephritis in children with and without associated reflux and obstruction. *Aust. N. Z. J. Surg.* 35: 120.

Bill, A.H. Jr. and Johnson, R.J. (1958) Failure of migration of the rectal opening as the cause for most cases of imperforate anus. *Surg. Gynecol. Obstet.* 106: 643.

Blumberg, N. (1976) Ureteral triplication. *J. Pediatr. Surg.* 11: 589.

Blyth, H. and Ockenden, B.G. (1971) Polycystic disease of kidneys and liver presenting in childhood. *J. Med. Genet.* 8: 257.

Bodian, M. (1957) Some observations on the pathology of congenital idiopathic bladder neck obstructions (Marions' disease). *Br. J. Urol.* 29: 393.

Boggan, R.H. (1933) Polyorchidism. *Br. J. Surg.* 20: 630–639.

Boggs, L.K. and Kimmelsted, P. (1956) Benign multilocular cysts of the kidneys. *J. Pediatr. Surg.* 12: 749.

Boissonnat, P. (1961) Two cases of complete double functional urethra with a single bladder. *Br. J. Urol.* 33: 461.

Boissonnat, P. (1962) What to call hypoplastic kidney? *Arch. Dis. Childh.* 37: 142.

Boissonnat, P. and Duhamel, B. (1962) Congenital diverticula of the anterior urethra associated with aplasia of the abdominal wall in the male infant. *Br. J. Urol.* 34: 56.

Bors, E. and Comarr, A.E. (1954) Effect of pudendal nerve operations on the neurogenic bladder. *J. Urol.* **72**: 666.

Boulesteix, J. et al. (1971) Les ectopies rénales hautes chez l'enfant (á propos de deux observations). *Ann. Pediat. (Paris)* 18: 717.

Brent, L. and Stephens, F.D. (1976) Primary rectal ectasia: a quantitative study of smooth muscle cells in normal and hypertrophied human bowel. In *Progress in Paediatric Surgery*, P.P. Rickham, W.Ch. Hecker and J. Prevot (eds), pp. 9, 41. Munich: Urban and Schwarzenberg.

Bricker, E.M. (1950) Bladder substitution after pelvic evisceration. *Surg. Clin. N. Amer.* **30**: 1511.

Brockis, J.G. (1952) The development of the trigone of the bladder with a report of a case of ectopic ureter. *Br. J. Urol.* 24: 192.

Bronshtein, M., Yoffe, N., Brandes, J.M. and Blumenfeld, Z. (1990) First and early second-trimester diagnosis of fetal urinary tract anomalies using transvaginal sonography. *Perinatal Diagn.* 10: 653–666.

Brown, A.L. (1931) Analysis of the developing metanephros in mouse embryos with abnormal kidneys. *Am. J. Anat.* 47: 117.

Brown, M.D., Peterson, N.R. and Schultz, R.E. (1988) Ureteral duplication with lower pole ectopia to the epididymis. *J. Urol.* 140: 139–142.

Brown, T., Mandell, J. and Lebowitz, R.L. (1987) Neonatal hydronephrosis in the era of sonography. *Am. J. Roentgenol.* 148: 959–963.

Browne, D. (1936) An operation for hypospadias. *Lancet* 1: 141.

Browne, D. (1936) Congenital deformities of mechanical origin, *Proc. Roy. Soc. Med.* 29: 1409–1431.

Browne, D. (1949) Treatment of undescended testicle. *Proc. R. Soc. Med.* 42: 643.

Browne, D. (1950) *Hypospadias: Techniques in British Surgery*, p. 412. London and Philadelphia: W.B. Saunders.

Browne, D. (1951) Some congenital deformites of the rectum, anus, vagina and urethra. *Ann. R. Coll. Surg. (Engl.)* 8: 173.

Browne, D. (1955) Congenital deformities of the anus and rectum. *Arch. Dis. Childh.* 30: 37–42.

Browne, D. (1959) The pathology and classification of talipes. *Aust. N.Z. J. Surg.* 29: 85–91.

Browne, M.K. and Glashan, R.W. (1971) Multiple pathology in a unilateral supernumerary kidney. *Br. J. Surg.* 58: 73.

Bugden, W.F. (1950) Two cases of intra-thoracic kidney. *Dis. Chest* 17: 357.

Bulgrin, J.G. and Holmes, F.H. (1955) Eventration of the diaphragm with high renal ectopia: a case report. *Radiology* 64: 249.

Burger, R.H. (1972) A theory on the nature of transmission of congenital vesicoureteral reflux. *J. Urol.* 108: 249.

Burger, R.H. and Smith, C. (1971) Hereditary and familial vesicoureteral reflux. *J. Urol.* 106: 845.

Burke, E.C., Wenzl, J.E. and Utz, D.C. (1967) The intrathoracic kidney: report of a case. *Am. J. Dis. Childr.* 113: 487.

Burt, J.C., Lane, C.M. and Hamilton, J.L. (1970) An unusual anomaly of the upper urinary tract. *Br. J. Urol.* 42: 151.

Cain, M.P., Kramer, S.A., Tindall, D.J. and Husmann, D.A. (1994) Expression of androgen receptor protein within the lumbar spinal cord during ontologic development and following antiandrogen induced cryptorchidism. *J. Urol.* 152: 766–769.

Campbell, M.F. (1930) Renal ectopy. *J. Urol.* 24: 187.

Campbell, M.F. (1951) *Clinical Pediatric Urology*, eds. P.P. Kelalis, L.R. King and A.B. Belman (a) p. 295; (b) p. 277; (c) p. 219; (d) p. 218; (e) p. 227; (f) p. 187; (g) p. 29; p. 195. Philadelphia: W.B. Saunders.

Campbell, M.F. (1952) Primary megalo-ureter. *J. Urol.* 68: 584.

Campbell, M.F. (1970a) Anomalies of the ureter. In *Urology*, M.F. Campbell and J.H. Harrison (eds), 3rd edn., p. 248. Philadelphia: W.B. Saunders.

Campbell, M.F. (1970b) Anomalies of the kidney. In *Urology*, M.F. Campbell and J.H. Harrison (eds), 3rd edn., Vol. 2, Ch. 36, p. 1422. Philadelphia: W.B. Saunders.

Cantwell, F.V. (1895) Operative treatment of epispadias by transplantation of the urethra. *Ann. Surg.* 22: 689–694.

Carlson, H.E. (1950) Supernumerary kidney: a summary of fifty-one reported cases. *J. Urol.* 64: 224.

Cass, A.S. and Vitco, R.J. (1972) An unusual variety of crossed renal ectopy with only one ureter. *J. Urol.* 107: 1056.

Cass, A.S. and Stephens, F.D. (1975) Posterior urethral valves: diagnosis and management, *J. Urol.* 112: 519.

Casthely, S., Maheswarian. C. and Levy, J. (1974) Laparoscopy: an important tool in the diagnosis of Rokitansky-Kuster-Hauser syndrome. *Am. J. Obst. Gynec.* 119: 571.

Chantler, C. (1975) Syndromes with a renal component. In *Pediatric Nephrology*, M.I. Rubin and T.M. Barratt (eds), pp. 891–902. Baltimore: Williams and Wilkins.

Chantler, C. (1983) Syndromes with a renal component. In *Congenital Malformations of the Urinary Tract*, F.D. Stephens (ed.), Appendix 2, p. 538.

Chapple, C.C. and Davidson, D.T. (1941) A study of the relationship between fetal position and certain congenital deformities. *J. Ped.* 18: 483–493.

Chatten, J. and Bishop, H.C. (1977) Bilateral multilocular cysts of the kidneys. *J. Pediatr. Surg.* 12: 749.

Chatterjee, S.K. (1980) Double termination of the alimentary tract—a second look. *J. Pediatr. Surg.* 15: 623.

Chen, A., Francis, M., Ni, L., Cremers, C.W.R.J., Kimberling, W.J., Sato, Y., Phelps, P.D., Bellman, S.C., Wagner, M.J., Pembrey, M. and Smith R.J.H. (1995) Phenotypic manifestations of branchiootorenal syndrome. *Am. J. Med. Genet.* 58: 365–370.

Chisolm, T.C. (1979) Exstrophy of the urinary bladder. In *Conference Proceedings Children's Hospital Surgical Symposium. Long-Term Follow-up in Congenital Anomalies*, W.B. Kieswetter (ed.), pp. 32–41. Pittsburgh, PA.

Chwalle, R. (1927) The process of formation of cystic dilation of the vesical end of the ureter and of diverticula at the ureteral ostium. *Urol. Cutan. Rev.* 31: 499.

Chun, D. and Braga, C. (1965) Ectopic ureters with congenital absence of urethral sphincters. *Br. J. Urol.* 37: 320.

Clifford, A.B. (1908) Two cases of abnormal kidney. *U.S. Naval Med. Bull.* 2: 37. Cited by Geisinger (1937).

Cohen, M.M. Jr. (1981) Principles of syndromology. In *Associated Congenital Anomalies*, M. El Shafie and C.H. Klippel, Jr. (eds), p. 40. Baltimore: Williams and Wilkins.

Colosimo, C. (1938) Uretere doppio e uretere bifido (osservazioni su 50 casi). *Urologia* 5: 239.

Cook, W.A. and Stephens, F.D. (1977) Fused kidneys: morphologic study and theory of embryogenesis. In *Urinary System Malformations in Children*, D. Bergsma and J.W. Duckett (eds). New York: Alan R. Liss for the National Foundation, March of Dimes, BD: OAS XIII(5), 327.

Cook, W.A. and Stephens, F.D. (1988) Pathoembryology of the urinary tract. In *Urological Surgery in Neonates and Young Infants*, L.R. King (ed.), p. 1.23. Philadelphia: W.B. Saunders.

Coppoletta, J.M. and Wolbach, S.B. (1965) Body length and organ weights of infants and children. *Am. J. Pathol.* 9: 55, Table 1.

Coret, A., Morag, B., Katz, M., Lotan, D., Heyman, Z. and Hertz, M. (1994) The impact of fetal screening on indications for cystourethrography in infants. *Pediatr. Radiol.* 24: 516–518.

Cox, C.E., Lacy, S.S. and Hinman, F. Jr. (1968) The urethra and its relationship to urinary tract infection. The urethral flora of the female with recurrent urinary infection. *J. Urol.* 99: 622.

Creevy, C.D. (1970) The atonic distal ureteral segment (ureteral achalasia). *J. Urol.* 97: 457.

Cruickshank, G. (1952) Diaphragmatic herniation of the kidney. *Br. J. Tuberc.* 46: 223.

Culp, O.S. (1947) Ureteral diverticulum: classification of the literature and report of an authentic case. *J. Urol.* 58: 309.

Culp, D.A. (1964) The histology of the exstrophied bladder. *J. Urol.* 91: 538–548.

Cumes, D.M., Sanfelippo, C.J. and Stamey, T.A. (1981) Single ectopic ureter masquerading as ureterocele in incontinent male. *Urology* 17: 60–64.

Cunha, G.R., Alaird, E.T., Turner, T., Donjacour, A.A., Boutin, E.L. and Foster, B.A. (1992) Normal and abnormal development of the male urogenital tract: role of androgens, mesenchymal-epithelial interactions and growth factors. *J. Androl.* 13: 465–475.

Currarino, G. and Pinckney, L.E. (1981) Renal displacement caused by a supradiaphragmatic, paraspinal Ewing-like sarcoma and simulating an adrenal mass. *Radiology* 139: 603.

Currarino, G. and Stephens, F.D. (1981) An uncommon type of bulbar stricture, sometimes familial of unknown cause: congenital versus acquired. *J. Urol.* 126: 658.

Currarino, G., Votteler, T.P. and Kirks, D.R. (1978) Anal agenesis with rectobulbar fistula. *Radiology* 126: 457.

Cussen, L.J. (1967a) Dimensions of the normal ureter in infancy and childhood. *Invest. Urol.* 5: 164.

Cussen, L.J. (1967b) The structure of the normal ureter in infancy and childhood: a quantitative study of the muscular and elastic tissue. *Invest. Urol.* 5: 179.

Cussen, L.J. (1971a) The morphology of congenital dilatation of the ureter: intrinsic ureteral lesions. *Aust. N.Z. J. Surg.* 41: 185.

Cussen, L.J. (1971b) Cystic kidneys in children with congenital urethral obstruction. *J. Urol.* 106: 939.

Cussen, L.J. (1972) The effect of incomplete chronic obstruction on the ureteric muscle of the dog. *Invest. Urol.* 10: 208.

Cussen, L.J. (1974) Quoted by F.D. Stephens (1974). Idiopathic dilatations of the urinary tract. *J. Urol.* 112: 819.

Cussen, L.J. (1979) Normal position of the ureteral orifice in infancy and childhood: A quantitative study. *J. Urol.* 121: 646.

Da Carpi, J.B. (1522) Isogogae breves, Bologna. In *A Short Introduction to Anatomy*. L.R. Lind (transl.), 1959, Chicago: University of Chicago Press.

Darcoczi, J. (1956) Nierendystrophie in die Brusthöhle. *Z. Urol.* 49: 664.

Darmody, E.M., Offer, J. and Woodhouse, M.S. (1970) Toxic metabolic defect in polycystic disease of kidney, *Lancet* 1: 547.

Das, S. and Brosman, S.A. (1977) Duplication of the male urethra. *J. Urol.* 117: 452.

Datnow, B. and Daniel, W.W. Jr. (1976) Polycystic nephroblastoma. *J. Am. Med. Ass.* 236: 2528.

Daut, R.V., Emmett, J.L. and Kennedy, R.L.J. (1947) Congenital absence of abdominal muscles with urologic complications: report on patients successfully treated. *Proceedings of the Staff Meetings of the Mayo Clinic 22* (8 January), p. 8.

Debierre, Cited by Cobb, F. and Giddings, H.G. (1911) Supernumerary kidney, subject of cystadenoma. *Ann. Surg.* 53: 367.

DeCastro, F.J. and Schumacher, H. (1969) Asymptomatic thoracic kidney. *Clin. Pediat.* 8: 279.

Dees, J. (1941) Clinical importance of congenital anomalies of the upper urinary tract. *J. Urol.* 46: 659.

Dees, J.E. (1942) Epispadias with incontinence in the male. *Surgery* **12**: 621–630.

Dehner, L.P. (1973) Intrarenal teratoma occurring in infancy: report of a case with discussions of extragonadal germ cell tumors in infancy. *J. Pediatr. Surg.* 8: 369.

DeKlerk, D.P. and Scott, W.W. (1978) Prostatic maldevelopment in the prune belly syndrome: a defect in prostatic stroma-epithelial interaction. *J. Urol.* 120: 341.

DeKlerk, D.P., Marshall, F.F. and Jeggs, R.D. (1977) Multicystic dysplastic kidney. *J. Urol.* 118: 306.

Denny-Brown, D. and Robertson, E.G. (1933) on physiology of micturition. *Brain* 56: 149.

Devereux, M.H. and Williams, D.I. (1972) The treatment of urethral stricture in boys. *J. Urol.* 108: 489.

Devine, C.J. Jr. and Horton, C.E. (1973) Chordee without hypospadias. *J. Urol.* 110: 264–271.

De Vries, P.A. and Friedland, G.W. (1974) Congenital 'H-type' ano-urethral fistula. *Radiology* 113: 397–407.

Dewhurst, C.J. (1963) *Gynaecological Disorders of Infants and Children.* p. 25. London: Cassell.

Dickens, D.R.V. (1991) Orthopaedic abnormalities. In *Oesophageal Atresia,* S.W. Beasley, N.A. Myers and A.W. Auldist (eds), pp. 249–262. London: Chapman and Hall.

Dixon, A.F. (1910) Supernumerary kidney: the occurrence of three kidneys in an adult male subject. *J. Anat. Phys.* 45: 117. Cited by Geisinger (1937).

Donahoe, P.K., Ito, Y., Morikawa, Y. and Hendren W.H. III. (1977) Müllerian inhibiting substance in human testes after birth. *J. Pediatr. Surg.* 12: 323–330.

Dorairajan, T. (1963) Defects of spongy tissues and congenital diverticula of the penile urethra. *Aust. N.Z. J. Surg.* 32: 209.

Dougherty, J. (1954) Duplication of upper part of urinary tract. *J. Int. Coll. Surg.* 21: 160.

Downs, R.A. (1970) Congenital polyps of the posterior urethra: a review of the literature and report of two cases. *Br. J. Urol.* 42: 76.

Duckett, J.W. (1978) Epispadias. *Urol. Clin. N. Amer.* **5**: 107–126.

Duckett, J.W. Jr. (1976) The prune belly syndrome. In *Clinical Pediatric Urology,* Vol. 2, P.P. Kelalis, L.R. King and A.B. Belman (eds), p. 615. Philadelphia: W.B. Saunders.

Duckett, J.W. Jr. and Keating, M.A. (1989) Technical challenge of the megameatus intact prepuce hypospadias variant: the pyramid procedure. *J. Urol.* 141: 407–409.

Duckett, J.W. and Lotfi, A.H. (1993) Appendicovesicostomy (and variations) in bladder reconstruction. *J. Urol.* **149**(3): 567–569.

Duhamel, B. (1961) From the mermaid to anal imperforation: the syndrome of caudal regression. *Arch. Dis. Childh.* 36: 152.

Duhamel, B., Haegel, P. and Pages, R. (1966) *Morphogenése Pathologique des Monstruosités aux Malformations,* p. 151. Paris: Masson et Cie.

Dunlop, E.M. (1961) Incidence of urethral stricture in the male after urethritis. *Br. J. Vener. Dis.* 37: 64.

Dunn, N.R., Winnier, G.E., Hargett, L.K., Schrick, J.J., Fogo, A. and Hogan B.M.L. (1997) Haploinsufficient phenotypes in Bmp4 heterozygous null mice and modification by mutations in Gli3 and Alx4. *Dev. Biol.* 188: 235–247.

Dunn, P.M. (1976) Congenital postural deformities. *Br. Med. Bull.* 32: 71–76.

Dwoskin, J. (1976) Sibling uropathology. *J. Urol.* 115: 726.

Dwoskin, J.Y. and Perlmutter, A.D. (1973) Vesicoureteral reflux in children: a computerized review. *J. Urol.* 109: 888.

Eagle, J.F. Jr. and Barrett, G.S. (1950) Congenital deficiency of abdominal musculature with associated genito-urinary abnormalities: syndrome, report of nine cases. *Pediatrics* 6: 721.

Edling, N.P.G. (1953) The radiologic appearance of diverticula of the male cavernous urethra. *Acta Radiol.* 40: 1.

Effman, E.L., Lebowitz, R.L. and Colodny, A.H. (1976) Duplication of the urethra. *Radiology* 119: 179–185.

Eisendrath, D.R. (1938) Ectopic ending of ureter. *Urol. Cutan. Rev.* 42: 404.

Eklof, O. and Ringertz, H. (1976) Kidney size in children: a method of assessment. *Acta Radiol. (Diagn.)* 17: 617, Fig. 3.

Elbadawi, A. (1972) Anatomy and function of the ureteral sheath. *J. Urol.* 107: 224.

Elbadawi, A., Amaku, E.D. and Frank, I.N. (1973) Trilaminar musculature of submucosal ureter. Anatomy and functional implications. *Urology* 2: 409.

Elder, J.S. (1989) Laparoscopy and Fowler-Stephens orchiopexy in the management of the impalpable testis *Urol. Clin. N. Am.* 16: 399–411.

Elias, S. and Simpson, J.L. (1992) Amniocentesis. In *Genetic Disorders and the Fetus,* 3rd edn., A. Milinsky (ed.), p. 33–57. Baltimore: Johns Hopkins University Press.

Elkin, M. (1980) *Radiology of the?????* Little, Brown.

Emmett, J.L. (1977) *Clinical Urography. An Atlas and Textbook of Roentgenologic Diagnosis,* Vol. 2, p. 596. Philadelphia: W.B. Saunders.

England, M.A. (1983) *A Colour Atlas of Life Before Birth. Normal Fetal Development.* London: Wolfe Medical.

Ericsson, N.O. (1954a) Ectopic ureterocele in infants and children: a clinical study. *Acta Chir. Scand. (Suppl.)* 197: 12.

Ericsson, N.O. (1954b) Ectopic ureterocele in infants and children: a clinical study. *Acta Chir. Scand.* 197: 27.

Ericsson, N.O. and Ivemark, B.I. (1958a) Renal dysplasia and pyelonephritis in infants and children: I. *Arch. Pathol. Lab. Med.* 66: 255.

Ericsson, N.O. and Ivemark, B.I. (1958b) Renal dysplasia and pyelonephritis in infants and children: II. *Arch. Pathol. Lab. Med.* 66: 264.

Exley, M. and Hotchkiss, W.S. (1944) Supernumerary kidney with clear cell carcinoma. *J. Urol.* 51: 569.

Fallat, M.E., Hersh, J.H. and Hutson, J.M. (1992) Theories on the relationship between cryptorchidism and arthrogryposis. *Pediatr. Surg. Int.* 7: 271–273.

Feldman, K.W. and Smith, D.W. (1975) Fetal phallic growth and penile standards for newborn male infants. *J. Pediatr.* 86: 395.

Felix, W. (1912) Development of the urogenital organs. In *Manual of Human Embryology,* F. Kiebel and F.P. Hall (eds), Vol. 2, pp. 752–979. (a) p. 880; (b) p. 842; (c) p. 879; (d) p. 954; (e) p. 773. Philadelphia: Lippincott.

Fenger, C. (1894) Operation for the relief of valve formation and stricture of the ureter in hydro- or pyonephrosis. *J. Am. Med. Ass.* 22: 335.

Fentener van Vlissingen, J.M., van Zoelen, E.J.J., Ursem, P.J.F. and Wensing, C.J.G. (1988) *In vitro* model of the first phase of testicular descent: identification of a low-molecular weight factor from fetal testis involved in proliferation of gubernacular testis cells and distinct from specified polypeptide growth factors and fetal gonadal hormones. *Endocrinology* 123: 2868–2877.

Fetterman, G.H., Shuplock, N.A., Philipp, F.J. and Gregg, H.S. (1965) The growth and maturation of human glomeruli and proximal convolutions from term to adulthood; studies by microdissection. *Pediatrics* 35: 601.

Field, P.L. and Stephens, F.D. (1974) Congenital urethral membranes causing urethral obstruction. *J. Urol.* 111: 250.

Filmer, R.B. and Taxy, J.B. (1976a) Cysts of the kidney, renal dysplasia and renal hypoplasia. In *Clinical Pediatric Urology*, P.P. Kelalis, L.R. King and A.B. Belman (eds), Vol. 2, p. 713. Philadelphia: W.B. Saunders.

Filmer, R.B. and Taxy, J.B. (1976b) Glomerulocystic kidney: report of a case. *Arch. Pathol. Lab. Med.* 100: 186.

Filmer, R.B., Taxy, I.B. and King, L.R. (1974) Renal dysplasia: clinicopathological study. *Trans. Amer. Assoc. Genitourin.* 66: 18.

Fischer, K. and Rosenloecher, R. (1925) Ueber einem Fall von dritter Niere met selbstaendigen Harnleiter. *Z. Urol. Chir.* 17: 61. Cited by Geisinger (1973).

Flateau, E., Josefsberg, Z., Reisner, S.H., Bialik, O. and Zaron, Z. (1975) Penile size in the newborn infant. *J. Pediatr.* 87: 663.

Fleischner, F., Robins, S.A. and Abrams, M. (1950) High renal ectopia and congenital diaphragmatic hernia. *Radiology* 55: 24.

Fobi, M., Mahour, G.H. and Isaacs, H. Jr. (1979) Multilocular cyst of the kidney. *J. Pediatr. Surg.* 14: 282.

Fourie, T. (1981) A free supernumerary kidney. A case report. *S. Afr. Med. J.* 60: 251.

Fowler, R. and Stephens, F.D. (1959) The role of testicular vascular anatomy in the salvage of high undescended testes. *Aust. N.Z. J. Surg.* 29: 92–106.

Fowler, R. and Kesavan, P. (1977) Extravesical reconstruction for ureterovesical obstruction in childhood. *J. Urol.* 118: 1050.

Franciskovic, V. and Marincic, N. (1959) Intrathoracic kidney. *Br. J. Urol.* 31: 156.

Franco, B., Guioli, S., Pragliola, A., Incerti, B., Bardoni, B., Tonlorenzi, R., Carrozo, R., Maestrini, E., Pieretti, M., Tiallon-Miller, P., Brown, C.J., Willard, H.F., Lawrence, C., Persico, M.G., Camerino, G. and Ballabio, A. (1991) A gene deleted in Kallmann's syndrome shares homology with neural cell adhesion and axonal path-finding molecules. *Nature* 353: 529–536.

Frank, R.T. (1938) The formation of an artificial vagina without operation. *Am J. Obst. Gynec.* 35: 1053.

Frazer, J.E. (1931) *A Manual of Embryology* (a) p. 438; (b) p. 437; (c) p. 427; (d) p. 431. London: Bailliére, Tindall and Cox.

Frazer, J.E. (1953) *A Manual of Embryology*, 3rd edn., p. 432. London: J.S. Baxter, Bailliére, Tindall and Cox.

Fried, A.M., Oliff, M., Wilson, E.A. and Whisnant, J. (1978) Uterine anomalies associated with renal agenesis: role of Gray scale ultrasonography. *Am J. Roentgen.* 131: 973.

Friedland, G.W. and Cunningham, J. (1972) The elusive ectopic ureteroceles. *Am. J. Roentgenol. Radium Ther. Nucl. Med.* 116: 792.

Friedland, G.W. and De Vries, P. (1975) Renal ectopia and fusion. *Urology* 5: 698.

Fujita, J. (1980) Transverse testicular ectopia. *Urology* 16: 400–401.

Fuzione, D. and Molnar, W. (1966) Anomalous pulmonary venous return, pulmonary sequestration bronchial atresia, aplastic right upper lobe, pericardial defect and intrathoracic kidney. *Am. J. Radiol.* 97: 350.

Gasc, J.M., Shanmugam, S., Sibony, M. and Corvol, P. (1994) Tissue-specific expression of type 1 angiotensin II receptor subtypes. An in situ hybridization study. *Hypertension* 24: 531–537.

Gauderer, M.W.L., Erisoni, E.R., Stellato, T.A., Ponsky, J. and Izant R.J. Jr. (1982) Transverse testicular ectopia. *J. Pediatr. Surg.* 17: 43–47.

Gearhart, J.P. and Jeffs, R.D. (1988) Augmentation cystoplasty in the failed exstrophy reconstruction. *J. Urol.* 139: 790–793.

Gearhart, J.P., Forschner, D.C., Jeffs, R.D., Ben-Chiam, J. and Sponseller, P.D. (1996) A combined vertical and horizontal pelvic osteotomy approach for primary and secondary repair of bladder exstrophy. *J. Urol.* 155: 689–693.

Gehring, G.G., Vietenson, J.H. and Woodhead, D.M. (1973) Congenital urethral perineal fistulas. *J. Urol.* 109: 419.

Geisinger, J.G. (1937) Supernumerary kidney. *J. Urol.* 38: 331.

Gibbons, M.D., Cromie, W.J. and Duckett, J.W. Jr. (1978) Ectopic vas deferens. *J. Urol.* 120: 597.

Gibbons, M.D., Cromie, W.J. and Duckett, J.W. Jr. (1979) Management of the abdominal undescended testicle. *J. Urol.* 122: 76–79.

Gibson, T.E. (1957) A new operation for ureteral ectopia. Case report. *J. Urol.* 77: 414.

Gill, B., Kogan, S., Starr, S., Reda, E. and Levitt, S. (1989) Significance of epididymal and ductal anomalies associated with testicular maldescent. *J. Urol.* 142: 556–558.

Gill, R. (1952) Triplication of the ureter and renal pelvis. *J. Urol.* 68: 140.

Gil-Vernet, S. (1948) *Diverticulos Vesicales*. Barcelona: Editorial Modesto Uson.

Girotti, M. and hauser, G.A. (1969) Sindrome di Mayer-Rokitansky-Kuester. Nuovi aspetti del quadro simtomatologico. *Riv. Ital. Ginec.* 53: 124.

Glassberg, K.I., Stephens, F.D., Lebowitz, R.L., Braren, V., Duckett, J.W., Jacobs, E.C., King, L.R. and Perlmutter, A.D. (1987) Renal dysgenesis and cystic disease of the kidney: a report of the Committee on Nomenclature and Classification, Section on Urology, American Academy of Pediatrics. *J. Urol.* 138: 1085–1092.

Glenister, T.W. (1954) The origin and fate of the urethral plate in man. *J. Anat.* 88: 413–425.

Glenister, T.W. (1956) A consideration of the processes involved in the development of the prepuce in man. *Br. J. Urol.* 28: 243–249.

Glenister, T.W. (1958) A correlation of the normal and abnormal development of the penile urethra and of the infra-umbilical abdominal wall. *Br. J. Urol.* 30: 117–126.

Glenn, J.F. (1959) Analysis of 51 patients with horseshoe kidney. *N. Engl. J. Med.* 261: 684.

Gockels, C. L. (1686) De vesica spongiosa extra abdomen posita cum defectu penis. Misc. Acad. Nat. Curiosa. Nurnberg Decad. ii, anno V, 1686. Abstr. Abhaandl. Rom-Kais. Akad. Naturf. Nurnberg, XV:83, 1766. Quoted in The History of Urology, (1972), Murphy, L. J. T. (ed.), Springfield Ill: Charles C. Thomas.

Goh, D.W., Momose, Y., Middlesworth, W. and Hutson, J.M. (1993) The relationship between CGRP, androgen and gubernacular development in three animal models of cryptorchidism. *J. Urol.* 150: 571–573.

Goh, D.W., Farmer, P.J. and Hutson, J.M. (1994a) Absence of normal sexual dimorphism of the genitofemoral nerve spinal nucleus in the mutant cryptorchid (TS) rat. *J. Reprod. Fertil.* 102: 195–199.

Goh, D.W., Middlesworth, W., Framer, P.J. and Hutson, J.M. (1994b) Prenatal androgen blockade with flutamide inhibits masculinization of the genitofemoral nerve and testicular descent. *J. Pediatr. Surg.* 29: 836–838.

Golomb, J. and Ehrlich, R.M. (1989) Bilateral ureteral triplication with crossed ectopic fused kidneys associated with the VACTERL syndrome. *J. Urol.* 141: 1398.

Gomez, F. and Stephens, F.D. (1983) Cecoureterocele: morphology and clinical correlations. *J. Urol.* 129: 1017.

Gosalbez, R.J., Gosalbez, R., Pero, C., martin, J.A. and Jimeniz, A. (1991) Ureteral triplication and ureterocele: report of 3 cases and review of the literature. *J. Urol.* 145: 105–108.

Graves, F.T. (1954) The anatomy of the intrarenal arteries and its application to segmental resection of the kidney. *Br. J. Surg.* 42: 132.

Graves, F.T. (1956) The aberrant renal artery. *J. Anat.* 90: 553.

Graves, F.T. (1971) *The Arterial Anatomy of the Kidney.* (a) p. 28; (b) p. 29; (c) p. 7. Baltimore: Williams and Wilkins.

Gray's Anatomy (1980) P.L. Williams and R. Warwick (eds), 36th edn., p. 1408. Philadelphia: W.B. Saunders.

Greef, E. (1982) Uber Drei Fälle von Missbildung Durch ambiotische stränge [Thesis], p. 21. Kiel K. Biernatscki. (Quoted by Torpin, 1968).

Griffin, J.E. (1992) Androgen resistance: the clinical and molecular spectrum. *N. Engl. J. Med.* 326: 611–618.

Griffin, J.E., Edwards, C., Madden, J.D., Harrod, M.J. and Wilson, J.D. (1976) Congenital absence of the vagina. The Mayer-Rokitansky-Kuster-Hauser syndrome. *Ann. Intern. Med.* 85: 224.

Griffiths, A.L., Middlesworth, W. and Hutson J.M. (1993) Exogenous calcitonin gene-related peptide (CGRP) causes gubernacular development in neonatal mice with complete androgen resistance (TFM). *J. Pediatr. Surg.* 28: 1028–1030.

Grocock, C.A., Charlton, H.M. and Pike, M.C. (1988) Role of the fetal pituitary in cryptorchidism induced by exogenous maternal oestrogen during pregnancy in mice. *J. Reprod. Fertil.* 83: 295–300.

Gross, R.D. (1953) *The Surgery of Infancy and Childhood*, p. 660. Philadelphia and London: W.B. Saunders.

Gross, R.D. and Clatworthy, W.H. (1950) Ureterocele in infancy and childhood. *Pediatrics* 5: 58.

Gruber, C.C.M. (1929) A comparative study of the intravesical ureters (uretero-vesical valves) in man and in experimental animals. *J. Urol.* 21: 567.

Gruenwald, P. (1941) The relation of the growing müllerian duct to the wolffian duct and its importance for the genesis of malformations. *Anat. Rec.* 81: 1.

Gruenwald, P. (1943) The normal changes in the position of the embryonic kidney. *Anat. Rec.* 85: 163.

Guérin, A. (1864) *Elements de Chirurgie Opératoire, 3rd edn.*, p. 587. Paris: F. Chamerot.

Gutierrez, R. (1931) The clinical management of horseshoe kidney. *Am. J. Surg.* 14: 657.

Gutierrez, R. (1944) Double kidney as a source of impaired dynamism: its surgical treatment by heminephrectomy. *Am. J. Surg.* 65: 256.

Gwinn, J.L. and Fletcher, H.D. (1968) Radiological case of the month, denoucment and discussion: superior renal ectopia (thoracic kidney). *Am. J. Dis. Childr.* 116: 301.

Habib, R. (1979) Pathology of renal segmental corticopapillary scarring in children with hypertension: The concept of segmental hypoplasia. In *Reflux Nephropathy*, J. Hodson and P. Kincaid-Smith (eds), p. 220. New York: Masson.

Hadziselimovic, F., Duckett, J.W., Snyder, H.M., Schnaufer, L. and Huff, D. (1987) Omphalocele, cryptorchidism and brain malformations. *J. Pediatr. Surg.* 22: 854–856.

Hahn (1938) quoted by Torpin (1968; no reference given in Torpin's book).

Hamilton, W.J., Boyd, J.D. and Mossman, H.W. (1978) *Human Embryology*, 4th edn. (a) p. 354; (b) p. 396; (c) p. 397; (d) p. 433. London: Macmillan.

Hanley, H.G. (1942) Horseshoe and supernumerary kidney; triple kidney with horseshoe component. *Br. J. Surg.* 30: 165.

Hanley, H.G. (1945) Blind-ending duplication of the ureter. *Br. J. Urol.* 17: 50.

Hanna, M.K. and Wyatt, J.K. (1975) Primary obstructive megaureter in adults. *J. Urol.* 113: 328.

Hanna, M.K., Jeffs, R.D., Sturgess, J.M. and Barkin, M. (1976) Ureteral structure and ultrastructure. II. The congenital uretero-pelvic junction obstruction and primary obstructive megaureter. *J. Urol.* 116: 725.

Hannan, Q.H.A. and Stephens, F.D. (1973) The influence of trigonectomy on vesicoureteral reflux in dogs. *Invest. Urol.* 10: 469.

Harley, L.M., Chen, Y. and Rattner, W.H. (1972) Prune belly syndrome. *J. Urol.* 108: 174.

Harris, A. (1937) Ureteral anomalies with special reference to partial duplication with one branch ending blindly. A report of two cases with renal obstruction cured by surgical resection. *J. Urol.* 38: 442.

Harrow, B.R. (1966) Peri-anal micturition due to congenital posterior urethral fistula. *J. Urol.* 96: 328.

Hartman, G.W. and Hodson, C.J. (1969) The duplex kidney and related abnormalities. *Clin. Radiol.* 20: 387.

Hatch, D.A., Maizels, M., Zaontz, M.R. and Firlit, C.F. (1989) Hypospadias hidden by a complete prepuce. *Surg. Gynec. Obstet.* 169: 232–234.

Hauser, G.A. and Schreiner, W.E. (1961) Mayer-Rokitansky-Kuester syndrome. Rudimentary solid bipartite uterus with solid vagina. *Schweiz. Med. Wsch.* 91: 381.

Hawthorne, A.B. (1936) The embryologic and clinical aspect of double ureter. *J. Am. Med. Ass.* 106: 189.

Heale, W.F. (1979) Personal communication.

Heale, W.F., Shannon, F.T., Utley, W.L.F. and Rolleston, G.L. (1979) Familial and hereditary reflux nephropathy. In *Reflux Nephropathy*, J. Hodson and P. Kincaid-Smith (eds), p. 49. New York: Masson.

Heikel, P.E. and Parkkulainen, K.V. (1966) Vesicoureteral reflux in children. A classification and results of conservative treatment. *Ann. Radiol.* 9: 37.

Hein, L., Barsh, G.S., Pratt R.E., Dzau, V.J. and Kobilka, B.K. (1995) Behavioural and cardiovascular effects of disrupting the angiotesin II type-2 receptor gene in mice. *Nature* 377: 744–747.

Hendren, W.H., Donahoe, P.K. and Phister, R.C. (1976) Crossed renal ectopia in children. *J. Urol.* 7: 135.

Henley, W.L. and Hyman, A. (1953) Absent abdominal musculature, genitourinary anomalies and deficiency in pelvic autonomic nervous system. *Am J. Dis. Childr.* 86: 795.

Henneberry, M.O. and Stephens, F.D. (1980) Renal hypoplasia and dysplasia in infants with posterior urethral valves. *J. Urol.* 123: 912.

Hertz, A. and Schahn, N. (1969) Ectopic thoracic kidney. *Israel J. Med.* 5: 98.

Heyns, C.F. (1987) The gubernaculum during testicular descent in the human fetus. *J. Anat.* 153: 93–112.

Heyns, C.F. (1990) Exstrophy of the testis. *J. Urol.* 144: 724–725.

Heyns, C.F. and Hutson, J.M. (1995) The history of theories on testicular descent. *J. Urol.* 153: 754–767.

Hicks, C.C., Boehm, G.A.W., Sybers, R.G., Stone, H.H. and O'Brien, D.P. (1976) Traumatic rupture of horseshoe kidney with partial ureteral duplication associated with supernumerary kidney. *Urology* 8: 149.

Higginbottom, M.C., Jones, K.L., Hall, B.D. and Smith, D.W. (1979) The amniotic band disruption complex: timing of amnion rupture and variable spectra of consequent defects. *J. Pediatr.* 95: 544–549.

Higgins, T.T., Williams, D.I. and Nash, D.F. (1951) *The Urology of Childhood*, p. 8. London: Butterworth.

Hill, J.E. and Bunts, R.C. (1960) Thoracic kidney: case reports. *J. Urol.* 84: 460.

Hodson, C.J. (1979) Reflux nephropathy: scoring and damage. In *Reflux Nephropathy*, J. Hodson and P. Kincaid-Smith (eds), p. 29. New York: Masson.

Hodson, C.J., Drewe, J.A., Karn, M.N. and King, A. (1962) Renal size in normal children: a radiographic study during life. *Arch. Dis. Childh.* 27: 616.

Hogan, B.L.M. (1996) Bone morphogenetic proteins: multifunctional regulators of vertebrate development. *Genes Dev.* 10: 1580–1594.

Hohenfellner, K., Hunley, T.E., Schloemer, C., Brenner, W., Yerkes, E., Zepp, F., Brock, III J.W. and Kon, V. (1999) Angiotensin type 2 receptor is important in the normal development of the ureter. *Pediatr. Nephrol.* 13: 187–191.

Howard, E. (1981) Personal communication.

Hutch, J.A. (1958) *The Ureterovesical Junction*, p. 68. Berkeley and Los Angeles: University of California Press.

Hutch, J.A. (1961a) Saccule formation at the uretero-vesical junction in smooth walled bladders. *J. Urol.* 86: 390.

Hutch, J.A. (1961b) Theory of maturation of the intravesical ureter. *J. Urol.* 86: 534.

Hutch, J.A. (1972) *Anatomy and Physiology of the Bladder, Trigone and Urethra*, p. 81. (a) p. 24; (b) p. 130. New York: Meredith, Appleton-Century-Crofts.

Hutch, J.A. and Amar, A.D. (1972) *Vesicoureteral Reflux and Pyelonephritis*. New York: Education Division, Meredith, Appleton-Century-Crofts.

Hutson, J.M. (1985) A biphasic model for the hormonal control of testicular descent. *Lancet* 2: 419–421.

Hutson, J.M. (1986) Testicular feminization. A model for testicular descent in mice and men. *J. Pediatr. Surg.* 21: 195–198.

Hutson, J.M. and Beasley, S.W. (1987) The aetiology of prune belly syndrome. *Aust. Paediatr. J.* 23: 309.

Hutson, J.M. and Beasley, S.W. (1989) Why testicular descent may be impaired in cloacal exstrophy. *Pediatr. Surg. Int.* 4: 122–123.

Hutson, J.M. and Beasley, S.W. (1992) *Descent of the Testis*. London: Edward Arnold.

Hutson, J.M. and Donahoe, P.K. (1986) The hormonal control of testicular descent. *Endocr. Rev.* 7: 270–283.

Hutson, J.M., Chow, C.W. and Ng, W.D. (1987) Persistent müllerian duct syndrome with transverse testicular ectopia. *Pediatr. Surg. Int.* 2: 191–194.

Hutson, J.M., Beasley, S.W. and Bryan, A.D. (1988) Cryptorchidism in spina bifida and spinal cord transection: a clue to the mechanism of transinguinal descent of the testis. *J. Pediatr. Surg.* 23: 275–277.

Hutson, J.M., Watts, L.M., Montalto, J. and Greco, J. (1990) Gonadotropin fails to reverse estrogen-induced cryptorchidism in fetal mice: evidence for non-androgenic control of testicular descent in the fetus. *Pediatr. Surg. Int.* 5: 13–18.

Hutson, J.M., Baker, M.L., Griffiths, A.L., Momose, Y., Goh, D.W., Middlesworth, W., Zhou, B. and Cartwright, E. (1992) Endocrine and morphological perspectives in testicular descent. *Reprod. Med. Rev.* 1: 165–177.

Hutson, J.M., Davidson, P.M., Reece, L.A., Baker, M.L. and Zhou, B. (1994) Failure of gubernacular development in the persistent müllerian duct syndrome allows herniation of the testes. *Pediatr. Surg. Int.* 9: 544–546.

Hutson, J.M., Terada, M., Zhou, B. and Williams, M.P.L. (1995) Normal testicular descent and the aetiology of cryptorchidism. *Adv. Anat. Embryol. Cell Biol.* (in press).

Ichiki, T., Labosky, P.A., Shiota, C., Okuyama, S., Imagawa, Y., Ichikawa, I., Hogan, B.L.M. and Inagami, T. (1995) Hypertension and reduced exploratory behavior in mice lacking angiotensin II type 2 receptor. *Nature* 377: 748–750.

Immergut, M.A. and Wahman, G.E. (1968) The urethral caliber of female children with recurrent urinary tract infection. *J. Urol.* 99: 189.

Immergut, M., Culp, D. and Flocks, R.H. (1967) The urethral caliber in normal female children. *J. Urol.* 97: 693.

Ireland, E.F.J. and Chute, R. (1955) A case of triplicate-duplicate ureters. *J. Urol.* 74: 342.

Isaja, A. (1921) Rene sopranumerario constato duranti la vita. *Ann. del. r. 1st. di. chil. Chir. di. Roma.* 4: 369. Cited by Geisinger (1937).

Israel, I. (1918) Diagnose und Operation einer ueberzaehligen Niere. *Berl. Klin. Wschr.* 55: 1081. Cited by Geisinger (1937).

Ives, E.J. (1974) The abdominal muscle deficiency triad syndrome–experience with 10 cases. In *Birth Defects*, D. Bergsma (ed.) Baltimore: Williams and Wilkins for the National Foundation, March of Dimes BD: OAS X(4): 127.

Jeffs, R.D. (1983) Complications of exstrophy surgery. *Urol. Clin. N. Amer.* **10**(3): 509–518.

Jeffs, R.D. (1986) Exstrophy of the urinary bladder. In Pediatric Surgery, K.J. Welch, J.G. Randolph, M.M. Ravich, J.A. O'Neill and M.I. Rowe (eds), p. 1216. Chicago: Yearbook Medical.

Johnston, J.H. (1960) Vesical diverticula without urinary obstruction in children. *J. Urol.* 84: 535.

Johnston, J.H. (1972) Problems in pediatric urology. *Excerpta Medica.* Amsterdam: Excerpta Medica.

Johnston, J.H. and Davenport, T.J. (1969) The single ectopic ureter. *Br. J. Urol.* 41: 428–433.

Johnston, J.H. and Coimbra, J.A.M. (1970) Megalourethra. *J. Pediatr. Surg.* 5: 304.

Johnston, J.H. and Kogan. S.J. (1974) The exstrophic anomalies and their surgical reconstruction. *Current Problems in Surgery Year Book.* Chicago: Medical Publishers

Johnston, J.H., Evans, J.P., Glassberg, K.I. and Shapiro, S.R. (1977) Pelvic hydronephrosis in children: a review of 219 personal cases. *J. Urol.* 117: 97–101.

Johnston, T.B. and Whillis, J. (eds) (1954) *Gray's anatomy*, 31st edn., pp. 597, 598. London: Longmans, Green.

Jones, F. (1902) Section of an early human embryo. *J. Anat.* 36: 5.

Jones, F.W. (1904) The nature of malformations of the rectum and the urogenital passages. *Br. Med. J.* 2: 1630.

Jones, K.L. (1988) Early amnion rupture sequence. In *Smith's Recognizable Patterns of Human Malformation*, 4th edn., pp. 576–577. Philadelphia: W.B. Saunders.

Jorulf, H., Nordmark, J. and Jonsson, A. (1978) Kidney size in infants and children assessed by area measurement. *Acta Radiol. (Diagn.)* 19: 154, Fig. 3.

Jorup, S. and Kjellberg, S.R. (1948) Congenital valvular formations in the urethra. *Acta Radiol. (Stockh.)* 30: 197.

Josso, N., Lamarre, I., Picard, J-Y, Berta, P., Davies, N., Morichon, N., Peschanski, M. and Jeny, R. (1993a) Anti-müllerian hormone in early human development. *Early Human Devel.* 33: 91–99.

Josso, N., Cate, R.L., Picard, J-Y; Vigier, B., Di Clemente, N., Wilson, C., Imbreaud, S., Pepinsky, R.B., Guerrier, D., Boussin, L., Legeai, L. and Carre-Eusebe, D. (1993b) Anti-müllerian hormone: the Jost factor. *Rec. Progr. Hormone Res.* 49: 1–59.

Kadowaki, K., Koshiba, K., Ao, T. and Kanzaki, M. (1983) Right intrathoracic kidney. *Urology* 21: 79.

Kakuchi, J., Ichiki, T., Kiyama, S., Hogan, B.L.M., Fogo, A., Inagami, T. and Ichikawa, I. (1995) Developmental expression of renal angiotensin II receptor genes in the mouse. *Kidney Int.* 47: 140–147.

Kalousek, D.K., Fitch, N. and Paradice, B.A. (1990) Amnion rupture sequence and limb body wall complex. In *Pathology of the Human Embryo and Pre Viable Fetus—An Atlas*, pp. 142–147. New York: Springer Verlag.

Kambayashi, Y., Bardhan, S., Takahashi, K., Tsuzuki, S., Inui, H., Hamakubo, T. and Inagami, T. (1993) Molecular cloning of a novel angiotensin II receptor isoform involved in phosphotyrosine phosphatase inhibition. *J. Biol. Chem.* 268: 24543–24546.

Kandzari, S.J., Cha, E.M. and Milam, D.F. (1972) Solitary fused kidney with a single Y-shaped ureter. *West Virginia. Med. J.* 68: 181–183.

Kangarloo, H. et al. (1977) Ultrasonographic evaluation of juxta-diaphragmatic masses in children. *Radiology* 125: 785.

Kaplan, G.W. (1979) Myelomeningocele. In *Campbell's Urology*, J.H. Harrison, R.F. Gittes, A.D. Perlmutter, T.A. Stamey and P.C. Walsh (eds), 4th edn., Vol. 2, p. 1787. Chicago: Year Book.

Kaplan, G.W. and Lamm, D.L. (1975) Embryogenesis of chordee. *J. Urol.* 114: 769–772.

Kaplan, L.M., Koyle, M.A., Kaplan, G.W., Farrer, J.H. and Rajfer, J. (1986) Association between abdominal wall defects and cryptorchidism. *J. Urol.* 136: 645.

Katz, A., Sombolos, K. and Oreopoulos, D.G. (1987) Acquired cystic disease of the kidney in association with chronic ambulatory peritoneal dialysis. *Am. J. Kidney Dis.* 9: 166–171.

Katzan, P. and Trachtman, B. (1954) Diagram of vaginal ectopic ureter by vaginogram. *J. Urol.* 72: 808.

Kaufmann, E. and Knochel, W. (1996) Five years on the wings of fork head. *Mech. Dev.* 57: 3–20.

Keibel, F. and Mall, F.P. (1912) *Manual of Human Embryology*, Vol. 2. (a) p. 322; (b) p. 773. Philadelphia: Lippincott.

Kelalis, P.P., Malet, R.S. and Segura, J.W. (1973) Observations on renal ectopia and fusion in children. *J. Urol.* 110: 588.

Keller, H., Neuhauser, G., Durkin-Stamm, M.V., Kaveggia, E.G., Schaaff, A. and Sitzmann, F. (1978) 'ADAM Complex' (amniotic deformity, adhesions, mutilations)—a pattern of craniofacial and limb defects. *Am. J. Med. Genet.* 2: 81–98.

Kelly, H.A. and Burnam, C.F. (1914) *Diseases of the Kidneys, Ureters and Bladder*, Vol. 1, p. 582. New York: Appleton.

Kelly, H.A. and Dumm, W.M. (1914) Urinary incontinence in women without manifest injury to the bladder. *Surg. Gynecol. Obstet.* 18: 444.

Kelly, J.H. (1995) Vesical exstrophy: repair using radical mobilization of soft tissues. *Pediatr. Surg. Int.* 10: 298–304.

Kelly, J.H. and Eraklis, A.J. (1971) A procedure for lengthening the penis in boys with exstrophy of the bladder. *J. Ped. Surg.* 6: 645.

Kennedy, L.A. and Persaud, T.V. (1977) Pathogenesis of developmental defects induced in the rat by amniotic sac puncture. *Acta Anat.* 97: 23–35.

Kenney, P.J., Spirt, B.A. and Leeson, M.D. (1984) Genitourinary anomalies: radiologic-anatomic correlations. *Radiographics* 4: 233.

Kerr, A.T. (1911) Complete double ureter in man. *Anat. Rec.* 5: 55.

Kesavan, P., Ramakrishnan, M.S. and Fowler, R. (1977) Ectopia in unduplicated ureters in children. *Br. J. Urol.* 49: 481.

King, P.A. and Stephens, F.D. (1977) Ureteral muscle tone in prevention of vesicoureteral reflux. *Invest. Urol.* 14: 488.

Kirschenbaum, A.S., Puri, H.C. and Rao, B.R. (1981) Congenital intrathoracic kidney. *J. Urol.* 125: 412.

Kitchen, P.R.B. and Stephens, F.D. (1971) A study of the surgical anatomy of congenital recto-bulbar fistula. *Aust. N.Z. J. Surg.* 40: 248.

Kjeilberg, S.R., Ericsson, N.O. and Rudhe, U. (1957) *The Lower Urinary Tract in Childhood*, p. 188. Chicago: Year Book.

Klauber, G.T. and Reid, E.C. (1972) Inverted Y reduplication of the ureter. *J. Urol.* 107: 362.

Klauber, G.T. and Crawford, B.D. (1980) Prolapse of ectopic ureterocele and bladder trigone. *Urology* 15: 164.

Knutrud, O. (1983) Personal communication.

Koff, A.K. (1933) Development of the vagina in the human fetus. *Carnegie Contributions to Embryology*, Vol. 24, pp. 61–69. Carnegie Institution of Washington Publications.

Koff, S.A., Thrall, H.H. and Keyes, J.W., Jr. (1979) Diuretic radionuclide urography: a non-invasive method for evaluating nephroureteral dilatation. *J. Urol.* 122: 451.

Koff, S.A., Thrall, H.H. and Keyes, J.W., Jr. (1980) Assessment of hydroureteronephrosis in children using diuretic radionuclide urography. *J. Urol.* 123: 531.

Kohri, K., Nagai, N., Kaneko, S., Igushi, M., Kadowaki, T., Akiyama, T., Yachiku, S. and Kurita, T. (1978) Bilateral trifid ureters associated with fused kidney, ureterovesical stenosis, left cryptorchidism and angioma of the bladder. *J. Urol.* 120: 249–250.

Kolln, C.P., Boatman, P.L., Schmidt, J.D. and Flocks, R.H. (1972) Horseshoe kidney: review of 105 patients. *J. Urol.* 107: 203.

Koyanagi, T., Hisajima, S., Goto, T., Tokunaka, S. and Tsuji, I. (1980) Everting ureteroceles: radiographic and endoscopic observation, and surgical management. *J. Urol.* 123: 538.

Kretschmer, H.L. (1929) Supernumerary kidney, report of a case with review of the literature. *Surg. Gynec. Obstet.* 49: 818.

Kretschmer, H.L. (1933) Duplication of ureters at their distal ends, one pair ending blindly; so-called diverticula of the ureters. *J. Urol.* 30: 61.

Kreuger, R.P., Hardy, B.E. and Churchill, B.M. (1980) Cryptorchidism in boys with posterior urethral valves. *J. Urol.* 124: 101–102.

Kumar, De. S., Chandra, Roy, S., Mohon Das. M. and Chatterjee, B.P. (1968) Thoracic kidney. *J. Indian Med. Assoc.* 50: 316.

Kume, T., Deng, K. and Hogan, B.L.M. (2000) Murine forkhead/winged helix genes *Foxc1* (*Mf1*) and *Foxc2* (*Mfh1*) are required for the early organogenesis of the kidney and urinary tract. *Development* 127; 1387–1395.

Kume, T., Deng, K.Y., Winfrey, V., Gould, D.B., Walter, M.A. and Hogan, B.L.M. (1998) The forkhead/winged helix gene *Mf1* is disrupted in the pleiotropic mouse mutation congenital hydrocephalus. *Cell* 93: 985–996.

Kuster, H. (1910) Uterus bipartitus solidus rudimentarius cum vagina solida. *Z. Geb. Gyn.* 67: 692.

Larkins, S.L., Williams, M.P.L. and Hutson, J.M. (1991) Localization of calcitonin gene-related peptide within the spinal nucleus of the genitofemoral nerve. *Pediatr. Surg. Int.* 6: 176–179.

Latarjet, M., Galy, P., Brune, J. and Cuche, P. (1970) Un cas de rein gauche intra-thoracique. *Lyon chirurgical* 66: 144.

Lattimer, J.K. (1958) Congenital deficiency in the abdominal musculature and associated genitourinary anomalies: a report of twenty-two cases. *J. Urol.* 79: 343.

Lau, F.T. and Henline, R.B. (1931) Ureteral anomalies. Report of a case manifesting three ureters on one side with one ending blindly in an aplastic kidney and a bifid pelvis with a single ureter on the other side. *J. Am. Med. Am.* 96: 587.

Laumonier, M. *et al.* (1957) Ectopie thoracique de rein droit. *Poumon. Coeur.* 13: 119.

Laurence, K.M. (1974) Letter to Editor. *Lancet* 11: 1120.

Lawrence, D., Howard, E.R. and Harris, R. (1983) A case of congenital urethral duplication cyst and its embryological significance. *Br. J. Surg.* 70: 565–566.

Lawson, K.A., Dunn, N.R., Roelen, B.A., Zeinstra, L.M., Davis, A.M., Wright, C.V., Korving, J.P. and Hogan, B.L.M. (1999) *Bmp4* is required for the generation of primordial germ cells in the mouse embryo. *Genes Dev.* 13: 424–436.

Leadbetter, G.W.J. (1964) Surgical correction of total urinary incontinence. *J. Urol.* 91: 261–266.

Leduc, B., van Campenhout, J. and Simard, R. (1968) Congenital absence of the vagina. Observations on 25 cases. *Am J. Obst. Gynec.* 100: 512.

Lee, L.M., Johnson, H.W. and McLoughlin, M.G. (1984) Microdissection and radiographic studies of the arterial vasculature of the human testes. *J. Ped. Surg.* Vol 19, No 3: 287–301.

Lee, M.M. and Donahoe, P.K. (1993) Müllerian inhibiting substance: a gonadal hormone with multiple functions. *Endocrine Rev.* 14: 152–164.

Lee, P.A., Mazur, T., Danish, R., Amrhein, J., Blizzard, R.M., Money, J. and Migeon, C.J. (1980) Micropenis: I. Criteria, etiologies and classification. *Johns Hopkins Med. J.* 146: 156.

Lenaghan, D. (1962) Bifid ureters in children: an anatomical, physiological and clinical study. *J. Urol.* 87: 808.

Lenaghan, D., Cass, A.S. and Stephens, F.D. (1972a) Influence of partial division of the intravesical ureter on the occurrence of vesicoureteral reflux in dogs. *J. Urol.* 107: 580.

Lenaghan, D., Cass, A.S. and Stephens, F.D. (1972b) Long-term vesicoureteral reflux in dogs: I. Without urinary infection. *J. Urol.* 107: 758.

Lepor, H. and Jeffs, R.D. (1983) Primary bladder closure and bladder neck reconstruction in classical bladder exstrophy. *J. Urol.* 130: 1142.

Leung, A.K.C., Robson, W.L.M. and Tay-Uyboco, J. (1993) The incidence of labial fusion in children. *J. Paediatr. Child Health* 29: 235–236.

Levitt, S.B. (1981) Medical versus surgical treatment of primary vesicoureteral reflux. A prospective international reflux study in children. Report of the International Study Committee. *J. Urol.* 125: 277.

Lewis, L.G. (1948) Cryptorchidism. *J. Urol.* 60: 345–346.

Linberg, B.E. (1924) Zur Frage der Nierenanomalien. *Z. Urol. Chir.* 15: 315. Cited by Geisinger (1937).

Litvak, A.S., Morris, J.A. Jr. and McRoberts, J.W. (1976) Normal size of the urethral meatus in boys. *J. Urol.* 115: 736, Table 1.

Livaditis, A., Maurseth, K. and Skog, P.A. (1964) Unilateral triplication of the ureter and renal pelvis: report of a case. *Acta Chir. Scand.* 127: 181.

Ljungqvist, A. (1965) Arterial vasculature of the multicystic dysplastic kidney. *Acta Path. Microbiol. Scand.* 64: 309.

Louw, J.H. and Barnard, C.N. (1955) Congenital intestinal atresia: Observations on its origin. *Lancet* 2: 1065.

Lowsley, O.S. (1912) The development of the human prostate gland with reference to the development of other structures at the neck of the urinary bladder. *Am. J. Anat.* 13: 299.

Lowsley, O.S. (1914) Congenital malformation of the posterior urethra. *Ann. Surg.* 60: 733.

Lowsley, O.S. and Kirwin, T.J. (1944) *Clinical Urology*, 2nd edn., p. 617. Baltimore: Williams and Wilkins.

Lozano, R.H. and Rodriguez, C. (1975) Intrathoracic ectopic kidney. Report of a case. *J. Urol.* 114: 601.

Lund, A.J. (1949) Uncrossed double ureter with rare intravesical orifice relationship. Case report with review of literature. *J. Urol.* 62: 22.

Lundius, B. (1975) Intrathoracic kidney. *Am J. Radiol.* 125: 785.

Luthra, M. and Stephens, F.D. (1988) Embryogenesis of the hymen and caudal end of the vagina deduced from uterovaginal anomalies. *Pediatr. Surg. Int.* 3: 422–425.

Luthra, M., Hutson, J.M. and Stephens, F.D. (1989) Effects of external inguinoscrotal compression on descent of the testis in rats. *Pediatr. Surg. Int.* 4: 403–407.

Lyon, R.P. and Smith, D.R. (1963) Distal urethral stenosis. *J. Urol.* 89: 414; *Acta Pathol. Microbiol. Scand.* (A), 64: 309.

Lyon, R.P., Marshall, S. and Tanagho, E.A. (1969) The ureteral orifice: its configuration and competency. *J. Urol.* 102: 504.

MacKellar, A. and Stephens, F.D. (1960) Vesical diverticula in children. *Aust. N.Z. J. Surg.* 30: 20.

MacKelvie, A.A. (1955) Triplicate ureter: case report. *Br. J. Urol.* 27: 124.

Mackie, G.G. and Stephens, F.D. (1975) Duplex kidneys: a correlation of renal dysplasia with position of ureteral orifice. *J. Urol.* 114: 274–280.

Mackie, G.G., Awang, H. and Stephens, F.D. (1975) The ureteric orifice: the embryologic key to radiologic status of duplex kidneys. *J. Pediatr. Surg.* 10: 473.

Magee, M.C., Lucey, D.T. and Fried, F.A. (1979) A new embryologic classification for uro-gynecologic malformations: the syndromes of mesonephric duct induced müllerian deformities. *J. Urol.* 121: 265.

Magnus, R.V. (1968) Rectal atresia as distinguished from rectal agenesis. *J. Pediatr. Surg.* 3: 593.

Magnus, R.V. (1972) Congenital rectovesical fistula and its associated anomalies. *Aust. N.Z. J. Surg.* 42: 197.

Maizels, M. and Stephens, F.D. (1979) The induction of urologic malformations: understanding the relationship of renal ectopia and congenital scoliosis. *J. Invest. Urol.* 17: 209.

Maizels, M. and Stephens, F.D. (1980) Valves of the ureter as a cause of primary obstruction of the ureter: anatomic, embryologic and clinical aspects. *J. Urol.* 123: 742.

Maizels, M., Stephens, F.D., King, L.R. and Firlit, C.F. (1983) Cowper's syringocele: a classification of dilatations of Cowper's gland duct based upon clinical characteristics of 8 boys. *J. Urol.* 129: 111.

Manivel, J.C., Pettinato, G.P., Reinberg, Y., Gonzalez, R., Burke, B. and Dehner, L.P. (1989) Prune belly syndrome: clinico-pathologic study of 29 cases. *Ped. Path.* 9: 691.

Marion, G. (1933) De maladie du col vesical. *Rep. Int. Soc. Urol.* 1: 392.

Markland, C. and Hastings, D. (1974) Vaginal reconstruction using cecal and sigmoid bowel segments in transsexual patients. *J. Urol.* 111: 217.

Marshall, A.G. (1953) The persistence of foetal structures in pyelonephritic kidneys. *Br. J. Surg.* 41: 38.

Marshall, V.F. and Meucke, E.C. (1962) Variations in exstrophy of the bladder. *J. Urol.* 88: 766.

Marshall, V.F. and Muecke, E.C. (1968) Congenital abnormalities of the bladder. In *Encyclopedia of Urology*, Vol. 7, *Malformations*, Berlin: Springer-Verlag.

Marshall, V.F., Marchetti, A.A. and Krantz, K.E. (1949) The correction of stress incontinence by simple vesicourethral suspension. *Surg. Gynec. Obstet.* 88: 509.

Maximovitch, A.S. (1927) Case of accessory kidney. *Z. Urol.* 21: 801. Cited by Geisinger (1937).

Mayall, G.F. (1970) The incidence of medullary sponge kidney. *Clin. Radiol.* 21: 171.

Maydl, K. (1894) Über die Radikaltherapie der Ektopia vesicae urinariae. *Wien Med. Wschr.* 44: 1113, 1169, 1209, 1256, 1297.

Mayer A. (1952) Über Missbildungen infolge von Trayman während der Schwanger-schaft und über Versehen der Schangeren. *Geburtsh Irauenheuk* 12/12: 1075 (quoted by Torpin, 1968).

Mayer, C.A.J. (1829) Über Verdoppelungen des uterus und ihre Arten, nebst Bemerkungen über Hasenscharte and Wolfsrachen. *J. Chir. Auger.* 13: 525.

Mayo, C.H. (1908) Transperitonael removal of tumours of the bladder. *Ann. Surg.* 48: 105.

Mazel, E. (1899) Über Blasenektopie und deren operative Behandlung. *Beitr. Klin. Chir.* 23: 444.

McArthur, L.L. (1908) Some renal anomalies. *St. Paul Med. J.* 10: 440. Cited by Geisinger (1937).

McClone, D.E. and Stpehens, F.D. (1990) Amniotic constraints as a cause of embryonic neural deformation. In *Concepts in Pediatric Neurosurgery*, A.E. Marlin (ed.), Vol. 10, pp. 22–29. Basel: Karger.

McCredie, J. (1974) Embryonic neuropathy, a hypothesis of neural crest injury as the pathogenesis of congenital malformations. *Med. J. Aust.* 1: 159–163.

McCrory, W.W. (1978) Embryologic development and prenatal maturation of the kidney. In *Pediatric Kidney Disease*, C.M. Edelman, Jr. (ed.), p. 23. Boston: Little, Brown.

McGovern, J.H. and Marshall, V.F. (1959) Congenital deficiency of the abdominal musculature and obstructive uropathy. *Surg. Gynec. Obstet.* 108: 289.

McIndoe, A. (1950) Treatment of congenital absence and obliterative conditions of the vagina. *Br. J. Plast. Surg.* 2: 254.

McKusick, V.A., Bauer, R.L., Koop, C.E. and Scott, R.B. (1964) Hydrometrocolpos as a simply inherited malformation. *J. Am. Med. Ass.* 189: 813–816.

Merei, J., Hasthorpe, S., Farmer, P. and Hutson, J.M. (1998) Relationship between esophageal atresia with tracheooesophageal fistula and vertebral anomalies in mammalian embryos. *J. Pediatr. Surg.* 33: 58–63.

Mering, J.H., Steel, J.F. and Gittes, R.F. (1972) Congenital ureteral valves. *J. Urol.* 107: 737.

Meyer, R. (1946) Normal and abnormal development of the ureter in the human embryo: a mechanistic consideration. *Anat. Rec.* 96: 355.

Meyer-Ruegg (1939) Quoted by Torpin, 1968: Zur pathogenese de gravitas extra-amnialis. *Zentralbl. Gynaek.* 68: 594.

Michon, J. (1978) Rétrécissement 'familial' de l'urétre. *J. Urol. Nephrol.* 84: 107.

Mikulicz-Radecki, F.V. (1922) Ein Beitrag zur Kongenitalen, intrathorakalen Nierendystrophie. *Zbl. Gynäk.* 46: 1718.

Miller, A. (1958) The aetiology and treatment of diverticulum of the bladder. *Br. J. Urol.* 30: 43–56.

Miller, M.E. Graham, J.M., Higginbottom, M.C. and Smith, D.W. (1981) Compression related defects from early amnion rupture: evidence for mechanical teratogenesis. *J. Pediatr.* 98: 292–297.

Milliken, L.D. and Hodgson, N.B. (1972) Renal dysplasia and urethral valves. *J. Urol.* 108: 960.

Mills, J.C. (1939) Complete unilateral duplication of ureter with analysis of literature. *Urol. Cutan. Rev.* 43: 444.

Mills, W.M. (1911) A case of supernumerary kidney. *J. Anat. Physiol.* 46: 313.

Mininberg, D.T., Montoya, F., Okada, K., Galioto, F. and Presutti, R. (1973) Subcellular muscle studies in the prune belly syndrome. *J. Urol.* 109: 524.

Mitrofanoff, P. (1980) Cystomie continente trans-appendiculaire dans le traitement des vessies neurologiques. *Chir. Pediatr.* 21: 297.

Miyazaki, Y., Oshima, K., Fogo, A., Hogan, B.L.M. and Ichikawa, I. (2000a) Bone morphogenetic protein 4 regulates the budding site and elongation of the mouse ureter. *J. Clin. Invest.* 105: 863–873.

Miyazaki, Y., Oshima, K., Fogo, A. and Ichikawa, I. (2000b) BMP4 is a multipotent regulator for the kidney and urinary tract development [abstract]. *J. Am. Soc. Nephrol.* 11: 379A–380A.

Moazzenzadeh, A.R., Khodadadian, P. and Potter, R.T. (1977) The intrathoracic kidney. *J. Thorac. Cardiovasc. Surg.* 73: 480.

Moerman, P., Fryns, J.P., Goddeeris, P. and Lauweryns, J.M. (1984) Pathogenesis of the prune belly syndrome: A fractional urethral obstruction caused by prostatic hypoplasia. *Pediatrics* 73: 470–75.

Mollard, P., Mouriquand, P.D.E. and Buttin X. (1994) Urinary continence after reconstruction of classic bladder exstrophy (73 cases). *Br. J. Urol.* 73: 298.

Momose, Y., Griffiths, A.L. and Hutson, J.M. (1992) Testicular descent. III. The neonatal gubernaculum shows rhythmic contraction in organ culture in response to calcitonin gene-related peptide. *Endocrinology* 131: 2881–2884.

Momose, Y., Goh, D.W., Watts, L.M. and Hutson, J.M. (1993) Calcitonin gene-related peptide stimulates motility of the gubernaculum via cyclic adenosine monophosphate. *J. Urol.* 150: 571–73

Monie, I.W. and Sigurdson, L.A. (1950) A proposed classification for uterine and vaginal anomalies. *Am. J. Obst. Gynec.* 59: 696.

Monti, P.R., Lara, R.C., Dutra, M.A. and de Carvalho J.R. (1997) New techniques for reconstruction of efferent conduits based on the Mitrofanoff principle. *Urology* 49: 112–115.

Moore, K.L. (1977) *The Developing Human*, 2nd edn., p. 60. Philadelphia: W.B. Saunders.

Morgagni, J.B. (1719) *Adversaria Anatomica Omnia*, Part 1, Article 10, p. 5. Padua: J. Cominus.

Moskowitz, P.S., Newton, N.A. and Lebowitz, R.L. (1976) Retention cysts of Cowper's ducts. *Radiology* 120: 377.

Mowat, J. (1747) An account of a child born with the urinary and genital organs preternaturally formed. *Medical Essays and Observations*. Published by a society in Edinburgh. 3:220, 1747 Quoted in The History of Urology (1972), L.J.T. Murphy (ed.). Springfield Ill: Charles C. Thomas.

Moynihan, B.G.A. (1906) Extroversion of the bladder—Relief by transplantation of the bladder into the rectum. *Ann. Surg.* 43: 237.

Müller, P. (1968) Malformations génitales et urinaries associees chez la femme. *Gynaecologia* 165: 285.

Murnaghan, G.F. (1957) Experimental investigation of the dynamics of the normal and dilated ureter. *Br. J. Urol.* 29: 403.

Murphy, L.J.T. (1972) *The History of Urology*. Springfield, Ill: Charles C. Thomas.

Najmaldin, A., Burge, D.M. and Atwell, J.D. (1990) Reflux nephropathy secondary to intrauterine vesicoureteric reflux. *J. Pediatr. Surg.* 25: 387–390.

Nakala, H. and Sakaguchi, T. (1977) Thoracic kidney presenting as a mass in the base of the lung. *Chest. (Suppl.)* 71: 123.

Nation, E.F. (1944) Duplication of kidney and ureter. A statistical study of 230 new cases. *J. Urol.* 51: 456.

Neinstein, L.S. and Castle, G. (1983) Congenital absence of the vagina. *Am. J. Dis. Childr.* 137: 669.

Nesbitt, T.E. (1955) Congenital megalourethra. *J. Urol.* 73: 839.

Neuhauser, E.B.D. (1970) Right diaphragmatic hernia with thoracic kidney. *Postgrad. Med.* 48: 57.

Newman, H. and Ditchek, T. (1969) Triplication of the ureter. *J. Urol.* 101: 692.

Newman, L.B., McAlister, W.H. and Kissane, J. (1974) Segmental renal dysplasia associated with ectopic ureteroceles in childhood. *Urology* 3: 23.

N'Guessen, G. and Stephens, F.D. (1983) Supernumerary kidney. *J. Urol.* 130: 649–653.

N'Guessen, G., Stephens, F.D. and Pick, J. (1984) Congenital superior ectopic (thoracic) kidney. *Urology* 24: 219–228.

Nini, W. (1961) Le rein intrathoracique. *Bull. Soc. Int. Chir.* 20: 548.

Nishimura, H., Yerkes, E., Hohenfellner, K., Miyazaki, Y., Ma, J., Hunley, T.E., Yoshida, H., Ichiki, T., Schulman, M., Kon, V., Phillips, III J.A., Hogan, B.M.L., Fogo, A., Brock, J.W., Inagami, T. and Ichikawa, I. (1999) Role of the angiotensin type 2 receptor gene in congenital anomalies of the kidney and urinary tract, CAKUT, of mice and men. *Mol. Cell* 3: 1–10.

Noordijk, J.A. (1967) Ungewöhnliche Zwerchfellhernien. *Arch. Klin. Chir.* 39: 740.

Normand, C.S. and Smellie, J.M. (1979) Vesicoureteric reflux: the case for conservative management. In *Reflux Nephropathy*, J. Hodson and P. Kincaid-Smith (eds), p. 281. New York: Masson.

Notley, R.G. (1972) Electron microscopy of the primary obstructive megaureter. *Br. J. Urol.* 44: 229.

Nunn, I.N. (1964) Bladder neck obstruction. *J. Urol.* 93: 693.

Nunn, I.N. and Stephens, F.D. (1961) The triad syndrome: a composite anomaly of the abdominal wall, urinary system and testes. *J. Urol.* 86: 782–794.

Ong, T.H., Ferguson, R.S. and Stephens, F.D. (1974a) The pattern of intrapelvic pressures during vesicoureteral reflux in the dog with normal caliber ureters. *J. Urol.* 11: 347.

Ong, T.H., Ferguson, R.S. and Stephens, F.D. (1974b) The pattern of intrapelvic pressures during vesicoureteral reflux in the dog with megaureters. *J. Urol.* 11: 352.

O'Rahilly, R. (1977) The development of the vagina in the human. In *Morphogenesis and Malformation of the Genital System*. R.J. Blandau and D. Bergsma (eds), pp. 123–136. National Foundation, March of Dimes XIII. BD:OAS(2)XIII. New York: Alan R. Liss.

Oshima, K., Miyazaki, Y., Brock, III J.W., Adams, M.C., Ichikawa, I. and Pope, IV J.C. (2000) Effects of angiotensin type-2 receptor (AT2) activation on ureteral budding [abstract]. *J. Am. Soc. Nephrol.* 11: 380A.

Osler, W. (1901) Congenital absence of the abdominal muscles with distorted and hypertrophied urinary bladder. *Johns Hopkins Hosp. Bull.* 22 (128): 331.

Ostling, K. (1942) The genesis of hydronephrosis: particularly with regard to the changes at the ureteropelvic junction. *Acta Chir. Scand. (Suppl.)* 86: 72.

Page, R.E. (1981) Hypospadias revisited. *Br. J. Plastic Surg.* 34: 149–151.

Pagon, R.A., Smith, D.W. and Shephard, T.H. (1979) Urethral obstruction malformation complex: a cause of abdominal muscle deficiency and the 'prune belly'. *J. Pediatr.* 94: 900–906.

Panarolus (1654) Quoted by H.A. Wilmer (1938. Unilateral fused kidney: A report of four cases and a review of the literature. *J. Urol.* 40: 551.

Paquin, A.J. Jr. (1959) Ureterovesical anastomosis: the description and evaluation of a technique. *J. Urol.* 82: 573.

Paquin, A.J. Jr., Marshall, B.F. and McGovern, J.H. (1960) The megacystis syndrome. *J. Urol.* 83: 634.

Park, W-H and Hutson, J.M. (1991) The gubernaculum shows rhythmic contractility and active movement during testicular descent. *J. Pediatr. Surg.* 26: 615–617.

Parker, R.M., Pohl, D.R. and Robison, J.R. (1970) Ureteral triplication with ectopia. *J. Urol.* 103: 727.

Parvenin, T. (1976) Complete ureteral triplication. *J. Pediatr. Surg.* 11: 1039.

Patel, N.P. and Lavengood, R.W. Jr. (1975) Triplicate ureter. *Urology* 5: 242.

Pathak, I.G. and Williams, D.I. (1964) Multicystic and cystic dysplastic kidneys. *Br. J. Urol.* 36: 318.

Patten, B.M. (1947) *Human Embryology*, 2nd edn. (a) p. 570; (b) p. 585; (c) p. 571; (d) p. 570. New York: McGraw-Hill.

Patten, B.M. and Barry, A. (1952) The genesis of exstrophy of the bladder and epispadias. *Am. J. Anat.* 90: 35.

Paul, A.T.S., Uragoda, O.G. and Jayewardene, F.L.W. (1960) Thoracic kidney with a report of a case. *Br. J. Surg.* 47: 395.

Paul, M. and Kanageruntheram, R. (1957) The congenital diaphragmatic hernia of Bochdalek. *Thorax* 12: 203.

Pelander, W.M., Luna, G. and Lilly, J.R. (1978) Polyorchidism: case report and literature review. *J. Urol.* 119: 705–706.

Penso, C.A. Sandstrom, M.M., Garber, M.F., Ladoulis, M., Stryker, J.M. and Benacerraf, B.B. (1990) Early amniocentesis: report of 407 cases with neonatal follow-up. *Obstet. Gynecol.* 76: 1032–1036.

Perkins, P.J., Kroovand, R.L. and Evans, A.T. (1973) Ureteral triplication. *Radiology* 108: 533.

Persky, L., Izant, R. and Bolande, R. (1967) Renal dysplasia. *J. Urol.* 98: 431.

Pescione, F. (1957) High renal ectopy: a contribution to the knowledge of the so-called 'thoracic kidney'. *Urol. Int.* 4: 142.

Peters, C.A., Carr, M.C., Lais, A., Retik, A.B. and Mandell, J. (1992) The response of the fetal kidney to obstruction. *J. Urol.* 148: 503–509.

Petrovc[v]ic['], F. and Milic['], N. (1956) Horseshoe kidney with crossed ureter condition after right nephrectomy. *Br. J. Radiol.* 29: 114.

Pfister, R.C., McLaughlin, A.P. III and Leadbetter, W.F. (1971) Radiological evaluation of primary megaloureter. *Radiology* 99: 503.

Pichel, J.G., Shen, L., Sheng, H.Z., Granholm, A.C., Drago, J., Grinberg, A., Lee, E.J., Huang, S.P., Saarma, M., Hoffer, B.J., Sariola H. and Westphal H. (1996) Defects in enteric innervation and kidney development in mice lacking GDNF. *Nature* 382: 73–76.

Piekarski, D.H. and Stephens, F.D. (1976) The association and embryogenesis of tracheo-esophageal and anorectal anomalies. In *Progress in Paediatric Surgery*. P.P. Rickham, W. Ch. Hecker and J. Prevot (eds), pp. 9, 63. Munich: Urban and Schwarzenberg.

Pinsky, L. (1974) A community of human malformation syndromes involving the mülleria ducts, distal extremities, urinary tract, and ears. *Teratology* 9: 65.

Pinter, A.B., Shafer, J. and Varro, J. (1982) Two supernumerary kidneys with ureteral atresia. *J. Urol.* 127: 119.

Popek, E.J., Tyson, R.W., Miller, G.J. and Caldwell, S.A. (1989) Phosphate development in prune belly syndrome (PBS) and posterior urethral valves (PUV): etiology of PBS-lower urinary tract obstruction or primary mesenchymal defect? *Lab. Invest.* 60: 73A.

Poppert, P. (1896) Üeber eine Methode zur Erzielung eines normalen Blasenverschlusses bei angeborener Blasen- und Harnrohrenspalte. *Arch. Klin. Chir.* **53**: 454.

Possoegel, A.K., Diez-Pardo, J.A., Morales, C., Navarro, C. and Tovar, J.A. (1998) Embryology of esophageal atresia in the adriamycin rat model. *J. Pediatr. Surg.* 33: 606–612.

Poswillow, D. and Roy, L.J. (1965) The pathogenesis of cleft palate. An animal study. *Brit. J. Surg.* 52: 902–913.

Potampa, P.B., Hyman, M.D. and Catlow, C.E. (1949) An unusual renal anomaly: combined tandem and horseshoe kidney. *J. Urol.* 61: 340.

Potter, E.L. (1972) *Normal and Abnormal Development of the Kidney.* (a) p. 163; (b) p. 3; (c) p. 18; (d) p. 73; (e) p. 141; (f) p. 109; (g) p. 213; (h) p. 182; (i) p. 229. Chicago: Year Book.

Potter, E.L. and Craig, J.M. (1975) *The Pathology of the Fetus and Infant.* 3rd edn., p. 434. Chicago: Year Book.

Prader, A. (1954) Der Genitalbefund beim Pseudohermaphroditismus Femininus des kongenitalen adrenogenitalen Syndromes. Morphologie, Haufigkeit, Entwicklung und Vererbung der verschiedenen Genital-formen. *Helv. Pediatr. Acta* 9: 231-248.

Qi, B.Q. and Beasley, S.W. (1999) Relationship of the notochord to foregut development in the fetal rat model of esophageal atresia. *J. Pediatr. Surg.* 34: 1593–1598.

Quan, L. and Smith, D.W. (1973) The VATER association, Vertebral defects, Anal atresia, T-E fistula with esophageal atresia, Radial and Renal dysgenesis: a spectrum of associated defects. *J. Pediatr.* 82: 104–107.

Raffensperger, J.G. and Ramenofsky, M. (1973) The management of a cloaca. *J. Pediatr. Surg.* 8: 647.

Ramos, A.J., Slovis, T.L. and Reed, J.D. (1979) Intrathoracic kidney. *Urology* 13: 14.

Ransley, P.G., Duffy, P.G. and Woolin, M. (1988) Bladder exstrophy closure and epispadias repair. In *Paediatric Surgery*, L. Spitz and H.H. Nixon (eds), P. 620. London: Butterworths.

Ransley, P.G., Vordermark, J.S., Caldamone, A.A. *et al.* (1984) Preliminary ligation of the gonadal vessels prior to orchiopexy for the intra-abdominal testicle: a staged Fowler-Stephens procedure. *World J. Urol.* 2: 266–268.

Rao, K.G. (1975) Congenital proximal bulbar stricture in adults. *Urology* 6: 576.

Ratner, I.A., Fisher, J.H. and Swenson, O. (1961) Double ureters in infancy and childhood. *Pediatrics* 28: 810.

Rattner, W.H., Meyer, R. and Bernstein, J. (1963) Congenital abnormalities of the urinary system: IV. Valvular obstruction of the posterior urethra. *J. Pediatr.* 63: 84.

Reboud, E. and Bernard, R. (1958) Un nouveau cas d'ectopie rénale intrathoracique. *Poumon. Coeur.* 14: 597.

Redman, J.F. and Fraiser, L.P. (1979) Apparent congenital anterior urethral strictures in brothers. *J. Urol.* 122: 707.

Reinberg, Y., Shapiro, E., Manimel, J.C., Manley, C.B., Pettinato, G. and Gonzalez, R. (1991) Prune belly syndrome in females: a triad of abdominal musculature deficiency and anomalies of the urinary and genital systems. *J. Ped.* 118: 395.

Renfree, M.B., Wilson, J.D., Short, R.V., Shaw, G. and George F.W. (1992) Steroid hormone content of the gonads of the Tammar Wallaby during sexual differentiation. *Biol. Reprod.* 47: 644–647.

Riba, L.W., Schmidlapp, C.J. and Bosworth, N.L. (1946) Ectopic ureter draining into seminal vesicle. *J. Urol.* 56: 332.

Rice, P.B., Holder, T.M. and Ashcraft, K.W. (1978) Congenital posterior urethral perineal fistula: a case report. *J. Urol.* 119: 416.

Rich, M.A., Heimler, A., Waber, L. and Brock, W.A. (1987) Autosomal dominant transmission of ureteral triplication and bilateral amastia. *J. Urol.* 137(1): 102–105.

Rickham, P.P. (1956) The use of the isolated ileal loop in paediatric urology. *Br. J. Urol.* **28**: 394.

Ringer, M.G. Jr. and MacFarlane, S.M. (1964) Complete triplication of the ureter: a case report. *J. Urol.* 92: 429.

Risdon, R.A. (1971) Renal dysplasia: I. A clinico-pathological study of 76 cases. *J. Clin. Pathol.* 24: 57.

Risdon, R.A., Young, L.W. and Crispin, A.R. (1975) Renal hypoplasia and dysplasia: a radiological and pathological classification. *Pediatr. Radiol.* 3: 213.

Roberts, J.B.M. (1961) Congenital anomalies of the urinary tract and their association with spina bifida. *Br. J. Urol.* 108: 823.

Rock, J.A. and Jones, H.W. Jr. (1980) The double uterus associated with an obstructed hemivagina and ipsilateral renal agenesis. *Am J. Obst. Gynec.* 138: 339.

Rognon, L.M. (1960) Ectopie haute de rein. *J. Urol. (Paris)* 66: 516.

Rokitansky, K. (1838) Über die sogenannten Verdoppelungen des Uterus. *Med. Jahrb. Ost. Staat.* 26: 39.

Rolleston, G.L. (1970) The significance and management of vesico-ureteric reflux in infancy. Part 2: Radiological aspects. In *Renal Infection and Renal Scarring*. P. Kincaid-Smith and K.F. Fairley (eds), p. 246. Melbourne: Mercedes Press.

Rolleston, G.L., Shannon, F.T. and Utley, W.L.F. (1970) Relationship of infantile vesicoureteric reflux to renal damage. *Br. Med. J.* 1: 460.

Rose, G. and Vaughan, E.D. Jr. (1975) Common renal pelvis: a case report. *J. Urol.* 113: 234–235.

Rosenberg, H.K., Udassin, R., Howell, C., Betts, J. and Schnauffer, L. (1982) Duplication of the uterus and vagina, unilateral hydrometrocolpos, and ipsilateral renal agenesis: sonographic aid to diagnosis. *J. Ultrasound Med.* 1: 289.

Rowsell, A.R. and Morgan, B.D.E. (1987) Hypospadias and the embryogenesis of the penile urethra. *Br. J. Plastic Surg.* 40: 201–206.

Rubin, J.S. (1948) Supernumerary kidney with aberrant ureter terminating externally. *J. Urol.* 60: 405.

Rundle, J.S.H., Primrose, D.A. and Carachi, R. (1982) Cryptorchidism in cerebral palsy. *Br. J. Urol.* 54: 170–171.

Rutkowski, M. (1899) Zur Methode der Harnblasenplastik. *Zentral. bl Chir.* 26: 473.

Saccone, A. and Hendler, H.B. (1934) Supernumerary kidney: report of a case and a review of the literature. *J. Urol.* 31: 711. Cited by Geisinger (1937).

Sainio, K., Suvanto, P., Davies, J., Wartiovaara, J., Wartiovaara, K., Saarma, M., Arumae, U., Meng, X., Lindahl, M. and Pachnis, V. (1997) Glial-cell-derived neurotrophic factor is required for bud initiation from ureteric epithelium. *Development* 124: 4077–4087.

Samarakkody, U.K.S. and Hutson, J.M. (1992) Intrascrotal CGRP(8-37) causes a delay in testicular descent in mice. *J. Pediatr. Surg.* 27: 874–875.

Sampson, J.A. (1903) Ascending renal infection: with special reference to the reflux of urine from the bladder into the ureters as an etiological factor in its causation and maintenance. *Johns Hopkins Hosp. Bull.* 14: 344.

Samuels, A., Kern, H. and Sachs, L. (1922) Supernumerary kidney with ureter opening into vagina. *Surg. Gynec. Obs.* 35: 599. Cited by Geisinger (1937).

Sanchez, M.P., Silos-Santiago, I., Frisen, J., He, B., Lira, S.A. and Barbacid, M. (1996) Renal agenesis and the absence of enteric neurons in mice lacking GDNF. *Nature* 382: 70–73.

Sandegard, E. (1958) The treatment of ureteral ectopia. *Acta Chir. Scand.* 115: 149.

Sanyanusin, P., Schimmenti, L.A., McNoe, L.A., Pierpont, M.E., Sullivan, M.J., Dobyns, W.B. and Eccles, M.R. (1995) Mutation of the PAX2 gene in a family with optic nerve colobomas, renal anomalies and vesicoureteral reflux. *Nat. Genet.* 9: 358–363.

Sarto, G.E. and Simpson, J.L. (1978) Abnormalities of the müllerian and wolffian duct systems. *Birth Defects* 14(C): 37.

Sasidharan, K., Babu, A.S., Rao, M.M. and Bhat, H.S. (1976) Free supernumerary kidney. *Br. J. Urol.* 48: 388.

Saxen, L. (1987) *Organogenesis of the kidney*. Cambridge: Cambridge University Press.

Schapira, E., Fishel, E. and Levin, S. (1965) Intrathoracic kidney in a premature infant. *Arch. Dis. Childr.* 40: 86.

Scheffer, I.E., Hutson, J.M., Warne, G.L. and Ennis, G. (1988) Extreme virilization in patients with congenital adrenal hyperplasia fails to induce descent of the ovary. *Pediatr. Surg. Int.* 3: 165–168.

Schenk von Grafenberg, J. (1644) *Observationum medicarum, rariorum Libri VII*, Lugduni, 1644 Quoted in *The History of Urology* (1972), L.J.T. Murphy (ed.), Springfield, Ill: Charles C. Thomas.

Schmeller, N.T. and Schermer, H.K.A. (1982) Trifurcation of the urethra. A case report. *J. Urol.* 127: 545, Fig. 2c.

Schonfeld, W.A. and Beebe, G.W. (1942) Normal growth and variation in the male genitalia from birth to maturity. *J. Urol.* 48: 759.

Schuchardt, A., D'Agati, V., Pachnis, V. and Costantini, F. (1996) Renal agenesis and hypodysplasia in ret-k-mutant mice result from defects in ureteric bud development. *Development* 122: 1919–1929.

Schwarz, R.D. and Stephens, F.D. (1978) The persisting mesonephric duct: high junction of vas deferens and ureter. *J. Urol.* 120: 592.

Schwarz, R.D., Stephens, F.D. and Cussen, L.J. (1981) The pathogenesis of renal dysplasia. I, II and III. *J. Invest. Urol.* 19: 94–101.

Schwarzt, A. and Frankel, M. (1952) High renal ectopia, detected on routine chest examination. *Acta. Radiol.* 37: 583.

Scott, J.E.S. (1981) The single ectopic ureter and the dysplastic kidney. *Br. J. Urol.* 53: 300.

Scott, J.E.S. (1987) The Hutson hypothesis. A clinical study. *Br. J. Urol.* 60: 74–76.

Scott, R. (1970) Triplication of the ureter. *Br. J. Urol.* 42: 150.

Scott, W.W. (1960) Two unusual urethroplasties. *Am. Surg.* 26: 196.

Seftel, A.D., Resnick, M.I. and Boswell M.V. (1994) Dorsal nerve block for the management of intraoperative penile erection. *J. Urol.* 151: 394.

Shane, J.H. (1942) Supernumerary kidney with vaginal ureteral orifice. *J. Urol.* 47: 344.

Shapiro, E., Lapor, H. and Jeffs, R.D. (1984) The inheritance of classical bladder exstrophy. *J. Urol.* 132: 308–310.

Shokeir, M.H.K. (1978) Aplasia of the müllerian system: evidence for probable sex-limited autosomal dominant inheritance. *Birth Defects* 14(C): 147.

Shono, T. and Hutson, J.M. (1994) Capsaicin increases the frequency of cryptorchidism in flutamide-treated rats. *J. Urol.* 152: 763–765.

Shono, T., Goh, D.W., Momose, Y. and Hutson, J.M. (1995) Physiological effects *in vitro* of calcitonin gene-related peptide (CGRP) on gubernacular contractility with or without denervation. *J. Pediatr. Surg.* 30: 591–595.

Shopfner, C.E. and Hutch, J.A. (1967) The trigonal canal. *Radiology* 88: 209.

Shrom, S.H., Cromie, W.J. and Duckett, J.W. Jr. (1981) Megalourethra. *Urology* 17: 152–156.

Siegel, M.J. and McAlister, W.H. (1980) Simple cysts of the kidney in children. *J. Urol.* 123: 75.

Silverman, F.N. and Huang, N. (1950) Congenital absence of the abdominal muscles, associated with malformation of the genitourinary and alimentary tracts: report of cases and review of literature. *Am. J. Dis. Childr.* 80: 91.

Sinclair, A.H. (1994) The cloning of SRY. In *Molecular Genetics of Sex Determination*, S.S. Wachtell (ed.), pp. 23–42. New York: Academic Press.

Singh, M. and Blandy, J.P. (1976) The pathology of urethral stricture. *J. Urol.* 115: 673.

Smellie, J.M. (1967) Medical aspects of urinary infection in children. *J. R. Coll. Phys. (Lond.)* 1: 189.

Smellie, J.M. and Normand, I.C.S. (1979) Reflux nephropathy in childhood. In *Reflux Nephropathy*, John Hodson and P. Kincaid-Smith (eds), p. 14, New York: Masson.

Smellie, J.M., Hodson, C.J., Edwards D. and Normand. J.C.S. (1964) Clinical and radiological features of urinary infection in childhood. *Br. Med. J.* 2: 1222.

Smith, D.W. (1981) Recognizable patterns of human deformation. In *Major Problems in Clinical Pediatrics*, Vol. 21. A.J. Shaffer and M. Markoritz (eds), p. 1. Philadelphia: W.B. Saunders.

Smith, D.W. (1981) Small uterine cavity deformation: malformed uterus, uterine fibroids, small uterus. In *Major Problems in Clinical Paediatrics, Vol. XXI, Recognizable Patterns of Human Deformation*, A.J. Schaffer and M. Markowitz (eds), p. 81. Philadelphia: W.B. Saunders.

Smith, D.W. (1982a) Early amniotic rupture. In *Recognizable Patterns of Human Malformation: Genetic, Embryologic and Clinical Aspects*, 3rd edn., p. 488. Philadelphia: W.B. Saunders.

Smith, D.W. (1982b) Recognizable patterns of human malformation. In *Major Problems in Clinical Pediatrics, Genetic, Embryologic and Clinical Aspects*, 3rd edn., Vol. 7, p. 482. Philadelphia: W.B. Saunders.

Smith, E.D. (1965) *Spina Bifida and the Total Care of the Child*, p. 109. Springfield: Charles C. Thomas.

Smith, E.D. (1968) Urinary anomalies and complications in imperforate anus and rectum. *J. Pediatr. Surg.* 3: 337.

Smith, E.D. (1977) Report of working party to establish an international nomenclature for the large ureter. In *Urinary System Malformations in Children*. D. Bergsma and J.W. Duckett (eds). New York: Alan R. Liss for the National Foundation, March of Dimes, BD:OAS, 5: 3.

Smith, E.D. (1980) Malformations of the bladder and urethra, and hypospadias. In *Pediatric Surgery*, T.M. Holder and K.W. Ashcraft (eds), p. 769. Philadelphia: W.B. Saunders.

Smith, I. (1946) Triplicate ureter. *Br. J. Surg.* 34: 182.

Smith, J.A., Hutson, J.M., Beasley, S.W. and Reddihough, D.S. (1989) The relationship between cerebral palsy and cryptorchidism. *J. Pediatr. Surg.* 23: 275–277.

Smith, N.M., Chambers, H.M., Furness, M.E. and Haan, E.A. (1992) The OEIS complex (omphalocele-exstrophy-imperforate anus-spinal defects): recurrence in sibs. *J. Med. Genet.* 29: 730–732.

Soderdahl, D.W., Shiraki, I.W. and Schamber, D.T. (1976) Bilateral ureteral quadruplication. *J. Urol.* 116: 255.

Sommer, J.T. and Stephens, F.D. (1980) Dorsal urethral diverticulum of the fossa navicularis: symptoms, diagnosis and treatment. *J. Urol.* 124: 94.

Sommer, J.T. and Stephens, F.D. (1981) Morphogenesis of nephropathy with partial obstruction and vesicoureteral reflux. *J. Urol.* 125: 67.

Soubottine, M. (1901) Intrarectal urethra for exstrophy of the bladder [Abstract]. *J.A.M.A.* **36**: 636.

Spangler, E.B. (1963) Complete triplication of the ureter. *Radiology* 80: 795.

Spasov, S.A., Dokumov, S.I., Diankov, L.A., Balkov, I.M. and Sarkanyatz, A.M. (1976) Efficacy of pneumogynecography in the diagnosis of Mayer-Rokitansky-Kuster-Hauser syndrome. *Am. J. Roentgen.* 126: 413.

Speert, H. (1958) Essays in eponymy. In *Obstetric and Gynecologic Milestones*. New York: Macmillan.

Spence, H.M. (1962) Congenital hydrocolpos. A review with emphasis on urologic aspects and a report of four additional cases. *J. Am. Med. Ass.* 180: 1100.

Spence, H.M., Baird, S.S. and Ware, E.W. Jr. (1957) Cystic disorders of the kidney: classification, diagnosis, treatment. *J. Am. Med. Ass.* 163: 1466.

Spillane, R.J. and Prather, E.C. (1952) Right diaphragmatic eventration with renal displacement. *J. Urol.* 62: 804.

Squiers, E.C., Morden, R.S. and Bernstein, J. (1987) Renal multicystic dysplasia: an occasional manifestation of the hereditary renal dysplasia syndrome. *Am. J. Med. Genet.* (Suppl.) 3: 279–284.

Stecker, J.F., Rose, J.G. and Gillenwater, J.Y. (1973) Dysplastic kidneys associated with vesicoureteral reflux. *J. Urol.* 110: 341.

Stephens, F.D. (1953a) Congenital imperforate rectum: Recto-urethral and recto-vaginal fistulae. *Aust. N.Z. J. Surg.* 22: 161.

Stephens, F.D. (1953b) Malformations of the anus. *Aust. N.Z. J. Surg.* 23: 9.

Stephens, F.D. (1954) Megaureter. *Aust. N.Z. J. Surg.* 23: 197.

Stephens, F.D. (1956a) Double ureter in the child. *Aust. N.Z. J. Surg.* 26: 81.

Stephens, F.D. (1956b) Megaureter. *Med. J. Aust.* 1: 233.

Stephens, F.D. (1957) The management of double ureters in children. *Med. J. Aust.* 2: 679.

Stephens, F.D. (1958a) Anatomical vagaries of double ureters. *Aust. N.Z. J. Surg.* 28: 27.

Stephens, F.D. (1958b) Ureterocele in infants and children. *Aust. N.Z. J. Surg.* 27: 288.

Stephens, F.D. (1963) *Congenital Malformations of the Rectum, Anus, and Genito-urinary Tracts* (a) p. 186; (b) p. 187; (c) p. 149. Edinburgh: Livingstone.

Stephens, F.D. (1964) Intramural ureter and ureterocele. *Postgrad. Med. J.* 40: 179.

Stephens, F.D. (1966) Urethro-vaginal malformations. *Aust. N.Z. J. Obstet. Gynec.* 6: 64.

Stephens, F.D. (1968) The female anus, perineum and vestibule: embryogenesis and deformities. *Aust. N.Z. J. Obstet. Gynec.* 8: 55.

Stephens, F.D. (1970a) Preliminary follow-up of 101 children with reflux treated conservatively. In *Renal Infection and Renal Scarring*, P. Kincaid-Smith and K.F. Fairley (eds), p. 283. Melbourne: Mercedes Press.

Stephens, F.D. (1970b) a form of stress incontinence in children another method of bladder neck repair. *Aust. N.Z. J. Surg.* 40: 124.

Stephens, F.D. (1971) Caecoureterocele and concepts on the embryology and aetiology of ureteroceles. *Aust. N.Z. J. Surg.* 40: 239.

Stephens, F.D. (1974) Idiopathic dilatations of the urinary tract. *J. Urol.* 112: 819.

Stephens, F.D. (1978) The normal and abnormal ureterovesical hiatus: methods of correction of vesicoureteral reflux and paraureteral diverticula. *J. Cont. Ed. Urol.*

Stephens, F.D. (1979a) The vesicoureteral hiatus and paraureteral diverticula. *J. Urol.* 121: 786.

Stephens, F.D. (1979b) In *Campbell's Urology*, J.H. Harrison, R.F. Gittes, A.D. Perlmutter, T.A. Stamey and P.C. Walsh (eds), Vol. 2, p. 1618. Philadelphia: W.B. Saunders.

Stephens, F.D. (1979c) Bifid and double ureters, ureteroceles and fused kidneys. In *Pediatric Surgery*. M.M. Ravitch, K.J. Welch, C.D. Benson, E. Aberdeen and J.G. Randolph (eds), 3rd edn., p. 1188. Chicago: Year Book.

Stephens, F.D. (1979d) Cystoscopic appearances of the ureteric orifices associated with reflux nephropathy. In *Reflux nephropathy*. J. Hodson and P. Kincaid-Smith (eds), pp. 119–125. Paris: Masson.

Stephens, F.D. (1981) Associated urological and vertebral anomalies in imperforate anus. In *Associated Congenital Anomalies*, M.E. Shafie and C.H. Kleppel (eds), p. 189. Baltimore: Williams and Wilkins.

Stephens, F.D. (1982) Ureterovascular hydronephrosis and the 'aberrant' renal vessels. *J. Urol.* 128: 984.

Stephens, F.D. (1983a) *Congenital Malformations of the Urinary Tract.* (5i) 200–201; (5ii) 286–292; (5iii) 194–195. New York: Praeger.

Stephens, F.D. (1983b) *Congenital Malformations of the Urinary Tract.* (a) p. 286; (b) p. 350. New York: Praeger.

Stephens, F.D. (1983c) Malformations of the external cloaca. In *Congenital Malformations of the Urinary Tract.* New York: Praeger.

Stephens, F.D. (1983d) Duplex ureters. In *Congenital Malformations of the Urinary Tract.* F.D. Stephens (ed.), p. 297. New York: Praeger.

Stephens, F.D. (1988) Embryology of the cloaca and embryogenesis of anorectal malformations. In *Anorectal Malformations in Children. Update* (1988). F.D. Stephens, E.D. Smith and N.W. Paul (eds), p. 187–209. New York: Alan R. Liss.

Stephens, F.D. (1993) Embryology and pathoembryology of the urinary tract. In *Reconstructive Urology*, Vol. 1. G. Webster, R. Kirby, L. King and B. Goldwasser (eds). 93: 104.

Stephens, F.D. (1994) Paediatric Surgery. III. Embryology of the upper genitourinary tract. In *Paediatric Urology*, 3rd edn., B. O'Donnell, and S. Koff (eds), London: Butterworths (in press).

Stephens, F.D. (1995) Pathoembryology of hypospadias. In *Reconstructive Surgery of the External Genitalia*, C.E. Horton, Sr. and J.S. Elder (eds). Boston: Little, Brown (in press).

Stephens, F.D. (1992) Triplication of the ureter. In *The Ureter*. J.M. Fitzpatrick and E.D. Vaughan, Jr. (eds). London: Springer-Verlag. (in press).

Stephens, F.D. and Lenaghan, D. (1962) The anatomical basis and dynamics of vesicoureteral reflux. *J. Urol.* 87: 670.

Stephens, F.D. and Smith, E.D. (1971) *Anorectal Malformations in Children*, p. 272. Chicago: Year Book.

Stephens, F.D. and Donnellan, W.L. (1977) 'H-type' urethroanal fistula. *J. Pediatr. Surg.* 12: 95.

Stephens, F.D. and Fortune, D. (1993) Pathogenesis of megalourethra. *J. Urol.* 149: 1512–1516.

Stephens, F.D. and Gupta, D. (1994) Pathogenesis of the prune belly syndrome. *J. Urol.* 152: 2328–2331.

Stephens, F.D. and Smith, E.D. (1971) *Anorectal Malformations in Children*, p. 282. Chicago: Year Book.

Stephens, F.D., Joske, H.A. and Simmons, R.T. (1955) Mega-ureter with vesicoureteric reflux in twins. *Aust. N.Z. J. Surg.* 24: 192.

Stevenson, E.D. (1972) Extra vertebrae associated with oesophageal atresia and tracheo-esophageal fistulas. *J. Pediatr.* 81: 1123–1129.

Stolpe, Y., King, L.R. and White, H. (1967) The normal range of renal size in children. *J. Urol.* 4: 600.

Stumme, E.G. (1903) Quoted by Silverman and Huang (1950) Über die symmetrischer, kongenitalen Bauchmuskeldefekte und über die kombination derselben mit anderen Bildungsanomalien des Rumpages (hochstand, Hypertrophie, und Dilation der Blase, Ureterendilation Kyrtorchismus, Furchen-nabel, Thoraxdeformität, u.z.w.). *Mitt. Brenzgeb. Med. Chir.* 11: 584.

Subbiah, N. and Stephens, F.D. (1972) Stenotic ureterocele. *Aust. N.Z. J. Surg.* 41: 257.

Sutliff, K.S. and Hutchins, G.M. (1994) Septation of the respiratory and digestive tracts in human embryos: crucial role of the tracheo-esophageal sulcus. *Anat. Record* 238: 237–247.

Supernumerary kidney (1838) *London Med. Gaz.* 2: 127. Cited by Kretschmer (1929).

Sweetser, T.H., Chisolm, T.C. and Thompson, W.H. (1952) Exstrophy of the urinary bladder: discussion of anatomic principles applicable to its repair, with preliminary report of a case. *Minn. Med.* **35**: 654.

Swenson, O., MacMahon, H.E., Jaques, W.E. and Campbell, J. (1951) New concept of the pathology of megaloureters. *Bull. N. Engl. Med. Cent.* 13: 157.

Sykes, D. (1964) The morphology of renal lobulations and calyces: their relationship to partial nephrectomy. *Br. J. Surg.* 51: 294.

Tada, Y., Kokado, Y., Hashinaka, Y., Kadowaki, T., Takasugi, Y., Shin, T. and Tsukaguchi, I. (1981) Free supernumerary kidney: a case report and review. *J. Urol.* 126: 231.

Tamura, E. *et al.* (1970) The thoracic kidney. *Paediat. Univ. Tokyo* 17: 49.

Tanagho, E.A. (1972) Surgically-induced partial urinary obstruction in the fetal lamb: III. Ureteral obstruction. *Invest. Urol.* 10: 35.

Tanagho, E.A. (1976) Embryogenic basis for lower ureteral anomalies: a hypothesis. *Urology* 7: 451.

Tanagho, E.A. and Pugh, R.C.B. (1963) The anatomy and function of the ureterovesical junction. *Br. J. Urol.* 35: 151.

Tanagho, E.A., Hutch, J.A., Meyers, F.H. and Rambo, O.N. Jr. (1965) Primary vesicoureteral reflux: experimental studies of its etiology. *J. Urol.* 93: 165.

Tanagho, E.A., Guthrie, T.H. and Lyon, R.P. (1969) The intravesical ureter in primary reflux. *J. Urol.* 101: 824.

Tanagho, E.A., Smith, D.R. and Guthrie, T.H. (1970) Pathophysiology of functional obstruction. *J. Urol.* 104: 73.

Tang, M-J., Worley, D., Sanicola, M. and Dressler, G.R. (1998) The RET-glial cell-derived neurotrophic factor (GDNF) pathway stimulates migration and chemoattraction of epithelial cells. *J. Cell Biol.* 142: 1337–1435.

Tank, E. (1981) Personal communication.

Tarry, W.F., Duckett, J.W. and Stephens, F.D. (1986) The Mayer-Rokitansky syndrome: pathogenesis, classification and management. *J. Urol.* 136: 648.

Taxy, J.B. and Filmer, R.B. (1976) Glomerulocystic kidney: report of a case. *Arch. Pathol. Lab. Med.* 100: 186–188.

Tayakkanonta, K. (1963) The gubernaculum testis and its nerve supply. *Aust. N.Z. J. Surg.* 33: 61–67.

Tench, E.M. (1936) Development of the anus in the human embryo. *Am. J. Anat.* 59: 333.

Terada, M., Goh, D.W., Farmer, P.J. and Hutson, J.M. (1994a) Calcitonin gene-related peptide receptors in the gubernaculum of normal rat and two models of cryptorchidism. *J. Urol.* 152: 759–762.

Terada, M., Goh, D.W., Farmer, P.J. and Hutson, J.M. (1994b) Ontogeny of gubernacular contraction and effect of calcitonin gene-related peptide in the mouse. *J. Pediatr. Surg.* 29: 609–611.

Terada, M., Hutson, J.M., Farmer, P.J. and Goh, D.W. (1995) The role of the genitofemoral nerve and calcitonin gene-related peptide in congenitally cryptorchid mutant TS rats. *J. Urol.* 154: 734–737.

Terada, M., Hutson, J.M., Watts, L.M. (1995) Characterization of the gubernacular contractile response to calcitonin gene-related peptid in the mouse. *J. Ped. Surg.* 30: 730–733.

Thevathasan, C.O. (1961) Accessory urethra in the male child: Report of two cases. *Aust. N.Z. J. Surg.* 31: 134.

Thielman, cited by Neckarsulmer, K. (1914) Ueber Beinieren. *Berl. Klin. Wschr.* 51: 1641. Cited by Geisinger (1937).

Thiersch, K. (1876) Ein operierter Fall von Epispadie mit Blasenspalte. *Zentral bl. Chir.* **3**: 504.

Thomas, K.B. (1964) The eponyms of James Douglas. In *James Douglas of the Pouch and his pupil William Hunter*, p. 194. Springfield: Charles C. Thomas.

Tokunaka, S., Gotoh, T., Koyanagi, T. and Tsuji, I. (1981) The morphological study of ureterocele: a possible clue to its embryogenesis as evidenced by a locally arrested myogenesis. *J. Urol.* 126: 726.

Tolmatschew, von N. (1870) Ein Fall von semilunaren Klappen der Harnohre und von vergrösserter Visicula Prostatica. *Virchows Arch. (Pathol.)* 49: 348.

Torbey, K. and Leadbetter, W.F. (1963) Innervation of the bladder and lower ureter: studies on pelvic nerve section and stimulation in the dog. *J. Urol.* 90: 395.

Torpin, R. (1965) Amniochorionic mesoblastic fibrous strings and amniotic bands: associated constricting fetal malformations or fetal death. *Am. J. Obstet. Gynecol.* 91: 65–75.

Torpin, R. (1968) *Fetal Malformations Caused by Amnion Rupture during Gestation* pp. 87–97. Springfield: Charles Thomas.

Tran, D., Picard, J-Y, Vigier, B., Berger, R. and Josso, N. (1986) Persistence of müllerian ducts in male rabbits passively immunized against bovine anti-müllerian hormone during fetal life. *Dev. Biol.* 116: 160–167.

Trelstad, R.L., Hayashi, A., Hayashi, K. and Donahoe, P.K. (1982) The epithelial-mesenchymal interface of the male rat müllerian duct: loss of basement membrane integrity and ductal regression. *Devel. Biol.* 92: 27–40.

Trendelenberg, F. (1892) De la cure opératoire de l'exstrophie vésicale et de l'épispadias. *Arch. Klin. Chir.* **43**: 394.

Trendelenberg, F. (1906) The treatment of ectopia vesicae. *Ann. Surg.* **44**: 281–289.

Turner, W.R., Jr. (1983) Personal Communication.

Uhlenhuth, E., Hunter, de W.T., Jr. and Leochel, W.E. (1953) *Problems in the Anatomy of the Pelvis.* (a) p. 36; (b) 179; (c) p. 47. Philadelphia: Lippincott.

Uson, A.C. (1961) A classification of ureteroceles in children. *J. Urol.* 85: 732.

Uson, A.C., Rosario, C.D. and Melicow, M.M. (1960) Wilms' tumor in association with cystic renal disease. *J. Urol.* 83: 262.

Van der Schoot, P. (1993) Doubts about the 'first phase of testis descent' in the rat as a valid concept. *Anat. Embryol.* 187: 203–208.

Van der Schoot, P. and Elgar, W. (1992) Androgen-induced prevention of the outgrowth of cranial gonadal suspensory ligaments in fetal rats. *J. Androl.* 13: 534–542.

Veran, P., Moigneteau, C.R. and Auvigne, J. (1958) Opacité de la base droite par malformation rénale. *Poumon. Coeur.* 14: 763.

Vitko, R.J., Cass, A.S. and Winter, R.S. (1972) Anomalies of the genitourinary tract associated with congenital scoliosis and congenital kyphosis. *J. Urol.* 108: 655.

Viville, Ch., Thomas, M., Jaeck, D. and Berger, J. (1971) Une maladie rare: la stenose apparemment congenitale de l'uréthre perineal chez l'homme. Á propos de deux observations. *J. Urol. Nephrol.* 77: 715.

Von Hansemann (January 1897) Ueberzachlige Nieren. *Berl. Klin. Wschr.*, p. 81. Cited by Geisinger (1937).

Waldeyer (1982) Quoted by A. Elbadawi (1972). Anatomy and function of the ureteral sheath. *J. Urol.* 107: 224.

Way, R.A. and Popper, H. (1946) Four urological anomalies in one person. *J. Urol.* 55: 454.

Weigert, C. (1877) Uber einge Bildungsfehler der Ureteren. *Virchows Arch. (Pathol. Anat.)* 70: 490.

Weigert, C. (1878) Nachtrag zu dem Aufsatze 'Ueber Einige Bildungsfehler der Ureteren' (Bd. 70) und Erwiderung auf die Bemerkung des Herrn Prof. Hoffmann zu obigem Aufsatze (Bd. 71s. 408). *Virchows Arch. (Pathol. Anat.)* 72: 130.

Weinberg, R.W. (1968) Complete triplication of the ureter. *S. Afr. Med. J.* 42: 531.

Wensing, C.J.G. (1973) Testicular descent in some domestic mammals. III. Search for the factors that regulate the gubernacular reaction. *Proc. Kon. Ned. Akad. Wetensch.* (Series C) 76: 196–202.

Welch, K.J. (1979) Abdominal musculature deficiency syndrome (prune belly). In *Pediatric Surgery*, 3rd edn., Vol. 2, M.M. Ravitch, K.J. Welch, C.D. Benson, E. Aberdeen and J.G. Randolph (eds), p. 1220. Chicago: Year Book.

Whitaker, J. and Danks, D.M. (1966) A study of the inheritance of duplication of the kidneys and ureters. *J. Urol.* 95: 176.

Whitaker, J. and Johnston, G.S. (1966) Urinary flow rate with two techniques of bladder pressure measurement. *Invest. Urol.* 4: 235.

Whitaker, J. and Johnston, G.S. (1969) Correlation of urethral resistance and shape in girls. *Radiology* 91: 757.

Whitaker, J., Johnston, G.S. and Lawson, J.D. (1969) Urinary outflow resistance estimation in children. *Invest. Urol.* 7: 127.

Whitaker, R.H. (1973) Diagnosis of obstruction in dilated ureters. *Ann. R. Coll. Surg. (Engl.)* 53: 153.

Wickramasinghe, S.F. and Stephens, F.D. (1977) Paraureteral diverticula: associated renal morphology and embryogenesis. *Invest. Urol.* 14: 381.

Wigger, H.J. and Blanc, W.A. (1977) The prune belly syndrome. *Pathol. Ann.* 12: 17.

Williams, D. (1952) The development and abnormalities of the penile urethra. *Acta Anat.* 15: 176–187.

Williams, D.I. (1958a) Congenital anomalies of the lower urinary tract. In *Urology in Childhood: Handbuch der Urologie*, Bd. 15, p. 68. Berlin-Göttingen-Heidelberg: Springer-Verlag.

Williams, D.I. (1958b) Megaureter. *Postgrad. Med. J.* 34: 159.

Williams, D.I. (1968) *Paediatric Urology*, 1st edn., p. 35. London: Butterworths.

Williams, D.I. (1979) Prune belly syndrome. In *Campbell's Urology*, 4th edn., J.H. Harrison, R.F. Gittes, A.D. Perlmutter, T.A. Stamey and P.C. Walsh (eds), Vol. 2, p. 143. Philadelphia: W. B. Saunders.

Williams, D.I. and Savage J. (1966) Reconstruction of the exstrophied bladder. *Br. J. Surg.* **53**: 168.

Williams, D.I. and Royle, M. (1969) Ectopic ureter in the male child. *Br. J. Urol.* 41: 421.

Williams, D.I. and Mikhael, R.B. (1971) Urethritis in male children. *Proc. R. Soc. Med.* 64: 133.

Williams, D.I. and Lightwood, R.G. (1972) Bilateral single ectopic ureters. *Br. J. Urol.* 44: 267.

Williams, D.I., Fay, R. and Lillie, G.G. (1972) The functional radiology of ectopic ureterocele. *Br. J. Urol.* 44: 417.

Williams, P.L. and Warwick, R. (1980) (eds) *Gray's Anatomy*, 36th edn. p. 550. Philadelphia: W.B. Saunders.

Wilmer, H.A. (1938) Unilateral fused kidney: a report of five cases and a review of the literature. *J. Urol.* 40: 551.

Wilson, J.D., George, F.W. and Griffin, J.E. (1981) The hormonal control of sexual development. *Science* 211: 1278–1284.

Wilson, W.A. and Littler, J. (1953) Polyorchidism: a report of two cases with torsion. *Br. J. Surg.* 41: 302–307.

Winnier, G., Blessing, M., Labosky, P.A. and Hogan, B.L.M. (1995) Bone morphogenetic protein-4 is required for mesodermal formation and patterning in the mouse. *Genes Dev.* 9: 2105–2116.

Winter, J.S., Kohn, G., Mellman, W.J. and Wagner, F. (1968) A familial syndrome of renal, genital, and middle ear anomalies. *J. Pediatr.* 72: 88.

Witschi, E. (1970) Development and differentiation of the uterus. In *Prenatal Life*, ed. H.C. Mack (ed.), Ch 1, p. 11. Detroit: Wayne State University Press.

Wofromm, G. (1940) Situation du rein dans d'eventration diaphragmatique droite. *Mem. Acad. de Chir.* 66: 41.

Wolff, E.T., Wolff, E.M. and Bishop-Calame, S. (1969) Enplants of embryonic kidney: technique and applications. In *The Kidney: Morphology, Biochemistry, Physiology*, C. Rouiller and A.F. Muller (eds), Vol. 2, p. 1. New York: Academic Press.

Woodburne, R.T. (1964) Anatomy of the ureterovesical junction. *J. Urol.* 92: 431.

Woodruff, S.R. (1941) Complete unilateral triplication of the ureter and renal pelvis. *J. Urol.* 46: 376.

Wright, H.B. and MacFarlane, D.J. (1955) Unilateral triplication of the ureter: report of a patient with three renal and three ureteral orifices. *J. Am. Med. Ass.* 158: 1166.

Wulfekuhler, W.F. and Dube, V.E. (1971) Free supernumerary kidney: report of a case. *J. Urol.* 106: 802.

Wulfsohn. M.A. (1980) Pyelocaliceal diverticula. *J. Urol.* 123: 1.

Xia, H., Migliazza, L., Montedonico, S., Rodriquez, J.I., Diez-Pardo, J.A. and Tovar, J.A. (1999) Skeletal malformations associated with esophageal atresia: clinical and experimental studies. *J. Pediatr. Surg.* 34: 1385–1392.

Yamanaka, J., Metcalfe, S.A., and Hutson, J.M. (1992) Demonstration of calcitonin gene-related peptide receptors in the gubernaculum by computerized densitometry. *J. Pediatr. Surg.* 27: 876–878.

Yamanaka, J., Metcalfe, S.A., Hutson, J.M. and Mendelsohn, F.A.O. (1993) Testicular descent. II. Ontogeny and response to denervation of calcitonin gene-related peptide receptors in neonatal rat gubernaculum. *Endocrinology* 132: 1–5.

Yang, S.S., (1990) ADAM Sequence and innocent amniotic band: manifestations of early amnion rupture. *Am. J. Med. Genet.* 37:

562–568.Young, H.H. and Davis, D.M. (1926) *Young's Practice of Urology*, Vol. 2. Philadelphia: W.B. Saunders.

Yang, C.C. and Bradley, W.E. (1998) Peripheral distribution of the human dorsal nerve of the penis. *J. Urol.* **159**(6): 1912–1917.

Young, H.H. (1922) An operation for the cure of incontinence associated with epispadias. *J.Urol.* **7**: 1–32.

Young, H.H. (1942) Exstrophy of the bladder: the first case in which a normal bladder and urinary control have been obtained by plastic operations. *Surg. Gynecol. Obstet.* **74**: 729–737.Young, H.H., Frontz, W.A. and Baldwin, J.C. (1919) Congenital obstruction of the posterior urethra. *J. Urol.* 3: 289.

Zimmerman, H. and Milderberger, H. (1980) Posterior urethral duplication and triplication in the male. *J. Pediatr. Surg.* 15: 212.

Zorgniotti, A.A. (1991) Temperature and environmental effects of the testis. *Adv. Exp. Med. Biol.*, Vol. 286. pp. 1–335. New York: Plenum Press.

Index

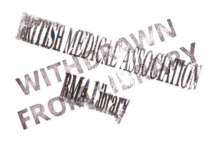